Comprehensive
WOUND MANAGEMENT

SECOND EDITION

Comprehensive WOUND MANAGEMENT

SECOND EDITION

Glenn L. Irion, PhD, PT, CWS

University of South Alabama
Mobile, Alabama

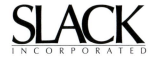

SLACK
INCORPORATED

www.slackbooks.com

ISBN: 978-1-55642-833-3

Comprehensive Wound Management, Second Edition Instructor's Manual is also available from SLACK Incorporated. Don't miss this important companion to *Comprehensive Wound Management, Second Edition*. To obtain the Instructor's Manual, please visit http://www.efacultylounge.com.

The procedures and practices described in this book should be implemented in a manner consistent with the professional standards set for the circumstances that apply in each specific situation. Every effort has been made to confirm the accuracy of the information presented and to correctly relate generally accepted practices. The authors, editor, and publisher cannot accept responsibility for errors or exclusions or for the outcome of the material presented herein. There is no expressed or implied warranty of this book or information imparted by it. Care has been taken to ensure that drug selection and dosages are in accordance with currently accepted/recommended practice. Due to continuing research, changes in government policy and regulations, and various effects of drug reactions and interactions, it is recommended that the reader carefully review all materials and literature provided for each drug, especially those that are new or not frequently used. Any review or mention of specific companies or products is not intended as an endorsement by the author or publisher.

SLACK Incorporated uses a review process to evaluate submitted material. Prior to publication, educators or clinicians provide important feedback on the content that we publish. We welcome feedback on this work.

Published by: SLACK Incorporated
                       6900 Grove Road
                       Thorofare, NJ 08086 USA
                       Telephone: 856-848-1000
                       Fax: 856-853-5991
                       www.slackbooks.com

Contact SLACK Incorporated for more information about other books in this field or about the availability of our books from distributors outside the United States.

Library of Congress Cataloging-in-Publication Data

Irion, Glenn
    Comprehensive wound management / Glenn L. Irion. -- 2nd ed.
         p. ; cm.
    Includes bibliographical references and index.
    ISBN 978-1-55642-833-3
    1. Wounds and injuries--Treatment. 2. Wound healing. I. Title.
    [DNLM: 1. Wounds and Injuries--diagnosis. 2. Wounds and Injuries--therapy. 3. Wound
Healing--physiology. WO 700 I68c 2010]
    RD93.I75 2010
    617.1--dc22
                                        2009025821

Printed in the United States of America

Last digit is print number: 10   9   8   7   6   5   4   3   2   1

DEDICATION

This textbook is dedicated to my children, Lindsay, Kyle, Christina, Phillip, and Connor, and my wife Jean. I also wish to dedicate this to the many patients who inspired me to create a second edition that might better help others improve the lives of their patients.

Contents

Instructors: *Comprehensive Wound Management, Second Edition* Instructor's Manual is also available from SLACK Incorporated. Don't miss this important companion to *Comprehensive Wound Management, Second Edition* available at http://www.efacultylounge.com.

ACKNOWLEDGMENTS

The author wishes to acknowledge individuals who contributed to the production of the second edition. Many of my recent patients happily consented to be photographed for this second edition knowing that other patients might be helped through publication of their images in this textbook. Their gratitude for any knowledge or skill that I was able to use for their benefit was great inspiration as each sentence, paragraph, and section was being crafted for the second edition. Mobile Infirmary Medical Center was instrumental in allowing me the opportunity to continue my clinical practice and meet these individuals. The University of South Alabama; my Physical Therapy Department Chairman, Dennis Fell; and College of Allied Health Professions Dean, Rick Talbott, have been supportive of my clinical practice and other professional development that have contributed to the improvements in the second edition. The assistance of those at SLACK Incorporated, including Brien Cummings, Debra Steckel, and John Bond, is appreciated.

ABOUT THE AUTHOR

Dr. Irion is certified as a Wound Specialist through the American Academy of Wound Management and is Associate Professor at the University of South Alabama where he teaches integumentary, cardiovascular and pulmonary, and basic physical therapy skills. He practices wound management at Mobile Infirmary Medical Center. The author received a PhD in Physiology at Temple University School of Medicine and furthered his research skills during postdoctoral fellowships at the Medical College of Virginia (Virginia Commonwealth University) and the University of Cincinnati/Cincinnati Children's Hospital. He is the author of more than 40 research articles, and co-editor with his wife, Jean, of *Women's Health in Physical Therapy*.

PREFACE

The text is divided into 5 units in an effort to develop a systematic understanding of normal and abnormal integumentary physiology, factors involving the patient, causes of wounds, and to develop a rational plan of care based on this understanding. For the most part, this process is described in the *Guide to Physical Therapist Practice* (the *Guide*). The *Guide* is divided into a description of the physical therapist and physical therapist practice. Emphasis is placed on a systematic approach to patient care. Part B of the *Guide* describes preferred practice patterns in 4 practice areas: musculoskeletal, cardiopulmonary, neuromuscular, and integumentary, with several patterns described within each practice area. Emphasis is placed on using a systematic approach to take a history, perform a physical examination, and perform special tests based on data collected from the history and physical examination. An assessment of the patient's condition and a diagnosis are developed based on the results, along with a prognosis. A plan of care is developed based on subjective report, objective findings and the unique set of circumstances of the patient, including occupation, social support, dwelling, level of understanding of the condition and its care.

Similar in organization to the *Guide*, the first unit of *Comprehensive Wound Management* consists of a description of the anatomy and physiology of the skin, normal wound healing, abnormal wound healing, and nutrition. The second unit addresses characteristics of the patient. Chapters in this unit review history taking and physical examination. The third unit is focused on the wound and consists of chapters on etiology of wounds, including acute wounds, neuropathic ulcers, pressure ulcers, vascular insufficiency, and a chapter on assessment of wounds. When these concepts are understood, a plan of care can be developed. For this reason, the fourth unit addresses the interventions carried out in the plan of care. These include infection control, pain control, wound bed preparation, dressings, scar management, adjuncts, thermal injuries, and special cases. The fifth unit consists of issues indirectly related to patient care, including chapters on plan of care, documentation, and administrative concerns.

The hope of the author is that the readers of this text will learn to develop a systematic approach based on history, physical examination, special tests, and assessment for each individual patient, rather than relying on referral-diagnosis driven protocols, and that the reader will learn to adjust the plan of care as the patient and the wound change.

Glenn L. Irion, PhD, PT, CWS

Basic Science

The first unit of the book focuses on the anatomy and physiology related to wounds and their healing. The chapters consist of normal anatomy and physiology of the skin, normal wound healing, abnormal wound healing, and nutrition as a specialized area of physiology. The information discussed in this unit will be used in subsequent chapters. The purpose of this unit is to give background information that will guide history taking and physical examination to develop an assessment, diagnosis, prognosis, and plan of care. As in chess, we wish to understand the layout of the board, the pieces, and the moves that are allowed. To continue with this analogy, in chess we are allowed many possible moves, but based upon the opposition, certain moves will be more fruitful than others. Understanding normal anatomy and physiology of skin, how unimpeded wound healing occurs, and understanding common problems with healing will help us make the right moves for our patients.

Anatomy and Physiology of Skin

1

OBJECTIVES

- Describe the functions of the skin and its appendages.
- Identify the layers of the skin and subcutaneous tissues, and their roles in health.
- Identify the components of the epidermis, including cells, accessory structures, and layers.
- Identify the components of the dermis, including cells, fibers, ground substance, and other structures.
- Describe changes in the skin of the elderly.

The skin is the largest organ of the body. The average person is enclosed in approximately 2 m^2 of skin, with an average thickness of 2 mm. Despite its seemingly simple appearance and role as a protective cover for the body, a large number of important physiological processes occur to maintain the integrity of the skin. In some cases, seemingly trivial insults to the anatomy or physiology can produce profound effects. A working knowledge of the components of the skin is necessary not only for the discussion of wound healing, but also in the diagnosis and prognosis of impairments of integumentary integrity. Knowledge of anatomy and physiology will also be used in the development of a plan of care and monitoring the patient's progress.

PHYSIOLOGY

The physiology of the skin may be divided into 3 main categories—protection, immunity, and thermoregulatory.

Each of these topics is described below. In addition to these functions, skin has a role in calcium metabolism through the effect of sunlight on the activation of vitamin D.

Passive Protection

Skin has the obvious role of providing passive protection of the body by keeping elements of the environment from entering the body and preventing the uncontrolled loss of water and other critical substances from the body. In addition, the immune system has a variety of components that act at the skin surface, the first line of defense.

Skin acts as a physical barrier against microorganisms, trauma, ultraviolet light, and loss of body fluid to the environment. The acidic nature of the skin's surface eliminates a number of bacteria. The skin consists of two primary layers, the epidermis and dermis (Figure 1-1). A subcutaneous fat layer is also critical to skin function. Subcutaneous fat increases the thermal insulation of the skin and protects skin

Irion G.
Comprehensive Wound Management, 2nd ed. (pp 3-14)
© 2010 SLACK Incorporated

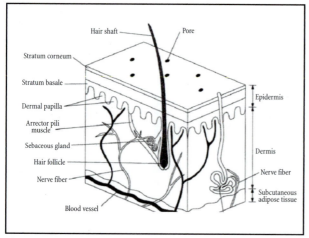

Figure 1-1. Components of the skin, including accessory structures of the epidermis. Note how deeply the hair follicles and sweat glands are surrounded by dermis.

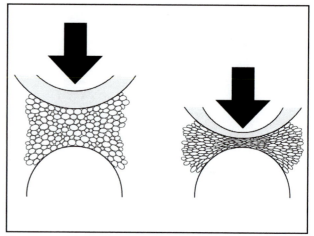

Figure 1-2. The cushioning effect of subcutaneous fat. Pressure and shearing forces between the skin and bony prominences are dissipated by deformation of subcutaneous fat before damage to the skin and subcutaneous tissues would otherwise occur.

from injury by pressure or shearing forces between support surfaces and the body's bony prominences as depicted in Figure 1-2. Below subcutaneous fat, other structures including muscle, tendon, ligaments, and bone may be found. The epidermis consists of organized layers of stratified epithelium with a well-defined transition of cell shape and structure as cells proceed from deeper layers to more superficial layers. The epidermis is generally 75 to 150 µm thick, but becomes 400 to 600 µm thick in palms and soles, which have an epidermal layer not found in other parts of the body. The dermis is much thicker than the epidermis, but is not as regularly organized. Within the dermis, one finds dense fibroelastic connective tissue that encloses accessory structures of the epidermis, fibrous bands that connect to fascia and bone, and below it, a subcutaneous loose areolar or fatty connective tissue.

Immunity

The variety of immune components ranges from simple chemical characteristics to adaptive components of the immune system. The skin has cellular and humoral components of the immune system and a variety of molecular defense systems against microorganisms. Additionally, molecular components called defensins bind certain bacteria, facilitating the immune system's response. Resident macrophages called Langerhans cells nonselectively destroy bacteria and present antigen to T cells, allowing the immune system to generate a specific response against cells bearing the antigen used to select T cells. Mechanisms involved in the immune response are described more fully in Chapter 9. Unfortunately, the immune system on occasion is a source of injury to the skin and may cause devastating loss of skin integrity in diseases such as Stevens-Johnson syndrome and pemphigus.

Thermoregulatory

The skin receives much more blood flow than required for its metabolic needs. Blood is warmed by passing through metabolically active tissues. The skin in contact with the external environment serves as a radiator from which the warm blood passing through the skin heats the air. Heat exchange between the skin and air depends on the difference in temperature between the blood and the air. To increase loss of heat to the environment, blood flow is increased through the skin. As the body's central core becomes warmer, blood vessels in the skin dilate, allowing more heat to pass through the skin and into the environment. Conversely, in a cold environment, blood vessels of the skin constrict, which reduces the loss of heat to the environment. The ability of the skin to exchange heat with the environment is enhanced by the tufts of capillaries within the papillary dermis (described below) and the large number of veins in the skin. Additionally, sweat glands release water onto the skin. Evaporation of water enhances the loss of heat carried by the blood to the environment. The function of sweat glands is described further below.

ANATOMY

The anatomy of the skin is divided into its superficial layer, the epidermis, and the deeper layer, the dermis. The cells and layers of the epidermis are described, followed by the skin's appendages. Then the 2 layers of the dermis and its structures are described. The subcutaneous fat layer has been described above.

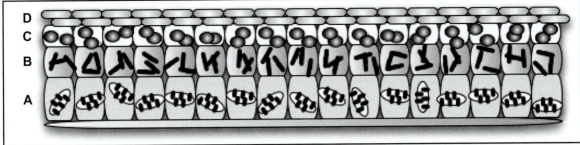

Figure 1-3. Cells and layers of the epidermis. The epidermis consists of 4 layers: (A) stratum basale, (B) stratum spinosum, (C) stratum granulosum, (D) stratum corneum. See text for details about each layer. Each stratum consists of several layers of cells. Figure is simplified for clarity.

Epidermis

Although the epidermis appears to be a simple passive covering for the skin, the epidermis is a dynamic tissue composed of cells that continue to develop as they migrate outwardly. The epidermis also lines the accessory structures (appendages) of the skin. The cells, layers, and accessory structures are described below.

Cells

The epidermis consists of 3 major cell types. The keratinocytes are the most abundant cells of the epidermis. Two other types of cells, melanocytes and Langerhans cells, migrate into the epidermis during development from the same source as the nervous system and from the immune system. Immigrant cells include melanocytes (neural crest cells), Langerhans cells (immune cells), and Merkel cells (sensory receptors).

Keratinocytes

Keratinocytes are the predominant cells in terms of number and function in the epidermis (Figure 1-3). They are considered by researchers to be the native cells of the epidermis to distinguish them from cells believed to migrate into the outer layer of skin during development. The cells are termed *keratinocytes* due to their production of filaments made of keratins (in addition to other proteins). The keratinocytes provide the physical barrier of the skin, which includes waterproofing. The epidermis is composed of layers of keratinocytes that change in structure and function as they migrate from the basement membrane (basal layer) outward.

Melanocytes

Pigmentation of the epidermis is achieved through the actions of the melanocytes. These cells produce the pigment melanin and distribute it to surrounding cells. Melanocytes are derived from cells that develop in the nervous system and they share some properties with neurons. In particular, melanocytes like neurons, have dendrites, move substances throughout the cells, and release vesicles that interact with surrounding cells. Melanin is packaged into melanosomes, which are transported via dendritic processes to approximately 30 surrounding cells. Melanosomes are then taken up by surrounding keratinocytes, resulting in skin pigmentation. Production of melanosomes is increased by exposure to ultraviolet light. Melanin provides protection of the genetic material of the keratinocytes as excessive exposure to ultraviolet light can potentially damage the epidermal cells resulting in loss of skin elasticity and skin cancers.

Langerhans Cells

The resident macrophages of the epidermis are called Langerhans cells. These cells originate as monocytes in the blood. As macrophages, Langerhans cells are responsible for eliciting T cell responses as well as nonspecific attacks on foreign matter, including bacteria. Antigens from foreign matter are presented to T cells, producing a delayed response. However, Langerhans cells are also responsible for mounting attacks against trivial matter such as plant oils, materials used in manufacturing clothing, and so forth, producing injury to the skin. Exposure to poison ivy is an example of such a response. The response of Langerhans cells is also the basis of the test for exposure to the organism that causes tuberculosis. Purified protein derivative (PPD) is injected subcutaneously. If a person has been exposed to *Mycobacterium tuberculosis*, T cells programmed to attack the antigen will produce an erythematous area around the injection.

Different individuals become sensitized to a variety of foreign antigens, some of which are presented by Langerhans cells and manifest themselves as type IV immune reactions (delayed hypersensitivity). In addition to skin rash, molecules associated with latex-derived materials can be involved in more immediate and serious immune response. Latex, in particular, is a major concern in wound management and will be addressed extensively in Chapter 9.

Merkel Receptors

Merkel receptors consist of a separate receptive element at the junction of the epidermis and dermis and a sensory neuron, whereas other mechanoreceptors consist of a specialized ending on the neuron. Other sensory neurons carrying pain and temperature have nonspecific endings. The Merkel receptor adapts slowly to stimuli and has a small receptive field. These properties make the Merkel receptor particularly useful for localizing constant pressure on the skin.

Layers

Upon inspection of the epidermis by microscopy, distinct layering can be observed. From deep to superficial, the layers are termed the *stratum basale* (basal layer), *stratum spinosum* (spiny layer), *stratum granulosum* (granular layer), and *stratum corneum* (the horn-like layer). In addition, a layer termed the *stratum lucidum* (clear layer) is observed in the palms and soles, creating a much thicker epidermal layer. The stratum lucidum increases resistance to shear stress and decreases the apparent pigmentation in the soles and palms. These layers are depicted in Figure 1-3.

Stratum Basale

The stratum basale consists of cuboidal/low columnar epithelium and is considered the germinative layer of the epidermis. It creates an undulating layer that rides along the surface of the dermis. This undulation increases the surface of contact between the dermis and epidermis and improves resistance to shear stress. These areas are sometimes termed *rete pegs*. The height of these undulations on palms and soles produces the unique patterns of fingerprints and footprints. Excessive shearing forces between the dermis and epidermis damage this area creating blisters (Figure 1-4).

With age, the height of the rete pegs decreases, increasing the susceptibility of the skin to tearing. As the germinative layer of the epidermis, markers of cell replication are abundant, as well as organelles of active cells, including mitochondria, Golgi apparatus, endoplasmic reticulum, and ribosomes. As the cells mature, they migrate superficially.

Stratum Spinosum

The stratum spinosum consists of several layers of cells with keratin aggregation observed in bundles. As cells migrate through the stratum spinosum, they become progressively flatter and begin to produce intracellular granules. The aggregation of filaments gives these cells the appearance for which they are named.

Stratum Granulosum

The next layer, the stratum granulosum, exhibits continued flattening with extrusion of granules into the intercellular space. The granules consist of a variety of lipid molecules. The lipid components of the extruded granules act as a permeability barrier between cells, similar to caulk or grout. As the cells continue to mature and migrate

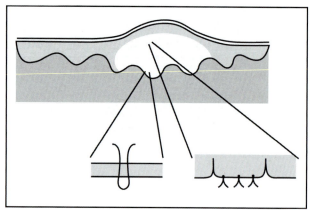

Figure 1-4. Formation of blisters. Fluid accumulation due to inflammation causes rupture of desmosomes and separation of epidermis from dermis.

through the stratum granulosum, one can observe an accumulation of keratohyaline on filament meshwork within the cells, which is most developed in the superficial layer, the stratum corneum.

Stratum Corneum

The stratum corneum is the outermost layer of the epidermis. Cells within this layer have lost most of their organelles, have become flatter, and overlap each other, producing the function of shingles on a roof. As cells mature and migrate outwardly toward the stratum corneum, gradual flattening and degradation of mitochondria, the nucleus, and other organelles of keratinocytes occur. On microscopy one can observe 15 to 20 layers of flattened cells filled with keratohyaline. The lower layers of cells demonstrate lipid layering and desmosomes, which provide physical linkage of adjacent cells. Upper cells of this layer, in contrast, demonstrate a loss of desmosomes and lipid layering. On average, approximately 14 days are required for a cell to migrate from the stratum basale to the stratum corneum and each cell lasts about 14 days within stratum corneum.

Cell Envelope

The cell envelope is a structure unique to keratinocytes. It develops beneath the cell membrane as cells mature and migrate superficially through the epidermis. It is constructed of several cross-linked proteins. These proteins are first detectable in the stratum spinosum. The envelope forms in the stratum granulosum and is complete in the stratum corneum. The enzymes required to synthesize the cell envelope develop as the cell matures.

Lipids

Lipids within the epidermis form the permeability barrier between adjacent keratinocytes. A distinct layering of lipid is observable in the stratum corneum. Sources of lipid within the stratum corneum include sebaceous glands, cell membranes, and lamellar granules. Lamellar granules develop in the stratum spinosum and are extruded in the stratum granulosum. The lack of essential fatty acids (discussed in Chapter 4) results in dry, scaly skin and increased skin permeability.

Growth Factors Affecting the Epidermis

A number of growth factors affect skin, including epidermal growth factor (EGF), acidic and basic fibroblast growth factor (aFGF and bFGF), insulin, insulin-like growth factor-1 (IGF-1), interleukin 2 (IL-2), colony-stimulating factors, nerve growth factor (NGF), platelet-derived growth factor (PDGF), and transforming growth factor beta (TGFβ). These growth factors have multiple sites of action. Receptors for EGF and TGFβ are found on basal keratinocytes, sweat duct cells, hair follicles, sheath cells, basal sebocytes, vascular smooth muscle cells, and arrectores pilorum muscle cells. EGF and FGF increase fibroblast number, TGFβ has been linked to angiogenesis and fibroplasia, and PDGF has been linked to chemotaxis, DNA synthesis, collagen deposition, and wound contraction. Experimentally, PDGF normalizes wound repair in diabetic animals, but is also suspected to be involved in atherosclerosis and neoplasia. Signals for release of growth factors have been studied. These include phospholipase C/protein kinase C, which is activated by bradykinin, histamine, thrombin, EGF, and PDGF. Phospholipase C/protein kinase C is implicated in both proliferation and differentiation of skin cells, the release of prostaglandins, and increased gene expression. Another signaling mechanism, tyrosine kinase, has been associated with TGFβ, insulin, and bFGF to promote proliferation of skin cells. Prostaglandins and leukotrienes are associated with inflammation, which, as discussed later, is an important component of normal healing, but if prolonged, impedes healing.

Normal skin appearance and function depend on a balance between cellular proliferation and differentiation. Scaling, plaques, and other disorders may result from an imbalance of these 2 processes. Production of the normal layering of epidermis requires both a sequence of timely production by mitotically active keratinocytes and subsequent differentiation of post-mitotic cells. In addition to skin's appearance, impaired wound healing and production of skin cancer may result from an imbalance. IGF-1 is an important regulator of cellular proliferation and differentiation. Both epidermal keratinocytes and dermal fibroblasts possess specific receptors for IGF-1. Binding of IGF-1 leads to proliferation of these cells. Lack of IGF-1 leads to thin, weak skin, whereas excessive quantities of IGF-1 may produce a range of effects from thickening to neoplasia. Excessive IGF-1 also inhibits normal differentiation of keratinocytes required for the normal layering of

epidermis. Alterations in the balance of different growth factors has been linked to several disorders, including psoriasis and scleroderma.

Accessory Structures

Accessory structures of the epidermis dwell in invaginations of epidermis into the dermis (see Figure 1-1). These structures may carry epidermal cells deeply into the dermis. The significance of the invagination of these structures is evident in partial-thickness burns. Although thermal injury may destroy the epidermis and some dermal depth, epidermal cells lining the accessory structures may provide cells to resurface the injured skin. These structures—hair follicles, nails, sebaceous glands, and sweat glands—are described below and are depicted in Figure 1-1.

Hair Follicles

Hairs are constructed of intermediate filaments, primarily keratins. This is basically the same material as nails, horns, and claws. Each hair consists of microfibrils embedded in a matrix. In turn, each filament consists of coils of polymerized alpha helices of protein molecules. Hairs grow cyclically with random cycles, so within a population of hairs, various hairs are at different phases at any given time. Hair follicles are dynamic tubular invaginations of epidermis lined with epithelial cells. Two major types of hairs are found on the human body. Vellus hairs are soft, unpigmented hairs that cover nearly the entire body and are often termed *under hairs*. The other type is the terminal hair, which is firm, long, coarse, pigmented, and observable easily with the unaided eye. These are found on the scalp of both sexes, and beginning with puberty with tremendous variability on the trunk and extremities, more so on men than women. During the growth cycle, hair follicles extend more deeply into the dermis, then gradually shorten as growth stops. The typical terminal hair grows about 0.5 mm/day on the head and about 0.4 mm/day on the body.

Nails

A nail plate is a densely compacted mass of keratinized cells sitting on a rectangular nail bed consisting of epithelial cells. This nail bed is located from the lunula (see next page) to the hyponychium, which is defined as the distal epithelium located beneath the free edge of the nail. Beneath the epidermal layer of the nail bed exists a thin dermal layer that adheres to the underlying bone. The nail bed contains longitudinally oriented blood vessels, which give rise to the longitudinal ridges observable in nails. These ridged surfaces, like the papillary dermis, interdigitate with the nail plate and provide adherence of the nail to the nail bed. In contrast to keratinocytes, no granular layer is present and keratinization is minimal in normal healthy nails. The nail itself, defined as devitalized cells, begins 7 to 8 mm proximal to the cuticle and the nail thickens as its plate migrates distally. The living cells develop in the matrix of the nail bed and then move from the matrix into the nail plate, losing their organelles and becoming hard and waterproof. Edges of the nail plate other than the free distal end are covered with a fold of skin called the nail folds. The cuticle is a specialized epidermis that seals the space between the nail fold and nail plate. The cuticle is continuous with digit epidermis and grows along with the nail.

The lunula represents the visible region of the nail matrix. As the name implies, it appears as a half-moon shaped area. The lunula is located under the proximal part of the nail plate and extends beyond the cuticle. Due to the small number of melanocytes in nail matrix epithelium, the nail beds are usually not pigmented. In some non-Caucasian individuals, a larger number of melanocytes within the nail matrix may lead to some pigmentation as either banded or diffuse pigmentation of the nail. Cells are moved in a diagonal manner from the matrix into the visible portion of the nail. The nail plate is moved forward at a rate of approximately 3 mm per month in the fingers and 1 mm per month in the toes. The proximal portion of the nail matrix gives rise to the superior surface of the nail and the distal portion gives rise to the lower surface.

Injury or disease affecting the proximal nail matrix manifests as abnormalities of the surface, and injury or disease affecting the distal matrix appears as an abnormal lower surface of the nail. Trauma may lead to production of keratohyaline granules (a granular layer) and increased keratinization in affected nail cells. Severe trauma may lead to permanent loss of the nail and less severe injury can produce continuous nail dystrophy. The granular layer produced in traumatized nail beds prevents normal adherence of the nail to the nail bed resulting in layering, separation (onychoschizia), and premature loss of the upper surface of the nails.

A number of disease states produce nail changes. Psoriasis frequently produces pitting. Banding (horizontal irregularities), splitting, and dystrophy may accompany other diseases. Thick, dark nails frequently occur with arterial disease of toenail beds along with fungal infections. Splinter hemorrhages occur as longitudinal markings caused by blood leaking from the longitudinally oriented nail bed blood vessels. Splinter hemorrhages are visible as the nail grows outwardly carrying coagulated blood with it. A fingernail will require 6 months to grow out completely and a toenail may require 1 to 1½ years to do so. Signs of trauma and disease, therefore, persist in the nail until the affected areas grow to the free, distal end of the nail.

Age and/or disease-related changes in nails may be manifested as a loss of the normal glossiness of the nails, more pronounced ridging, brittleness, and change in shape. Shape changes of the nails include flattening of the nails (platynychia), spooning (koilonychia) in which the nail's free end rises above the center of the nail, and clubbing. Normal nails have a curvature in only one plane, producing a cylindrical shape. The growth of nails with curvature in both planes produces a spherical nail. Cystic fibrosis, lung cancer, and other respiratory disorders often produce clubbing.

The hardness of nails is largely determined by their water content. Between 16% and 25% is considered normal water content. As water content decreases, nails become brittle; water content greater than normal produces softening of nails. With age, fingernails generally become thinner and more fragile, whereas toenails become thicker and harder. The term for excessively thickened nails is *onychogryphosis*. The great toenail is more prone to this condition, occurring in individuals with peripheral arterial disease and neuropathy, especially in diabetes mellitus. The nail folds that cover edges of the nail other than the free edge represents a space in which infection could spread. Injury to the nail folds, particularly from inappropriate nail trimming, may result in an infection that travels around the nail fold, under the cuticle. Acute paronychia is commonly caused by bacterial infection, whereas chronic paronychia is associated with fungal infection. Inflammation of the nail folds may also be caused by physical or chemical injury.

Sebaceous Glands

These glands are found everywhere on the body surface except on the palm, sole, and dorsum of the foot, producing the substance known as sebum. The glands are the densest and largest on scalp and face. These glands are not isolated but appear with and share a common opening onto the skin surface with hair follicles. Sebum flows through a short canal into the follicular canal, then onto skin. On mucus membranes the sebaceous glands open directly onto skin. These glands remain small until puberty. Within sebaceous glands, cells replicate at the base of the gland and migrate as lipid accumulation occurs within the duct. The cells themselves eventually become the excretory product (holocrine gland). Cells lose their nuclei and degrade, resulting in oil deposition onto the skin. The cells within the gland have a turnover time of 14 days. Although no short-term regulatory mechanisms are known, androgens increase sebum production and estrogens decrease production. The rapid increase in androgen production with puberty predisposes these glands to occlusion and infection, resulting in acne.

Sweat Glands

Two types of sweat glands are described. Eccrine glands have a thermoregulatory function, whereas apocrine glands have a social or emotional component. Both exist as coiled epithelial tubes. Apocrine glands are associated with hair follicles, whereas eccrine glands are distributed throughout the body surface. A tremendous variation in gland size

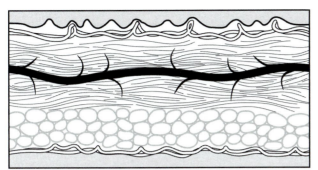

Figure 1-5. Structure of the dermis.

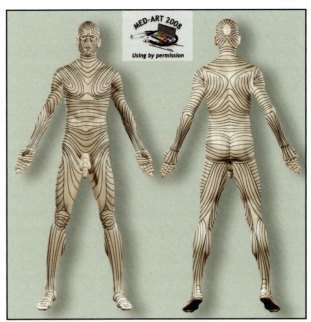

Figure 1-6. Langer's lines. These indicate lines of natural tension in the skin. A wound along these lines has little stress on it, whereas a wound running perpendicular to these lines will experience stress along its edges. (Used with permission of Davide Brunelli, MD. Available at www.med-ars.it/.)

and secretory rate exists from person to person. Centrally, sweating is stimulated at a threshold central temperature and increases with body temperature. Sweat glands also respond to local skin temperature. Central temperature is 9 times more effective in stimulating sweat production than local skin temperature. Eccrine glands are innervated by cholinergic sympathetic nerves. These glands initially secrete plasma-like fluid, but reabsorption of ions including sodium, chloride, and bicarbonate occurs along their length in response to aldosterone. Sweat is hypotonic at a low secretion rate, but increases in tonicity as sweat rate increases. Apocrine glands, in contrast, have adrenergic innervation and are stimulated by events that produce nonspecific activation of the sympathetic nervous system, including anxiety. These glands are found primarily in the axillary and perineal areas. The secretion of apocrine glands in certain animals is believed to be a chemoattractant. Whether this occurs in humans is still debated. As discussed in Chapter 7, these areas are prone to infection and may require surgical excision.

Dermis

The components of the dermis, the layers, ground substance, and fibers are discussed below.

Layers

The dermis consists of 2 major layers with important functional differences, and 3 basic components, which are depicted in Figure 1-5. Fibroblasts are the principal cells of the dermis. Although they are not tremendously numerous or active cells in stable skin, fibroblasts are capable of secreting important macromolecules during the healing process. Fibers, especially collagen and elastic fibers, are common in the dermis and are described further below. The third component is the ground substance, a gel of glycosaminoglycans and water.

Papillary Layer

The papillary dermis (pars papillaris) is thin and molded against the epidermal ridges/grooves. It consists of smaller, more loosely distributed collagen fibers than the deeper reticular dermis. In contrast to the reticular dermis, its fibers consist mainly of type III and IV collagen. The major feature of this layer is the network of blood and lymphatic vessels organized into plexuses. This layer is important in regulation of heat loss. Increased blood flow through the papillary dermis results in greater loss of heat to the environment.

Reticular Layer

This layer of dermis has a much greater thickness than the papillary layer and is relatively acellular and avascular compared with other tissues. It is characterized by denser fibers and less gel than the papillary layer and the presence of type I collagen that has a mesh-like organization with preferential direction. This organization of the reticular fibers gives rise to the structures know as Langer's lines, forming a grain-like nature to the skin. Langer's lines are important in performing body composition analysis with skin fold calipers. A proper skin fold results only when the skin is pinched such that Langer's lines run perpendicular to the calipers. They are also important in understanding preferential direction of skin contraction following injury. If possible, incisions for surgery are made parallel to Langer's lines to reduce the width of the resulting scar. The general directions of Langer's lines are depicted in Figure 1-6.

Ground Substance

Ground substance refers to the viscoelastic sol-gel of hydrophilic polymers found between cells and fibers of the dermis. The multiple branches of proteins with their charges are able to hold tremendous quantities of interstitial water in place. Overwhelming of the ground substance due to fluid balance derangement, ie, increased capillary pressure due to tissue injury or heart failure, produces free water movement in the interstitial space, which is manifested as pitting edema. Ground substance both lubricates and separates the fibers of the dermis, allowing them to move freely across each other. The binding of these molecules to collagen fibers also increases the tensile strength of collagen fibers. Glycosaminoglycans are the primary type of molecule in ground substance. These molecules consist of chains of polysaccharides linked to protein that are metabolized and degraded by fibroblasts. Different proportions of glycosaminoglycans are present in different tissues and contribute to the biomechanical properties of these tissues. The more common glycosaminoglycans are hyaluronic acid, chondroitin-4-sulfate, dermatan sulfate, and heparan sulfate. Different connective tissues of the body express different proportions of these specific molecules.

Fibers

Fibers give the dermis many of its characteristics, especially the ability to withstand stresses. The 3 basic types of fibers—collagen bundles, elastic fibers, and reticulin fibers—are discussed below.

Collagen Bundles

Collagen fibers (Figure 1-7) are the principal fibers of the dermis, representing 77% of fat-free, dry weight. Collagen provides tensile strength in many tissues, including the skin. Different types of collagen, based on subtle variations in the molecular structure of the individual collagen molecules, are found in the body. Type I is predominant in reticular dermis, providing high tensile strength (ability to withstand traction). Other types of collagen are characterized by their ability to withstand compression or are more elastic.

Elastic Fibers

Elastic fibers consist of a fibrillar component termed *fibrillin* and an amorphous component named *elastin*. Elastic fibers are characterized by their wavy nature and spring-like quality, thereby providing elasticity to skin. In Marfan's syndrome, fibrillin is defective, resulting in the physical characteristics of the disease as well as aortic insufficiency and risk of aortic aneurysm.

Reticulin Fibers

Reticular fibers are composed of type III collagen and form a meshwork over the papillary dermis. In contrast to the cable-like property of collagen fibers, reticular fibers are fine and interconnect creating a netlike appearance. These fibers allow the exchange of heat and materials between the dermis and epidermis and help

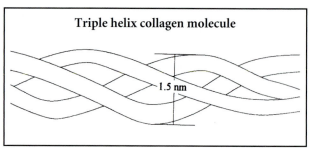

Figure 1-7. Structure of collagen fibers.

bind the dermis to the epidermis creating the rete pegs of the skin. The papillary layer of the dermis and the reticular fibers are damaged early in the process of pressure ulcers development.

Basal Lamina

The basal lamina is the junction of the dermis and epidermis. It consists of the clear, 20-nm-thick lamina lucida and the lamina densa. The 2 layers of the basal lamina are named based on their microscopic appearance. Within the lamina lucida, anchoring filaments pass from the basal layer. In the lamina densa filamentous glycoproteins and type IV collagen are found. To increase the adherence of the epidermis to the dermis, collagen fibers pass through loops of anchoring filaments within the lamina densa. In certain diseases, the filamentous attachments of the epidermis to the dermis are selectively destroyed resulting in a loss of large sheets of epidermis.

BIOMECHANICS OF SKIN

Skin is much more elastic than the dense connective tissue of bone, ligament, and tendon. Some of the differences are due to the components, and some are due to the arrangements of these components. Tendons are very stiff and elongate very little with applied force. This stiffness is primarily due to the parallel arrangement of very thick bundles of collagen, but as discussed above, tendons have different proportions of glycosaminoglycans than elastic cartilage or skin. In addition to its elastic nature, normal skin has tensile and viscous properties. Much of the elasticity comes from viscous elements; therefore, skin is described as having a viscoelastic property. In a simple model, collagen fibers may be ascribed the role of providing tensile strength, ie, the ability to resist lengthening. However, collagen fibers are both coiled and undulating. As stretch is applied to collagen fibers, they become straightened, and at several points along each bundle of collagen fibers, a number of elastic fibers attach to each other, and other collagen bundles. Further stretch straightens the alignment of collagen and elastic fibers. The 3-dimensional interaction of collagen fibers and the attachment of elastic fibers made of elastin provide the ability of the skin to recoil when a stretch is applied to it. Ground substance, made of glycosaminoglycans and water, also provides some elasticity to the skin. Dehydration of the skin, as occurs with aging, diminishes skin turgor and allows the fibers of the skin to become lax. This is manifested as tenting in which a pinch of skin does not recoil when released. The response of material to an applied force is graphically represented as a stress-strain curve (see Figure 1-8). The force applied to the tissue represents the stress (dependent variable on the y-axis) and the length of the tissue represents the strain as the independent variable plotted on the x-axis. Therefore, these measurements represent a measurement of force across the tissue as its length is changed.

Five areas subdivided within 2 major regions are characteristic of connective tissue. In the elastic region, no permanent change in tissue length occurs with stretch. If force is plotted with both increases and release of the stretch, a somewhat different path is followed. This phenomenon is termed *hysteresis* and is due chiefly to the viscoelastic nature of connective tissue.

The elastic region is divided into 3 phases. The compliant phase represents taking up of slack within individual fibers, and the force across the tissue changes very little. The second phase, the transition phase, has a greater slope, producing more, but still relatively little, force as it is lengthened. Within the first 2 phases of the elastic region, slope increases with increasing length, however, in the linear portion, the slope of the stress-strain relationship becomes linear due to the lattice of fibers becoming aligned with the force across it.

The plastic region represents a permanent change in tissue length once a certain length is achieved. This point at which the plastic region is reached is termed the *yield point* as the material yields to the force applied and tension actually falls with increasing length. At the microscopic level, attachments of fibers to each other are destroyed such that the 3-dimensional lattice of fibers is changed to more of a 1-dimensional arrangement parallel to the direction of applied force. Release of stretch leaves the tissue in an elongated and weakened state.

In the second yield region, individual fibers unravel further, yielding to the applied force up to the point of failure, manifested as tearing of the tissue. Loss of collagen and elastic fibers and dehydration cause skin to become less extensible and weaker (more brittle) with age. Skin tears, especially with the imprudent use of adhesives and multiple ecchymoses (bruises), become frequent in the elderly. On the other hand, prudent application of external forces can aid the repair of skin in a more functional way. Scar management will be discussed extensively in Chapter 13.

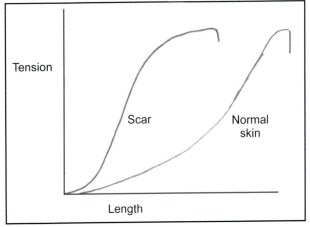

Figure 1-8. Stress-strain relationship of tendon and skin. Note 4 regions: In the first region, lengthening occurs with little stress. In the second region, a linear relationship between lengthening and stress can be observed. With further stress, fibers are damaged and elasticity is lost. Also note the greater extensibility of skin for a given stress. Scar tissue extensibility is similar to tendon.

BIOMECHANICS OF SCAR TISSUE

Scar tissue differs from normal skin in several ways. The collagen is a different type and the ground substance has different proportions of the component molecules. In scar tissue, collagen is primarily type IV, which is stiffer than type I. In normal skin, hyaluronic acid, chondroitin sulfate, and dermatan sulfate represent about 42%, 5%, and 54% of the glycosaminoglycans. In scar tissue, hyaluronic acid decreases dramatically, and chondroitin sulfate increases to proportions similar to those of tendon and bone. Because of these changes, scar tissue is much stiffer than normal skin. Because all the skin is contiguous, the entire mass acts as a reservoir of elasticity. Therefore, flexing the fingers tightens the skin on the dorsum of the hand as well as that on the forearm. The effect of finger flexion is much greater on the hand, but even the opposite hand or foot has some of the elastic reservoir taken away. Under normal circumstances this example has no practical application. However, when a large proportion of the skin is injured as in a burn, we see loss of range of motion not only at the joint involved in the burn, but also in diminishing fashion in adjacent joints. A burn that causes extensive scarring at the elbow leads to profound loss of range of motion at the elbow, but also decreases range of motion at the wrist, hand, and shoulder. A more extensive burn could also limit range of motion at the neck as well. Interventions directed toward maintaining range of motion following burn injuries are covered in Chapter 15.

SENSORY RECEPTORS

Receptors present in the skin include mechanoreceptors sensitive to touch, particularly to vibration, thermoreceptors sensitive to warmth and cold, and nociceptors sensitive to painful stimuli and particular types of chemicals. The 4 major receptors involved in producing the simple sensation of touch are depicted in Figure 1-9. These include Pacinian corpuscles, Meissner's corpuscles, Ruffini's corpuscles, and Merkel's disks. Pacinian corpuscles and Meissner's corpuscles are rapidly adapting receptors with specialized endings. Pacinian receptors are found deep in the skin and respond to high frequency vibration within a range of 60 to 500 Hz and to deep pressure. Pacinian corpuscles are particularly important in the evaluation of thermal injuries. The ability to detect deep pressure following deep burns indicates the survival of the deepest region of the dermis, whereas anesthesia to pinprick indicates a full-thickness injury. Meissner's corpuscles respond to lower frequency vibration up to 80 Hz and may be used to detect movement of the skin. Meissner's corpuscles are located in non-hairy (glabrous) skin. On hairy skin, the Meissner's corpuscle is replaced by hair receptors with similar properties to the Meissner's corpuscle. Ruffini's corpuscles and Merkel's disks are slowly adapting receptors. As described above, Merkel's disks have small receptive fields, are superficial, and are useful for localizing continuous pressure. Ruffini receptors are found deep in the skin and respond to deep pressure and stretch. These receptors are also directionally sensitive and are useful in proprioception and kinesthesia.

Thermoreceptors are found both peripherally in the skin and within deep structures. Skin thermoreceptors provide information used to sense environmental temperature, to determine the level of thermal comfort, and to regulate body temperature. Cutaneous receptors serve as warnings to avoid damaging the skin and feed information forward concerning the environmental temperature so that the thermoregulatory system can prevent excessive rises or falls in internal temperature. Both cold and warm sensations are derived from neurons without specialized end-organs. Temperature information is transmitted by slowly conducting C and Aδ neurons. Warmth and cold receptors are slowly adapting so they can convey both changes in temperature and develop a steady action potential frequency when temperature is held constant. Cold receptors respond within a range of approximately 5°C with a peak action potential frequency of about 25°C. Warm fibers respond within a range of about 30°C with a peak response at about 42°C. A combination of information from both types of receptors is necessary to detect temperature over a range of 5°C. Very high or low temperatures stimulate pain receptors and, therefore, give the same sensation.

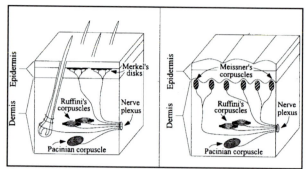

Figure 1-9. Sensory receptors of the skin.

Nociceptors are receptors for noxious stimuli. They have no specialized endings and are distributed throughout the skin, muscle, bones, joints, dura, and capsules of organs. Two different types of neurons transmit different types of pain information. Neurons of the Aδ class transmit pain information that is localized, graded to intensity, and lasts as long as the stimulus is applied. The more primitive type of neuron, the C fiber, transmits a more diffuse, poorly localized, and persistent pain associated with tissue damage or inflammation. These receptors respond to a number of chemical messengers including capsaicin, substance P, potassium, serotonin, bradykinin, histamine, and prostaglandins. Nociceptors also convey discomfort in response to ischemia that motivates individuals to unconsciously shift weight. The lack of nociception places individuals at risk for pressure ulcers on skin beneath weight-bearing bony prominences. Capsaicin is the active ingredient in hot peppers, producing a sensation of warmth and pain due to binding to receptors. Although capsaicin may produce a burning sensation, it does not damage tissues as heat would. Menthol, an ingredient in mints, activates the same receptors as cold, resulting in a cool sensation.

AGING SKIN

A number of aspects of the gross morphology of aging skin are evident. These include decreased moisture content manifested as greater roughness and scaliness of the skin, decreased elasticity manifested as wrinkling and laxity, the accumulation of benign neoplasms, and increased risk of malignant neoplasms. Some of these effects, however, do not simply appear to be the effect of aging, but the accumulation of sun damage. At the microscopic level, flattening of the dermal-epidermal junction can be observed with effacement of dermal papillae. The height of dermal papillae decreases 55% from 3rd to 9th decades. As these changes occur, the surface between the vascularized dermis and the epidermis decreases. Several changes observed in the skin of the elderly result from the decreased contact between these layers. The area available for nutrient transfer, the number of cells within the stratum basale, and resistance to shearing are decreased due to this loss of contact surface between the dermis and epidermis.

Aging Epidermis

The thickness of the stratum corneum remains unchanged with aging, but an increased size and variability of cells are observed. In addition, the number of melanocytes decreases at a rate of about 10% to 20% per decade. Consistent with the decline in the number of melanocytes is a decreased number of nevi. As a result of the decline in the number of melanocytes, the skin has a progressively decreased protection from UV light. In addition, the resident macrophages of the epidermis, the Langerhans cells experience a 20% to 50% decrease.

Aging Dermis

As opposed to the epidermis, the dermis experiences a significant decrease in its thickness, averaging about 20%. This decrease in thickness produces the transparent appearance of elderly skin. Due to a 30% decrease in mast cells, less inflammation results from UV exposure. In addition, regression of the dermal vascular bed and decreased blood flow to appendages leads to gradual atrophy and fibrosis of appendages. A remodeling of elastic fibers into thicker, disorganized elastic fibers results in diminished elasticity and increased risk of tearing.

Functional Changes in the Skin

A 30% to 50% decrease in epidermal turnover has been described from the third to the eighth decade. In addition, a decreased repair rate has been quantified as both decreased wound tensile strength and collagen deposition. Dry, inelastic skin, with larger, more irregular epidermal cells leads to decreased barrier function. Moreover, decreased sensory perception increases the risk of injury to skin by mechanical forces such as pressure. Decreased sebum, estimated to decline by 23% per decade, allows the skin to become dry. Due to decreased numbers of Langerhans cells, immunity within the skin declines, putting the skin at higher risk of infection. Due to the more rigid, less elastic, drier nature of elderly skin with decreased contact area between the dermis and epidermis, the skin of elderly individuals tears and bleeds easily. Skin tears and multiple ecchymoses are commonplace in the skin of the elderly, especially those with multiple intra-venous lines, and with the use of harsh adhesives on tape used to hold IV lines in place.

SUMMARY

Skin consists of 2 primary layers and a subcutaneous fat layer. The epidermis consists primarily of keratinocytes and waterproofs the skin. Distinct layers of cells support the function of the epidermis as the cells mature and migrate toward the surface. Langerhans cells provide an immune function and melanocytes protect the skin from ultraviolet radiation. The dermis consists of a papillary layer that attaches to and nourishes the epidermis and a reticular layer. The dermis consists of fibroblasts within a sea of collagen and elastic fibers and ground substance. Both the structure of the fibers within the dermis and their arrangement provide tensile strength and elasticity of the dermis. Excessive stretch applied to the skin results in tearing. Tearing occurs much more readily in the skin of the elderly. Subcutaneous fat provides thermal insulation and cushions bony prominences. Emaciated individuals are at much higher risk of pressure ulcers because of the lack of soft tissue between the bony prominences and skin.

QUESTIONS

1. List the functions performed by the skin.
2. Contrast the complexity and thickness of the dermis and epidermis.
3. Contrast the functions of the papillary and reticular dermis.
4. How does knowledge of the layers of the skin assist in determining the depth of skin injury?
5. In terms of healing, what is the benefit of the depth of the appendages of the skin?

BIBLIOGRAPHY

Brunelli, D. Langer's Lines. Available at http://www.med-ars.it/. Accessed September 9, 2009.

Irion G. *Physiology: The Basis of Clinical Practice*. Thorofare, NJ: SLACK Incorporated; 2000.

Sadagurski M, Yakar S, Weingarten G, et al. Insulin-like growth factor 1 receptor signaling regulates skin development and inhibits skin keratinocyte differentiation. *Molec Cell Biol.* 2006;26(7):2675-2687.

Normal Wound Healing 2

OBJECTIVES

- Identify the important aspects associated with the 4 phases of normal wound healing, including wound closure and ultimate healing.
- List the phases of normal wound healing and their time frames.
- List the 6 processes occurring in a healing wound.
- Describe events of the inflammatory (lag) phase, including hemostasis and roles of immune cells.
- Describe the events of granulation tissue formation.
- Describe the need for coordination of granulation tissue formation and re-epithelialization.
- Describe the events of the remodeling phases and factors determining wound strength.
- Contrast the injury and healing of superficial, partial-thickness, and full-thickness wounds with subcutaneous tissue involvement.
- Discuss the roles of oxygen in wound healing.
- Describe features distinguishing fetal wound healing from adult wound healing.

NORMAL TISSUE HEALING

Upon injury, a stereotypical sequence of events occurs, leading to the bridging of the defect and resurfacing. The depth of injury to the skin determines the sequence of events. Wounds may be limited to the epidermis (superficial), some of the depth of dermis (partial-thickness), or the wound may involve the complete thickness of the wound (full-thickness) and even extend into subcutaneous tissue. Most, but not all, of the wounds referred to individuals reading this text will involve full-thickness with

subcutaneous involvement and healing by the secondary intent. The bulk of this chapter is a discussion of secondary intent. Following a full-thickness injury, a programmed sequence of events unfolds, which the clinician may either facilitate or disturb with interventions. In this chapter, a description of these events is given. In subsequent chapters, the ways we can facilitate and avoid interfering with the processes will be described. In sequence, these phases of normal wound healing by secondary intent are hemostasis, inflammation, proliferation, and remodeling (Figure 2-1). During these phases an overlapping, orderly sequence of

Irion G.
Comprehensive Wound Management, 2nd ed. (pp 15-24)
© 2010 SLACK Incorporated

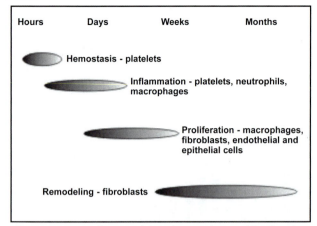

Figure 2-1. Time frames of the phases of wound healing by secondary intention. The relative length of each phase is depicted as the length of each ellipse. Note the time scale, the overlapping of phases, and the cells responsible for each phase.

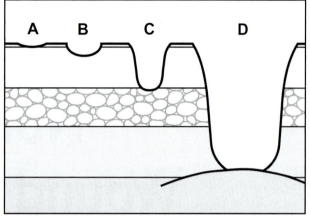

Figure 2-2. Skin structures involved in different depths of wounds.

6 processes occurs: activation of hemostasis, activation of inflammation, re-epithelialization, granulation tissue formation, contraction, and remodeling.

TYPES OF WOUND HEALING

Superficial thickness wounds are caused by shearing, friction, and mild burn (first degree). Healing occurs by regeneration of epithelial cells on the wound surface due to loss of contact inhibition and migration of epidermal cells across the surface. Because no defect in skin continuity occurs, this type of healing does not cause scars, and accessory structures remain intact (Figure 2-2A). However, a serious deep injury may be identified incorrectly as a superficial wound. In many cases of pressure and shear injury, necrotic tissue may be hidden below an injured, but still intact epidermis. Erosion through the remaining thickness of the skin (iceberg/volcano analogy) may lead to expulsion of necrotic tissue, creating a large void.

Partial-thickness wounds (Figure 2-2B) heal in a means similar to superficial thickness wounds. Damage to the dermis occurs, but accessory structures are spared. Eschar may form on the wound (desiccated necrotic tissue, similar to a scab). Partial-thickness wounds have similar causes as superficial wounds, but generally with greater intensity of insult and may also be caused by pressure. Full-thickness wounds (Figure 2-2C) and wounds with subcutaneous involvement (Figure 2-2D) may be closed by primary intent, delayed primary intent (also known as tertiary intent), or by secondary intent. Although inflammation is usually associated with deeper injuries, even superficial wounds will generate some inflammation due to release of chemical messengers that promote inflammation diffusing from damaged epider-

mis into the vascularized tissue below. The processes used for wound closure are described below.

Primary Intention

Primary closure can be accomplished by suturing, stapling, or the use of adhesives. This type of closure (Figure 2-3A) is used for surgical or traumatic wounds that have clean, smooth edges and minimal subcutaneous tissue loss. Attempts to close wounds that do not have these characteristics increase the risk of infection or may cause cosmetic problems. When appropriate, primary closure results in faster healing and less scarring than secondary or delayed primary closure. Epithelialization begins within the first 24 hours if the edges of the wound are apposed and may be complete within 48 to 72 hours. Delayed primary closure uses sutures or staples later, often after irrigation and drainage of an abscess or osteomyelitis (Figure 2-3C). This type of closure is chosen when contamination, tissue loss, or risk of infection is present.

Secondary Intention

Healing by secondary intention refers to allowing wounds to close on their own, as opposed to closing them directly. Ideally, the primary way of closing a surgical wound is by sutures, staples, or adhesives. Should primary intention not be a good option, one goes to the secondary intention. Delayed primary may also be termed *tertiary intention*, the third choice.

Secondary intent (Figure 2-3B) is used for wounds with tissue loss, irregular edges, tissue necrosis, high microbial count, or presence of other debris. The phases of healing by secondary intent are described below.

Hemostasis and Inflammation

The first phase, hemostasis and inflammation, is initiated with blood vessel disruption and the extravasation of

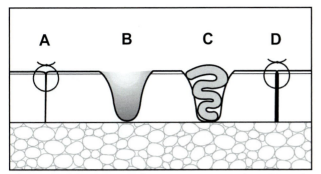

Figure 2-3. Comparison of primary (A), secondary (B), and delayed primary or tertiary (C and D) healing. C depicts packing of wound to be closed later, D depicts wound in C closed with sutures. Note the clean edges and minimal granulation tissue of primary healing. Secondary healing is characterized by the production of granulation tissue and wound contraction. Delayed primary healing may be associated with some amount of granulation tissue and contraction depending on the amount of tissue lost to necrosis.

blood constituents. Injury to blood vessels is followed rapidly by activation of platelet aggregation and the coagulation cascade, resulting in the formation of the insoluble fibrin molecule and hemostasis. During this process, activation of complement occurs, leading to the sequence of events of inflammation, including the recruitment of macrophages and neutrophils. Afterward, blood flow to the area is restored by mechanisms described below.

Platelets

With tissue injury, platelets are activated by collagen and thrombin. A positive feedback of secretion and aggregation ensues, amplifying the platelet response to injury. With platelet activation, PDGF release occurs. As discussed in Chapter 1, PDGF plays a major role in healing and is frequently defective in poorly controlled diabetes mellitus. PDGF also stimulates release of other growth factors such as vascular endothelial growth factor (VEGF) and bFGF.

Coagulation Cascade

The series of chemical reactions leading to the production of fibrin is stimulated by the Hageman factor, which is activated either by exposure to collagen or by the release of tissue factor by injured cells. In addition, complement and other proteins activated by Hageman factor intensify the inflammatory response to injury. The coagulated region of injury will become the site on which macrophages and fibroblasts are attracted and granulation will be activated with deposition of collagen and matrix.

Neutrophils

An influx of white cells begins with neutrophils early and macrophages later. Neutrophils migrate into the area within the first 24 hours of wounding and may persist for several hours to days. Neutrophils increase the permeability of undamaged vessels, causing the leakage of plasma and proteins, and the swelling associated with inflammation. The basic sequence used by neutrophils to clear bacterial contamination consists of opsonization of bacteria by complement, generation of chemotactic factors, adhesion of white blood cells to endothelium, and emigration of white blood cells through vessels, attachment of opsonized bacteria to white blood cells, phagocytosis, and killing and digestion of bacteria.

Due to the nonspecific nature of neutrophil action, neutrophil recruitment also leads to tissue damage from release of enzymes and free radicals. Neutrophils are recruited by numerous factors related to the injury and, under normal circumstances, they largely leave the area of injury when bacteria and dead cells are removed. The activation of neutrophils causes release of elastase and collagenase, which degrade the connective tissue surrounding the injury. Their primary function in an injury site is the destruction of bacteria via phagocytosis and enzyme and free radical release. Neutrophil infiltration ceases in a few days if a wound becomes clean.

At this time programmed death of the neutrophils (apoptosis) occurs, which limits the destruction of cells in the area of injury. The appearance of spent neutrophils phagocytized by macrophages marks the end of early inflammation. However, contamination of wounds causes persistence of neutrophil immigration. Foreign surfaces initiate complement activity; therefore, repeated trauma by harsh treatment of wounds may also cause persistence of neutrophils.

Macrophages

Macrophages have the dual roles of destruction of nonviable material and the stimulation of new tissue growth. Unlike other cells in the healing process, macrophages are present across all phases of healing. The accumulation of macrophages continues regardless of neutrophil activity due to the presence of selective chemoattractants for macrophages. Macrophages, like neutrophils, also release proteases to aid in the degradation of devitalized tissue. The presence of macrophages is necessary for both the initiation and propagation of granulation tissue.

Initially, macrophages are responsible for phagocytosis of bacteria, spent neutrophils, and cell debris. In addition, they release numerous substances, including prostaglandins and leukotrienes, a variety of chemoattractants for cells to repair the defect, and the release of the growth factors including PDGF, bFGF, tumor necrosis factor (TNF), and TGFß. The transition from the inflammatory phase to the proliferative phase is dependent on the effectiveness of the macrophage to clean an area of debris and release growth factors.

Mast Cells

Recently, mast cell-nerve interaction has drawn attention in wound healing and various other signaling mechanisms. During trauma, mast cells are degranulated, causing the release of a large number of chemical signals. Degranulation appears to be mediated by both an immediate sensory nerve-mediated response to injury and direct trauma. The importance of mast cell degranulation and release of substances including histamine, heparin, bFGF, IL-4, and TNF is maintaining the viability of the tissue surrounding the injury. In the immediate area of the wound, hemostasis prevents the loss of fluid, cells, and proteins; however, thrombosis of vessels may interfere with supply of nutrients to surrounding areas and increase the necrosis of tissue beyond the area of injury. Histamine produces vasodilation and increased permeability, thereby maintaining blood flow to adjacent tissue, as well as allowing cells responsible for immunity and repair into the area of injury. Heparin controls hemostasis, preventing excessive coagulation and thereby limiting damage to surrounding tissue. Basic FGF stimulates attraction and reproduction of epidermal cells, IL-4 increases synthesis of types I and III of collagen, laminin, and fibronectin. Mast cell release of TNF provides a strong stimulus for the production of collagen. Capsaicin, the active ingredient of chili peppers, has been studied as a means of decreasing pain through the release of substance P and the down regulation of capsaicin receptors. Release of substance P and related compounds causes degranulation of mast cells and release of endothelial adhesion molecules and other cytokines that promote healing. Release of molecules such as histamine, bradykinin, and prostaglandins produces vasodilation in the injured area, leading to increased blood flow, increased pressure within the capillaries which, coupled with the increase in permeability caused by these chemical signals, allows the loss of plasma, plasma proteins, and cells into the wounded area. For these reasons, swelling and pain are experienced in the wounded and surrounding area in addition to the erythema and warmth associated with inflammation. Inflammation in acute wounds should last 3 to 7 days; a longer period of inflammation is predictive of slow healing.

Proliferative Phase

During the proliferative phase (Figure 2-4), both re-epithelialization and granulation tissue formation occur. In some types of wounds, wound contraction also occurs. Re-epithelialization begins within 24 hours, although it may not be observable for the first 3 days. This perceived delay at the macroscopic level is the basis for the term *lag phase*, which is sometimes used in the place of the term *inflammatory phase*. Granulation tissue formation begins in 3 to 5 days. During this time, re-epithelialization and granulation occur concurrently. Re-epithelialization pro-

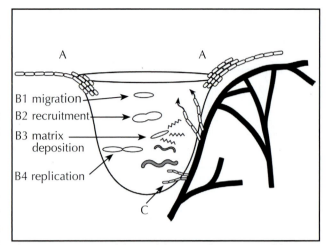

Figure 2-4. Events of the proliferative phase. (A) Proliferation and migration of epithelial cells from wound margins. (B) Proliferation of fibroblasts and production of collagen fibers. (C) Proliferation of angioblasts and angiogenesis.

vides protection, whereas granulation and contraction fill defects in tissue. A variety of signals for initiation of new tissue growth are responsible for the proliferative phase, including chemotactic factors and growth factors released by the accumulation of macrophages and degranulation of mast cells in the injured tissue. In addition, the loss of neighboring cells (loss of cell restraint or contact inhibition) stimulates the replication of epidermal cells. The proliferation of cells needed for repair is dependent on a balance of growth factors and proteolytic enzymes, especially matrix metalloproteinases. The factors that promote and inhibit tissue growth are regulated by redundant controls to provide the proper amount of proliferation, such as tissue inhibitors of metalloproteinases (TIMPs). Imbalance of these molecules results in problematic healing. Abnormal healing is discussed in the Chapter 3.

Granulation Tissue Formation

The production of granulation tissue is dependent on macrophage accumulation. Macrophages stimulate fibroblast ingrowth, deposition of loose connective tissue, and angiogenesis (formation of new capillaries in the wound). These processes, termed *fibroplasia* and *angiogenesis*, are stimulated by chemotactic factors released by platelets, in addition to those of the macrophages. Stimulation of fibroblasts by growth factors results in proliferation of fibroblasts, migration of fibroblasts to the area of injury, connective tissue matrix deposition, and wound contraction. Granulation tissue formation is stimulated by low levels of bacteria in the wound, but inhibited by high levels of bacteria.

Connective Tissue Matrix

The connective tissue matrix deposited by macrophages provides substrate for migration into the wound by other macrophages, angioblasts (immature cells of capillary walls), and fibroblasts. Angiogenesis is the process of forming new blood vessels, in this case, in the area of a wound. During angiogenesis, endothelial cells respond to chemotactic and growth factors, and enzymes are released to degrade the basement membrane of existing blood vessels. As angioblasts are attracted to the distal end of blood vessels, they are stimulated to extend pseudopods through existing vessels, leading to the migration of angioblasts. The proliferation of angioblasts to form tube-like extensions from existing capillaries creates new capillaries. These new vessels allow healing to continue by supplying cells with nutrients to support increased metabolic rate and materials to construct granulation tissue. The loops of vessels and matrix produce a shiny, reddish-pink tissue into pebbly mounds, which leads to the term *granulation tissue*. Initially granulation tissue may appear pink. As blood vessels continue to develop, the granulation tissue should become red. Failure of granulation tissue to become redder is a possible indicator of arterial disease preventing adequate blood flow through the new granulation tissue.

Re-epithelialization

Resurfacing of the injured tissue is accomplished by the movement of keratinocytes from free edges, including those surrounding hair follicles and sweat glands, into the wound. As new cells are formed at the wound's edge in response to release of IL-1 and epidermal growth factor, they adhere to the granulation tissue beneath, and replicated cells migrate by a means called epiboly that has been described as a leap frog, pouring over cells to reach the advancing wound edge (see Figure 2-4). With the loss of contact inhibition and the presence of growth factors, an alteration of the phenotype of cells occurs. A retraction of internal keratin filaments occurs along with dissolution of desmosomes to allow mobility of keratinocytes toward the wound edge. The newly unrestrained keratinocytes develop actin filaments and mobility, they lose apical/basal polarity and extend pseudopods toward the wound. These cells will produce a provisional matrix consisting of fibrin, fibronectin, and type V collagen if the basement membrane is damaged. Cells also change the composition of undamaged basement membrane by incorporating more fibronectin as it is stimulated by the release of TGFß. Cells are transformed to a normal phenotype when the wound is covered, and the keratinocytes are again constrained. Normal composition of the basement membrane is restored and desmosomes are reestablished to secure keratinocytes through the basement membrane to the dermis.

Fibroplasia and Contraction

Fibroblasts undergo a phenotypic change following injury. Their migration into the wound is aided by fibronectin. The molecules deposited by fibroblasts, in particular fibronectin, result in production of a loose extracellular matrix. Amplification of granulation tissue growth results as fibronectin allows fibroblast movement across it, fibronectin links multiple fibroblasts into the network and greater quantities of matrix molecules are released into the wound site. As fibroblasts release the precursors to collagen fibers and collagen fibers develop, wound strength increases. The processes involved in producing collagen fibers are oxygen-dependent. Hydroxyproline produced by the fibroblasts aggregates in a triple helix forming procollagen, which is released into the extracellular space. Procollagen molecules are further processed in the extracellular space into tropocollagen. The tropocollagen molecules aggregate to form an initial unorganized network of collagen fibers, providing the limited tensile strength of the immature wound. Wound strength cannot develop without the angiogenesis necessary to supply oxygen and amino acids needed to form hydroxyproline, the precursor to collagen.

Contraction of the wound occurs as fibroblasts retract their endoplasmic reticulum and Golgi bodies and begin to synthesize large quantities of collagen. The formation of actin filaments transforms fibroblasts into myofibroblasts. The process of contraction produces radial movement of intact skin around the wound toward the center of the wound. Contraction of full-thickness wounds reduces the quantity of new tissue required to fill the wound. Examples of wound contraction are shown in Figure 2-5. To avoid contraction that may lead to functional limitations, a strategy of allowing the wound bed to fill with granulation tissue, then covering it with a skin graft may be used. Skin grafts are further discussed later in the chapter. The presence of even a split thickness of skin may be sufficient to minimize wound contraction is many cases.

Remodeling

The process of remodeling is typically thought of as a long-term response to wounding. However, extracellular matrix changes continually. Extracellular matrix and fibroblasts control each other until a stable matrix is formed in months to years. As a result, the extracellular matrix is different in the periphery and the center of a wound. Although wound strength increases with deposition of collagen, strength increases by a greater magnitude than what can be attributed to the accumulation of collagen. The reasons suggested for this phenomenon include selective degradation of unstressed collagen fibers, reinforcement of stressed fibers, and reinforcement of collagen fibers by glycosaminoglycans.

Healing

When granulation, re-epithelialization, and contraction are complete, the wound may be covered, but the skin has not yet recovered. Re-epithelialized skin has

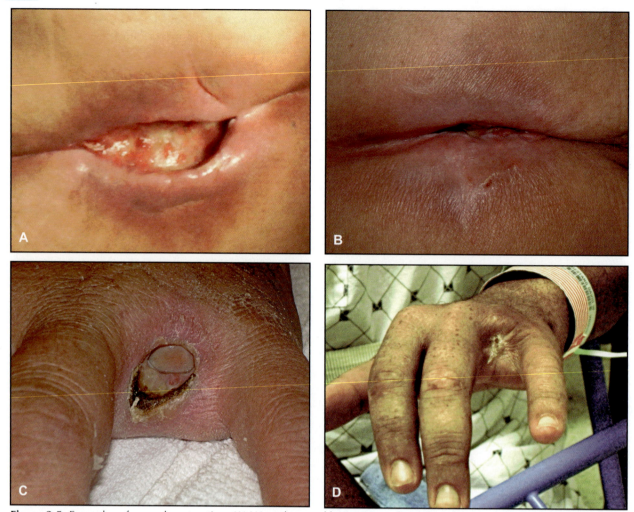

Figure 2-5. Examples of wound contraction. (A) Wound created by excision of rectal carcinoma. (B) Same wound following granulation, re-epithelialization, and contraction. (C) Wound caused by amputation of fourth finger of left hand due to ischemic necrosis. (D) Same wound following granulation, epithelialization, and wound contraction. In both B and D, note the tension placed on surrounding skin by the contraction and the uneven nature of the contraction.

strength approximately 15% of normal and reaches about 80% of normal strength when remodeling is complete. The increase in strength from 15% to 80% comes largely from the remodeling process. A newly covered wound must still be protected from even minor trauma to prevent chronic inflammation, which may lead to unnecessary thickening of the skin and further loss of elasticity. Moreover, the site of the wound influences the extent to which the skin will regain its normal function. Certain areas of skin are prone to stresses because of their location over joints or the shape of what lies below the skin. A wound on the elbow, knee, or dorsum of the hand or foot is subjected to the stresses of joint structures moving below. Areas such as the bridge of the nose, the buttocks, or heels have skin pulled around them tightly. Relatively flat areas without structures moving below them are more likely to recover strength and elasticity.

Tertiary Intention

Tertiary intention or delayed primary intention refers to leaving a wound open until closing it becomes prudent. Closing a wound that is likely to harbor harmful bacteria may lead to sepsis or death. Therefore, such wounds are initially allowed to stay open as they would be with secondary intention. However, with tertiary intention, the wound is not allowed to granulate in completely and re-epithelialize. Instead, when the wound is deemed clean and stable and therefore unlikely to pose a significant risk of infection, it is closed with sutures or staples as it would be with primary intention. In some cases, sutures are placed across the wound, but the edges are not opposed. As the ends of the wound granulate in, sutures are tied off until the wound is closed.

Healing by tertiary intention is appropriate in cases such as those described for secondary intention. If tissue loss occurs in wounding, granulation tissue can be allowed to fill the void and then closure is performed. In wounds at high risk of infection, the wound is cleansed or debrided until the wound is unlikely to become infected. This procedure is most commonly done following incision and drainage of abscesses. Dead space of the wound is filled with suitable materials to prevent premature closure of the wound.

EFFECTS OF OXYGEN

Oxygen is believed to be important to several aspects of wound healing, including the competence of the immune cells, development of new blood vessels, and the production of collagen. Tissue partial pressure of oxygen (PO_2) has been shown to vary with distance from a wound from a value close to 0 mmHg at the wound site and areas of vessel injury and to a value near arterial PO_2 nearby uninjured vessels. Although hypoxia and acidosis attract neutrophils to the site of a wound, hypoxia along with hypercapnia (excessive carbon dioxide) and acidosis may impair both immunity and collagen synthesis. Hypoxia is also a strong stimulus for angiogenesis. Lactate produced by either aerobic or anaerobic metabolism stimulates angiogenesis. Because macrophages produce lactate even under aerobic conditions, the stimulation of angiogenesis occurs even in a normoxic condition. Restoration of blood flow through angiogenesis provides a better environment for the immune cells attracted to the area. Much of the antimicrobial effect of immune cells is mediated by oxidative killing by neutrophils. The rate of oxidative killing by neutrophils is directly dependent on the production of superoxide radicals from molecular oxygen, which in turn is dependent on the PO_2 of tissue surrounding the neutrophil. The presence of neutrophils also enhances the effectiveness of antimicrobial drugs. If the site of bacterial entry remains hypoxic, bacteria may proliferate too quickly for neutrophils to prevent infection. The greater the arterial oxygenation during surgery, the less likely the patient is to experience a postoperative infection.

Oxygen also has a potentially deleterious effect through the process of reperfusion injury. Neutrophils in an injured area are stimulated to produce free radicals such as superoxide as part of the process of destroying microbes in an injured area. With a sudden increase in blood flow carrying oxygen to the injured area, free radical generation may become severe enough to injure otherwise healthy cells, including the endothelium of the vessels supplying the area. Additionally, neutrophils that are activated to produce free radicals cannot deform and may plug the microcirculation. As a result of the injured endothelium and neutrophil plugging, tissue death in the injured area exceeds what it would have been without reperfusion.

FETAL WOUND HEALING

Differences in fetal incisional wound healing have been described for several years. Incisional wounds heal rapidly, with normal skin morphology and without scarring. Other features of scarless fetal repair include a lack of neutrophils and acute inflammation, rapid epithelialization, low vascularity, highly organized collagen and a hyaluronan-rich matrix. Discovery of the exact mechanism allowing scarless healing is hoped to lead to application to abnormal wound healing in the adult. One factor that is clearly delineated is the rich hyaluronic acid environment of the fetal wound. Hyaluronidase introduced into a fetal wound results in fibrosis and angiogenesis characteristic of adult wound healing. Thus, a high level of hyaluronic acid and low hyaluronidase may be necessary for scarless healing. Adult skin transplanted to a fetus, and then wounded, heals with scarring. Fetal tissue transplanted to a subcutaneous location on an adult and wounded heals without scarring, but when transplanted to a cutaneous location does scar. When transplanted to a subcutaneous location, the graft heals with collagen generated by the fetal fibroblasts, whereas the cutaneous transplants heal with collagen from the host, leading to scarring. Moreover, adult skin transplanted to fetuses heals with scar formation, indicating that fetal cells, not the environment of the wounded tissue, determines whether scarring occurs. As the fetus approaches full-term, wounds heal with inflammation, granulation tissue formation, wound contraction, and scarring. Excisional wounds differ from incisional wounds in that tissue must be generated to fill a gap between edges of the wound. With this type of wound, both the size and gestational age increase the likelihood of adult-like scar formation. The most promising strategy to mimic fetal healing at this time is manipulation of TGFß. This cytokine has several roles in wound healing, particularly as a chemoattractant for cells involved in inflammation. TGFß does not increase with fetal wounding as it does in adults. Moreover, the addition of antibodies to TGFß significantly reduces scarring in adult skin, whereas application of TGFß increased scarring.

OPERATIVE REPAIR

If possible, direct closure of an acute wound is preferable to prevent contamination and chronic inflammation. Indications for direct closure include lacerations with minimal tissue loss, surgical wounds and other incisions. Regardless of the cause of the wound, for direct closure to be the method of choice, the wound must be clean and likely to heal. Prior to direct closure, the site must be irrigated and debrided of any foreign material or necrotic tissue. A surgeon may choose delayed primary closure (tertiary closure) if significant undermining or contamination is present. Should direct closure be chosen, deep sutures are placed in the depth of the wound to decrease stress on the skin's surface. Surgical staples or adhesives (glue) may be used in the place of sutures. A number of techniques are available to plastic surgeons to close even complicated wounds with minimum evidence of scarring. In some cases, however, primary closure is not sufficient and grafts are required.

Grafts

In the event that sufficient skin is unavailable to close wounds optimally, tissue may be transplanted from one part of the body to another. Types of grafts used in plastic surgery include skin grafts, which have no blood supply, and flaps that are transplanted with a blood supply.

Skin Grafts

Skin grafts are indicated for wounds that are not expected to close spontaneously in a reasonable time frame, provided the patient has suitable graft donor sites with sufficient vascularity to be invaded by blood vessels within the site that will be receiving the graft. Skin grafts are only indicated if the site has no need for subcutaneous tissue to act as padding. Additional considerations include aesthetics of the healed graft site. Either split thickness or full-thickness grafts may be used, depending on the area to be covered. The advantage of a split thickness skin graft is its ability to cover a larger area due to meshing, which allows a surface area approximately 3 times as large to be covered as the donor area and the ability to reharvest the same donor site. A meshed split thickness graft also has the advantage of allowing fluid to escape rather than accumulate under the graft and prevent adherence. The stretching of the meshed graft has the important effect of converting a single large defect in the skin into multiple small wounds that can heal by re-epithelialization more rapidly that a single large wound of the same cumulative surface area. As the donor site heals by re-epithelialization, it can be reharvested after 10 to 14 days to provide a graft for another area of the body. Drawbacks of split thickness grafts include cosmetic problems and function on flexor surfaces. Certain areas of the body such as the face, hands, and flexor surfaces may require a full-thickness graft. Full-thickness grafts have sufficient strength to function on flexor surfaces such as the anterior elbow, axilla, and posterior knee, and are much more cosmetically acceptable than the residual diamond effect left in a healed meshed split thickness skin graft. However, full-thickness skin grafts can only cover 1/3 of the area that a split thickness graft can and the available surface area for taking full-thickness grafts may be limited. Cultured skin is another way of covering a wound. A small piece of skin is harvested from the patient and grown under optimal conditions in a laboratory setting. After several weeks, a piece of skin originally only a few cm^2 may reach a size approaching a square meter. Precautions following successful grafting include the risk of infection, protecting the graft from the effect of shear for 7 to 14 days and the need for lubrication.

Flaps

In certain cases, flaps are preferable to grafts. Benefits of a flap include better quality skin cover, sensation is more likely to remain intact with a flap, the provision of padding, the ability to cover exposed anatomic structures and prostheses, the ability to maintain blood supply, cosmesis, and the possibility of functional restoration. Flaps are classified based on the type of tissue grafted and the anatomic relationship between the donor and graft site of the flap. Tissue type may include skin and subcutaneous tissue, muscle with or without overlying skin, or bone with or without original overlying tissue. The anatomic relationship between the donor and graft site may be classified as local, in which the tissue harvested is adjacent to the defect to be filled; distant, in which the harvested tissue is attached temporarily to its original site until vascularization occurs at the new location; and a free flap, which has been removed from its donor site, but blood vessels are anastomosed to blood vessels in the new location.

Skin Flaps

Although the purpose of using a skin flap rather than a skin graft is the presence of intact blood vessels, blood supply to the skin flap can be unpredictable. If blood vessels are identifiable within the flap, the preference is for a flap with an axial, arterial supply running the length of flap. An axial supply can provide a larger flap than a flap with a horizontal blood supply.

Muscle Flaps

This type of flap can be done without overlying skin, but if overlying skin is not used, then it must be covered with a split thickness skin graft. As with the skin flap, an axial blood supply is preferred with perforating blood vessels to revascularize skin. In contrast to skin flaps, muscle flaps provide padding. Good blood supply decreases risk of infection or failure of graft to take.

Free Flaps

To perform a free flap, the surgeon must be able to identify vessels to anastomose in both the flap and recipient site. If this vessel anastomosis can be done, the free flap provides well-vascularized tissue to a site that does not have a good local blood flow. In addition, a skilled surgeon may be able to anastomose a nerve. Other specialized flaps exist and the reader is directed toward texts covering these flaps.

Living Skin Equivalents

The types of biosynthetic skin known as living skin equivalents (LSEs) are based on dermal-derived and epidermal/dermal-derived processes. Cells harvested from neonatal foreskins are used to avoid rejection. The material is grown in culture without immune markers or accessory structures of the skin.

Apligraf (Organogenesis, Canton, MA) is a bilayered material marketed as "living bilayered, cell therapy." It consists of human keratinocytes and fibroblasts in addition to bovine type I collagen. As such it is not considered a graft, but a temporary covering that allows the recipient to eventually replace the applied product with his/her own skin. This product contains matrix, cytokines, and growth factors normally found in human skin. The presence of growth factors and cytokines is believed to be responsible for the patient's ability to regenerate new skin to gradually replace the product. However, Apligraf does not contain any melanocytes, immune cells, blood vessels, nerves, or accessory structures (sweat glands, hair follicles, sebaceous glands). Apligraf is currently approved for venous and neuropathic ulcers (diabetic foot ulcers). Apligraf is packaged as a disk 75 mm in diameter and 0.75 mm thick.

When applied, Apligraf can be fenestrated ("windows" cut into it) or meshed to avoid fluid buildup under the product to improve its adhesion to granulation tissue. It can be affixed with tape, sutures, staples, Steri-Strips, or skin adhesive. A secondary dressing and compression are applied. The patient is to avoid activities that could either lead to edema in the area or shear the material from the wound. Dressings directly in contact with Apligraf need to be left in place at least 5 to 7 days to avoid damaging the material. Outer dressings may be changed more frequently as needed (3 to 5 days).

Other available LSEs consist of different materials: fibroblasts embedded in nylon and porcine collagen (TransCyte, Smith & Nephew, St Petersburg, FL); acellular dermal matrix (Alloderm, LifeCell Corporation, Branchburg, NJ); bovine collagen, chondroitin-6-sulfate and silicone (Integra, Integra Lifesciences Corporation, Plainsboro, NJ); human fibroblasts in a bioabsorbable polyglactin mesh scaffold that produces human collagen, matrix proteins, growth factors, and cytokines (Dermagraft, Advanced BioHealing, Westport, CT). Other LSEs are likely to be developed in the future along with guidelines of which product may be most suitable for different applications. LSEs do not always take, and may need to be reapplied, especially in cases of arterial disease or excessive edema of the application site. Even with good results, additional applications may be required. Application of LSEs is limited to physicians at this time.

SUMMARY

Normal wound healing differs with the depth of injury. Simple partial-thickness wounds heal by re-epithelialization, whereas full-thickness wounds may heal by either primary intention or secondary intention. Primary intention refers to surgical closure of clean, narrow wounds. Delayed primary or healing by third intent is used after a wound is sufficiently clean and narrow to be closed later. Healing by secondary intent requires a coordination of hemostasis, inflammation, re-epithelialization, production of granulation tissue, wound contraction, and remodeling of the scar tissue. Fetal incisional wounds heal without scarring, although the risk of scarring increases with both the size of the wound and age. The greater proportion of hyaluronic acid and lower TGFß activity appear to be important in scarless fetal wound healing. Transplant studies indicate that the cells active in healing, rather than the wound environment, determine whether scarless healing occurs.

QUESTIONS

1. Contrast healing of superficial and partial-thickness wounds to full-thickness wounds.
2. Why does inflammation only occur in vascularized tissues?
3. Why might harsh treatment of wounds resulting in bleeding slow wound healing?
4. What benefit does exercise provide in preventing loss of range of motion following large full-thickness skin injuries?

BIBLIOGRAPHY

Agren MS, Karlsmark T, Hansen JB, Rygaard J. Occlusion versus air exposure on full-thickness biopsy wounds. *J Wound Care.* 2001;10:301-304.

Allen DB, Maguire JJ, Mahdavian M, et al. Wound hypoxia and acidosis limit neutrophil bacterial killing mechanisms. *Arch Surg.* 1997;132:991-996.

Baserga R, Hongo A, Rubini M, Prisco M, Valentinis B. The IGF-I receptor in cell growth, transformation and apoptosis. *Biochim Biophys Acta.* 1997;1332:F105–F126.

Bauer O, Razin E. Mast cell-nerve interactions. *News in Physiological Sciences.* 2000;15:213-218.

Byl NN, Hopf H. The use of oxygen in wound healing. In: McCulloch JM, Kloth LC, Feedar JA, eds. *Wound Healing: Alternatives in Management.* 2nd ed. Philadelphia, PA: F.A. Davis; 1995.

Cass DL, Meuli M, Adzick NS. Scar wars: implications of fetal wound healing for the pediatric burn patient. *Pediatr Surg Int.* 1997;12:484-489.

Cass DL, Bullard KM, Sylvester KG, Yang EY, Longaker MT, Adzick NS. Wound size and gestational age modulate scar formation in fetal wound repair. *J Pediatr Surg.* 1997;32:411-415.

Cohen PR. The lunula. *J Am Acad Dermatol.* 1996;34:943-953.

Estes JM, Adzick NS, Harrison MR, Longaker MT, Stern R. Hyaluronate metabolism undergoes an ontogenic transition during fetal development: implications for scar-free wound healing. *J Pediatr Surg.* 1993;28:1227-1231.

Fleckman P. Anatomy and physiology of the nail. *Dermatol Clin.* 1985;3:373-381.

Fusenig N, Limat A, Stark HJ, Breitkreutz D. Modulation of the differentiated phenotype of keratinocytes of the hair follicle and from epidermis. *J Dermatol Sci.* 1994;7(Suppl.):S142–S151.

Gottwald T, Coerper S, Schäffer M, Köveker G, Stead RH. The mast cell-nerve axis in wound healing: a hypothesis. *Wound Repair Regen.* 1998;6:8-20.

Greif R, Akca O, Horn E-P, Kurz A, Sessler DI. Supplemental perioperative oxygen to reduce the incidence of surgical-wound infection. *N Engl J Med.* 2000;342:161-167.

Iizuka H, Takahashi H, Honma M, Ishida-Yamamoto A. Unique keratinization process in psoriasis: late differentiation markers are abolished because of the premature cell death. *J Dermatol.* 2004;31:271–276.

Longaker MG, Whitby DJ, Ferguson MW, Lorenz HP, Harrison MR, Adzick NS. Adult skin wounds in the fetal environment heal with scar formation. *Ann Surg.* 1994;219:65-72.

Lorenz HP, Lin RY, Longaker MT, Whitby DJ, Adzick NS. The fetal fibroblast: the effector cell of scarless fetal skin repair. *Plast Reconstr Surg.* 1995;96:1251-1259.

Martin P. Wound healing—aiming for perfect skin regeneration. *Science.* 1997;276:75–81.

Mehrel T, Hohl D, Rothnagel JA, et al. Identification of a major keratinocyte cell envelope protein, loricrin. *Cell.* 1990;61:1103–1112.

Miki H, Yamauchi T, Suzuki R, et al. Essential role of insulin receptor substrate 1 (IRS-1) and IRS-2 in adipocyte differentiation. *Mol Cell Biol.* 2001;21:2521-2532.

Raja, Sivamani K, Garcia MS, Isseroff RR. Wound re-epithelialization: modulating keratinocyte migration in wound healing. *Front Biosci.* 2007;12:2849-2868.

Sayama K, Yamasaki K, Hanakawa Y, et al. Phosphatidylinositol 3-kinase is a key regulator of early phase differentiation in keratinocytes. *J Bio Chem.* 2002;277:40390–40396.

Shah M, Foreman DM, Ferguson MWJ. Neutralisation of TGFβ-2 or exogenous addition of TGF-β to cutaneous rat wounds reduces scarring. *J Cell Sci.* 1995;108:985-1002.

Wakita H, Takigawa M. Activation of epidermal growth factor receptor promotes late terminal differentiation of cell-matrix interaction-disrupted keratinocytes. *J Biol Chem.* 1999;274:37285–37291.

West DC, Shaw DM, Lorenz P, Adzick NS, Longaker MT. Fibrotic healing of adult and late gestation fetal wound correlates with increased hyaluronidase activity and removal of hyaluron. *Int J Biochem and Cell Biology.* 1997;29:201-210.

Winter GD, Scales JT. Effect of air drying and dressings on the surface of a wound. *Nature.* 1963;197:91-92.

Yuspa SH, Hawley-Nelson P, Koehler B, Stanley JR. A survey of transformation markers in differentiating epidermal cell lines in culture. *Cancer Res.* 1980;40:4694-4703.

Abnormal Wound Healing

3

OBJECTIVES

- Discuss the clinical significance of local, systemic, and comorbid factors that affect healing.
- Define abnormal wound healing; list common causes.
- List signs of infection.
- Describe the appearance of necrotic tissue and its influence on wound healing.
- Describe the appearance of epiboly, the problems it causes with healing, and means of correcting it.
- Define maceration; describe its appearance, list its cause and means of correcting it.
- Define desiccation; discuss its impact on healing, and list means of correcting it.
- Describe the appearance of wounds with chronic inflammation and chronic proliferation.

Abnormal wound healing refers to the failure of a wound to progress through the phases of wound healing in a timely manner. Problems include the potential failure of inflammation, re-epithelialization, granulation tissue formation, and remodeling. Abnormal healing may manifest itself as chronicity of the phases of either inflammation or proliferation. Other manifestations may include abnormal granulation, re-epithelialization, or remodeling.

FACTORS AFFECTING HEALING

Many potential factors may interfere with timely progression of a wound through the phases of healing. For the sake of explanation, these can be divided into systemic, local, and iatrogenic factors. The term *systemic factor* implies a process that affects the patient in ways beyond slowing of wound healing. Local factors are limited to the area of the wound, although they could be manifested in other areas based on properties of the affected body parts. For example, unrelieved pressure over the greater trochanter, or arterial disease affecting the feet are local factors.

One important indicator of faulty healing is the early rate of healing. Wound area measurements after 4 weeks of care for diabetic foot ulcers, and repeated measurements at 12 weeks, indicate that those with a greater reduction in wound size after 4 weeks were much more likely to close wounds at 12 weeks than those with less wound area reduction. For those with a healing rate at 4 weeks faster than the median rate, 58% close at 12 weeks, whereas only 9% of those who heal more slowly than the median at 4 weeks heal at 12 weeks. For wounds that close at 12 weeks, the percentage of change in wound area at 4 weeks is 82%,

Irion G.
Comprehensive Wound Management, 2nd ed. (pp 25-36)
© 2010 SLACK Incorporated

but is only 25% on average after 4 weeks in those who fail to attain wound closure by 12 weeks.

Systemic

Global factors impeding wound healing include any break in the chain of nutrients reaching the wound site. Nutrition and hydration affect the patient as a whole and are discussed in the Chapter 4. Comorbidities such as congestive heart failure, respiratory disease, diseases preventing the gastrointestinal tract from absorbing nutrients are also considered systemic factors. Patients may also be immunosuppressed due to inherited diseases that produce deficiency of certain aspects of the immune system (primary immunodeficiency), or secondary immunodeficiencies that may include diseases such as AIDS, diabetes mellitus and other diseases that affect the immune system, burn injury, certain types of cancer, and consumption of tobacco, alcohol, and other drugs. Aging may also be considered as a systemic factor for slow healing. Infection may be either a systemic or local influence on wound healing as are sensation and functional mobility. Ability to reposition one's self decreases the risk of pressure ulcers in particular. Inability to feel mechanical factors that may be damaging the skin could result from a systemic process such as a stroke, or a more localized factor such as a peripheral nerve injury. Incontinence may be considered a systemic factor, although its effect is mainly on the perineum.

Local

The division into local and systemic factors is not always clear and perhaps does not need to be. However, the term *local* is generally interpreted as processes that do not affect the entire body such as diseases including diabetes mellitus do. Examples of local factors include hypergranulation, localized reduction in perfusion and oxygenation of tissues due to arterial disease or other types of occlusion. Other possible local factors include infection (including cellulitis), edema, pressure, friction, shear, moisture, localized neuropathy, hyperkeratosis (callus formation), and epiboly.

Iatrogenic

Iatrogenic causes of abnormal wound healing include medications and surgery, but also include harsh or inappropriate wound care. Drugs that affect inflammation, immunity, hemostasis, or cell growth in general may cause healing problems. Anti-inflammatory drugs, including over the counter medications, are very common. Some patients may take large quantities of over-the-counter anti-inflammatory drugs and forget to mention them when a history is taken. Two basic classes are non-steroidal anti-inflammatory drugs (NSAIDs) and glucocorticoids. These drugs may be used for a variety of ailments including chronic

muscle or joint pain. Glucocorticoids are used for conditions such as arthritis, asthma, lupus, scleroderma, and other autoimmune diseases characterized by inflammation. Another class of drugs blocks the effects of leukotrienes, which mediate much of the inflammation associated with asthma. The immune system may be deliberately suppressed to prevent rejection of transplants or to treat autoimmune diseases such as lupus, scleroderma, psoriasis, rheumatoid arthritis, and others that do not respond sufficiently to anti-inflammatory drugs. Drugs that suppress the immune system may have their effects on leukocytes or more specific elements of the immune system, eg, tumor necrosis factor.

Cancer chemotherapeutic agents that affect the production of new cells such as cells of the hair follicles, lining of the gastrointestinal tract, and the hematologic and immune systems, will also inhibit the growth of cells required for wound healing. Many patients may be taking drugs to prevent coagulation or platelet aggregation. Warfarin, heparin, and low-molecular-weight heparins are anticoagulants. Other drugs affecting hemostasis include aspirin and other drugs affecting cyclooxygenase, ADP receptor inhibitors (Clopidogrel, Ticlopidine), phosphodiesterase inhibitors (Cilostazol), glycoprotein IIB/IIIA inhibitors (Abciximab, Eptifibatide, Tirofiban), and adenosine reuptake inhibitors (Dipyridamole).

Skin may also be damaged by procedures performed on the patient. Examples include surgical incisions, long surgical procedures with unrelieved pressure on the same areas of the body leading to pressure ulcers, and infiltration of IV or dialysis lines into the interstitial space leading to substantial swelling and injury to the skin. Another cause is irradiation used primarily to treat neoplastic disease. A given patient may have radiation treatments to avoid surgery, have a poor response, and then have a surgical incision made in radiation-damaged skin. Radiation skin damage is dose-dependent; therefore, efforts are made to irradiate tumors from different directions (see Figures 2-5A and 2-5B). Skin damage caused by radiation is discussed further in Chapter 7.

Some of the treatments provided as wound care or wound prevention may result in damage to the wound bed and surrounding skin. Excessively vigorous removal of necrotic tissue includes use of wet-to-dry dressings, which generally consist of moistened gauze placed in a wound, allowed to dry into the necrotic tissue, and pulled out. Evaporation from wet-to-dry dressings decreases the temperature of the wound bed, slowing growth of tissue and decreasing the release of oxygen from hemoglobin to the tissue. Even appropriate dressings applied with tape or other adhesives may damage skin. Irrigation with excessive pressure can damage a wound bed, and allowing a body part to remain in water, especially in a whirlpool tank, will cause maceration. Hydrotherapy and excessive

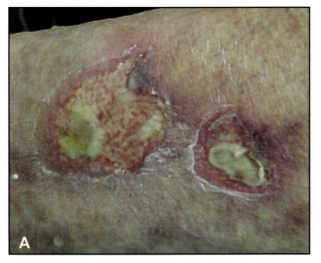

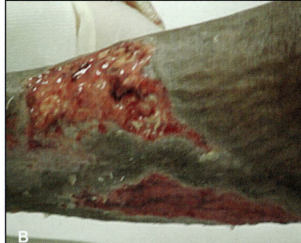

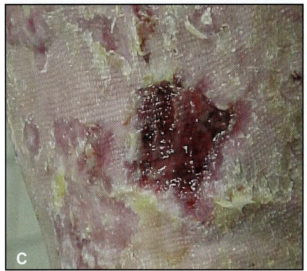

cleaning of the skin leads to loss of skin oil and drying of the skin. Attempts to prevent skin damage that could be caused by incontinence of the bowel or bladder may instead cause skin damage. Cleaning with hot water-soaked rough washcloths and harsh soaps or chemicals may damage the perineum.

CHRONIC INFLAMMATION

Chronic inflammation is characterized by discoloration of the surrounding skin with evidence of microvascular bleeding such as hemosiderin staining, ecchymosis, and induration, with possible undermining or tunneling (these terms will be further discussed later in this chapter). The wound itself will consist of necrotic tissue, fibrinous eschar, and will produce moderate to maximum drainage (see Figure 3-1). The fluid present in chronic wounds promotes inflammation. This fluid applied to otherwise healthy cells inhibits growth of endothelial cells, keratinocytes and fibroblasts. Analysis of chronic wound fluid reveals high levels of inflammatory cytokines, matrix metalloproteinases (MMPs), and low levels of growth factors.

Chronic inflammation generally results from the failure to optimize the wound and surrounding skin environment, and to protect the wound from the forces that initially produced the wound. The inability to remove necrotic tissue from a wound, clear infection, prevent repeated trauma to a wound, failure to optimize wound and skin moisture, and introduction of foreign materials such as gauze are likely causes of chronic inflammation. These problems arise because of insufficient debridement (removal of dead tissue), incorrect use of wound care products, failure to protect the wound, and failure to correct the underlying causes of the wound, such as arterial insufficiency, venous hypertension, pressure, and shear.

Chronic inflammation may also be caused by repeated trauma due to inadequate occlusion or protection.

Figure 3-1. Chronic inflammation. (A) Failure to debride necrotic tissue has maintained inflammation. (B) Inflammation caused by untreated venous disease. (C) Close-up of skin affected by venous disease.

Occlusion of a wound refers to the process of creating a separate environment around the wound (a microenvironment) by using special moisture retentive dressings that can retain the optimal combination of fluid, macromolecules, and heat within the wound. Protection may be achieved by simple dressings, bulky bandages, or splints, depending on the location and extent of the wound.

LACK OF INFLAMMATION

Because the initial phase of wound healing is dependent on inflammation to prepare the wound site, anti-inflammatory and other drugs that decrease the effectiveness of the immune system, such as anticancer drugs, chelating drugs (drugs that bind metal ions), and immunosuppressive drugs

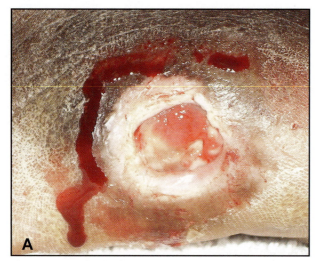
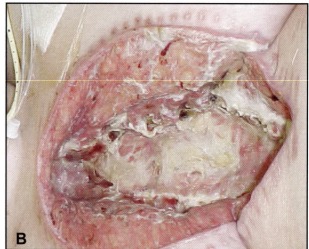

Figure 3-2. Lack of inflammation. (A) Despite presence of wound, the patient fails to mount a normal inflammatory response. (B) Lack of inflammation in a wound with desiccated necrotic tissue.

used for either preventing transplant rejection or for treating autoimmune diseases delay wound healing. Individuals with compromised immunity due to either a primary immunodeficiency (one of several genetic diseases), or secondary immune deficiency—eg, poorly controlled diabetes mellitus, alcoholism, and AIDS—may lack the inflammation necessary to start the healing process. These wounds may also have damage to the surrounding skin with hemosiderin staining and ecchymosis. Because the lack of inflammation is often associated with arterial insufficiency, the surrounding skin may be an ashen gray or even a purple color. A wound lacking inflammation will be dry and cool, covered in eschar, usually hard and black, with little or no drainage (Figure 3-2). Accompanying insufficient blood flow, ischemic injury, free radical injury (including reperfusion injury), and imbalance of cytokines and proteases prevent transition to the proliferative phase. Diminished blood flow also interferes with the removal of necrotic cells, creating a physical barrier to angiogenesis needed for tissue repair.

INFECTION

Infection refers to the unchecked replication of microorganisms. Normally, small quantities of a number of bacteria and fungi may be present on the surface of a wound. However, in analogy to a community aquarium, the proper mix and amounts of different bacteria and fungi are usually benign. With introduction of a new species, or even strains of bacteria or fungus, or a change in the microenvironment of a wound, a particular type of microorganism may grow out of control. Generally, clinical infection capable of slowing wound healing has been defined by the presence of greater than 100,000 organisms per gram.

Infection is also characterized by invasion of tissue below wound surfaces. Degrading the tissue beneath the skin surface produces the phenomena of undermining, tunnels, and sinus tracts, which are depicted in Figure 3-3. Undermining is the development of a wound configuration in which the size of the wound beneath the skin exceeds the opening of the visible wound. This is determined by probing the wound during the physical examination. A sinus tract is caused by the degradation of subcutaneous tissue in a linear manner with another wound opening at the other end of the tunnel. Tunneling usually implies a blind linear area of subcutaneous necrosis without a wound opening at the other end of the tunnel.

In the case of the acute wound, the presence of bacteria is believed to be the reason for wounds becoming chronic. Persistence of bacteria in an acute wound is believed to increase the production of inflammatory cytokines such as IL-1 and TNF-α. Treatment of wound infection is accomplished by restoring the balance of bacteria in the wound through debridement, drainage, and appropriately-timed wound closure. Closure of a wound with greater than 100,000 bacteria per gram is nearly certain to result in infection in adults in most areas of the body, although well-vascularized tissues, such as the face, are able to tolerate a greater bacterial burden. Necrotic tissue, hematoma, and foreign bodies, including sutures, may need to be removed to restore a proper balance of bacteria in an infected wound.

Certainly in the acute wound, infection is the major concern in terms of delayed wound healing. Unfortunately, many topical (locally applied) treatments to control wound infection are cytotoxic (poisonous to cells) and by themselves delay wound healing. Povidone-iodine and Dakins solution, in particular, have been discouraged for use in pressure ulcers because of their cytotoxicity. Although infection can delay wound healing, treating a wound that

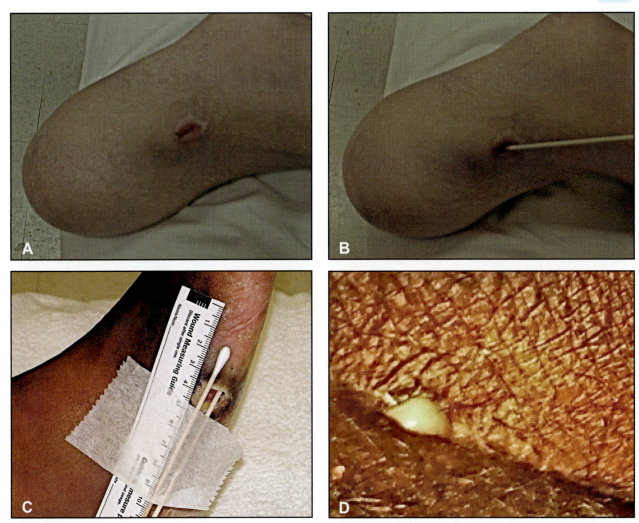

Figure 3-3. Subcutaneous tissue defects. (A) Superficially, this wound appears to be closed. (B) The same wound with a cotton-tipped applicator inserted 1.5 cm into a tunnel caused by infection of a wound produced by prosthesis injury. (C) Undermining of the same wound shown in 3-2A. This wound has 1.8 cm of undermining detected by careful palpation and probing of the wound. (D) Example of a wound with a very small opening (1 mm diameter) with a subcutaneous defect 1 cm around the opening and 4 mm deep. This wound continued to produce purulent drainage until the subcutaneous defect filled with granulation tissue. Special effort was needed to prevent completion of re-epithelialization until the subcutaneous defect was filled with granulation tissue.

is not infected as if it were is not harmless, but significantly delays what could otherwise be normal healing.

Signs of Infection

One of the major problems in diagnosing wound infection is that the same characteristics are present in both infection and inflammation. Both infection and inflammation are characterized by heat, tenderness, erythema, and swelling. Part of the problem is that release of cytokines occurs in response to the presence of both necrotic tissue and bacteria. Several descriptions of wound infections exist in the literature. In surgical wounds, a definitive diagnosis of infection requires the presence of purulent drain-

age or inflammation spreading beyond what is expected of normal healing. Additionally, a quantitative culture obtained by tissue biopsy demonstrating greater than 100,000 organisms per gram or the presence of β-hemolytic streptococci may be necessary to diagnose a wound infection. A rule of thumb often used clinically is the failure of surrounding warmth and erythema to recede by 4 days postop indicates infection, or other disturbance with the transition from inflammation to proliferation. A wound that proceeds from warm to cold is suggestive that cell death has occurred in the inflamed area. Palpation should also be done to examine the surrounding skin for any induration or edema, especially if the tissue becomes tense and painful. The expression of purulence from a wound is often taken as a certain sign of infection. Palpation may reveal a hardened or boggy area that has become sealed off from the open area of the wound that is visible. Careful probing with a cotton-tipped applicator or other appropriate device may be necessary to identify these areas. The bursting of these "pus pockets" during examination is another good reason to use standard precautions and personal protective equipment when examining wounds.

For surgical wounds, the prevailing belief is that a wound that heals primarily without discharge is uninfected, and is infected if purulent discharge occurs. The problem with culturing the purulent discharge is that bacteria may not be detected because the purulent drainage consists of dead bacteria, neutrophils, and tissue debris. Biopsy cultures of the wound, as opposed to the swab cultures, are more likely to contain the bacteria causing the infection. In chronic wounds, infection may sometimes be detected visually as a dark discoloration (often brown) surrounded by normal reddish tissue, indicating invasion of healthy surrounding tissue by bacteria (Figure 3-4). Infection can cause necrosis of what had been healthy tissue, degrading it, and expanding the size of the wound. This is particularly apparent in the case of what have been termed *flesh-eating bacteria* that spread along fascial planes, destroying healthy tissue.

Recommendations for treatment of infected pressure ulcers include the use of systemic antibiotics and a trial of topical antibiotics, which must be prescribed by a physician. The persistence of inflammation occurs in the presence of either necrotic tissue or bacteria. Cytokines such as IL-1 and tumor necrosis factor increase in response to bacteria in a wound, increase matrix metalloproteinases and inhibit growth factors. Another risk factor for wound infection is the innervation of the tissue. Experimentally, the loss of innervation increases the bacterial growth in a wound 100-fold. Denervation also appears to decrease leukocyte function and increase the number of septic areas within the wound. Therefore, wounds accompanied by nerve injuries can be expected to have a higher risk of infection. A critical cause of delayed wound healing that can be addressed by the therapist or nurse is the presence of necrotic tissue. Necrotic tissue causes the mutual problems of increased risk of infection and slow wound healing. By their natures, infection increases the risk of delayed healing, and delayed healing increases the risk of infection. Debridement of necrotic tissue removes much of the risk of infection. In the case of infected wounds, nonocclusive wound dressings are recommended. Moisture retentive dressings are conducive to cell growth and replication. Unfortunately, this may include bacteria; therefore, nonocclusive dressings and frequent cleansing are recommended for infected wounds.

MOISTURE

Maceration (Figure 3-5) is the result of excessive moisture on epithelial surfaces, giving the appearance of a tissue that is swollen and "bleached out." Normal skin may become macerated even under seemingly trivial circumstances such as swimming or staying in a bathtub too long. During maceration, swelling of epithelial cells with disruption of desmosomes, and death or loss of attachment of epithelial edges occurs. Application of a protective substance such as barrier cream or skin sealant on the surface of the wound can often protect the surrounding skin from maceration. Using a dressing with increased absorbency to keep moisture off the surrounding skin or more frequent dressing changes may also reduce maceration. Decreasing the handling of a wound to minimize trauma and inflammation may reduce the amount of fluid released from the wound, thereby decreasing the risk of maceration.

Desiccation is the drying out of a wound (Figure 3-6). It is caused by one or more of the following in combination: dressings that allow fluid to evaporate uncontrollably from a wound, excessive dressing changes with loss of fluid from the wound, or fluid disorders. Desiccation can be prevented by using a moisture-retentive dressing over the wound, decreasing the frequency of dressing changes, or the use of a hydrogel filler or sheet (a gel substance) that can release moisture into a wound. When treating desiccation, however, one must be alert to the possibility of causing maceration of surrounding skin. During the course of treatment, different types of dressings may be required to optimize a wound's moisture.

WOUND EDGES

Epiboly is a condition in which the epithelial edge of a wound rolls under itself (Figure 3-7). When the margin of a wound rolls under itself, epithelial cells contact each other, causing contact inhibition and the cessation of re-epithelialization. Epiboly is corrected by burning with silver nitrate or cutting the rolled edges from the wound to re-establish a free edge, and optimizing the wound environment.

MISMATCH OF GRANULATION AND RE-EPITHELIALIZATION

Under normal circumstances, granulation tissue fills a wound from the bottom and sides. Meanwhile, re-epithelialization moves across the granulation tissue just as it reaches the height of the surrounding epidermis. A mismatch may occur in which re-epithelialization occurs too quickly relative to granulation. In the mildest case, the closed wound exhibits a depression where the wound had been. A more serious concern is the bridging over a subcutaneous defect,

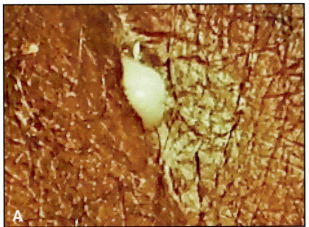

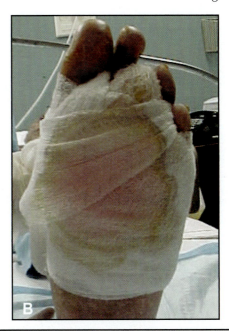

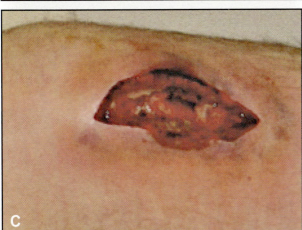

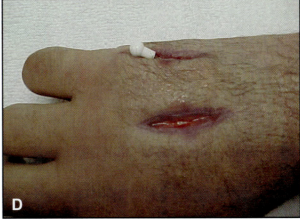

Figure 3-4. Signs of wound infection. (A) Expression of purulence from same wound as Figure 3-3D. (B) Drainage from wound indicative of infection by *Pseudomonas aeruginosa*. Both blood and green drainage can be seen on dressing (serosanguinous drainage with greenish tint). (C) Four classic signs of inflammation are demonstrated—induration (hardness), fever (heat), edema, and erythema are present. Induration and fever are detectible with palpation. The original width of this wound was the width of a scalpel blade used to drain the purulence. The edema has produced the gapping shown here. In addition, the presence of stringy yellow slough in the wound, black eschar in the wound and on some of the edges, and hemosiderin in the surrounding skin are indicative of infection. This wound and similar wounds are generally accompanied by rapid and seemingly sudden swelling and pain, and in some cases the expression of purulence. In other cases, purulence is not released until surgical incision and drainage. (D) Failure of wound to close in timely manner and continued edema in metacarpal fracture fixation. Pin was removed from fourth metacarpal. (E) Classic signs of infection of right leg and foot with induration, fever, erythema, and edema. Tissue necrosis is present without purulence. Surgical removal of the necrotic skin was required.

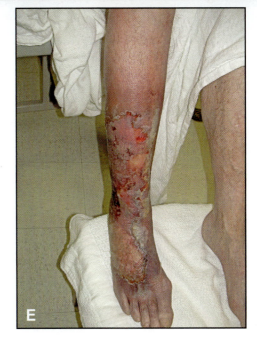

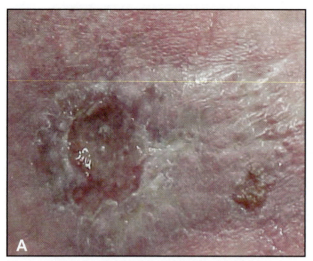

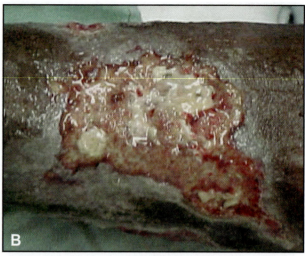

Figure 3-5. Maceration. (A) Excessive drainage allowed to accumulate on skin has injured surrounding skin with swelling and loss of pigmentation. (B) Untreated venous hypertension leading to copious serous drainage accumulating on surrounding skin. In this example, heavily pigmented skin has lost its color from moisture damage to skin.

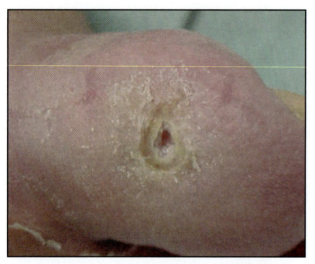

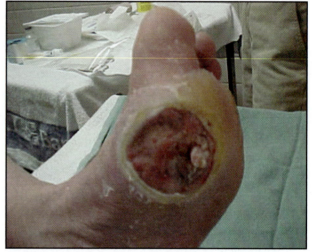

Figure 3-6. Desiccated wound secondary to diabetic neuropathy. Lack of moisture and callus formation produce a dry wound bed that will be slow to heal without intervention.

Figure 3-7. Wound on same foot displays a number of issues related to slow healing. Epiboly is seen on lateral wound edge and thick callus is seen around most of the wound edge. Pink, uneven granulation tissue is seen within the wound bed, indicative of diminished arterial supply and likely wound infection.

especially if the wound continues to exhibit purulent drainage (pus). In this case, bacteria and devitalized tissue are enclosed in the subcutaneous tissues with high likelihood of infection occurring, or in the case of an abscess that had been opened to drain, chronic infection of the site may occur.

Two basic options to slow the progression of re-epithelialization are filling the wound's opening with packing strip or other suitable material or by burning the epithelial edge with silver nitrate. Silver nitrate sticks are available for this purpose (Figure 3-8). The ends of these sticks need to be moistened with normal saline before application, and the wound needs to be flushed with normal saline to prevent burning other areas of the wound.

Another approach is to determine the cause of delayed granulation and correct it. Possibilities include optimizing the environment for granulation by using an appropriate moisture-retentive to retain not only moisture content, but also temperature and growth factors within the wound microenvironment. Fibroblast activity is greatest at normal body temperature and decreases in either warmer or cooler temperatures. Uncontrolled evaporation of wound fluid can decrease temperature several degrees and require hours for normal temperature to be achieved after the wound is covered by materials that adequately insulate

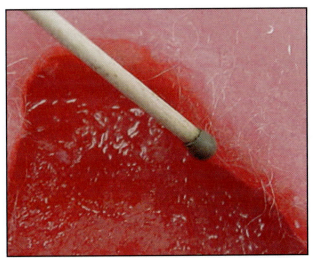

Figure 3-8. Silver nitrate stick, which may be used to burn rolled-over edges to aid epithelialization in a wound slowed by epiboly.

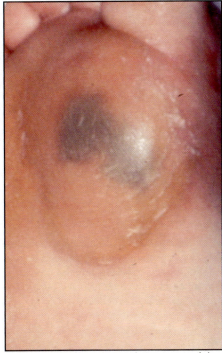

Figure 3-9. Subcutaneous hematoma of the forefoot. The clinician cannot determine the extent of the subcutaneous necrosis (if any) in this case.

the wound. A related complication of wound healing is subcutaneous hematoma due to chronic insult to underlying tissue (Figure 3-9). With this condition, the extent of necrosis cannot be determined easily.

Hypergranulation

Hypergranulation refers to growth of granulation tissue in excess of the surface of the wound (Figure 3-10). Hypergranulation is frequently caused by interference with re-epithelialization of wounds due to epiboly, maceration, or unrelieved physical stresses on the surrounding skin. Hypergranulation allows the base of the wound to exceed the height of the surrounding skin, producing a cosmetically unacceptable scar. Steps may be taken to correct slow epithelialization by protecting the wound margin from maceration (see below), removing any rolled over edges (epiboly) by burning the affected wound margin by a silver nitrate stick, or cutting the epiboly by a surgeon.

Chronic proliferation occurs frequently with venous insufficiency. Damage to periwound skin with hemosiderin staining or ecchymosis and contraction of the skin from previous venous ulcers is frequently observed. In venous insufficiency, the granulation tissue is a bright, healthy, red color. Treatment of venous disease (see Chapter 7) is necessary to improve the health of the surrounding skin. Chronic proliferation attributable to arterial insufficiency is obvious from the pink color of the granulation tissue. Note, however, that arterial insufficiency can be concurrent with venous insufficiency, resulting in chronic proliferation of pink granulation tissue with damaged surrounding skin. Generally, little is available to treat arterial disease other than drugs used to either dilate arterial

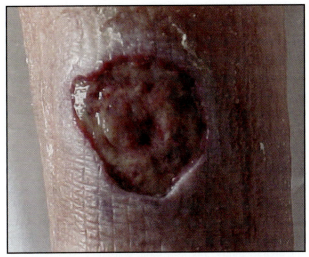

Figure 3-10. Hypergranulation of a leg wound. Note maceration of surrounding skin and granulation exceeding the height of the surrounding skin. Injury to the surrounding skin, fungal infection, or carcinoma are potential causes.

vessels or improve the flow of blood through narrowed vessels, and surgical procedures to repair or bypass narrowed arterial vessels. Arterial insufficiency, as discussed previously, frequently fails to produce inflammation or proliferation in addition to a failure of re-epithelialization.

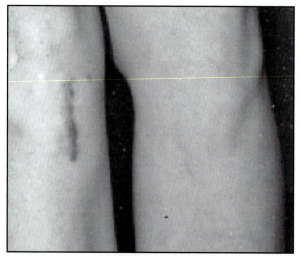

Figure 3-11. Hypertrophic scarring produced by hardware removal several months following anterior cruciate repair. Note the presence of faint white resolved hypertropic scars from original surgical procedure.

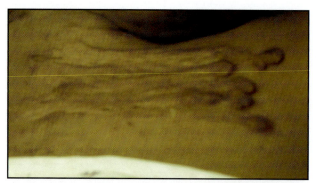

Figure 3-12. Keloid scar on chest. Note the raised nature and the extension of keloid beyond the original sternotomy incision.

Other causes of hypergranulation include fungal infection and neoplastic disease. In these cases, the granulation tissue has a fungating appearance characterized by a highly irregular surface of the granulation tissue in terms of the depth (or height) of the wound base. These will be discussed further in Chapter 16.

OVERREPAIR

Classically, 2 types of overrepair have been described: hypertrophic scars (Figure 3-11) and keloids (Figure 3-12). These phenomena result in susceptible individuals following wounding and are often discussed as part of the remodeling process of normal wound healing. These responses to wounding are due to failure to terminate the remodeling of a wound. Both types of wounds have a characteristic gross appearance described as red, raised, and rigid. Several important differences distinguish hypertrophic scarring and keloid formation. Keloids are more persistent, tend to regrow if excised, and extend beyond the area of injury. Hypertrophic scars may rise above the level of the surrounding skin, but generally do not extend beyond the area of injury. With time, hypertrophic scars decrease in size, height, and vascularity. In many cases, hypertrophic scars become white, flat, and avascular after several weeks to months. Keloid scars have been associated with diminished levels of interferon alpha and gamma and increased levels of IL-6 and TNF-α, which is consistent with loss of inhibition on fibroblast metabolism and runaway collagen accumulation. Recently, a differentiation has been made between hypertrophic scars caused by surgical wounds and proliferative scars associated with burn injuries. Proliferative scarring associated with burn injuries does not appear until the patient is healthy and reaches a normal immunocompetence. Individuals susceptible to proliferative scarring following burn injury demonstrate increased IL-1, IL-6, TNF-α and TGF-α activity in blood cells. In particular, TGF-β stimulates a number of processes related to excessive repair and inappropriate scarring in a number of conditions in addition to proliferative scarring. Treatment of proliferative scarring is described in Chapter 15.

NEUROPATHY

Injury to the nervous system leads to problems in terms of causing and slowing wound healing. Peripheral neuropathy associated with diabetes mellitus and unrelieved pressure caused by spinal cord or other injuries or diseases resulting in lack of sensation are discussed in Chapter 7. In addition to being a causative factor of wounds, neuropathy results in slower wound healing. Some of the impairment in healing in diabetes can be linked to metabolic issues, yet healing is also slowed in other neurologic injuries and diseases. Collagen breakdown is increased and synthesis is decreased, resulting in weaker skin that increases the risk of future breakdown of closed wounds. A type of sensory nerve receptor is altered in basal keratinocytes with nerve injury and diabetic neuropathy. The connection between neural activity and integumentary integrity has not been elucidated, but appears to involve vanilloid receptors and nerve growth factor.

Stress and activation of the sympathetic nervous system affect wound healing. In rats, chemically induced sympathetic denervation increases the rate of wound contraction and myofibroblastic differentiation, but decreases the rate of mast cell migration, and delays re-epithelialization. If inflammation is allowed to occur before chemically-induced sympathetic denervation, wound contraction does not occur as rapidly as it does if denervation precedes wounding. The neurogenic component of inflammation presumably delays wound contraction, but later on, increases re-epithelialization.

SUMMARY

Wound healing can be delayed by a number of factors either due to the patient's condition or due to inappropriate care of the wound. The wound fails to progress through its normal sequence in the proper time frame due either to chronicity of a phase or failure of a phase to begin. Conditions that either prevent or sustain inflammation are common culprits. These include the presence of necrotic tissue, infection, placing gauze or cytotoxic agents in the wound, rough handling, and compromised immunity. Undermining, tunneling, and sinus tracts may occur as a result of compromised healing. Optimal care is provided by maintaining a moist wound bed at normal body temperature and keeping the surrounding skin dry. Failure to do these slows wound healing, causing desiccation, hypergranulation, or maceration. Excessive moisture caused by venous insufficiency needs to be addressed by appropriate compression therapy. Lack of inflammation due to arterial insufficiency needs to be addressed by a vascular surgeon.

QUESTIONS

1. If infection is a cause of slow wound healing, why are we so concerned about the effects of topically-applied antimicrobial agents to wounds?

2. Why do wounds with epiboly fail to re-epithelialize and often have hypergranulation?

3. Why must the excessive moisture of venous insufficiency be treated to optimize wound healing?

4. Why does inflammation often fail in the presence of arterial insufficiency?

5. What products are available to keep surrounding skin dry in the presence of high levels of drainage?

BIBLIOGRAPHY

Alison WE, Phillips LG, Linares HA, et al. The effect of denervation on soft tissue infection pathophysiology. *Plast Reconstr Surg.* 1992;90:1031-1035.

Bayat A, Bock O, Mrowietz U, Ollier WE, Ferguson MW. Genetic susceptibility to keloid disease and hypertrophic scarring: transforming growth factor beta1 common polymorphisms and plasma levels. *Plast Reconstr Surg.* 2003;111:535-543.

Himel HN. Wound healing: focus on the chronic wound. *Wounds.* 1995; 7(5)(suppl A):70A-77A.

Hui P-S, Pu LL, Kucukceleki A. et al. The effect of denervation on leukocyte function in soft tissue infection. *Surgery.* 1999;126:933-938.

Ladwig GP, Robson MC, Liu R, Kuhn MA, Muir DF, Schultz GS. Ratios of activated matrix metalloproteinase-9 to tissue inhibitor of matrix metalloproteinase-1 in wound fluids are inversely correlated with healing of pressure ulcers. *Wound Repair Regen.* 2002;10:26-37.

McCarthy DJ. Anatomic considerations of the human nail. *Clin Podiatr Med Surg.* 1995;12:163-181.

McCauley RL, Chopra V, Li YY, Herndon DN, Robson MC. Altered cytokine production in black patients with keloids. *Journal of Clinical Immunology.* 1992;12:300-308.

Polo M, Ko F, Busillo F, Cruse CW, Krizek TJ, Robson MC. Cytokine production in patients with hypertrophic burn scars. *J Burn Care Rehabil.* 1997;18:477-482.

Robson MC. Wound infection. A failure of wound healing caused by an imbalance of bacteria. *Surg Clin North Am.* 1997; 77:637-650.

Robson MC, Mannari, RJ, Smith PD, et al. Maintenance of wound bacterial balance. *Am J Surg.* 1999;178:399-402.

Sheehan P, Jones P, Caselli A, Giurini JM, Veves A. Percent change in wound area of diabetic foot ulcers over a 4-week period is a robust predictor of complete healing in a 12-week prospective trial. *Diabetes Care.* 2003;26:1879–1882,

Souza BR, Cardoso JF, Amadeu TP, Desmouliere A, Costa AM. Sympathetic denervation accelerates wound contraction but delays reepithelialization in rats. *Wound Repair Regen.* 2005;13:498-505.

Trengove NJ, Stacey MC, MacAuley S, et al. Analysis of the acute and chronic wound environments: the role of proteases and their inhibitors. *Wound Repair Regen.* 1999;7:442-452.

Winter GD, Scales JT. Effect of air drying and dressings on the surface of a wound. *Nature.* 1963;197:91-92.

Yang L, Scott PG, Giuffre J, et al. Peripheral blood fibrocytes from burn patients: identification and quantification of fibrocytes in adherent cells cultured from peripheral blood mononuclear cells. *Lab Invest.* 2002;82:1183-1192.

Yang L, Scott PG, Dodd C, et al. Identification of fibrocytes in post-burn hypertrophic scar. *Wound Repair Regen.* 2005;13:398-404.

Wang J, Jiao H, Stewart TL, Shankowsky HA, Scott PG, Tredget EE. Improvement in postburn hypertrophic scar after treatment with IFN-alpha2b is associated with decreased fibrocytes. *J Interferon Cytokine Res.* 2007;27:921-930.

Nutrition

4

OBJECTIVES

- Describe the essential nutrients to prevent wounds and promote healing.
- Describe the need for caloric intake to prevent wounds and how the need increases with integumentary injury.
- Describe normal protein requirement and how it needs to change to promote healing.
- Describe the roles of fatty acids, trace elements, and vitamins in wound prevention and healing.
- Discuss the relationships among obesity, wound healing, and weight loss.
- Discuss means of supplementing nutrition to promote wound healing.

Nutrition may break down at many levels, putting a person at increased risk of developing wounds, or of slow healing of existing wounds. In the healthy individual, many of these potential pitfalls are taken for granted. An individual needs the cognitive abilities to choose appropriate foods, the cognitive and physical ability to prepare it, and the desire to consume it. Once consumed, proper functioning of the digestive system is needed. The person must be able to mechanically reduce the food to digestible forms, secrete enzymes into the gastrointestinal tract, and absorb the reduced forms. After absorption, the simple nutrients require processing, metabolic control, and delivery to cells. With delivery to cells, the nutrients derived from food need other nutrients to provide energy and structures for the cell. Disease or aging of the gastrointestinal tract, liver, heart, blood vessels, and respiratory system, and diabetes mellitus can undermine optimal diet. Elderly individuals living alone with poor mobility and diminished cognition are at tremendous risk of malnourishment and development of wounds.

NUTRIENTS

The components of nutrition are termed *nutrients*. These include both the chemical structure and the energy that can be derived from the chemical structure so that ATP can be regenerated. In general, protein is discussed in the sense of structures, and carbohydrates and fat as sources of energy. The picture is somewhat more complex. Vitamins (from the term *vital amine*) are required for a number of processes, including facilitation of the processes necessary to allow the use of molecules derived from food to be used to generate energy or create structures. Other substances are termed *micronutrients*. These are generally minerals needed for enzymatic processes. Discussion of nutrients will include the potential energy content of food measured in calories, and

Irion G.
Comprehensive Wound Management, 2nd ed. (pp 37-44)
© 2010 SLACK Incorporated

the intake of protein, vitamins, and micronutrients needed to facilitate use of the other nutrients.

Calories

The amount of energy that can be derived from food has historically been quantified in calories. A calorie is defined as the amount of energy necessary to increase the temperature of 1 g of water by 1°C. This unit is quite small relative to what can be obtained from food, so the term *kilocalorie* (kcal) is used instead. Calorie spelled with an upper case C may be used to indicate a kilocalorie (the amount of energy necessary to raise the temperature of 1 kg of water by 1°C). Therefore, nutritional information is provided as kcal or Calories. Regardless of the source, energy to regenerate ATP from chemical bonds of ingested foods is required. Calories can be obtained from carbohydrates, protein, and fat. Fat is the most efficient source of calories. Other metabolic products such as ketones and lactic acid can be salvaged as sources of calories.

Protein

Protein is a critical source of structures in the body, particularly of fat-free body mass. Proteins are also used to create many of the chemical signals, components of the immune system, and the plasma proteins that allow water to remain within blood vessels in spite of the hydrostatic pressure within them. Protein can also be used as a source of energy. The consequences of inadequate protein consumption are described below. Proteins are chains of amino acids. The amino acids are harvested from proteins by the digestive system, providing cells with the opportunity to assemble necessary proteins from amino acids present in the bloodstream.

Amino acids are composed of nitrogen in addition to carbon, hydrogen, and oxygen atoms. Nitrogen atoms are removed as amino groups (NH3) to provide simpler molecules that can be used to provide energy through oxidative metabolism. The amino groups are converted to urea and excreted from the body primarily in the urine.

Amino acids may be divided into the groups of essential and nonessential. Nonessential amino acids can be synthesized from other amino acids. Essential amino acids cannot be synthesized by rearranging the molecules of nonessential amino acids. Therefore, ingesting them as components of proteins is essential, whereas nonessential amino acids do not need to be provided directly through the diet. Meat sources contain essential amino acids; diets that exclude meat must be adjusted or supplemented to provide essential amino acids. Of the 20 amino acids, 9 are essential—isoleucine, leucine, lysine, threonine, tryptophan, methionine, histidine, valine, and phenylalanine. If a specific amino acid must not be ingested, eg, phenylalanine in phenylketonuria, other amino acids (in this

example, tyrosine) can become essential. The other 11 amino acids can be synthesized by rearrangement of other ingested amino acids, except in newborns, who cannot synthesize histidine and arginine. In a stressed state, glutamine may also become an essential amino acid. Patients in a stressed state, eg, major burns, recover better with diets higher in glutamine.

Protein nutrition is complicated in renal disease. Protein is lost in the urine in nephrotic syndrome and ingestion may need to be supplemented. Patients with renal insufficiency or renal failure may be required to limit protein consumption as part of their therapy. Consultation with a dietician may be necessary to ensure that the patient receives sufficient amounts of essential amino acids without further injury to the kidneys.

Essential fatty acids, like essential proteins, cannot be synthesized from other building blocks, but must be ingested. Essential fatty acids include omega-3 and omega-6 fatty acids. Essential in this sense refers to fatty acids needed for purposes other than regeneration of ATP. Lack of essential fatty acids leads to a number of problems. Eicosanoids and other factors involved in either inflammation or regulation of inflammation require essential fatty acids for their production. Lack of essential fatty acids diminishes inflammation and cellular proliferation.

Vitamins

Vitamins as originally described were the presumed fat-soluble factor (vitamin A) and water-soluble factor (vitamin B) necessary for health. Following the discovery of different components of water-soluble vitamins, terminology was altered. The B vitamins may be termed by a subscript following the B, or given their own names. For example, vitamin B_{12} is also termed *cyanocobalamin*. The discovery of more vitamins follows the same lettering from C, D, E, then skipping to vitamin K. Historically, all of the letters from A to K have been used, but F, G, H, I, and J have been abandoned because of the discovery of the actual nature of the substance so named. K also stands for coagulation, spelled in German with a K. In addition to B, water soluble vitamins also include C. Excessive quantities of water soluble vitamins are excreted in the urine and cannot be stored for long periods of vitamin unavailability from the diet. In contrast, fat-soluble vitamins can be stored in fatty tissue and released as their concentration in the blood falls. However, excessive consumption of fat-soluble vitamins can produce toxicity. The fat-soluble vitamins are A, D, E, and K. These vitamins can be supplemented specifically for individuals who digest fat poorly, particularly many people with cystic fibrosis.

Vitamin A (retinol) is stored in the liver and obtained in the diet as beta-carotene from plants and retinyl esters from animals. Retinoic acid binds to receptors to affect gene expression. Vitamin A acts as a morphogen to regulate epidermal development and is teratogenic. Pregnant women must avoid exposure to the high doses of vitamin A and its analogs, eg, tretinoin topical used for treating skin disorders such as acne. Retinol suppresses the maturation of keratinocytes. Excess retinol causes thinning and drying of the skin. Deficiency of vitamin A causes hyperkeratosis and metaplasia of glands of the epidermis. Retinol and chemicals of similar structure are used therapeutically to treat acne through the suppression of oil production by sebaceous glands. Deficiency of vitamin A has been shown to delay wound healing as well as increase susceptibility to infection, presumably because of a requirement of vitamin A by the immune system.

The B vitamins are necessary for energy metabolism and synthesis of DNA. Deficiency of niacin produces pellagra, a condition characterized by hyperkeratotic eruptions of sun-exposed skin and damage to other organs. Deficiency of vitamin B_6 (pyroxidine) or essential fatty acids causes scaling. Both riboflavin and thiamine are required for collagen synthesis, but no links have been shown between deficiencies of these vitamins and impairment of wound healing.

Vitamin C is essential for collagen development. Vitamin C deficiency (scurvy) causes diminished tensile strength of connective tissues and slows wound healing, but does not prevent wound healing. Vitamin C deficiency in Western civilization is rare, and supertherapeutic doses of vitamin C have not been demonstrated to enhance healing of either acute or chronic wounds.

Vitamin D is related to calcium metabolism. Sunlight reaching the skin converts vitamin D into a more active form.

Vitamin E has been attributed antioxidant properties and is thought to have a protective effect on the skin by reducing sun and other types of damage. It is frequently used as an additive to over-the-counter skin products with a suggestion of improved skin integrity. However, vitamin E has also been shown to decrease wound healing, possibly by interference with collagen synthesis, and vitamin E has not been demonstrated to be important to wound repair.

Vitamin K is responsible for producing the active form of several of the coagulation factors in the blood (II [prothrombin], VII, IX, X, protein C, protein S, and protein Z). Deficiency of this vitamin increases coagulation time and leads to excessive bleeding with trauma. Warfarin is a drug used to interfere with the recycling of vitamin K, leading to its depletion, which in turn decreases the risk of excessive coagulation therapeutically. This drug is used by individuals at risk for myocardial infarction and stroke and in other conditions such as heart valve replacement and atrial fibrillation, which may stimulate coagulation. Patients using warfarin or other anticoagulation medica-

tions may bleed excessively during debridement. History taking should include questions about the patient's use of anticoagulants, vitamin K deficiency, or other conditions leading to excessive bleeding.

Minerals/Trace Elements

Several minerals are required in low concentrations for healthy skin. Copper, manganese, and iron, although appearing to be necessary for tissue regeneration, have not been directly related to impaired wound healing. Selenium is part of an enzyme system (glutathione) that reduces oxidative damage by free radicals. Zinc is a part of many metalloenzyme systems, notably DNA and RNA polymerase. Zinc deficiency leads to dermatitis and slow healing. Supplemental zinc, however, has not been shown to aid wound healing in those without demonstrable zinc deficiency and excessive zinc may slow healing as well as have deleterious effects on immune function and copper metabolism. Unna's boots applied directly over venous insufficiency ulcers have been demonstrated to slow healing, which may be attributable to the zinc oxide in the material. Copper is also essential to the production of collagen, as well as elastin and melanin. It is present in the enzymes that produce cross-linking of collagen, elastin, and keratin. Supplementation of selenium, copper, and zinc may be critical for patients with major burns due to their roles in antioxidant mechanisms.

Water

Although not often considered a nutrient, adequate hydration is necessary for normal wound healing. Water represents a large fraction of body weight, dependent on lean body mass. Water represents about 2/3 of body mass. This number is higher in lean individuals and may approach 75%. In obese individuals, the percentage of body weight may be substantially lower than 60%. A general guideline for water consumption is 30 ml of water per day per kg body weight. In general, water ingestion is encouraged because excess water can be excreted in the urine without harm to the patient, but dehydration can lead to significant electrolyte disturbances. Although excessive water consumption is difficult to achieve, extreme consumption can lead to water intoxication with cerebral swelling as the most serious consequence. Because intact skin acts as a barrier for water loss, large open wounds, especially burns, can require greater consumption of water. Heavily draining wounds, vomiting, diarrhea, and use of specialty beds that cause suction or evaporation of fluid from wounds will require increased water consumption. All patients, however, should not be encouraged to drink water; those with congestive heart failure, pulmonary edema, or other disease characterized by water retention may have input/output of fluid monitored carefully. In such cases, any water intake restrictions should be communicated clearly to all healthcare providers and visitors to ensure adherence to fluid intake restrictions.

MALNUTRITION

A person not meeting dietary needs may be classified as at risk or malnourished. Nutritional screening is used to determine whether a given person is at risk for malnutrition; further testing is needed to determine if malnutrition exists and what interventions are required.

Dietary needs may be divided into 3 basic categories: energy quantified by the number of calories consumed; protein to regenerate necessary enzymes and other structures; and cofactors necessary for metabolism, notably vitamins and trace minerals. Nutrition of the skin requires a healthy vascular supply through the dermis, which provides a rich supply to the papillary dermis. Blood flow through the papillary dermis provides nourishment to the metabolically active stratum basale where new cells of the epidermis are generated. Diffusion of nutrients occurs from the papillary dermis to stratum basale to support its metabolic needs. In addition, these plexuses are involved in thermoregulation. However, the blood supply to the relatively acellular reticular dermis is rather low due to its low metabolic rate. Nutrition is frequently poor in ill or injured individuals with an estimated 30% to 55% rate of malnutrition in the hospital patient population. Impaired nutritional intake, lower dietary protein intake, impaired ability to feed oneself, and recent weight loss have been shown to be independent predictors of pressure ulcer development. Moreover, these factors are likely to occur in combination in many individuals. Even individuals receiving nutritional support may develop hospital-induced malnutrition. Patients on total parenteral nutrition (TPN) for extended periods will have difficulty receiving nutrients that cannot be adequately supplied through this means. A key question is how common malnutrition may be for others with some of the risk factors listed above related to obtaining, preparing, digesting, and delivering nutrients to cells. Clearly, malnutrition is a major risk factor for pressure ulcers and delayed wound healing.

Two basic types of malnutrition described in the literature are Marasmus (total calorie malnutrition) and Kwashiorkor (hypoalbuminemia, protein malnutrition). In addition, cachexia represents a generalized wasting of the body associated with disseminated cancer. Marasmus and Kwashiorkor are associated with children weaned from breastfeeding and provided with poor diets. Marasmus presents as long-term inadequate intake with chronic weight loss and wasted adipose and muscle tissue, but intact visceral protein stores. Historically, Kwashiorkor describes malnourished children weaned from breastfeeding and fed diets consisting of carbohydrates and lack-

ing protein. Kwashiorkor results in generalized edema, including ascites.

In adults who have access to food, hypoalbuminemia is generally a result of an acute insult such as surgery or illness. Protein malnutrition may have a rapid onset and may be difficult to detect without appropriate lab tests. Hypoalbuminemia is characterized by a preservation of fat and somatic protein. Combination malnutrition generally results from an underlying chronic malnourishment with a superimposed acute insult, resulting in loss of fat, muscle, and visceral protein. Any given individual may experience a number of deficiencies in the diet, whether due to lack of food in general, disease of the digestive system, or lack of particular nutrients.

ASSESSING NUTRITION

Nutritional status may be assessed by a combination of anthropometric and biochemical data. Additionally, several patient characteristics are known risk factors for under- or malnutrition. These factors are listed in Table 4-1.

Anthropometric

These methods rely on body measurements such as height and weight. Based on normative data, one can estimate whether a patient is adequately nourished. Ideal body weight is commonly used as a basis for comparison. A patient's body weight is compared with normative data to determine the percentage of ideal body weight. A person who is malnourished would likely have a body weight less than 100% ideal body weight, although an overweight person may be malnourished because of a deficiency of specific nutrients in spite of adequate caloric intake.

Ideal Body Weight

Ideal body weight (IBW) may be computed in a number of ways. A commonly used set of equations is as follows. For men the equation is 106 pounds for the first 5 feet, plus 6 pounds for each additional inch above 5 feet of height (106# for 5' + 6# per inch). For women the equation is 100 pounds for the first 5 feet and 5 pounds for each additional inch (100# for 5' + 5# per inch). Adjustments are made for body types by subtracting 10% for a small frame and adding 10% for a large frame. For example a 6'1" man has an ideal body weight of 106 + (6 x 13) = 184 pounds and a 5'3" woman has an ideal body weight of 100 + (5 x 3) = 115 pounds. Computing the percentage of IBW provides an index of risk of either malnutrition or overnutrition. Overnutrition is also an important risk factor due to the relationships among obesity, type 2 diabetes mellitus, and atherosclerosis. Percentage of IBW is computed by dividing current body weight (CBW) by IBW as: percent IBW = CBW/IBW x 100. Normal is considered to be between 90%

Table 4-1

Risk Factors for Malnutrition

- Report of poor intake by patient, family, or caregivers
- Weight less than 80% of ideal body weight
- Loss of greater than 10% of usual body weight within last 6 months
- Alcoholism
- Advanced age
- Impaired cognitive status
- Malabsorption syndromes
- Renal failure or nephrotic syndrome
- Heavily draining wounds
- Multiple trauma
- Edema not attributable to congestive heart failure or venous disease

and 110% IBW. A value of 80% to 90% is considered to be underweight and a value of 79% or less defines Marasmus.

Other anthropometric analyses might include body mass index (BMI), waist circumference, and hip-to-weight ratio. Body mass index is computed as mass in kg divided by the square of height in meters (BMI = mass (kg) / ht (m)^2. To convert from pounds and inches, multiply the number of pounds by 703 and divide by the square of height in inches. (180 x 703/742) = 23. A value between 19 and 25 for BMI is considered healthy. A value of 25 to 30 is considered overweight; 30 to 40 is considered obese. Greater than 40 is considered clinically significantly obese (morbid obesity). Guidelines for bariatric surgery restrict gastric bypass to those with a BMI greater than 50, or greater than 40 if the body weight is associated with significant morbidity such as refractory hypertension. A value of BMI less than 19 is considered underweight. Although BMI may give misleading results for people with large muscle mass, it is a quick and reliable means for the general population. A waist circumference greater than 40 inches for men and 35 inches for women is considered a risk factor for cardiovascular disease. Greater than 43.5 inches for women and greater than 47 inches for men is considered to be very high risk. Waist-to-hip ratio is an indicator of where fat is deposited in the body. A high waist-to-hip ratio (greater than 0.95 for men and greater than 0.86 for women, represents the apple shape and greater risk of cardiovascular disease than a low ratio, represented as the pear shape, which is less of a cardiovascular risk. Although weight loss for obese patients is generally encouraged to improve overall health, loss of weight while a person has a significant wound is discouraged. Gastric bypass surgery is discussed further in Chapter 16.

Biochemical

A number of lab tests may be used to assess whether nutritional needs are being met adequately. Three tests are related directly to protein: albumin, prealbumin, and nitrogen balance. Other tests used to assess nutrition include blood work such as hematocrit, hemoglobin concentration, and white blood cell count.

Albumin

Albumin is considered the gold standard for assessing protein malnutrition. A normal value of albumin is considered to be 3.5 to 5.0 g/dL. Moderate depletion is considered to be a value between 3.2 and 3.5 g/dL, and severe hypoalbuminemia is defined as a value less than 2.8 g/dL. Evaluation of albumin is particularly important for the person with a chronic wound due to the potential for albumin and other plasma proteins to be lost in wound exudate. The problem with low albumin is compounded by its effect on fluid distribution. Albumin loss leads to edema, which in turn, causes decreased diffusion of nutrients through the interstitial space. In acute protein malnutrition, however, albumin may not have fallen yet and would not be indicative of an inadequate intake.

Prealbumin

For an indicator of short-term protein intake, prealbumin is measured. Mild, moderate, and severe depletion are defined as less than 17 g/dL, less than 12 g/dL, and less than 7 g/dL of prealbumin, respectively. A decline in prealbumin will occur prior to a decline in albumin in acute protein malnutrition.

Nitrogen Balance

Under normal circumstances, the amount of nitrogen entering the body in the form of proteins is equal to the amount of nitrogen excreted in the urine as urea. A positive nitrogen balance indicates accumulation of nitrogenous compounds in the body as would occur with an increase in fat-free mass. If a person does not take in sufficient calories, protein is broken into amino acids and deaminated for regenerating ATP, which results in excess excretion of nitrogen through the urine. When more nitrogen goes out in the urine than comes into the body by ingestion of protein, the patient has a negative nitrogen balance. Adequate protein intake should result in a positive nitrogen balance unless the caloric intake is excessively low.

COMPUTING NUTRITIONAL REQUIREMENTS

Both total calories and protein intake need to be computed to meet an individual's nutritional needs. If at all possible, a thorough assessment by a licensed clinical dietician should be done. A simple guideline is to provide 30 to 35 Calories per kg to maintain current body weight and 40 to 45 Calories per kg to promote anabolism. For a more precise determination of the nutritional requirements, the Harris-Benedict equation is frequently used. The equation for basal energy expenditure (BEE) for men is as follows: BEE (kcal) = 66 + (13.7 x mass in kg) + (5 x ht in cm) - (6.8 x age in years). For women, the equation is: BEE (kcal) = 665 + (9.6 x mass in kg) + (1.8 x ht in kg) - (4.7 x age in years). To calculate total daily expenditure, one must take account for the patient's activity (activity factor) and severity of injury (injury factor). The basal energy expenditure is adjusted to derive total daily expenditure as: BEE x AF x IF, where AF is activity factor, which ranges from 1.2 for bed rest to 2.0 for an extremely active person and IF is injury factor, which ranges from 1.2 for minor surgery to 2.5 for extreme thermal injury. Using the conversions of 2.54 cm per inch and 2.2 lbs per kg, the following examples are given. Example 1: 160 lb male, 73 inches tall, 40 years old, low activity: 30-35 kcal/kg x 160 lbs/2.2 kg/lb = 2182 - 2545 kcal/day or using the Harris Benedict formula: = (66 + 996.4 + 927.1 - 272) x 1.5 (AF) = 2576 kcal/day. Example 2: 120 lb female 63 inches tall, 38 years old, extremely active: 30-35 kcal/kg x 120lbs/2.2 kg/lb = 1636 - 1909 kcal/day or using the Harris Benedict formula: = (665 + 523.6 + 288.0 - 178.6) x 2 (AF) = 2596 kcal/day.

Required protein intake is computed as 0.8 to 2.0 g of protein per kg. The effectiveness of this intake can be monitored by calculating nitrogen balance. This is done by estimating the number of protein calories ingested in a 24-hour calorie count and the protein used for metabolism by calculating urine urea output. The appearance of urea in the urine indicates the use of protein for purposes other than replacing protein stores of the body, such as supplying energy after the protein is deaminated and urea is produced. A greater intake of protein than urea would indicate storage of protein in the body, generally as increased muscle mass. A positive nitrogen balance is desired in the person who is recovering from an injury.

Assessing the diet is not just an issue for undernourished individuals. Anyone who has been injured will have increased nutritional needs. Although weight reduction is an important long-term goal to maintain overall health, the person with a wound should not be placed on a weight reduction diet until the person is no longer at risk for developing a wound or having slow wound healing. Therefore, adjusting the diet to promote weight loss should not be a goal during wound healing. Even the obese individual needs a positive nitrogen balance, sufficient calories, and trace elements to promote wound healing.

DIETARY SUPPLEMENTATION

Depending on several factors, notably the ability to ingest adequate calories and protein, the diet may need to be manipulated by the clinician. The least invasive dietary intervention sufficient for some patients is to increase food intake by increasing intake of nutrient dense foods such as cheese, nuts, peanut butter, eggs, ice cream, and milkshakes. A further step is the use of commercial supplements such as Sustacal (Mead Johnson, Glenview, IL) and Ensure (Ross Products, Columbus, OH). More extreme and invasive interventions include enteral and parenteral feeding.

Enteral Feeding

Enteral feeding refers to the delivery of nutrients artificially to the gastrointestinal tract, usually utilizing a pump and a line placed into the gastrointestinal tract. For short-term feeding, a tube may be placed through the nose into the stomach (nasogastric tube). Long-term feeding requires a surgically placed tube either through the skin into the stomach or into the jejunum. A line placed into the stomach is called a PEG tube (percutaneous endoscopic gastrostomy). A J tube is surgically placed into the jejunum to provide nutrients for the individual who cannot ingest a sufficient diet. The placement of the feeding tube will be determined by a number of factors, including the patient's tolerance. For example, a tube may be placed into the duodenum if the patient does not tolerate a nasogastric tube.

Parenteral Feeding

Introduction of nutrients directly to the bloodstream, bypassing the gastrointestinal tract is termed *parenteral feed-*

ing. Because nutrients are dissolved in water, provision of adequate nutrition would cause fluid overload if the fluid were isotonic. Nutrients must be concentrated in parenteral feeding, resulting in hypertonic fluid that would damage a peripheral vein. For this reason, parenteral feeding must be delivered by a central venous line directly into the right atrium where the fluid can be immediately diluted by the entire cardiac output. Another problem with parenteral feeding is providing fat-soluble nutrients and lipids. In the short term, provision of water-soluble nutrients can be adequate because of storage of fat and fat-soluble vitamins in adipose tissue. If needed, a short-term solution for feeding using a 5% dextrose (D5W) solution can be used. Over a longer time, lipids and fat-soluble vitamins will also need to be provided.

SUMMARY

Adequate nutrition depends on a chain of factors including financial and other resources for obtaining food, cognition, taste, choice of appropriate food, ability to prepare meals, gastrointestinal function, and diseases that alter appetite and cardiovascular function. Both caloric and protein consumption need to be assessed. Equations are available for determining appropriate intake of protein and calories. Assessment of nutritional status can be determined many ways, including simple anthropometric calculations and biochemical tests. The function of key vitamins and minerals for wound healing are discussed.

QUESTIONS

1. Why must both caloric and protein intake be considered in the assessment of nutrition?

2. Why do diseases such as cancer and infectious disease retard wound healing?

3. How does arterial insufficiency produce malnutrition at the cellular level?

4. How does cognitive status affect nutrition?

5. Describe how a patient may enter a vicious cycle of poor nutrition and immobility.

BIBLIOGRAPHY

Berger MM, Baines M, Raffoul W, et al. Trace element supplementation after major burns modulates antioxidant status and clinical course by way of increased tissue trace element concentrations. *Am J Clin Nutr.* 2007;85:1293-1300.

Boyce ST, Supp AP, Swope VB, Warden GD. Vitamin C regulates keratinocyte viability, epidermal barrier, and basement membrane in vitro, and reduces wound contraction after grafting of cultured skin substitutes. *J Invest Dermatol.* 2002;118:565-572.

Shils ME, Olson JA, Shine M, Ross AC, eds. *Modern Nutrition in Health and Disease.* 9th ed. Baltimore, MD: Lippincott Williams & Wilkins; 1999.

Thomas DR. Specific nutritional factors in wound healing. *Adv Wound Care.* 1997;10:40-43.

The Patient

A patient is wheeled up to the whirlpool. The dressing is removed and the wound is measured. A few observations are made and a few questions are asked about how the wound came about. The wound is put in the whirlpool every day for 2 months and never gets better. What went wrong? A wound represents an impairment of the integumentary system. What occurs within the patient/client happens to the wound. A host of problems, some of which might seem remote to the cause of the wound, led to the wound or its slow healing. If the unique characteristics of the patient/client and lifestyle are not understood, optimizing wound healing cannot be understood. This unit is focused on discovering characteristics of the patient/client that either contribute to the etiology of the wound or impair wound healing. This unit includes 2 chapters that describe the vital information to prevent wounds from occurring and optimizing healing.

History Taking and Tests and Measures

OBJECTIVES

- Describe the 5 integumentary patterns described in the *Guide to Physical Therapist Practice*.
- List critical elements in taking a history to aid in diagnosis and prognosis.
- List risk factors for developing and slow healing of wounds that may be elicited by a history.
- Describe lab studies that may aid in the development of a diagnosis and prognosis.
- Describe the impact of social and work history on wound management.
- Describe how mobility impacts wound management.
- Describe how various types of equipment may affect wound management.

This chapter is the beginning point of intervention with the patient. Although a patient may be referred to us with a specific diagnosis and the patient exhibits all of the characteristics associated with the referring diagnosis, we may still not understand important aspects of the patient's life that change the risk to integumentary integrity and may affect wound healing. Even with a complete description of the patient, we need to know what the patient does at work, home, and during recreational activities. Many times the referring diagnosis is insufficient or not germane to the interventions we may use for treatment. History taking and physical examination go hand-in-hand throughout our interaction with the patient. What we learn from the patient by asking questions will refine our physical examination of the patient; what we learn from the physical examination may lead us to ask for more information, or may uncover inconsistencies that may be due to the patient not understanding our questions, the patient trying to give us answers he or she thinks we should hear, or the patient concealing information because of embarrassment, moral or legal issues, or other reasons. In some cases, we will continue to learn important information about the patient throughout the episode of care, or the patient's circumstances or resources may change.

THE *GUIDE TO PHYSICAL THERAPIST PRACTICE*

The *Guide to Physical Therapist Practice* (the *Guide*) was published in its original form in the November 1997 issue of *Physical Therapy* as a means of improving the uniformity of physical therapist practice. The *Guide* consisted at that time of 2 parts: a description of the practice of physical

Irion G.
Comprehensive Wound Management, 2nd ed. (pp 47-56)
© 2010 SLACK Incorporated

therapy and a series of preferred practice patterns. The preferred practice patterns are grouped by body systems into musculoskeletal, neuromuscular, cardiopulmonary, and integumentary. Within each body system a different number of patterns are described. Musculoskeletal refers mainly to the areas typically described previously as orthopedic, including disease or injury to the muscles and their structural supports such as bone, ligament, and tendon. Neuromuscular includes a number of injuries or diseases of the nervous system, ranging from the input to the nervous system, processing of sensory input, and output to the effectors. Cardiopulmonary patterns (cardiovascular and pulmonary in the second edition) represent disease or injury affecting the heart, blood vessels, and lungs. The *Guide* was revised in 2001, with little change to the integumentary practice patterns, although lymphatic disorders were moved from integumentary to cardiovascular and pulmonary in the second edition.

The integumentary patterns include Pattern A: Primary Prevention/Risk Factor Reduction for Integumentary Disorders; Pattern B: Impaired Integumentary Integrity Secondary to Superficial Skin Involvement; Pattern C: Impaired Integumentary Integrity Secondary to Partial-Thickness Skin Involvement and Scar Formation; Pattern D: Impaired Integumentary Integrity Secondary to Full-Thickness Skin Involvement and Scar Formation; and Pattern E: Impaired Integumentary Integrity Secondary to Skin Involvement Extending into Fascia, Muscle, or Bone.

The *Guide* makes explicit use of terminology that had not been used uniformly by physical therapists. In particular, the terms *examination, evaluation, diagnosis, prognosis, plan of care, intervention,* and *outcomes* are defined in the *Guide* as used in physical therapy.

Examination

Examination includes taking a history from the patient/client verbally, on a history form, or a combination of the two. Taking a history is the major emphasis of this chapter. A physical examination guided by the history of the patient/client is then performed. The physical examination consists of a pertinent systems review examining components of the cardiopulmonary, neuromuscular, musculoskeletal, and integumentary systems, determining ability to communicate, and performing specific tests and measures as the history, systems review, and other tests and measures dictate. In the past, the terms *evaluation* and *assessment* have been used interchangeably. To some, the terms convey different meanings. According to the *Guide,* evaluation is the mental process by which the clinician makes judgments regarding diagnosis and prognosis. Diagnosis is an entity encompassing a cluster of signs and symptoms, syndromes, or categories based on the data collected from the examination. Typically, the diagno-

sis encompasses one of the preferred practice patterns. Rather than reiterating the referring diagnosis, which is pathology-driven, the process is meant to establish which preferred practice pattern best fits the individual patient/client to derive an impairment-driven diagnosis. In many cases, 2 or more patterns may seem to fit a given individual. However, we are usually able to select one pattern that includes the most appropriate outcomes for that individual. In certain cases, especially involving multiple trauma or multisystem involvement, 2 or more patterns may be necessary.

Prognosis

Prognosis refers to the clinician's estimate of optimal level of function that could be attained given the unique combination of diagnosis and characteristics of the individual patient/client. A prognosis also includes a time frame quantified either as a number of visits or number of weeks/months. A combination of time and visits may also be used. For example, one may have a prognosis that a wound will be clean and stable in 2 weeks, requiring 10 visits. The plan of care lists specifically the goals, expected outcomes, the interventions to be used, duration (a time frame), frequency of visits needed, and criteria for discharge.

Interventions

Interventions are divided among the 3 categories of 1) communication, coordination, and documentation; 2) patient/client education; and 3) procedural interventions such as debridement and dressing changes. Outcomes are the measurable or observable products of intervention and are generally related to goals and discharge criteria.

Integumentary Practice Patterns

Each pattern includes a uniform set of headings. The first heading is Patient/Client Diagnostic Group. Under this heading, a number of medical diagnostic categories are listed, followed by a listing of possible diagnoses included in and excluded from the specific pattern. Also given is a listing of possible ICD9 (International Classification of Disease, Version 9) codes that might apply to patients/clients described by the pattern. Examination is defined as the collection of information, which includes taking a history, performing a systems review, and performing tests and measures. Under the examination heading, an exhaustive listing of possible items to be discovered by the history is given. Systems review includes determination of the physiologic and anatomic status of the cardiopulmonary, integumentary, musculoskeletal, and neuromuscular systems and communication, affect, cognition, language, and learning style. An alphabetical listing of pertinent tests and measures for the practice pattern follows.

For the integumentary patterns one typically assesses integumentary integrity, orthotic, protective, and supportive devices, and pain. Tests and measures of ventilation, respiration, and circulation should also be done. The next major heading is Evaluation, Diagnosis and Prognosis. Each of these terms is defined, followed by a prognosis for the pattern based on an 80% confidence interval, ie, 80% of patients/clients described by a pattern will achieve the outcomes listed in the *Guide* within the time limits given. Also listed under this heading are factors that either may require a new episode of care or may modify the time limits stated in the prognosis. The next major heading is Intervention. Interventions are discussed throughout Unit IV of this text.

Pattern A is the primary prevention and risk factor reduction pattern. The primary health problems that fit this pattern include those with low or moderate risk assessment score (Braden or Norton scale, discussed in Chapter 7), amputations, diabetes mellitus, and spinal cord injury. Pattern B refers primarily to superficial wounds, including first degree (superficial) burns, grade 0 neuropathic ulcers (ulcers due to decreased sensation, motor, or autonomic nerve function), and stage I pressure ulcers. Pattern C deals with partial-thickness wounds and scar formation. This pattern is used mainly for patients with second degree (superficial partial-thickness) burns, certain blistering dermatologic disorders, grade 1 neuropathic ulcers, and stage II pressure ulcers. Pattern D progresses to full-thickness wounds and includes full-thickness burns, necrotizing fasciitis, grade 2 neuropathic ulcers, stage III pressure ulcers, venous insufficiency, abscess, and frostbite. Pattern E includes wounds with subcutaneous tissue involvement. These may include abscess; necrotizing fasciitis; grade 3, 4, or 5 neuropathic ulcers; stage IV pressure ulcers; surgical wounds; and wounds caused by arterial disease, acute amputation, electrical burns, and frostbite. Because each of these patterns deals with impairment of integumentary integrity, a large overlap occurs across patterns.

ELEMENTS OF A HISTORY

History must be sufficiently thorough to guide the clinician to the proper tests and measures to determine the cause of the wound and to identify any characteristics of the wound, patient, family, caregivers, living arrangements, work/school, and resources that would affect the outcomes of different intervention strategies so an optimal plan of care can be devised. Demographic data typically included are age, sex, height, weight, race/ethnicity, and primary language. Additional information could be derived from computing body mass index (BMI). The age of the patient has an impact on the rate of healing and the typical daily activities of the patient. Age and race may be related to the probability of certain etiologies of the

wound, eg, sickle cell disease. Hand and foot dominance are often overlooked unless the wound is located on a hand. With wounds on a hand or foot, the patient needs to be questioned about activities involving those extremities and possible alternatives for accomplishing tasks should any limitations be placed on the extremities. Knowing hand/foot dominance may also be important in terms of any home program to ensure that the patient has sufficient dexterity to perform self-care. Developmental history includes any disorders that may aggravate the wound, create difficulty in carrying out a home program, or impede the patient's ability to protect the wound.

Medications

Patients may be taking no medications or have a long list. A list of medications being taken for the current condition, as well as other conditions, is critical information. Many individuals will forget names and dosages of drugs, whereas some patients will carry a list of medications with them at all times. A strategy of asking the patient to bring all prescriptions can aid in producing an accurate list. Inpatient or home therapy can be easier because all medications will be listed in the patient's chart. Regardless of setting, patients may be taking nonprescription drugs, including over-the-counter, street drugs, herbs, or other substances that can also affect wound healing. Particularly important for the patient with a wound are corticosteroids, NSAIDs, other anti-inflammatory or immunosuppressant drugs, antibiotics, anticoagulants, chemotherapy, insulin, and oral glycemic drugs. In addition to prescription medications, determine whether the patient is using any herbal or home remedies. An issue related to medication is whether the patient is receiving other types of interventions such as radiation treatments for cancer and any allergies. Patients may be allergic to substances such as iodine, lidocaine, or specific antibiotics that may be used in their care.

History of Present Illness

A history of the present condition should include the date of onset (if known), course of events, pattern of symptoms, and what the patient thinks caused the wound. In the case of an acute wound, the cause is usually obvious, such as a burn or laceration. In the case of a chronic wound, knowing how the wound was managed previously is imperative. For example, was the underlying venous insufficiency treated? What preventive measures have been undertaken to alleviate pressure? Is the present treatment causing chronic inflammation? In the case of a wound that is not easily diagnosed, learning what interventions were tried and how well they worked may assist in the diagnosis as much as knowing the past medical history and medications being used. The history of the current condition needs to include prior therapeutic interventions and careful questioning to determine why previous therapy was ineffective. Was the underlying problem addressed? Was the intervention not carried through? Was the intervention performed incorrectly? These can be delicate questions, especially when the clinician thinks the cause of the wound is obvious. The clinician needs to be prudent in implying incompetence of other healthcare providers, especially before a clear diagnosis can be made.

The specific concerns that led the patient to seek services and concerns or needs of the patient need to be explored. The patient's goals for intervention also must be determined. The plan of care may need to be modified to match the priorities of the patient, rather than forcing the clinician's priorities on the patient. Many times optimal treatment for the wound is not the optimal treatment for the individual patient because of work, home, or other concerns. The plan of care will also need to accommodate the patient's, family's, and caregiver's emotional response to the current clinical situation and possible treatments.

Social History, Living, and Working Conditions

Social history consists of many factors related to the person's culture, resources, activities, and support system. Each patient has a unique combination of these factors that impact his or her risk for wounds and prognosis for healing. Over the course of an episode of care, one or more of these factors may change, so we must make an effort to keep up-to-date on these changes.

Social History

Cultural beliefs and behaviors may affect the patient's ability to heal from a wound profoundly and may also directly or indirectly be the cause of a wound. Some religious beliefs will limit the range of interventions available for a plan of care. Moreover, the use of home remedies that are a part of a person's heritage but are unknown to the clinician may affect wound healing. A frank discussion of family and caregiver resources, including time, not just financial resources, is important in determining what interventions are likely to be successful. Social interactions, social activities, and support systems may affect the patient's willingness to adhere to a treatment plan. Current and prior community and work (job/school) activities need to be analyzed in terms of possible causes of wounds and whether these activities are likely to help or hinder wound healing.

Social habits can be difficult to ascertain. Unfortunately many of these social habits profoundly slow wound healing. Habits such as exercise, smoking, alcohol consumption, and drug abuse are important pieces of information to allow the clinician to develop an appropriate plan of care.

Many patients will have a combination of social habits that are not conducive to wound healing. One should account for them when developing a prognosis, stating these issues explicitly in documentation. Efforts to change social habits may result in frustration and a patient may need to be referred to individuals trained specifically in this area.

Living Conditions

Living environment, community characteristics, and projected discharge destinations must be discussed. Frequently the living environment and discharge destinations must be considered together. A patient with little support and living in an environment that is physically challenging may need to be admitted to a facility that provides the necessary support, whereas a person living in a one-floor efficiency apartment on the ground floor may be discharged to home under identical clinical conditions. Discovering who will be assisting the patient, and determining whether that caregiver is able to deliver the assistance needed should be done as early as possible. Meeting with family members or volunteer or paid caregivers to discuss roles and what can be accomplished will often be critical to successful intervention. One should also try to ascertain the willingness of caregivers in addition to their abilities to avoid poor living conditions hampering the patient's recovery. Another issue to be explored is the patient's tidiness at home. One can get some idea from the patient's general appearance, but the patient may have hygiene problems related to pets or housecleaning that interfere with the treatment plan.

Working Conditions

Important questions related to occupation include what tasks the job entails, whether the wound will impede the patient's ability to work, or whether the tasks will prevent the wound from healing. If working is not appropriate, can the patient's work responsibilities be changed by work modification or reassignment to another job? For example, a patient with venous ulcers should be standing as little as possible and a person with foot ulcers should minimize walking. Does the wound present a risk to coworkers, eg, a wound infected with methicillin-resistant *Staphylococcus aureus*? As discussed with living arrangements, how tidy is the work environment? Some patients may be exposed to a work environment that is unsuitable for wound healing. For a number of these reasons, a patient may not be able to return to work as quickly as desired. Many patients will have short- and long-term disability plans, or sufficient sick days to stay home; however, many will lack financial resources and will feel compelled to return to work. Discussion of these issues with the patient is imperative. Rather than have the patient return to work without the healthcare provider's knowledge, adaptations to the plan of care may be possible to allow the patient to earn an income while recovering.

Family History

A number of health risks tend to occur in family members either because of genetic or lifestyle similarities. Type 2 diabetes, arterial disease, hypertension, sickle cell disease, cancer, and other diseases existing in the family may be undiagnosed in the patient. A history should include both the patient's and the patient's family's medical history.

Functional Status

The functional status and activity level prior to the problem, and expectation of return to this function and activity, are critical areas for an interview. Functional status and activity level may be a cause or complicating factor for a wound. For example, the person with a neuropathic ulcer on the plantar surface whose work requires walking or the person with venous insufficiency who is on her feet all day can both cause and slow healing of ulcerations. Determine the current and prior functional status in self-care and home management activities, including activities of daily living (ADL) and instrumental activities of daily living (IADL), and who at home is available to assist with activities if the patient is not able or needs to desist from the activities to allow wound healing. Moreover, recreational or leisure activities and degree of physical fitness need to be considered in both developing a diagnosis and tailoring a plan of care that matches the patient's needs.

Although a patient's current mobility will be explored as part of the physical examination, the patient's mobility history is important for several reasons. The patient needs to be both asked about mobility and to demonstrate mobility to the clinician. How mobile is the person in a bed or in a chair? Can the patient shift weight or get into and out of a bed or a chair independently or is assistance needed? Is a referral to physical therapy or occupational therapy needed to aid in the prevention of more wounds or to promote healing of existing ulcers? We also need to know how long the patient has had the current level of mobility. Did the person have a gradual decline or an abrupt decline in mobility? Were certain aspects of mobility affected earlier than others? Has the patient received intervention for mobility problems previously? For example, does the patient have experience using crutches? Reduced mobility limiting a patient to a bed or a chair represents a great risk for pressure ulcers. Not using an assistive device with neuropathic feet may be a risk factor as well. Any alteration in normal gait pattern also represents a risk of injury to the foot.

What equipment does the patient have? Does she know how to use it? Does the equipment suit the impairment or disability of the patient? For example, does a person with weightbearing restrictions use a rolling walker? Does a person with diminished vision or poor balance use a rolling walker or standard walker? Why was the patient given the equipment? In many cases, the patient may have borrowed a cane, walker, or crutches from a friend or family member without being instructed in its use and is simply using the wrong type of equipment because it was convenient. Patients may have a piece of equipment but not use it for cosmetic reasons or may forget to use it. Asking a patient why he was given a walker may elicit a response that the patient was supposed to have weightbearing restrictions that were not communicated to you.

Past Medical and Surgical History

Either before or during the interview a patient should be asked about health issues that occurred earlier. Although they may not be obvious contributors to the patient's current condition, access to medical and surgical history may assist in diagnosis of a wound or lead us to alter our plan of care for the patient. Depending on the cause of the wound, certain systems may become more important. Because of the prevalence of diabetes mellitus, all patients should be asked about endocrine/metabolic disease, especially diabetes. Patients with diabetes should also be asked about glucose control. Does the patient use insulin? What type and time of day? Does the patient manage diabetes with diet and exercise, or with oral glycemic drugs?

Cardiovascular disease is also common and should be addressed. Does the patient have a history of angina, shortness of breath, and surgical interventions such as coronary artery bypass grafting? The patient should also be asked about hypertension, arrhythmia, valve disease, and any treatment for these. Gastrointestinal disorders may lead to malnutrition, anemia, or bowel incontinence; genitourinary issues include bladder incontinence leading to injury to the skin. Questions related to the integumentary system include previous wounds, dermatologic conditions, and treatments for them. A history of musculoskeletal and neuromuscular disorders can produce abnormal forces on the skin and injury. These injuries or diseases may occur in the central or peripheral nervous systems. A general history of any hospitalizations and surgeries may be relevant to the patient's present condition or how the treatment plan is developed.

The risk factors listed above should always be explored. A simple means is to have the patient fill out a health history form. A thorough history should be available on the chart of an inpatient. Additionally, the medications taken by the patient may alert the clinician to a disease not uncovered during the history. Given the prevalence of diabetes mellitus and its impact on wounding and healing, every patient should be asked about diabetes and the family history for diabetes. Other health-related questions should include immune system status, which can allow wounds to develop and also impede wound healing. Some of these are discussed in greater detail above.

Neuropathy

Similar to mobility, we need to know the history of neuropathy. We will examine the patient to determine the extent of neuropathy, but will need to know the history of the neuropathy as well. Longer history of ambulation with neuropathy carries a greater risk of foot ulceration. We also need to know what interventions have been used such as off-loading devices and assistive devices. When discussing neuropathy, we should ask the patient appropriate questions about glycemic control. How often does the patient perform glucose monitoring? What are the numbers like? Does the patient know his or her HbA1c? How often does the patient see a healthcare provider about his or her foot care?

Vascular Disease

Questions about vascular disease will follow the same approach as mobility and neuropathy in that we want a history of the severity, duration, and any interventions that patient has received related to vascular disease. We will perform vascular testing as part of the physical exam (discussed in Chapter 6). Questions should be asked about any other issues related to arterial disease, such as ischemic heart disease, stroke, renal disease, amputations, and surgical interventions. A related issue is asking about any tobacco use.

Nutrition

Nutrition was discussed in the previous chapter. During a history, questions that will relate to the physical exam should be asked. Has the patient experienced recent weight gain or weight loss. What is the history of any weight changes? Has the patient made any changes to his or her diet? Depending on whether a dietician is available for nutrition screening, we may need to ask the patient about his or her diet.

Continence

Incontinence of the bladder or bowel is a risk factor particularly to the skin of the perineum. Any patient with erythema of the perineum and surrounding areas should be asked about incontinence and any interventions. Although this is particularly true for incontinence, we may need to discuss any of these risk factors with family or other caregivers if the patient is unable to provide the information. Many people are easily embarrassed and unwilling to discuss continence issues with others, so the healthcare provider must approach the topic tactfully. A simple approach is to discuss all the risk factors for skin injury, then ask whether the patient has any of them. If patients or caregivers know why the questions about incontinence are important, they may not be as reluctant to discuss incontinence as they would if they were asked without prefacing the question by discussing incontinence as a risk factor for skin injury.

Trauma

Injuries caused by trauma are often self-explanatory, yet some aspects of the injury could be missed if we do not ask appropriate questions. Depending on the circumstances of the injury, patients may have an emotional response, particularly if others were injured in the same incident. Traumatic injury may produce alterations in gait patterns or place unusual stress on other body parts. Questions may need to be asked as we examine different areas of the body as some more minor injuries or injuries occurring where the patient has limited sensation could be missed.

Lab Studies

Results from basic lab studies can be found on the charts of inpatients. Outpatients are unlikely able to provide much assistance to the clinician regarding results of lab studies. The results useful to the clinician include blood counts to determine if anemia, thrombocytopenia (lack of platelets), or leukopenia (lack of white blood cells) is present. Blood chemistry including electrolytes (potassium, sodium, chloride, and bicarbonate), blood urea nitrogen (BUN) and creatinine for renal function, and blood glucose should be present on the chart of an inpatient and may be available from the referring physicians.

Blood Counts

Both total white blood cell count (WBC) and differential white cell counts may be important in certain cases. In terms of risk for infection, or diagnosis of infection, neutrophil counts are also critical. Normal WBC counts range from 4,500-11,000/mm^3 in both men and women. Leukocytosis is a count exceeding this range. Of particular importance in the context of wound management is the diagnosis of infection. Other causes of leukocytosis that should be considered include leukemia or another form of cancer, tissue injury, and some other source of inflammation. Leukocytosis is frequently accompanied by fever, somnolence, and anorexia produced by elevated cytokines released in these conditions. As discussed in subsequent chapters, wound infection has a profound effect on decision-making. Leukopenia, defined as a count less than the range listed above, can be produced by a number of causes including bone marrow disease (aplastic anemia), viral infection, and cancer chemotherapy. As the white cell count falls, the clinician must become more careful with technique. A white cell count below 1,000 or neutrophil count below 500 usually requires reverse isolation with gloving, gowning, donning a mask, and sterile technique, even for routine wound care.

Neutrophils observed in a differential count may be termed either *segmented* (mature) or *bands* (immature). Neutrophil counts are generally elevated in the presence of bacterial infection. A large number of bands are particularly diagnostic of bacterial infection. Lymphocytes are categorized into B cells and T cells and then further classified into subcategories. B cells are responsible for antibody-mediated immunity, whereas T cells are involved in specific cell-mediated immunity against specific antigens. T cell-immunity is associated particularly with neoplasms and viral infection, but is involved in delayed hypersensitivity reactions, including skin reactions, eg, poison ivy. Monocytes are blood cells equivalent to the tissue macrophage. These cells are responsible for later destruction of marked cells and destruction of debris following neutrophil infiltration. Eosinophils are involved in defenses against worms and are implicated in allergic responses, including asthma. Basophils are the blood equivalent of mast cells, which release mediators of inflammation, particularly histamine. Normal differential counts are 50% to 60% neutrophils, 30% to 40% lymphocytes, 1% to 9% monocytes, 0% to 3% eosinophils, and 0% to 1% basophils. In addition, bands (immature neutrophils) range from 0% to 7%. Elevations in neutrophils, termed *neutrophilia*, and especially bands are usually indicative of infection by pyogenic organisms such as Staph or Strep species. Lymphocytosis (excessive B or T lymphocytes) is indicative of viral infection. Monocytosis (elevated monocyte count) may occur in severe infections. Excessive numbers of eosinophils (eosinophilia) are indicative of severe allergic reactions or worm infestation, and basophilia indicates parasitic infection or hypersensitivity reactions. Neutropenia, defined as a neutrophil count of less than 500, as with leukopenia, requires reverse isolation.

The normal red cell count is greater in men than women. For men, the normal ranges are 4.7 to 6.1 million per µL, a hematocrit of 42% to 52%, and a hemoglobin concentration of 14 to 18 g/dL. These ranges for women are 4.2 to 5.4 million per µL, 37% to 47%, and 12 to 16 g/dL, respectively. During pregnancy, these numbers decrease. The importance of red cell parameters, regardless of which is used, is the ability to transport oxygen to aid in wound healing. Elevations in red cell parameters (polycythemia) are rare, but clinically significant. Much more common are conditions that lower these numbers, producing anemia. Causes of anemia include bleeding, diseases of red cell production (aplastic anemia, pernicious anemia, iron and vitamin deficiencies), diseases characterized by excessive destruction of red cells (hemolytic anemias, including several autoimmune diseases and sickle cell anemia), and genetic diseases of hemoglobin synthesis (thalassemias). Several lab tests are available for determining the cause of anemia. Another major cause is cancer chemotherapy. Regardless of the cause of anemia, decreased oxygen transport capacity of blood has a deleterious effect on wound healing and elevating red cell parameters by correcting the cause, or transfusion or administration of erythropoietin is important to assist wound healing. Patients with renal disease or who are receiving cancer chemotherapy may be using exogenous erythropoietin to maintain red cell counts.

Platelets are fragments of cells called megakaryocytes. Platelets have a major role in hemostasis, which is usually the first step in acute wound healing. The normal range for platelets is 150,000 to 400,000 per µL. *Thrombocytosis* is the term for an elevated count, whereas a deficiency is termed *thrombocytopenia*. In terms of wound healing, the normal concern is thrombocytopenia, rather than thrombocytosis. Thrombocytopenia, like anemia and leukopenia, occurs with aplastic anemia and cancer chemotherapy. Platelets can be diminished by a number of autoimmune diseases or consumed in disseminated vascular coagulation. Thrombocytopenia reduces the initial reaction to wounding and proliferation by decreasing the availability of platelet derived growth factor. The effectiveness of platelets is also reduced in von Willebrand disease, a genetic disorder that prevents platelets from adhering at the site of injury. Tests related to hemostasis are the International Normalized Ratio (INR), prothrombin time (PT), and partial thromboplastin time (PTT). Inadequate hemostasis is a concern for several aspects of wound management and these values and their interpretation should be understood. Thrombin is produced in the coagulation cascade as the final enzyme of the processes, converting fibrinogen to fibrin, augmenting the strength of the platelet aggregate, and trapping red cells in the thrombus. PTT is an index of the effectiveness of the coagulation cascade only, whereas PT is affected by clotting factors, prothrombin, and fibrinogen. PT is prolonged with anticoagulation therapy, vitamin K deficiency, and genetic defects in the coagulation cascade such as hemophilia and von Willebrand disease. PT is tested both to screen for coagulation disorders and to determine the effectiveness of anticoagulation therapy. Because of variation in PT in different labs, the INR was developed. This index corrects for variations in testing materials and compares results of PT to reference values; therefore, INR should be identical in different labs for the same person. Normal values for PT range from 12 to 15 seconds, PTT ranges from 25 to 40 seconds and INR should be between 0.9 and 1.1. Note INR does not have units; it is a ratio of PT to PT reference values. Values of PT 1.5 to 2.5 times normal are desirable for patients with hypercoagulability concerns such as history of deep venous thrombosis, coronary artery disease, or cerebrovascular disease. A PT greater than 2.5 times normal presents a risk of spontaneous bleeding, but particular care must be taken even with a therapeutic PT. Using INR numbers, concern for bleeding occurs at a value greater than 2.0. A value of 3.0 places the patient at risk of spontaneous bleeding.

Basic Metabolic Profile and Comprehensive Metabolic Profile

The basic metabolic profile (BMP) and comprehensive metabolic profile (CMP) are common laboratory tests. BMP consists of measurements of important electrolytes, 2 indicators of renal function, and blood glucose. Any one or more of these tests might be performed separately. CMP consists of the same tests, but includes tests of liver and related function.

Electrolytes

The electrolytes routinely analyzed are serum sodium, potassium, chloride, bicarbonate, and sometimes calcium and magnesium. Because these are electrolytes, alterations from normal ranges can have profound effects on excitable tissues—muscle, nerve, and myocardial cells. Normal serum sodium has a range of 135 to 145 mEq/L, potassium is 3.5 to 5.0, chloride is 98 to 109, bicarbonate is 20 to 30, calcium is 9.0 to 10.5, and magnesium is 1.2 to 2.0 mEq/L. The amount of sodium in the body determines fluid volumes, and alterations can cause swelling or shrinkage of cells. Potassium is the primary determinant of membrane potentials. Excessive potassium in the extracellular fluid depolarizes cells, whereas depletion of extracellular potassium hyperpolarizes cells. In either case, serious, potentially life-threatening arrhythmias can develop with either hyper- or hypokalemia. Hypokalemia can produce muscle tetany due to depolarization of muscle and nerve cells, whereas hyperkalemia leads to hyperpolarization and muscle weakness. Alterations of chloride are diagnostic for fluid balance disorders, and bicarbonate changes are diagnostic of acid-base disorders. Both calcium and magnesium are intimately involved with neuromuscular function. Ionized calcium decreases the probability of neuromuscular excitation and, as such, both hypocalcemia and hypomagnesemia cause tetany and arrhythmias. Hypercalcemia and hypermagnesemia cause muscle weakness and arrhythmias.

Renal Function

The 2 lab values of BUN and creatinine are routinely measured. Normal kidney function eliminates these substances within a given range of these values. Failure of the kidneys to excrete them allows these substances to accumulate in the blood. Normal values of BUN range from 10 to 20 mg/dL in adults. Because BUN represents a balance between production of urea from breakdown of proteins and excretion by the kidney, a sharp increase in protein intake may increase BUN. Increased BUN may also result from gastrointestinal bleeding and dehydration. Decreases in BUN may be seen with liver disease because of a diminished ability of the liver to produce urea and

with overhydration. Creatinine is a product of muscle tissue. The normal range for creatinine is 0.5 to 1.2 mg/dL. Creatinine excretion decreases with renal disease causing plasma creatinine to increase above this concentration. Plasma concentration may decline with decreasing muscle mass or increase with muscle injury. Of concern with renal disease are the accompanying cardiovascular problems, including hypertension and anemia. Because erythropoietin is synthesized by renal cells, administration of exogenous erythropoietin may be used to treat the anemia of end stage renal failure

Blood Glucose

Normal fasting blood glucose is considered to be less than 110 mg/dL. Blood glucose rises with eating and decreases with insulin and exercise. A person with normal glucose metabolism will return blood glucose to the normal range within 2 hours of consumption of 75 g of glucose. Blood glucose of a person with diabetes mellitus will exceed 200 mg/dL at the end of the test and a person with impaired glucose tolerance will have a blood glucose value between 140 and 200 mg/dL. Either an oral glucose tolerance test or an elevated fasting blood sugar can be indicative of diabetes mellitus. By the older definition, hyperglycemia is present with blood glucose in excess of 150 mg/dL. Newer definitions have lowered the threshold. In 1998, the American Diabetes Association (ADA) defined a new category called impaired fasting glucose. Impaired fasting glucose is considered to exist at a value of 110 to 125 mg/dL. This condition has been referred to as a pre-diabetic state. Some experts suggest that interventions at this point might be able to prevent the development of type 2 diabetes. Blood glucose exceeding 126 mg/dL on at least 2 measurements is diagnostic of diabetes mellitus.

Impaired glucose metabolism is considered a risk factor for future diabetes mellitus and macrovascular disease. A person with fasting blood glucose between 120 and 150 mg/dL is considered to have impaired glucose tolerance. As such, clinicians should be concerned about wound management for an individual with any impairment in glucose uptake. Another test commonly performed is the 2-hour postprandial blood sugar. In this test, blood glucose is measured 2 hours after eating. A normal value should be obtained within this time frame. Short-term, elevated blood glucose values up to 250 mg/dL are not considered to be dangerous. When blood glucose concentration exceeds this level, the ability of the renal tubules to reabsorb glucose is saturated and glucose appears in the urine. Over the long-term, elevations of blood glucose above 120 mg/dL are considered a health risk. A means of monitoring long-term glucose control is to measure glycated hemoglobin. The percentage of glycated hemoglobin is an index of how well glucose has been controlled over the 120-day lifespan of the average red blood cell. Poor glucose control causes glycated hemoglobin (HbA1c) to exceed 9%. This corresponds to an average value for blood glucose greater than 210 mg/dL. Optimal control produces HbA1c values of less than 6.1%, which represents an average blood glucose value of less than 120 mg/dL.

An additional concern, and potential medical emergency, is hypoglycemia. Hypoglycemia results from imbalance of eating, insulin, and exercise and is not uncommon in ill individuals. Symptoms of hypoglycemia may manifest at a wide range of blood glucose values. At a value of 70 or less, corrective action should be taken, usually by providing oral carbohydrates in various forms such as sugar tablets, carbohydrate snacks, or concentrated sugar drinks such as orange juice, but not diet drinks. Symptoms of hypoglycemia are basically those of generalized sympathetic nervous system activation. This includes tachycardia, shaking, and excessive sweating. The patient may also complain of a headache or be apathetic and uncoordinated. Maintaining balanced eating, insulin, and activity needs to be stressed with a patient with diabetes, especially an individual who is sick or has wounds. Illness or surgery can lead to wild fluctuations in blood glucose. Frequently, stress elevates corticosteroids, which in turn elevate blood glucose. Insulin doses are increased, but often patients fail to eat regularly and blood glucose can plummet. Clinicians must be constantly aware of this possibility and should be able to test for blood glucose and take corrective action themselves in addition to reporting the episode to the physician responsible for managing the patient's diabetes.

CMP

More information can be obtained from a CMP, which consists of the tests included in the BMP with the addition of serum concentrations of markers of liver function. The tests performed as part of the CMP that are not part of the BMP may be done separately as a hepatic function panel, instead of performing them as part of the CMP.

The hepatic function panel consists of ALP (alkaline phosphatase), ALT (alanine amino transferase, formerly called SGPT), AST (aspartate amino transferase, formerly called SGOT), and bilirubin. The hepatic function panel is used to detect liver damage or disease. Alanine aminotransferase is an enzyme mainly found in the liver and as such is the primary test for detecting hepatitis. Alkaline phosphatase is related to the bile ducts and is increased when they are blocked and may indicate gall bladder, liver, and bile duct disease, but may also be elevated due to increased bone turnover in chronic renal failure. Aspartate aminotransferase is found in the liver, but also in the heart and skeletal muscles and historically had been used for differential diagnosis of chest pain. Bilirubin is measured as either total bilirubin or direct and indirect bilirubin. Elevated total bilirubin can be due to liver disease, bile duct occlusion, hemolytic anemia, or other causes. Measurements of direct and indirect bilirubin aid in determining the cause of elevated total bilirubin. Albumin and total protein reflect the ability of the liver to synthesize proteins.

Results of Diagnostic Imaging

Patients may have diagnostic imaging for a number of reasons. Most relevant to wounds is determining whether infection has spread to bone. Bones of the foot are most susceptible, particularly in those with diabetes mellitus. Osteomyelitis may show as localized destruction of bone. Free air produced by fermentation may be detected on x-ray due to deep infection with anaerobic bacteria. For example, a patient with a fracture of the humerus may develop free air around the fracture site due to *E. coli* infection from being catheterized.

SUMMARY

A number of factors related to the patient's health status and history can either cause a wound or impair the healing of a wound. Using the *Guide to Physical Therapist Practice* to structure the history and physical examination of the patient is an important factor. The terms *history, physical examination, review of systems, diagnosis, prognosis, plan of care,* and *outcomes* are defined. Deviations from normal lab values need to be interpreted for a potential influence on wound healing, especially blood cells and glucose. The clinician must also understand the social/work/play history of the patient and any medications, either prescribed by a physician or self-prescribed.

QUESTIONS

1. Why are we concerned about the use of anti-inflammatory drugs in wound management?

2. What is the importance of an elevated white cell count?

3. Contrast the pathology-driven medical diagnosis with the impairment-driven diagnosis described in the *Guide to Physical Therapy Practice.*

4. Why is having a patient show you all of the medications being taken important?

5. Why should you observe a patient using any assistive or adaptive devices?

BIBLIOGRAPHY

Garritan S, Jones P, Kornberg T, Parkin C. Laboratory values in the intensive care unit. *Acute Care Perspectives.* 1995;3(4):7-11.

Irion G. Lab values update. *Acute Care Perspectives.* 2004;13(1):1-5.

Irion GL, Goodman CC. Laboratory tests and values. In: Goodman CC, Fuller KS (eds). *Pathology: Implications for the Physical Therapist.* 3rd ed. Philadelphia, PA: W.B. Saunders; 2008:1637-1668.

Ramos Martínez A, Duca A, Muñez Rubio E, Valverde Herreros ML, Ramírez Feito C. Osteomyelitis due to Escherichia coli complicating a closed humeral fracture. *An Med Interna.* 2006;23(12):588-590.

Physical Examination

OBJECTIVES

- Describe changes in the gross appearance of an extremity that may be related to the etiology of a wound.
- Describe normal skin color, causes of variation in skin color, and how heavily pigmented skin differs from Caucasian skin.
- Describe changes in hair and nails that may be related to the cause of a wound.
- Discuss how temperature variations may be indicative of disease processes.
- List common accumulations in the skin and their associated conditions.
- Describe normal hydration, turgor, and elasticity of skin and possible causes of changes in hydration, turgor, and elasticity.
- Describe common vascular tests and interpret abnormal findings.
- Discuss the importance of testing strength, range of motion, sensation, reflexes, mobility, coordination, balance, and aerobic/cardiopulmonary testing.

The history helps direct the physical examination. A thorough physical examination may take several hours to complete; however, the history and careful observation should narrow the focus of the physical examination. For most patients, all aspects of the physical exam can be addressed within a few minutes if the history is done well. For other patients, a very thorough examination will be required even if the cause of the wound is very clear. An example is the patient with a history of diabetes mellitus. A very thorough examination of the strength and sensation of the lower extremities is in order, regardless of the physical appearance of the wound. On the other hand, a person with an acute wound of known etiology might be examined in 10 to 15 minutes.

REVIEW OF SYSTEMS

The review of systems includes the basic elements of the examination that pertain to all patients. For physical therapy, the review of systems is generally divided into integumentary, cardiovascular and pulmonary, musculo-skeletal, and neuromuscular. Each of these systems will be discussed below.

Integumentary

When inspecting the skin, one examines the gross appearance of representative or at-risk areas of skin. Skin coloration, temperature, texture, turgor, and elasticity also

Irion G.
Comprehensive Wound Management, 2nd ed. (pp 57-70)
© 2010 SLACK Incorporated

must be examined. In addition to the skin, much may be learned by examining the hair and nails, which reflect stresses that are likely to affect the skin as well.

Skin Color

Melanin and hemoglobin are the 2 primary determinants of skin color. Melanin is the brown pigment produced by melanocytes. In individuals of sub-Saharan African descent, melanin pigmentation may be so great that variation in hemoglobin content of the skin becomes obscured. Saturated hemoglobin with good arterial supply produces the pinkish hue typical of Caucasian skin. Differences in blood flow can vary skin color from a ghostly pallor to a bright red. Pallor suggests arterial insufficiency. Worse yet, is a purplish hue produced by the presence of desaturated hemoglobin circulating through an extremity. This indicates severe arterial insufficiency, severe congestive heart failure, or severe pulmonary disease. A bright red color is produced by hyperemia (excessive blood flow). Reddish color (erythema) is an indication of inflammation and perhaps infection. Because blood flow also brings warm blood from the body's core to the surface, erythema is usually accompanied by skin warmth, also an indication of inflammation or infection. In heavily melanin-pigmented skin, hyperemia produces a violet or eggplant color and increased warmth that may be missed by the inexperienced clinician. The loss of brown pigmentation may be manifested in two important ways. In vitiligo, patches of hypopigmented skin, usually a few centimeters across with somewhat irregular borders, are observed. Albinism produces a uniform hypopigmentation with accompanying hypopigmentation of the hair and irises of the eyes. Increased brown pigmentation occurs with stimulation of melanocytes with adrenocorticotrophic hormone (ACTH). The structure of ACTH closely resembles the hormone melanocyte stimulating hormone. High concentrations of ACTH occur with Addison's disease and pregnancy. In pregnancy, increased brown pigmentation occurs in characteristic locations such as the face, nipples, and the linea nigra, along the vertical centerline of the abdomen, extending to the umbilicus.

Temperature

As discussed above, skin temperature is altered by the magnitude of blood flow to the skin. Decreased skin temperature and pallor accompany lack of blood flow to the skin. The clinician must determine whether the diminished temperature is localized to an area of an extremity or perhaps to the entirety of the extremity by comparing 2 extremities and the length of each extremity. In addition, one must account for the ambient temperature, amount of clothing, and physical activity of the limb prior to examination. A single foot that feels cool compared with the other foot and the rest of the body is a clear sign of arterial insufficiency. At the other extreme, an area of skin that is warmer than expected based on a bilateral comparison, or, in the judgment of the clinician, warmer than it should be based on ambient temperature, clothing, and physical activity, is a sign of inflammation or infection and is usually accompanied by hyperemia. In many cases, temperature can be assessed easily by the clinician's touch. Very poor arterial circulation and fever are readily detected by most clinicians.

In some cases, quantification of local temperature is desirable. Tools available to perform this quantification include thermistors and radiometers. A thermistor is a temperature-sensitive probe that alters its resistance with changes in temperature. Typically a thermistor is plugged into a display unit with either an analog needle or digital display to allow temperature to be read in both Celsius and Fahrenheit scales (Figure 6-1). The probe is put in contact with the skin for a minimum of a few seconds (depending on the particular unit used, read instructions) to determine temperature. Thermistors are generally very accurate and reliable, but require direct contact with the tissue of interest. Radiometers are based on detection of infrared radiation emitted by the object of interest. Heat is exchanged from an object to surrounding objects that are not in direct contact by infrared radiation. The amount of infrared radiation is directly proportional to the temperature of the object. Therefore, a radiometer is capable of determining skin temperature without direct contact with a wound. However, these devices are used infrequently because of their price. In addition, the patient's body temperature should be measured using a device approved by the facility. Increased temperature is indicative of systemic infection. However, the clinician should be aware of factors that may affect temperature, including the temperature of the room, previous activity, excessive clothing, and recent exposure to a hot environment.

Accumulations

Various materials may accumulate in the skin as a result of disease processes. When these disease processes are also the causes of wounds, identification of the accumulation in the skin is useful in determining the etiology of a wound. Hemosiderin is a particularly important accumulation. Hemosiderin (literally blood iron) is an accumulation of iron that results from the degradation of red blood cells. Hemosiderin is a storage form of iron in the tissue. Macrophages eventually pick up hemosiderin from the tissues and recycle the iron to the bone marrow. Hemosiderin produces a brownish-yellow discoloration usually referred to as hemosiderin staining. Hemosiderin staining, particularly just superior to the medial malleolus, is very predictive of venous hypertension. Many chronic wounds will have hemosiderin accumulating in the skin

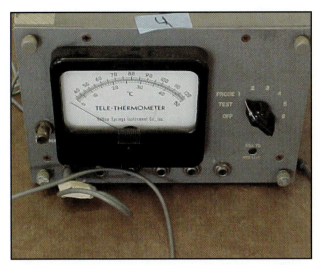

Figure 6-1. One type of instrument for use with a thermistor to detect skin temperature.

immediately adjacent to the wound due to repetitive trauma. Bilirubin and its precursor biliverdin are also the result of the breakdown of hemoglobin. Bilirubin and biliverdin are seen in bruises. Shortly after the loss of blood directly beneath the skin (eg, a contusion) the purplish hue is due to biliverdin. As biliverdin is broken down into bilirubin, the skin takes on a yellowish tint (jaundice). Later, as bilirubin is removed by the circulation from the site of injury, the brownish-yellow hemosiderin remaining at the site of injury becomes obvious. Generalized jaundice indicates systemic overload of bilirubin. Jaundice occurs frequently in newborns due to the destruction of red cells carrying fetal hemoglobin. In adults, jaundice represents the imbalance of hemoglobin breakdown and bilirubin excretion. Jaundice may result from either hemolytic anemia (excessive breakdown of hemoglobin), or the inability to excrete bilirubin due to hepatic disease (hepatitis) or biliary obstruction.

Lipodermatosclerosis

Lymphatic disease results in rough, tough skin with increased pigmentation. To some, the appearance resembles that of the skin of an orange, thus the term *peau d'orange*. The fluid and protein accumulating in the interstitial space causes fibrosis and puckering. In contrast to the mobilizable accumulation of fluid in venous insufficiency, lymphatic edema is difficult to mobilize. Lipodermatosclerosis may also occur in severe or long-standing venous insufficiency.

Hydration, Turgor, and Elasticity

These 3 are grouped together due to their association with the aging process. In senescent skin, a loss of all 3 occurs. With normal hydration, a firm gel is evident in the dermal portion of the skin. Hydration, turgor, and elasticity can be tested by pinching the skin. With a pinch, a firm rounded skin fold can be gently lifted from the surface. This skin fold immediately retracts to its former position when released.

In senescent skin, a dry, triangular skin fold can be observed, which does not immediately retract to its position upon release, but remains elevated in the shape of a tent, thus the term *tenting*. Tenting can be seen at certain locations, especially the neck, without pinching the skin. Turgor refers specifically to the firmness of skin as it is pinched. This firmness, or turgor, is caused by the gel-like property of a normally hydrated dermis, in which water molecules are trapped by the glycosaminoglycans of the ground substance of the dermis. With insufficient hydration, turgor is lost, as is the firm feel to the skin fold. Elasticity refers to the snapping back of healthy skin as the skin fold is released. It is partially due to skin turgor, but as the name implies is also due to the presence of elastic fibers constructed of the protein elastin in the skin. The number and thickness of elastic fibers decrease with age.

However, the skin of otherwise younger healthy skin can lose hydration, turgor, and elasticity in environments with low humidity, especially in the winter. Skin can rapidly lose moisture to dry, cold air and even crack in winter, requiring the use of moisturizers to maintain hydration, turgor, and elasticity.

Overhydrated skin occurs with derangements of fluid balance, resulting in edema. Edema can have many causes, but basically results from excessive hydrostatic pressure in capillaries or the imbalance of osmotic pressure across the capillary walls. Edema results from congestive heart failure, venous insufficiency, and hyperemia, producing excessive capillary hydrostatic pressure from excessive blood volume, failure to pump blood from veins back to the heart, or excessive dilation of arterial vessels. With vasodilation, pressure remains high as it enters capillaries, rather than dropping to manageable levels as blood moves into the capillaries and fluid is filtered into the interstitial space. Lack of plasma proteins secondary to lack of production in liver disease or malnutrition, or due to loss of plasma proteins by kidney disease, allows excessive movement of water out of capillaries. Excessive quantities of proteins in the interstitial space—whether due to injury, such as a burn, or due to very high capillary pressure—encourages the movement of water out of capillaries into the interstitial space, a phenomenon known as *third spacing*. Iatrogenic infiltration of fluid may occur when a line is assumed to be in a vein or a shunt used for hemodialysis and then the fluid is allowed to run into the limb. Fluid overload or edema results in damage to the epidermis and the peeling of the epidermis that resembles the result of sunburn.

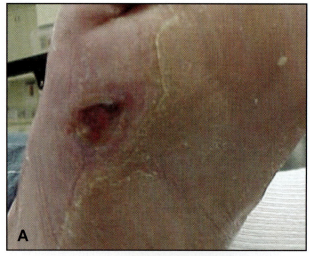

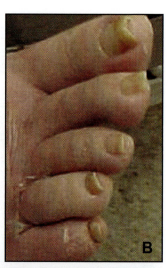

Figure 6-2. Appearance of diabetic skin and nails. (A) Thick callus on sole. (B) Fungal infection of the nails. (C) Spread of fungal infection through skin of toes and dorsum of foot. (D) Peeling thick callus. (E) Xerosis of skin extending onto patient's leg.

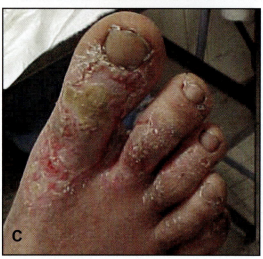

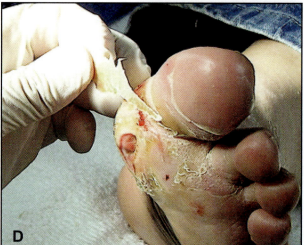

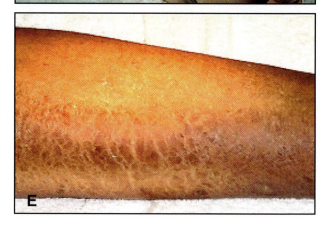

Hair and Nails

Loss of hair and thickening of nails are characteristic of arterial insufficiency, but also occur with aging. A change in hair and nail appearance can be established by asking the patient or comparing left and right sides. In the case of bilateral changes, the clinician may need to rely on patient recollection and personal judgment of normal hair and nail appearance. Thick, multilayered, yellowed nails are common with poorly controlled diabetes along with thick, rough skin on the soles (Figure 6-2).

Cardiovascular and Pulmonary

Components of the review of systems and common tests related to the cardiovascular and pulmonary systems are discussed below. Because many leg ulcers are related to arterial and venous disease, both vital signs and special tests related to them are included here.

Cardiac and Pulmonary Function

The review of systems related to cardiac function consists of vital signs. Heart rate and blood pressure should be measured at each opportunity; measurement with a pulse oximeter gives the opportunity to screen for breathing

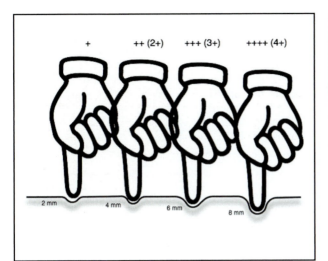

Figure 6-3. Quantification of pitting edema. (A) A pit of approximately 2 mm occurs with pressure in a limb with swelling that may not be obvious to an untrained examiner. The pit dissipates rapidly. (B) A pit of approximately 4 mm is produced in a limb that may look swollen to the patient, family, or caregivers. The pit will dissipate within a few seconds. (C) A pit of approximately 6 mm in a limb with an obvious change in contour. The pit will remain for several seconds. (D) A pit of approximately 8 mm is produced in a limb with gross deformity. The pit may last several minutes.

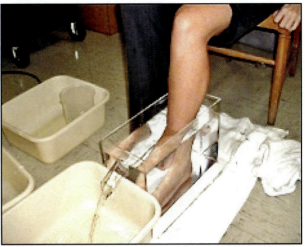

Figure 6-4. Use of a foot volumeter to quantify the effect of edema on lower extremity volume. The volumeter is filled to overflowing and the volume that overflows is discarded. The foot is gently placed in the volumeter with the foot flat, the ankle in neutral and the knee at 90 degrees of flexion. The volume that overflows is measured and used as a reference for comparison either to the contralateral limb or to the same limb to assess the effect of treatment or progression of edema.

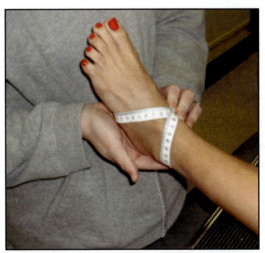

Figure 6-5. The figure-8 method used to assess for changes in foot/ankle volume. The tape is started at the insertion of the tibialis anterior, then placed over the landmarks of the head of the navicular, styloid process of the fifth metatarsal, medial malleolus, lateral malleolus, and back to the insertion of the tibialis anterior tendon, producing 2 loops. Serial measurements may be done to determine whether any changes in foot/ankle volume occur or to compare 2 extremities.

disorders as well as obtaining heart rate and blood pressure. Traditional tests associated with cardiovascular and pulmonary function include checking for clubbing, cyanosis, and edema. This is commonly denoted as CCE on a physical examination. As discussed in Chapter 1, clubbing represents a change in the shape of nails to spherical, as opposed to the normal cylindrical shape. Cystic fibrosis, lung cancer, and other cardiopulmonary diseases are associated with clubbing. However, clubbing is not very specific as many people with no underlying disease may have detectable clubbing. Cyanosis, a bluish tint to the skin, may be detected on the fingers, toes, around the mouth, or extend proximally if the cause is more severe. Causes may include respiratory disease, or low cardiac output as may occur in severe congestive heart failure. Edema may be detected in the dependent areas, chiefly the lower extremities, in congestive heart failure or other diseases that allow fluid to accumulate. Left-sided heart failure may lead to pulmonary edema, which may cause gurgling sounds with breathing, shortness of breath, frothy sputum, and orthopnea, the inability to breathe when lying flat due to pulmonary edema. Methods of assessing edema include checking for pitting (Figure 6-3) and measurements of edema. A foot volumeter may be used to compare the volume of 2 extremities and to detect changes in the volume of the same extremity (Figure 6-4). A quick and simple method that is sometimes used in place of volumetry is the figure-8 measurement shown in Figure 6-5. A tape measure is looped around the foot and ankle starting and finishing at the insertion of the tibialis anterior passing landmarks

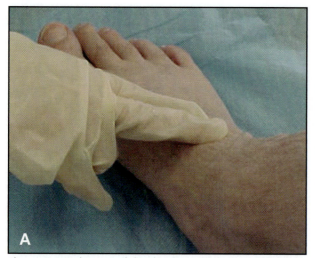
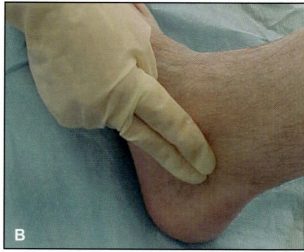

Figure 6-6. Palpation of distal pulses. (A) Location of the dorsalis pedis. (B) Location of the posterior tibial artery. Both of these should be tested bilaterally when performing ankle brachial index testing.

including the head of the navicular, the styloid process of the fifth metatarsal, medial, and lateral malleoli. Reliability of the measurement is improved by using a tape measure with a spring to ensure the same tension is placed on the tape with each measurement.

Additional tests of cardiac and pulmonary function may be performed in vascular and pulmonary function labs. Cardiac catheterization can provide information about the heart's pumping ability and valvular function as well as the integrity of the coronary vessels. Arterial disease, especially in patients with diabetes mellitus, is likely to affect coronary vessels as well as cerebral, and lower extremity arteries. Therefore, anyone with a history of disease in one of these areas is likely to have disease in others. For example, if a patient has a history of coronary bypass graft surgery, the patient is likely to be susceptible to arterial disease of the lower extremities, leading to arterial ulcers or slow healing. Pulmonary function testing may be used to determine the type and severity of pulmonary dysfunction as well as assessing the effectiveness of treatment. Diminished cardiac and pulmonary function will lead to slower healing. Additionally, impairment of these functions may cause patients to lose mobility and increase the risk of ulcerations caused by decreased mobility.

Vascular Testing

Because of the potentially serious nature of arterial insufficiency, and the treatments used for venous and lymphatic diseases, the importance of arterial testing cannot be overemphasized. Compression and elevation used to treat venous and lymphatic disease are likely to exacerbate the already compromised circulation. Several tests for arterial sufficiency are available and range from highly

sophisticated and expensive testing to cheap and easy, but questionably valid tests.

Simple tests that do not require any equipment may be used. The simplest is palpation of the dorsalis pedis and posterior tibial pulses (Figure 6-6) correlated with signs of arterial insufficiency already discussed, such as temperature and color of the limb, and the appearance of hair and nails on the extremity. This examination lacks both sensitivity and specificity. Moderate arterial disease can be overlooked easily (lack of sensitivity) and many individuals with perfectly fine lower extremity blood flow may have pulses that are difficult to palpate (low specificity). To improve sensitivity, a Doppler stethoscope may also be used to simply detect the presence of the lower extremity pulses. This is the same principle as palpating for a pulse, but is more likely to find the pulse than simple palpation.

A better test that quantifies arterial blood flow and is cost effective is measurement of the ankle brachial index (ABI), also called ankle pressure index (API) in some geographical regions. This test is based on the idea that obstruction of peripheral arteries diminishes the pressure of arterial blood as it passes distally into an extremity. Normal, healthy arteries produce little drop in arterial pressure, therefore, arterial pressure measured in the brachial artery is very close to aortic pressure. Even in the arteries of the legs, very little pressure is lost. This discussion assumes that pressure is measured at the same height. For example, when blood pressure is measured with a sphygmomanometer, the cuff is placed at the same level as the heart. By the same token, blood pressure measured in the leg needs to be done with the leg slightly elevated to raise it to the same level as the heart with the patient lying in supine. Unlike the brachial artery, which is sufficiently superficial to allow one to hear changes in flow pattern

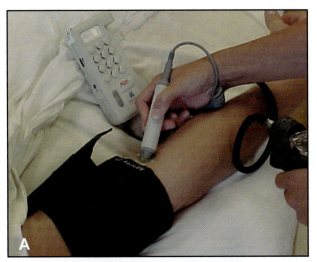 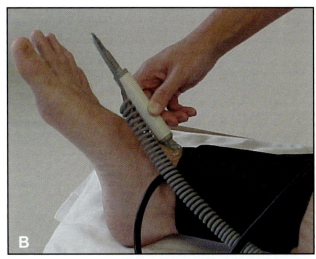

Figure 6-7. Performance of ankle brachial index testing. (A) Doppler probe is being held at a 45-degree angle over the brachial artery to determine systolic blood pressure of the arm. This should be done bilaterally. Some models of Doppler devices do not require the probe to be held at a specific angle. (B) Same technique being demonstrated over the dorsalis pedis artery of the right foot. Note the foot is elevated so the brachial and dorsalis pedis arteries are at the same height. When measuring systolic pressure of the posterior tibial arteries, the leg should be elevated to this same height. Measurements of systolic pressure should be made bilaterally on the brachial, dorsalis pedis, and posterior tibial arteries (total of 6 measurements).

with a stethoscope as vessels become occluded and free to flow, the vessels of the lower extremity are generally not amenable to this technique. In the arm, we can closely approximate true systolic pressure as the pressure in the cuff at the point that blood can be heard to spurt under the cuff only at the peak systolic pressure. The lack of noise heard through the stethoscope then approximates diastolic pressure when blood is free to flow under the cuff continually through the cardiac cycle.

For the lower extremities, an instrument called a Doppler stethoscope is used, typically over either the dorsalis pedis or posterior tibial arteries. The Doppler effect is typically described as the change in pitch made as a train approaches and then moves away. As the train approaches, sound waves are compressed, increasing frequency and as the train moves away, the sound waves are rarefied, decreasing frequency. A Doppler stethoscope emits ultrasound at 5 to 8 MHz. When the ultrasound strikes a moving medium, such as flowing blood, the shift in frequency is converted to a sound transmitted either to a speaker or earpieces. Older models used earpieces. Most modern devices have built-in speakers to allow the Doppler shift to be heard.

The technique involves finding either the dorsalis pedis (see Figure 6-6) or posterior tibial artery by palpation, then holding the probe at a 45-degree angle along the length of the artery as confirmed by a swishing sound. A blood pressure cuff is placed on the calf and inflated until the swishing sound is lost. The lack of sound indicates that arterial flow is occluded. The cuff is slowly deflated as is done in sphygmomanometry. Resumption of the swishing sound

indicates that pressure in the artery is just greater than pressure in the cuff. Note that the lack of a unique sound to indicate diastolic pressure. The Doppler stethoscope does not work on the principle of the Korotkoff sounds. It indicates either the presence or absence of blood flow; therefore, only systolic pressure can be determined.

The same technique with the Doppler device is done on both brachial arteries. If done at the same height relative to the heart, the values should be very close. Generally, the value in the leg is 5% to 10% greater due to the reflection of pressure waves along the longer vessels of the leg. Therefore, we expect the ABI to be 1.05 to 1.10 in a healthy person. When ABI falls below 0.8 (ankle systolic pressure is 80% of brachial systolic pressure) some experts recommend that compression therapy not be used. Other individuals are more liberal, using a limit of 0.7. A value of 0.75 to 0.9 is indicative of moderate arterial disease, a patient with an ABI of 0.5 to 0.75 is considered to have severe arterial disease and a value 0.5 or lower is considered dangerous for the health of the limb and requires referral to a vascular surgeon. The performance of ABI testing is shown in Figure 6-7. A value greater than 1.1 may indicate calcification of arterial vessels. Calcification prevents the collapse of arterial vessels when cuff pressure exceeds arterial pressure. Therefore, a value greater than 1.1 must be viewed with suspicion and other forms of arterial testing will be needed to conclusively diagnose arterial disease. Measurement of ABI should be performed using 6 locations—bilateral brachial arteries, dorsalis pedis, and posterior tibial arteries.

Other Arterial Tests

Pneumoplethysmography is a more sophisticated means of determining the same phenomenon as ABI. The principle underlying this technique is that diastolic pressure becomes insufficient to drive flow through diseased arteries. The technique measures relative blood flow during systole and diastole. As the ratio of systolic blood flow to diastolic blood flow increases, the risk to the limb increases. In severe disease, the ratio may become infinite as blood flow ceases during diastole with severe occlusion. The device consists of an air chamber surrounding the lower extremity and a device to measure changes in volume through the cardiac cycle. The device must be put through a calibration sequence and is expensive to obtain. This test is more likely to be performed by a vascular lab than in other clinical situations.

Transcutaneous oxygen ($tcPO_2$) measurements can be made in specialized vascular labs. The device, as the name implies, measures tissue oxygen through the skin. This measurement is performed with a special airtight sensor that heats the skin to 41°C to allow equilibration between capillary PO_2 and the sensor, taking approximately 20 minutes to perform. In particular, the device is used to determine appropriate amputation level, but can also be used to predict the likelihood of wounds healing. A value of less than 20 mmHg carries a poor prognosis for healing, whereas a value greater than 30 predicts healing. This information can also aid the decision to debride wounds. Using the same criteria, one may decide to debride a wound with a $tcPO_2$ reading of greater than 30 mmHg, but not if the surrounding skin produces a value of 20 mmHg. In any case, when in doubt, a vascular surgeon must be consulted.

An old standby test is the rubor of dependency test. It is based on gravitational challenge to the arterial circulation and observation. With the patient/client placed in supine (on the back), the lower extremity is raised 60 degrees for 1 minute. Signs of arterial insufficiency may be present in this first phase as complaints of pain with elevation and an ashen appearance to the extremity. In a healthy person, a decrease in the pinkness occurs and returns as the leg is lowered to the table. In a person with arterial disease, the color of the leg goes beyond the normal pink and becomes quite red due to the phenomenon termed *reactive hyperemia*. Reactive hyperemia refers to the dilation of vessels in response to occlusion of vessels. When the occlusion is released, blood flow is increased markedly above normal, producing the rubor of dependency. Rubor of dependency may be observed in some patients who are simply sitting. An example of rubor of dependency is shown in Figure 6-8.

Venous Tests

Several tests for venous insufficiency are also available. Often venous disease is obvious grossly by the presence

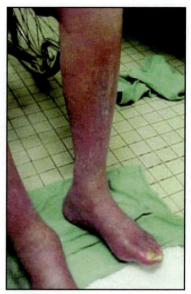

Figure 6-8. Rubor of dependency in an individual with peripheral arterial disease. Note the ruddy color of the lower half of both legs; shiny, hairless skin; and the thickened, yellow toenails. A similar coloration of the legs will occur with a positive rubor of dependency test.

of dilated superficial veins, especially if the dilated vessels are tortuous (following a twisting path, rather than a relatively straight line). Dilation of venous vessels occurs in response to increased pressure in them. Pressure within venous vessels is normally only a few mm Hg of pressure. Pressure is kept low even in the lower extremities by the presence of a venous pump. A pump in general consists of an energy source, valves to ensure one-way flow, and clear conduits to carry the flow to and from the pump. With this in mind, the causes of venous insufficiency become clear: occlusion of the vessels, failure of the valves, or loss of the source of energy for the pumping mechanism. Occlusion of venous vessels may occur from within, usually a blood clot or thrombus, or from outside the vessels by obesity, pregnancy, neoplasms, or improperly applied compression devices. Failure of venous valves is very common. The venous valves act to break the column of fluid into small columns. When one valve fails, the valve below is subjected to greater pressure than normal and is at risk for failure, thereby putting each valve below at great risk to fail. Neuromuscular diseases or injuries such as spinal cord injury, peripheral nerve injury, or immobilization of an extremity (for example following a fracture), decrease the ability of the calf muscle to exert pressure on the outside of leg veins to assist pumping of blood from the leg veins to maintain a low venous pressure. Leg vein pressure increases significantly as one changes from a sitting to standing posture, but decreases during walking to a pressure actually less than that measured in sitting.

Venous tests include the percussion test, venous filling time test, and venous plethysmography. The percussion test examines the patency of valves. A normal valve does not allow backflow from above the knee to below the knee. During this test, the examiner palpates a superficial vein below the knee and strikes the same vein above the knee. With normal valves, the pressure wave generated is baffled at the valve below. With insufficient valves, the pressure wave is transmitted distally and can be palpated below the knee. The venous filling time test superficially resembles the rubor of dependency test. The patient is placed in supine and the lower extremity is elevated to 60 degrees for 1 minute. The leg is massaged to reduce leg volume as much as possible. The patient is then asked to stand and the volume of the leg is observed. With normal circulation, the leg volume increases gradually through arterial inflow. Lack of filling within 10 to 15 seconds indicates arterial insufficiency. With venous insufficiency, leg volume increases rapidly through both arterial inflow and venous backflow. In addition, peripheral veins should become obvious. The Trendelenberg test is performed in a similar manner except for a tourniquet placed around the thigh, occluding venous but not arterial flow. The patient stands, and the examiner observes for filling of superficial veins. Immediate filling indicates incompetent valves of communicating veins. The tourniquet is then removed. Rapid filling of superficial veins demonstrates incompetence of the saphenous vein.

Venous plethysmography is a technological improvement of the venous filling time test. Similar to the arterial test, a plastic air chamber is placed over the lower extremity. A simple pressure-detecting device is attached to the chamber. The patient/client is asked to stand with the lower extremity in the chamber to provide a baseline volume. The decrease in volume that occurs in the supine position with the leg elevated is recorded. When a new baseline is reached, the patient/client is asked to stand rapidly. A progressive increase in lower extremity volume is considered normal. A rapid increase beyond the original standing baseline indicates venous insufficiency.

Imaging of Blood Vessels

Arterial blood vessels may be imaged through a number of modalities. Angiography is the use of radiopaque material injected into vessels so their presence can be viewed with routine x-ray technology. Although this is typically done for arterial vessels, it can also be used to image veins. Blood vessels may also be imaged with magnetic resonance imaging. Another technique is duplex ultrasound, which may be used for arterial or venous vessels. Any of these techniques can demonstrate occlusions of the vessels. Duplex ultrasound can also show velocity as different colors in the image. Ultrasound is a common test used when clots occluding the lower extremity wound are suspected.

Aerobic Capacity and Endurance

Every patient should be evaluated at least in terms of vital signs: heart rate, blood pressure, respiratory rate, and ideally oxyhemoglobin saturation using a pulse oximeter. Although expensive (~$600 to $1,000), when used on every patient/client entering the clinical facility, this measurement adds negligibly to the cost. Simple tests of aerobic function such as upper extremity ergometry or the Balke test may be used. The Balke test consists of setting a treadmill at 3.3 mph and increasing the grade of the treadmill 1% every minute. A treadmill test, whether the Balke, Bruce, or other protocol, is particularly useful for the patient with suspected arterial insufficiency. Intermittent claudication manifested as calf pain at a given intensity of exercise can be monitored through the course of treatment.

Musculoskeletal

The review of systems related to the musculoskeletal systems minimally consists of strength and range of motion testing. Additional testing may be done based on the results of this testing. Impairments in the musculoskeletal system may lead to abnormal forces being placed on the skin or the inability to shift pressure away from certain parts of the body.

Strength and Range of Motion

These tests are frequently ignored when focus is totally on the wound, rather than on the patient. We need to remember that we are working with a person who needs to function in a particular environment. For most patients, a rudimentary test can be conducted in less than 1 minute. Specific muscle tests can be performed as the examination or history dictates.

A brief sequence can consist simply of squeezing the examiner's hand, asking the patient/client to raise the arms over the head then back to shoulder level. The examiner then asks the patient/client to resist movement as the examiner attempts to move the shoulders, elbows, and wrists through the different possible planes of movement. The examiner then asks the patient to move the lower extremities through the normal range of motion and then to attempt to resist the examiner's attempts to move the hips, knees, and ankles through their available planes of movement (Figure 6-9).

Those with suspected neuropathy should be more carefully examined for strength, range of motion, and for deformities of the feet. Individuals with spinal cord injuries and other neuromuscular diseases or injuries should have a more thorough examination for range of motion

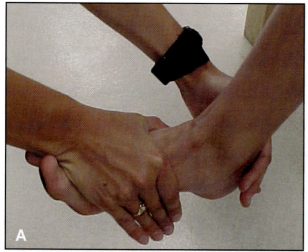
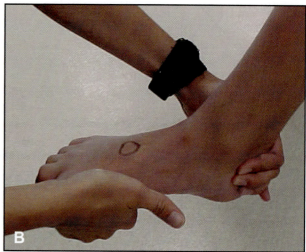

Figure 6-9. (A) Strength and range of motion testing of the foot and ankle. Long muscles innervated at the level of the leg are being tested. These muscles are less susceptible to diabetic neuropathy, but may become involved later in the course of the disease. (B) Intrinsic muscles of the foot are being tested. With their longer and smaller diameter neurons, these muscles are more susceptible to early diabetic neuropathy.

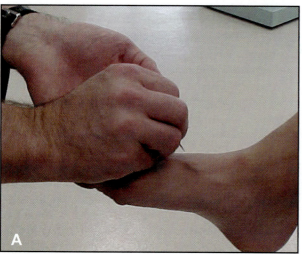
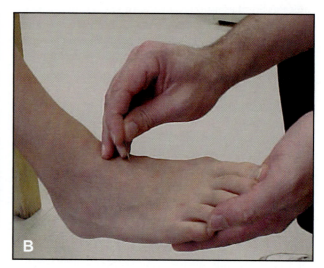

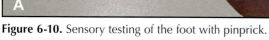

Figure 6-10. Sensory testing of the foot with pinprick.

and strength. Several textbooks are available for guiding a full strength and range of motion examination.

Neuromuscular

Components of the neuromuscular portion of the review of systems generally include sensory and reflex, in addition to the strength testing discussed above. A patient's balance, mobility, gait, and coordination should be tested as well. A patient may appear to be within normal limits for simple sensory, reflex, and strength testing but may not be able to perform higher-level tasks effectively. Balance, mobility, gait, and coordination problems may interfere with the healing of wounds and put other areas of the skin at risk.

Sensory Testing

Rudimentary sensory testing should also be done routinely with every patient. Again, more detailed testing of the distal extremities is required for anyone with suspected peripheral neuropathy or other neuromuscular diseases or injuries. Several textbooks are also available to provide a detailed approach. Often a simple test of light touch with a cotton-tipped applicator or pinprick (Figure 6-10) and the patient's eyes closed is sufficient to rule out sensory deficits.

Monofilament Testing

In addition to other tools used to determine sensory integrity, diabetic foot screening commonly uses Semmes-Weinstein monofilaments to assess risk of plan-

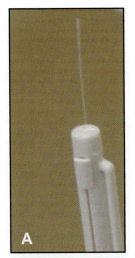

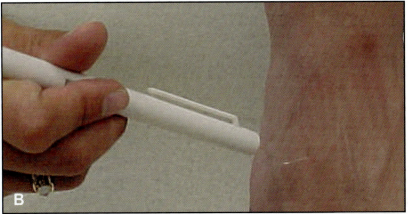

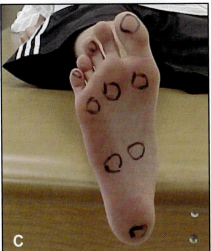

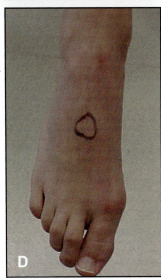

Figure 6-11. Sensory testing with monofilaments. (A) Example of a 10 g monofilament typically used for screening neuropathic feet. (B) Testing procedure showing bending of 10 g monofilament. Contact is made with the foot for ½ second, the monofilament is bent for ½ second, and then allowed to recoil for ½ second. The patient is prevented from seeing the monofilament; random order of test sites and random cadence of testing is used to prevent the patient from guessing. (C) Standardized locations for neuropathic foot testing on the plantar surface of the foot. (D) Standard testing location for neuropathic foot screening on the dorsum of the foot.

tar ulceration in ambulatory, sensory-impaired individuals. These special monofilaments are designed to bend at a calibrated force. Starting with the thinnest monofilament in the set, each monofilament is touched to skin for a total of 1 1/2 seconds: bending for 1/2 second, held bent for 1/2 second, and removed for 1/2 second (Figure 6-11). A person with normal sensation should feel a 10 g monofilament bend. Excessive callus on the foot will decrease the sensitivity of even normal feet. Once a person is able to feel a given monofilament, the clinician stops and records the value. In some cases, a clinician may wish to perform a more thorough test and actually map the entire foot. For a screening procedure, a single 10 g monofilament may be used for a prescribed number of standardized sites (see Figure 6-11). In addition, the clinician should check the foot for deformities and decreased strength, which may alter weight-bearing pattern and gait, and visually inspect the skin on each foot. Further sensory testing should be done to distinguish between small and large sensory neuron loss. Reflexes and vibration are carried by large neu-

rons. Loss of these functions indicates a greater degree of neuropathy because loss of neurons generally occurs first in small neurons, progressing to large neurons. Sensations such as temperature and pinprick are carried by smaller, more susceptible neurons. Loss of large neurons is particularly critical. Motor neurons and position sense are carried by large neurons. Loss of the position senses, proprioception, and kinesthesia are likely to exacerbate the problems caused by sensory neuropathy. A typical gait for a person with diminished proprioception includes short, slapping steps, and abnormal progression from heel strike to toe off.

Reflex Testing

Reflex testing includes the deep tendon reflexes of the biceps, triceps, brachioradialis for the upper extremities and quadriceps (knee jerk) and gastrocnemius/soleus (ankle jerk) with a reflex hammer (Figure 6-12). The Babinski hammer is recommended for this procedure for ease of use. The long handle and weighted head allow the hammer's head to be simply dropped onto the tendon

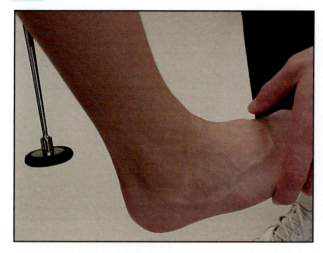 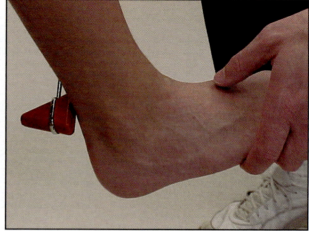

Figure 6-12. Reflex testing using the ankle jerk. (A) Babinski hammer. (B) Taylor hammer.

of interest as opposed to the Buck or Taylor (tomahawk) hammers, which require more skill in striking the tendon. In addition, testing the Babinski or related reflex on the sole may be necessary given a history of upper motor neuron lesion. Testing for resistance to quick movement, and the presence of clonus with quick movement of the wrists and ankles should also be done for individuals with upper motor neuron lesions. Increased tone manifested as either spasticity or rigidity predisposes this individual to pressure ulcers.

MOBILITY, COORDINATION, AND BALANCE

A brief assessment of the patient's bed mobility, transfers, and gait correlated with history including home and work environment is also commonly overlooked. Examine how the individual bears weight on different bony prominences when resting in bed, sitting, moving in bed, coming to sit, coming to stand, and when ambulating. Ask about the use of assistive devices and assess the patient's ability to use the assistive device. Inquire about weight-bearing restrictions, especially those involving the wounded body part. Discussion of footwear is also covered in Chapter 7. Poor balance or coordination may require compensations that have either created or exacerbated the wound. In some cases, simply providing a walker may alleviate the problem. Other cases may require more involved interventions such as the use of total contact casts (also discussed in Chapter 7). A patient with deficits in mobility should be referred to physical

therapy to improve mobility to the level consistent with the patient's desired lifestyle.

SUMMARY

Basic tests performed during the physical examination are described in this chapter. The selection of tests is driven by the history and review of systems. Four systems to be tested are the integumentary, cardiovascular and pulmonary, musculoskeletal, and neuromuscular. A general inspection of the skin is followed by more specific tests of the vascular system, sensation, strength, reflexes, and cardiovascular system. Tests are used to develop a diagnosis, and by using the information from the history, a meaningful prognosis is developed. An excessive focus on the wound instead of the patient leads to missing out on important information gathered from examining the rest of the skin and the other three systems.

QUESTIONS

1. Define skin turgor. What happens to skin turgor with age? Why does this happen?

2. What are the benefits of measuring skin temperature?

3. What does an elevated or depressed skin temperature indicate?

4. What other tests would confirm suspicions raised by a decreased skin temperature?

5. Name several tests available to test the neuromuscular aspects of the lower extremity.

BIBLIOGRAPHY

Carpenter JP. Noninvasive assessment of peripheral vascular occlusive disease. *Adv Skin Wound Care.* 2000;13:84-85.

Sieggreen MY, Maklebust J. Managing leg ulcers. *Nursing.* 1996;26(12):41-46.

Sloan H, Wills EM. Ankle-brachial index: calculating your patient's vascular risk. *Nursing.* 1999;29(10):58-59.

The Wound

Once an appropriate history and physical examination have been performed, the clinician next focuses on the wound itself. Although the cause of a wound is often readily identified, knowing the etiology of common types of wounds can be beneficial in several ways. The causes and characteristics of wounds are discussed to give perspective on how these tend to be managed and to understand how problems may develop requiring skilled services. In some cases of chronic wounds, the cause of the wound may be difficult to identify from the history. Chapter 7 addresses the etiology of chronic wounds caused by neuropathy, pressure, and vascular disease. In addition, wounds caused by trauma and infection, which may be acute or chronic, are also discussed. Burn rehabilitation and unusual wounds are discussed separately in Chapters 15 and 16. A care-

ful examination of the wound and understanding how different causes manifest themselves physically are often required to allow the clinician to identify the cause. The diagnostic process is critical because different etiologies may require very different interventions. Ideally, no two wounds should receive identical interventions, nor should any cookbook approach ever be taken. The characteristics of the wound and the lifestyle of the patient/client including home, work, family, and financial resources should dictate a unique plan of care for each patient/client. Chapter 8 addresses how to assess wounds based on the characteristics observed in the wound, regardless of etiology. Development of the plan of care and choosing interventions are described in more detail in later chapters.

Etiologies of Common Wounds

OBJECTIVES

- Differentiate among common types of wounds and correlate wound type with possible etiologies.
- Identify risk factors for development of pressure ulcers.
- Describe the components of tissue loads that place a person at risk for ulcer development: pressure, shear, friction, heat, and moisture.
- Describe the physiologic effects of tissue loading.
- List at-risk sites for development of pressure ulcers.
- List and discuss the relative efficacy of pressure redistribution devices.
- Discuss methods for offloading body segments.
- Demonstrate use of available tools for quantifying risk.
- Assess risk factors for neuropathic ulcers.
- Discuss control of diabetes mellitus.
- Discuss American Diabetes Association recommendations.
- List causes of Charcot foot and describe interventions to minimize its effects.
- Discuss how other complications of diabetes affect mobility.
- Discuss appropriate footwear for individuals with neuropathy.
- Discuss strategies for prevention of neuropathic ulcers.
- Identify risk factors for wounds caused by vascular diseases.
- Perform differential diagnosis of wounds caused by vascular diseases.
- List elements of a plan of care including direct interventions and patient education for a patient with wounds secondary to vascular diseases.
- List causes of traumatic wounds.
- Define the following terms and describe the mechanisms by which these wounds occur: lacerations, incisions, abrasions (road rash), and degloving (avulsion).

CONTINUED

Irion G.
Comprehensive Wound Management, 2nd ed. (pp 73-148)
© 2010 SLACK Incorporated

OBJECTIVES *CONTINUED*

- Discuss the complications of puncture wounds and bites.
- Discuss the complications involved in fractures; discuss pin care with external fixation.
- Describe the major types of gunshot wounds and contrast the injuries caused by bullets and shot.
- Describe the wounds caused by surgery, including amputations, and possible complications such as infection and dehiscence.
- Describe common types of skin and soft tissue infection, their causes, and treatment.
- List common pathologic skin conditions that produce open wounds and describe their etiologies.
- Describe injuries to the skin caused by thermal, chemical, and radiological burns and complications of burn injuries.

In many settings, the most common causes of chronic wounds are tissue loads over bony prominences, and lower extremity wounds secondary to neuropathy and venous hypertension. Occasionally, wounds due to ischemia may be seen. The ability to perform a good differential diagnosis between arterial, venous, and lymphatic disease becomes critical because the major interventions for correcting venous hypertension and lymphedema may be contraindicated in the presence of ischemia. Moreover, untreated lower extremity ischemia may become an emergent condition requiring surgery to prevent limb loss. Other settings may see a greater proportion of acute wounds, infections, and burn injuries. The etiologies of the most common wounds are described in this chapter. Wounds with unusual causes will be discussed separately in Chapter 16.

PRESSURE ULCERS

Pressure ulcers refer to wounds produced by injury of tissue between support surfaces and bony prominences. Pressure ulcers in immobile people with extreme obesity may occur in a somewhat different manner and will be discussed separately in Chapter 16. Pressure ulcers are among the most costly preventable injuries and, as such, various agencies including the National Pressure Ulcer Advisory Panel (NPUAP) and the Agency for Health Care Policy and Research (AHCPR) have published materials to develop a common language and guidelines for prevention and treatment of pressure ulcers. After these materials were published, the scope and mission of the AHCPR changed. The AHCPR became the Agency for Healthcare Research and Quality (AHRQ), but the original guidelines remain a valuable resource. Pressure ulcers have a high prevalence and incidence in acute and long-term care. Certain conditions are associated with a very high prevalence and incidence: quadriplegia (60% prevalence), femoral fractures (66% incidence), critical care (33% incidence, 41% preva-

lence) and a total cost of $1.335 billion. For the year 1992, a study performed for the AHCPR estimated an average of $21,000 per ulcer in hospital charges and $2,900 in physician charges; and additional charges by hospitals included $10,986 and $1,200 in physician charges for hip fractures due to pressure ulcers.

More recent data are available from the Healthcare Cost and Utilization Project at http://hcupnet.ahrq.gov/ for 2005. The Web site provides healthcare statistics gathered from states as part of the AHRQ. Queries can be performed based on diagnostic codes and other data of interest. Its data include hospitals and emergency departments and it allows trends to be analyzed. Data can be downloaded and analyzed in spreadsheets. Available data show 41,750 hospital admissions for ulcers in 2005 (not specified as pressure ulcers), with a mean length of stay of 9.4 days and median length of stay of 6 days. Mean cost was $26,104 and median cost was $14,720. For those admitted, 46% were from the emergency department, 10% from another hospital, and 3% from long-term care. Discharges included 29% routine, 4% to another hospital, 39% to a nursing home, rehab, or other facility, and 3% deaths. Home health was arranged for 23% of those admitted; 2% left against medical advice. These data suggest that the expense of ulcers extends beyond the hospital with admission to nursing homes and rehab facilities. For those returning home, a large proportion will require home health.

Types of Tissue Loads

Although this type of injury is termed a *pressure ulcer*, factors other than pressure are also responsible for the necrosis of tissue between a support surface and a bony prominence. *Tissue load* is more inclusive than pressure, although the term *pressure ulcer* and its predecessor *decubitus* are unlikely to be replaced by the term *tissue load ulcer*. Tissue loading is caused by pressure, friction, shear, and exacerbated by moisture and temperature (see Figure 7-1).

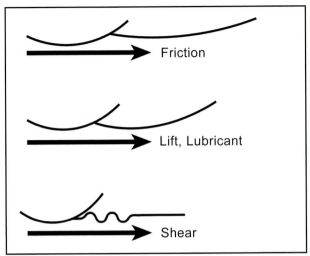

Figure 7-1A. Tissue loads other than pressure placing skin at risk.

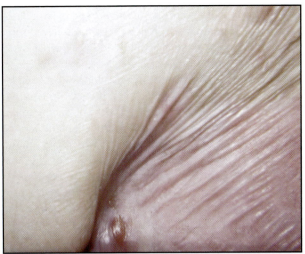

Figure 7-1B. Effect of shearing on the skin. Note the bunching effect of shearing forces on the skin. In this example, skin has been injured by the distortion of the skin superior to the gluteal cleft on the right side. Erythema of the injured skin is present along with small ulcers.

In many cases, shear is more of a problem than pressure, particularly in the individual left in a head up, reclining position greater than 30 degrees. Friction and shear are related but separate phenomena. Friction relates to the movement across a surface with a high coefficient of friction (generally a rough surface). The coefficient of friction and force used to move a person determine the amount of energy transferred into the skin as it is dragged across a support surface. Friction occurs as a patient is moved across the surface of a sheet. Repeated friction may then denude skin, producing a superficial skin injury.

Shear refers to a tangential force applied to a surface as is moved across a surface. Shear presents the same detrimental effects as friction on the skin with the additional component of blood vessel distortion causing ischemia in the sheared skin. Therefore, shear is a greater risk factor for tissue injury than friction alone and involves deeper tissues than friction. Shear commonly occurs in an individual sitting or lying in a position with the head elevated more than 30 degrees for a prolonged time. Prevention of pressure ulcers is accomplished by managing tissue loads by decreasing pressure, friction, and shear, by optimizing moisture and temperature, using proper positioning techniques, and using appropriate support surfaces. Different considerations are made for the patient in bed and the person in a chair.

Pathophysiology of Pressure Ulcers

Although pressure ulcers are described as injury resulting from forces between a support surface and skin over bony prominences, different mechanisms or combinations of mechanisms are possible. Classically, erythema of skin with insufficiently relieved pressure has been considered a heralding sign of tissue injury that could be prevented

as soon as nonblanchable erythema was detected through normally scheduled skin inspections. Mechanisms of injury include a mild surface injury resulting in erythema, deep tissue injury below the skin and likely beginning nearer the bone than the skin, friction injury by moving a patient across a surface resulting in superficial depth injury similar to abrasion discussed below as road rash, and superficial injury to the skin caused by chemical insult or inappropriate moisture. Using high resolution ultrasonography, one study showed that 80% of patients with an abnormal appearance of subcutaneous tissue suggestive of injury did not have erythema documented. This study strongly suggests that injury occurs first in the deep subdermal tissue, progressing to superficial dermal tissue before injury can be appreciated at the epidermal layer. Furthermore, dermal edema in this study was only observable when subdermal edema was already present. Although injury to skin due solely to chemical injury (urine or feces) gives a similar appearance to partial-thickness injury caused by friction, NPUAP now states specifically that this injury should not be considered a pressure ulcer. This injury may contribute to pressure ulcer development, but by definition, cannot be its sole cause.

Deep tissue injury appears to be produced by interrelated factors initiated by unrelieved pressure. Unrelieved pressure occluding venous vessels may lead to edema and occlusion of capillaries and lymphatics. Before the point of irreversible injury, those with normal sensation and mobility react by moving and relieving the pressure on the area due to stimulation of nociceptors caused by tissue insult. Without repositioning, thrombosis may begin in occluded capillaries and venous vessels. If pressure is relieved when cell injury is still reversible, reactive hyperemia aids in restoration of homeostasis. If pressure is not relieved soon enough, cell injury becomes irreversible as a vicious cycle of edema and occlusion occurs. Occlusion of both venules and lymphatics by increased interstitial pressure caused by unrelieved pressure allows interstitial pressure to continually increase and produce the equivalent of compartment syndrome in the affected area. Unlike the benefit derived from hyperemia in a reversible injury, hyperemia following irreversible injury can increase the size of the area of necrosis due to a phenomenon known as reperfusion injury. The ischemic injury stimulates the production of free radicals. With hyperemia and a tremendous increase in availability of oxygen, free radical production in an area of ischemic injury destroys cells that might otherwise have experienced only reversible injury.

Breakdown of tissue has been described as occurring in 4 stages. (Edberg et al). Hyperemia appears in 30 minutes or less. However, hyperemia will not be seen if the injury is too deep for visualization. This hyperemia lasts approximately 1 hour, providing the basis of the stage I pressure ulcer described below. Ischemic injury is proposed to occur within 2 to 6 hours of unrelieved pressure, depending on the site and amount of pressure. Erythema under this condition does not spontaneously regress for up to 36 hours. After 6 hours of unrelieved pressure, necrosis ensues with a blue to gray color (where visible) replacing the red color of hyperemia, and may be accompanied by induration due to edema. The fourth level of tissue injury described is ulceration, which may occur up to 2 weeks following the injury. The levels of tissue injury described are somewhat oversimplified, but give a rough estimate of the time frame of events. The times described will vary among individuals, areas of the body, and the time, distribution, and intensity of the unrelieved pressure. An important concern related to this description of injury is the necessity of instituting means of relieving pressure early when reversible injury and erythema that eventually resolves are present. A second concern is that the color changes described may occur too deeply to be appreciated before ulceration of skin and large areas of necrosis occur apparently without warning.

Definitions

The NPUAP defines a pressure ulcer "as any lesion caused by unrelieved pressure resulting in damage of underlying tissue. These usually occur over bony prominences and are staged to classify the degree of tissue damage observed."[1] The NPUAP has recently revised their definitions for pressure ulcer stages. The staging system refers to the depth of injury observed and does not necessarily correspond to an observable progression of tissue injury. In extreme cases, a deep wound may not be observable at all

until an ulcer progresses through subcutaneous tissue or the skin itself.[1]

Although the definitions are straightforward, some limitations need to be kept in mind. First, detection of stage I ulcers can be very difficult in darkly pigmented skin. Very careful observation needs to be performed, including detecting either an increase in temperature or a violescence (eggplant-like purple) compared with surrounding skin. Another issue with the terminology is that it suggests a sequence of I progressing to II, progressing to III, and then IV. However, this sequencing is unlikely to actually happen. Substantial damage to subcutaneous tissue has been observed with high resolution ultrasound in the absence of erythema. When eschar is present, accurate staging is not possible. Many clinicians may be tempted to guess at the extent of an ulcer. However, good practice dictates that staging not be done until eschar has been removed. Moreover, ulcers under casts, orthotic devices, and support stockings are difficult to assess and require extra work to remove the device to examine the skin on a regular basis.

A related problem is the insistence of certain agencies to reverse stage wounds as a means of documenting healing of a wound. The NPUAP has issued a position statement advising against this practice. A wound with subcutaneous involvement fills with granulation tissue and contracts; it does not fill with the same tissue that was originally in the wound. Therefore, once a wound is classified as a stage IV ulcer, it cannot be logically classified as a stage III, II, or I, because the tissue markers on which the definitions are based do not exist. Instead an appropriate description includes the original stage and the measurable depth of the current state of the wound.

Official definitions recently released by the NPUAP and their accompanying descriptions are described below. These definitions now address many of the deficiencies that existed in the previous definitions. The definitions are similar to the terminology used for wounds in general as partial-thickness, full-thickness, and partial-thickness with subcutaneous involvement. Definitions below also address the injury that may occur on the surface of intact skin and the situation in which injury to subcutaneous tissue may occur without a wound at the skin's surface.

Stage I

A stage I ulcer was initially defined as an area of a nonblanchable erythema of intact skin. This definition, however, proved inadequate for heavily pigmented skin. The definition has now been expanded to include increased warmth or altered coloration of skin (redness of Caucasian skin or purplish tint of more heavily pigmented skin). Stage I is now defined by the NPUAP as "intact skin with nonblanchable redness of a localized area usually over a bony prominence. Darkly pigmented skin may not have visible blanching; its color may differ from the surround-

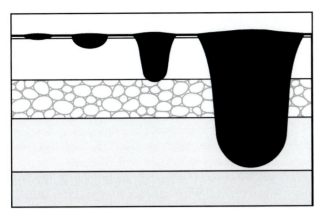

Figure 7-2A. Appearance of different stages of pressure ulcers. Stage I is characterized by nonblanchable erythema. Stage II demonstrates ulceration through the epidermis and partially into the dermis. Stage III extends through the entire dermis and may include injury to subcutaneous tissue down to the level of fascia. Stage IV ulcers include subfascial structures such as muscle, tendon, ligament, and bone.

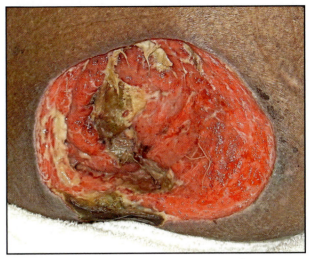

Figure 7-2B. Photo of stage IV pressure ulcer of right greater trochanter.

ing area."[1] Further, the NPUAP gives a description of a stage I ulcer as "the area may be painful, firm, soft, warmer or cooler as compared to adjacent tissue. Stage I may be difficult to detect in individuals with dark skin tones. May indicate 'at-risk' persons (a heralding sign of risk)."[1]

Deep Tissue Injury

The assignment of numbers to classify extent of the wound does not necessarily communicate the degree of ulcer severity. For example, a stage I ulcer may have very little tissue damage or it may have extensive necrosis beneath intact erythematous skin. Purple or maroon areas of seemingly intact skin or blood-filled blister may be present due to damage of tissue beneath the skin, which cannot be directly visualized. Extensive tissue necrosis may develop around a bony prominence and progress toward the skin. Discoloration may be the only indication of this process before erosion of the skin surface appears suddenly. Even when erosion of skin occurs, the true extent of the wound may not be appreciated without careful examination. A patient might present with a seemingly small diameter full-thickness injury, but actually have a more severe condition of no viable tissue down to the bone, undermining several centimeters under the opening and necrosis of the bone below. To address this situation, the NPUAP has defined a new category termed *deep tissue injury* (DTI). This injury is defined as: "The area may be preceded by tissue that is painful, firm, mushy, boggy, warmer or cooler as compared to adjacent tissue"[1] and the description given by the NPUAP is: "Deep tissue injury may be difficult to detect in individuals with dark skin tones. Evolution may be rapid exposing additional layers of tissue even with optimal treatment."[1]

Stage II

A stage II pressure ulcer had been defined as a partial-thickness wound involving epidermis, dermis, or both, but does not extend through the entire depth of the dermis (Figure 7-2A). The NPUAP also makes the distinction between pressure ulcers and other types of injuries of similar depth. This definition is now given as: "Partial-thickness loss of dermis presenting as a shallow open ulcer with a red or pink wound bed, without slough. May also present as an intact or open/ruptured serum-filled blister."[1] The official description is: "Presents as a shiny or dry shallow ulcer without slough or bruising. Bruising indicates suspected DTI. This stage should not be used to describe skin tears, tape burns, perineal dermatitis, maceration, or excoriation."[1]

Stage III

Once a wound extends into subcutaneous tissue, but not through the fascia, it is classified as a stage III ulcer. The NPUAP definition is now: "Full-thickness tissue loss. Subcutaneous fat may be visible but bone, tendon, or muscle are not exposed. Slough may be present but does not obscure the depth of tissue loss. May include undermining and tunneling."[1] The description is: "The depth of a Stage III pressure ulcer varies by anatomical location. The bridge of the nose, ear, occiput and malleolus do not have subcutaneous tissue and Stage III ulcers can be shallow. In contrast, areas of significant adiposity can develop extremely deep Stage III pressure ulcers. Bone/tendon is not visible or directly palpable."[1]

Stage IV

Any wound that extends through the fascia and deeper is classified as stage IV (Figure 7-2B). These full-thickness wounds may include damage to tissues such as muscle, bone, ligaments, or tendons. The NPUAP definition has been simplified to: "Full-thickness tissue loss with exposed bone, tendon, or muscle. Slough or eschar may be present on some parts of the wound bed. Often includes undermining and tunneling."[1] The description provided by the NPUAP is: "The depth of a Stage IV pressure ulcer varies by anatomical location. The bridge of the nose, ear, occiput and malleolus do not have subcutaneous tissue and these ulcers can be shallow. Stage IV ulcers can extend into muscle and/or supporting structures (eg, fascia, tendon or joint capsule) making osteomyelitis possible. Exposed bone/tendon is visible or directly palpable."[1]

Unstageable

Fascia is usually easily identifiable as a clear, smooth shiny layer, making distinction of stage II vs III and III vs IV fairly simple once the base of the wound is visible. For this reason, staging of pressure ulcers should not be done before the base of the wound is visible. For this circumstance, the NPUAP has created a new category called *unstageable*. This category is defined as: "Full-thickness tissue loss in which the base of the ulcer is covered by slough (yellow, tan, gray, green, or brown) and/or eschar (tan, brown, or black) in the wound bed."[1] The official description is: "Until enough slough and/or eschar is removed to expose the base of the wound, the true depth, and therefore stage, cannot be determined. Stable (dry, adherent, intact without erythema or fluctuance) eschar on the heels serves as 'the body's natural (biological) cover' and should not be removed."[1]

Prevention of Pressure Ulcers

Knowledge of risk factors allows the clinician and the caregivers to reduce the risk of developing pressure ulcers. Key among the risk factors is immobility or the lack of volition to move (see Table 7-1). In addition to immobility, risk factors include incontinence, malnutrition, and altered mental status. Mental status includes both level of consciousness and any psychological impairment that would decrease the person's awareness of the need to reposition. In the clinical situation, rather than simply assessing the risk factors informally, several tools have been developed in an attempt to quantify risk. Quantification allows clinicians and caregivers to speak a common language in terms of risk factors and also provides the clinician with an objective means of decision making. The goals of the tools described below are to identify individuals in need of prevention measures and address specific factors that put them at risk. Interventions may then follow directly from addressing the factors. Physical therapy may be prescribed to improve mobility and instruct the patient in the use of assistive and adaptive devices. Specialized support surfaces and orthoses may

be ordered. In addition, issues with incontinence may be addressed. The AHCPR recommends that bed- and chair-bound individuals, and anyone with an impaired ability to reposition, be systematically evaluated for risk factors. Furthermore, the AHCPR recommends that individuals be assessed on admission to acute care and rehabilitation hospitals, nursing homes, home care programs, and other healthcare facilities, and should be reassessed at periodic intervals. As recommended by the AHCPR, all assessments of risk should be documented. This not only provides legal protection for the clinician and the facility, but also allows changes in the patient's status to be evaluated easily. In addition to the ethical issues with prevention of pressure ulcers, a financial incentive has been put in place by the Center for Medicare and Medicaid Services (CMS). CMS will no longer provide additional payment for treatment of pressure ulcers not present on admission to a hospital. The admitting facility will be responsible for all additional treatment costs.

Risk Factors for Pressure Ulcers

One or a large number of factors may be responsible for the development of pressure ulcers in any given individual. Potential risks for development of pressure ulcers are listed in Table 7-1. Typically, a combination of lack of mobility, lack of cognition/motivation to move, and exacerbating factors of nutrition and incontinence are responsible. In particular, individuals with spinal cord injuries, diabetes mellitus, hip replacement surgery, femoral fractures, ICU patients with hypotension, and elderly patients with multiple diseases are at risk. In severe cases, prevention of pressure ulcers may become extremely difficult and perhaps impossible. The lack of volitional repositioning, whatever the cause, is associated with great risk of pressure ulcers. This was demonstrated in a paper published in 1961 (Exton-Smith and Sherwin) showing 90% of those with 20 spontaneous movements or fewer during sleeping hours developed pressure ulcers, whereas no subjects observed with greater than 50 spontaneous movements developed ulcers. A related problem is the failure to protect skin during prolonged surgical procedures.

At-Risk Areas

Statistically, 95% of reported pressure ulcers occur in 4 areas: sacral, ischial tuberosities, heels, and lateral malleoli. However, different circumstances may place different areas at risk. At-risk areas that need particular attention include heels, greater trochanters, sacrum, lateral malleoli, occiput, and epicondyles of the elbow in the person lying in bed. For anyone with any limitations of mobility, heel protection using pillows, splints, or heel lifts must be used ("floating the heels"). The sacrum is placed at great risk for a person reclining in either a bed or chair. For a person

Table 7-1

Risk Factors for Pressure Ulcers

Physical causes of immobility
Altered neuromuscular integrity
Diminished strength
Altered muscle tone (spasticity, rigidity, dystonia, athetosis, flaccidity, etc)

Altered musculoskeletal integrity
Decreased range of motion
Traumatic injury
Muscle disease
Other

Devices
Splints
Casts
Orthoses
Restraints

Cognitive causes of immobility
Altered state of consciousness, stupor, coma
Prolonged anesthesia
Diminished motivation to self-reposition

Diminished sensation
Spinal cord injury
Spina bifida
Head injuries
Peripheral neuropathy

Excessive moisture
Use of moisture resistant support surface
Urinary incontinence
Fecal incontinence

Emaciation
Malnutrition
Dehydration

Management
Inappropriate turning/repositioning schedule
Inappropriate support surface
Neglect of immobility issues
Failure to offload at-risk areas
Failure to clean following episodes of incontinence
Harsh cleaning procedures
Failure to moisturize/protect dry skin

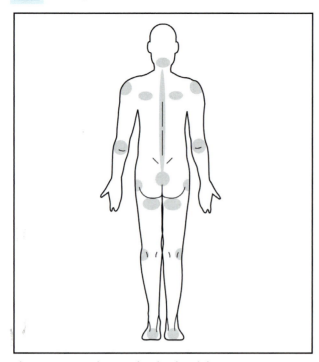

Figure 7-3. At-risk areas for skin breakdown.

sitting erect, the ischial tuberosities are placed at great risk (Figure 7-3). The occiput is easily neglected in a person with a head or neck injury. Too often necrosis of the skin over the occiput is not discovered in time to prevent injury in a person whose head is not repositioned due to fear of further injury to the head or spine by inspecting the occiput.

In addition, pressure ulcers can develop in a number of other locations with bony prominences particularly in those who are emaciated. These areas include the face, vertebral processes, ribs, the spine of the scapulae, the acromion processes, the iliac crests, posterior superior iliac spine, anterior superior iliac spine, the anterior, lateral and medial surfaces of the knee, the tibial crest, malleoli, the first and fifth metatarsals, and toes. The sacrum and heels are the most common locations (36% to 39% and 19% to 30%, respectively). The greatest numbers occur in the age group of 71 to 80, with a slightly lower number in 81 to 90, and somewhat less in the age group 61 to 70. Areas at risk and other characteristics of patients are likely to be different for different populations. One might surmise that a population that is primarily chairbound, rather than bedbound, would show fewer heel ulcers and more ischial ulcers and individuals unable to turn their heads would be at greater risk for occipital ulcers. Therefore, the clinician must be aware of particular areas at risk dependent on the circumstances of individual patients.

Skin Care

Those identified as having risk factors need interventions, including education of patient, family, and caregivers to maintain and improve tissue tolerance to pressure in order to prevent injury. The AHCPR recommends that all individuals at risk should have a systematic skin inspection at least once per day, paying particular attention to the bony prominences, and that the results of skin inspection should be documented. Historically, a process of trying to toughen the skin has been proposed as a means of increasing tissue tolerance to tissue load. To the contrary, this practice has been shown to cause damage rather than prevent injury. AHCPR guidelines state clearly that the practice of massaging over bony prominences should not be used.

Incontinence presents 2 problems. First is the presence of excessive moisture on the skin; second is the physical composition of urine and feces. Both are generally acidic. Urine pH can range from 6 to 3 and feces can contain a large quantity of bile acids. Because incontinence is such an important risk factor, skin cleansing should occur at the time of soiling and at routine intervals. Hot water and harsh detergents should not be used. Instead, many mild cleansing agents are available that can both minimize irritation and maintain appropriate moisture of the skin. Although removal of acidic urine and feces is important, minimizing force and friction applied to the skin is equally important to prevent skin injury. On the other hand, excessive skin dryness can also lead to injury.

Prevention of injury must also include minimizing low humidity (<40%) and exposure to cold. Moreover, dry skin should be treated with appropriate moisturizers. Various moisturizers are available. These moisturizers vary in their concentration of solids. Watery lotions with a low concentration of solids are not as effective as emollients with a higher concentration of oil and solids. An effective moisturizer will retain fluid within the skin, while protecting the skin from excessive external sources of moisture such as incontinence, perspiration, or wound drainage. Skin care products are discussed in Chapter 14. On occasion, sources of moisture may not be controllable. Various absorptive pads or garments may be necessary under these conditions. However, all underpads and briefs are not suitable for this purpose. Only those made of materials that absorb moisture and wick it away from the skin should be used. General purpose underpads may be suitable for those at low risk for a few days, eg, individuals at low risk for pressure ulcers after surgery with copious drainage from surgical wounds. Moisture barriers should be used for the individual who frequently has moisture on the skin. For the person at risk, extra care, including referral to physical therapy, becomes necessary to prevent skin injury due to friction and shear forces.

The patient, family, or caregivers should be instructed in proper positioning and transferring techniques. One may wish to use lubricants such as corn starch, and protective dressing materials, such as transparent film or hydrocolloid dressings, skin sealants, or protective padding. Because lack of mobility is the most important cause of pressure ulcers, referral to physical therapy to improve mobility should be made if potential for improvement exists and improved mobility is in accordance with patient and family goals. In some cases, maintaining current activity level, mobility, and range of motion is an appropriate goal, which may also require a course of physical therapy.

Support Surfaces

A large number of support surfaces have been created in a effort to reduce the risk of pressure ulcers. A number of terms associated with them are discussed below. The terms *pressure relief* and *pressure reducing* have been used in an effort to suggest appropriate use. A pressure-relieving surface provides an interface pressure measurement below 25 mmHg. Pressure-reducing devices provide an interface pressure of 26 to 32 mmHg. Interface pressure refers to the pressure measured between a support surface and bony prominences such as greater trochanters. The purpose of definitions based on 32 mm is to avoid pressures greater than the accepted standard for capillary closing pressure. This number is based on the assumption that an interface pressure greater than 32 mmHg deforms capillaries sufficiently to cut off blood supply to the tissue between the support surface and the bony prominence. This number is based on a 1930 study of healthy, younger men and may vary tremendously between men and women, and with age and cardiovascular status (Landis). More recently, the term *pressure redistributing* has been used to more adequately describe what the device can offer the patient.

A number of terms are used to evaluate support surfaces. Indentation load deflection is tested with specific equipment and testing procedures. A standard test of 25% indentation load deflection examines the load necessary to compress a surface to 75% of its original height. This load is expected to be within the range of 25 and 35 lbs. The 65% deflection is determined similarly. The ratio of the load necessary to compress the surface to 35% of its original height to the load necessary to compress the surface to 75% of its original height is termed the *support factor*. A high ratio indicates a surface that initially gives to provide comfort, but maintains firm support. Density of foam refers to the weight in pounds of a cubic foot of foam. Density should be greater than 1.8 lb/cubic foot to prevent bottoming out and premature fatigue of the foam. In addition, several terms are used to describe the performance of sup-

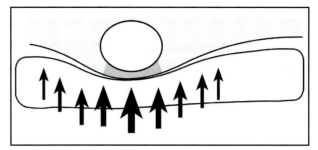

Figure 7-4. Pressure redistribution provided by a seat cushion.

port surfaces. *Immersion* allows bony prominences to sink into the support surface so that pressure can be borne by tissues surrounding the bony prominences (Figure 7-4). A support surface with low immersion places more pressure against a bony prominence as the surrounding tissues make little contact with the support surface. The term *envelopment* refers to the ability of the support surface to deform around any irregularities. Superficially, these 2 terms seem similar. Both are related to the property of deformation. Immersion refers more specifically to the "give" of the surface, whereas envelopment refers to the contouring of the surface to what is placed on it. A surface may have both good immersion and envelopment, or may be good in just one property. Postural stability refers to the ability of the patient to be held in place by the surface. A high immersion may provide good postural stability. However, a support surface with good envelopment provided by allowing material in the support surface to flow beneath the cover may produce poor postural stability. Many support surfaces may be constructed of combinations of materials to optimize these 3 characteristics.

To provide different properties, seat cushions may be created in several shapes other than flat. Precontouring a cushion to the general shape of a person's supporting tissues can provide more postural stability for a given amount of envelopment or immersion. A segmented cushion has the equivalent of cuts in both horizontal directions to allow movement among the different segments and provide better envelopment for a given immersion. A third strategy is cutting out a pressure relief area. The Isch-Dish (Span America, Greenville, SC) has a cutout area in the back of the cushion such that the sacrococcygeal region and ischial tuberosities are floated and more weight is borne on the posterior thighs, which can tolerate the pressure better than the skin over the bony prominences of the sacrococcygeal spine and ischial tuberosities. Covers used on the support surface influence the overall performance of the support surface. A tight cover reduces both immersion and envelopment. A cover designed to lower friction and shear may reduce postural stability.

Moisture and temperature control may also be important considerations. Certain materials have a low heat transfer rate, which allows retention of heat by the skin surface. Other materials may have a high heat transfer rate, which reduces the skin/body temperature. The process of draining heat from the body is known as heat sink. Moisture vapor transmission rate refers to the movement of moisture through the surface. The ability of specific materials to allow accumulation of moisture should also be taken into account when determining the most appropriate support surface for a given individual. Choice of support surface may become an exercise in compromise as a support surface with one good characteristic may become less useful because of a poor characteristic. For example, some materials used in fluid-filled cushions can provide excellent envelopment but provide poor postural stability, and cause retention of heat and moisture.

Pressure Redistributing Devices

Any individual assessed to be at risk for developing pressure ulcers should be placed on a pressure redistributing device (PRD) appropriate for the individual's amount of time sitting on a chair or lying in bed. These devices may be discussed as pressure-reducing devices or pressure relief devices. These devices do not actually reduce or relieve pressure across the support surface as a whole. Instead, pressure in areas that might be injured is reduced by redistributing it to areas that are able to withstand a greater pressure. For example, a cushion might be created that decreases pressure on the ischial tuberosities by redistributing some of the pressure to the posterior and some of the medial and lateral surfaces of the thigh. Pressure relief may be produced by cutting an area from a cushion (or other device) such that the body part does not contact a support surface. This procedure of removing material from a specific location is also known as *cutting a relief* in the device. Unless otherwise specified by the characteristics of a device as a pressure relief or pressure reducing device, PRD will imply pressure redistribution through exploiting some of the properties of available materials.

Anyone determined to be at risk for developing pressure ulcers should avoid uninterrupted sitting in a chair or wheelchair. Appropriate cushions or chair bottom should be supplied commensurate with risk. For the individual with musculoskeletal injuries of the lower extremities but otherwise able to reposition, a simple wheelchair with a sling seat may be sufficient. At the other extreme, a person with quadriplegia who is unable to reposition and lacks sensation should have a specialized pressure-redistributing cushion. In addition to redistributing pressure, seating arrangements must also take into consideration postural alignment, distribution of weight, balance and stability. The AHCPR guidelines recommend that an individual should be repositioned, shifting the points under pressure

at least every hour or be put back to bed if consistent with overall patient management goals. However, allowing a person to remain in bed also carries the risk of pressure ulcers. Some areas at risk in sitting will have pressure reduced, but lying in bed may continue to place pressure or shear on some of the same locations as sitting, particularly the sacrum. Moreover, lying in bed presents a tremendous risk to general health, including risk of thromboembolism, pneumonia, gastrointestinal, and renal disease and bone demineralization. Individuals should be taught to shift weight every 15 minutes if they have the physical and cognitive abilities, and a written plan for the use of positioning devices should be supplied and reviewed with each individual. A patient who has a pressure ulcer on a sitting surface should avoid sitting. If pressure on the ulcer can be relieved, limited sitting may be allowed.

A number of classifications of PRDs have been described. Surfaces can be categorized by their mechanisms as alternating pressure pads, beds, mattress overlays, mattress replacements, and enhanced overlays and mattresses. Alternating pressure pads consist of pumps that periodically direct air to one set of cells while simultaneously allowing air to be released from another set, resulting in alternating pressure points over a given time. To be effective, these devices must be at least 2 inches in depth. Beds, by definition, are integrated systems including a frame and any control devices for the support surface (Figure 7-5). These may be further categorized as air-fluidized beds, low-air-loss beds, and low-air-loss beds with adjuvant features. Air-fluidized beds consist of a tank filled with silicone microspheres that are circulated with an air pump and a sheet to contain the microspheres. The features of this support surface are described in greater detail below as a pressure-relieving device. Low-air-loss beds consist of interconnected air cells that are monitored for pressure and allow air to be lost as pressure increases within a cell. An air pump replaces air as needed when weight is shifted from a cell. These have a minimum depth of 5 inches and may require a stool to allow the patient to move in and out of the bed. Low-air-loss with adjuvant features are basically the same type of support surface, but include features such as vibration or periodic movement of a patient across the surface in an effort to reposition the patient to maintain airway clearance. Mattress overlays fit over a standard mattress. These include air, foam, gel, or water. Air overlays should be at least 3 inches in depth. Foam features include a density of 1.35 to 1.8 lb/cubic foot and a 25% indentation load deflection of 25 to 35 lb. A waterproof and friction-reducing cover should be part of the overlay. A minimum depth of 2 inches is recommended for gel overlays and 3 inches for water. Mattress replacements are designed to fit into standard bed frames, replacing a standard mattress, as opposed to an overlay or dedicated bed. These, like overlays, may be air, foam, gel, or water. Because they

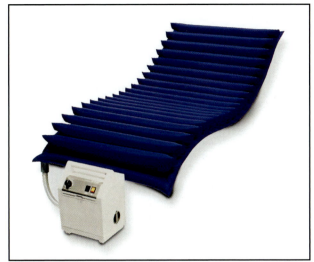

Figure 7-5A. Acucair® Continuous Airflow Therapy Surface powered, dynamic air overlay. © 2010 Hill-Rom Services, Inc. Reprinted with permission. All rights reserved.

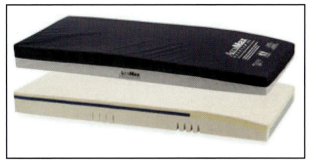

Figure 7-5B. AccuMax Quantum™ VPC, non-powered dynamic air overlay. © 2010 Hill-Rom Services, Inc. Reprinted with permission. All rights reserved.

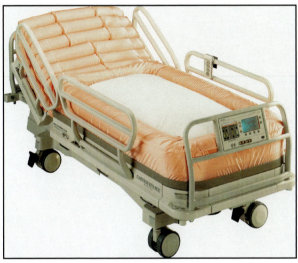

Figure 7-5C. Clinitron II RiteHite Air Fluidized Bed. © 2010 Hill-Rom Services, Inc. Reprinted with permission. All rights reserved.

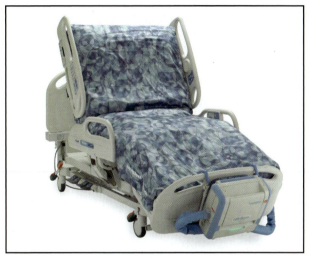

Figure 7-5D. Envision E700 low-air-loss bed. © 2010 Hill-Rom Services, Inc. Reprinted with permission. All rights reserved.

replace a mattress, the recommended thickness is greater than that of an overlay. For air it is 3 inches; foam is 5 inches and includes the features also mentioned for the overlay. Recommended gel depth is 5 inches, which is also recommended for water mattress replacements. At this time, enhanced overlays and mattresses include alternating pressure mattresses, low-air-loss overlays, nonpowered adjustable zone overlays, low-air-loss mattresses, and low-air-loss mattresses with adjuvant features. Classes of support surfaces are listed in Table 7-2.

Support surfaces may also be categorized by the materials used in them (Figure 7-6). Elastic foam is designed to deform to accommodate a load placed on the support surface and may consist of a series of layers, may be contoured, or may be combined with another material such as gel or air-filled chambers. A combination of foam and either gel or air chambers allows postural stability because of properties of immersion and envelopment of the gel or air chambers. Foam alone loses its resilience and bottoms out as the foam degrades with time, a property called *impression set*, and foam has a limited ability to envelope and allow immersion. Foam is absorbent, so it can retain heat and moisture against the skin, and become contaminated. A porous cover and construction with open cell foam allows some moisture to move through the surface away from the skin. Foam cushions and mattress overlays are useful only for comfort in patients at low risk of developing ulcers; they should never be used for a patient with any ulcers present. The stiffness of foam must strike a compromise between envelopment of soft foams and bottoming out. Precontouring a foam support surface provides immersion and envelopment with improved postural stability.

Table 7-2

Classes of Support Surfaces

Alternating pressure pads

Beds

   Air-fluidized beds
   Low-air-loss beds
   Low-air-loss beds with adjuvant features

Mattress overlays

   Air
   Foam
   Gel
   Water

Mattress replacements

   Air
   Foam
   Gel
   Water

Enhanced overlays and mattresses

Alternating pressure mattresses

Low-air-loss overlays

Nonpowered adjustable zone overlay

Low-air-loss mattress

Low-air-loss mattress with adjuvant features

Viscoelastic foam is constructed of open cell foam and is temperature sensitive. The foam nearest the skin becomes softer due to the increased temperature of the foam. The viscoelastic nature helps the foam conform to the body surface and reduce interface pressure. Solid gel support surfaces function in the same way as viscoelastic foam, but gel has the disadvantages of retaining heat if the surface is used for more than 2 hours and retaining moisture on the skin.

Fluid-filled support surfaces have the advantage of being deformable without the large restoring force of surfaces such as foams. This property allows very low interface pressures to occur if the surface is maintained properly. Fluid-filled support surfaces may be filled with air, water, or viscous fluid materials and may have interconnected chambers. Pressure is redistributed by the flow of the fluid between chambers permitting envelopment and immersion. Proper redistribution only occurs with proper filling; over- or underfilling negates their effectiveness. Moreover, their effectiveness for sufficient pressure reduction at the greater trochanters and heels is questionable. They tend to bottom-out easily and may become cold or leak. Like foam, water flotation is useful for lower risk, and only if the ulcer is not on the heel or

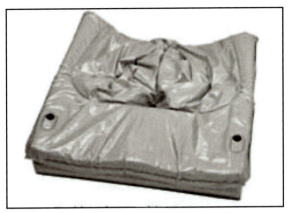

Figure 7-6A. Support surface for a chair: Jay J2 Deep Contour gel cushion (Sunrise Medical, Longmont, CO).

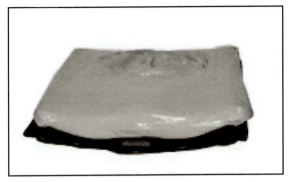

Figure 7-6B. Support surface for a chair: Jay J2 gel cushion (Sunrise Medical, Longmont, CO).

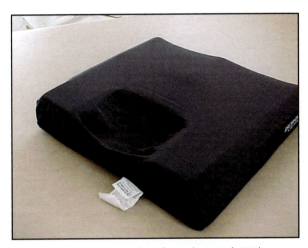

Figure 7-6C. Support surface for a chair: Isch-Dish (Span-America Medical Systems, Inc., Greenville, SC).

greater trochanter. They should be reserved for patients who are independent in mobility and weight shifting. Air-filled cushions must also be inflated optimally to prevent bottoming out with underinflation and excessive pressures with overinflation.

Gel overlays and seat cushions are more useful than foam and water flotation. In particular, these overlays are capable of dispersing both pressure and shearing forces. However, these overlays and cushions are costly, heavy, and allow moisture to accumulate. Gel overlays are useful for minimal to moderate risk patients and patients with manageable ulcers and independent mobility. They are frequently used on operating tables for prevention during long procedures that carry risk of pressure ulcers. Although gel seat cushions (Figures 7-6A and 7-6B) can be very expensive, they can be very effective for the person with a spinal cord injury or other loss of sensation below the waist. Gel-filled surfaces may periodically require redistribution of the gel through the surface to prevent bottoming out.

The most effective type of PRD for seat cushions is static air. These devices allow movement of air among channels to redistribute pressure and, to some extent, shear. Drawbacks include the potential for over- or underfilling, the potential for seams to fatigue and leak, and accidental puncture. Static air cushions and bed overlays can be useful for minimal to moderate risk patients and patients with manageable ulcers and independent mobility. They are easy to clean and transport, as opposed to water flotation and gel PRDs.

Dynamic air systems consist of adjacent compartments that alternately inflate and deflate, reducing the time that any area is exposed to a high pressure. These can be very useful for moderate risk, mobility-dependent patients and those with manageable ulcers. Dynamic air systems may take the form of a specialty bed or an overlay system placed upon a standard bed. Specialty beds consist of

either low air loss or air-fluidized or combination units (see Figure 7-5). These beds or overlays are recommended for stage III or IV ulcers on multiple turning surfaces. Because of the expense of providing support surfaces, most facilities have developed specific criteria for determining medical necessity, such as a specific score on one of the risk assessment tools or the guidelines elaborated in the AHCPR publication. Low-air-loss devices are now available in overlays as well as the traditional bed. In either case, the unit consists of compartments inflated separately with sensors and a pump to maintain proper pressure in each segment as air is lost slowly through the compartments to dissipate pressure. The cover is water vapor permeable; therefore, clinical decisions for managing wound drainage must take into account the greater evaporation of moisture from the wound. Pressure and airflow may be adjustable for individual compartments.

Some higher-end units provide airway clearance by either vibrating or rotating through an arc of movement to reduce time any given lung segment is left in a dependent position. Low-air-loss beds are very expensive; large hospitals may own a small number or they may be rented for hospital or home use. These devices are particularly useful for mobility-dependent, moderate to maximal risk patients and patients with difficult to manage ulcers. The compressibility of the air segments would make mobility and cardiopulmonary resuscitation (CPR) difficult without the safety mechanisms built into the units. Air can be let out rapidly in emergency situations by use of a CPR switch. Deflating the bed can be useful for transfers into and out of the bed, depending on the patient's height. Mobility can be improved by temporarily increasing the pressure within the segments by using a "maximum inflation" or equivalent function. Deflation of the bed is generally more useful for shorter patients and maximum inflation for taller patients.

Air-fluidized beds are the only true PRDs. These beds consist of a tank containing ceramic silicon-coated soda lime beads, a pump to drive air through the beads, and controlling mechanisms including temperature control. A vapor-transmitting sheet is placed over the beads in the tank. Because the beads in the tank are 1.5 times as dense as water, the suspended beads cause the patient to be floated, actually reducing pressure between the body and support surface. The bed is also designed to minimize friction, shear, and maceration. Body fluids drain into the tank, clumping the beads, which then settle out and can be removed. Moreover, drainage causes sodium ion release from the beads, rendering the medium bacteriostatic. In addition, the temperature of the microspheres is controllable. Appropriate dressings need to be placed on the wound to avoid desiccation that can occur due to the loss of fluid from the wound into low-air-loss and air-fluidized beds. Because these beds support the patient with the least pressure, they are indicated for patients with the greatest risk of developing pressure ulcers or for patients whose pressure ulcers may not be able to heal due to problems with positioning. These problems may include the inability to be repositioned or the presence of pressure ulcers on multiple turning surfaces, eg, pressure ulcers on both greater trochanters and the sacrum. As with low-air-loss beds, air flow can be turned off for emergency situations, such as administration of CPR. A combination of air-fluidized and low-air-loss bed is available from Hill-Rom Services Inc. (Batesville, IN). The upper section uses low air loss and the lower section uses an air fluidized tank. The upper section protects the upper body from pressure, while the lower section provides optimum pressure relief where pressure ulcers are most likely to develop. Air-fluidized beds may also be used for patients with extensive burns to promote healing of burned posterior regions and graft donor sites, Stevens-Johnson syndrome, necrotizing fasciitis, and other skin conditions that will be discussed below, and may be used for end-stage cancer.

Selection of Pressure Redistributing/ Reducing/Relief Devices

The selection criteria that the AHCPR suggests for making decisions on support surfaces include providing an increased support area, low moisture retention, reduced heat accumulation, shear reduction and pressure reduction properties. Other properties to be considered are the dynamic vs static properties and cost per day. The panel recommended that clinicians assess all patients with existing pressure ulcers to determine their risk for developing additional pressure ulcers. If the patient remains at risk, a pressure-reducing surface should be used. Static support surfaces are recommended for patients who are able to assume a variety of positions, those who can stay off the ulcer, and those who do not cause the device to bottom out. *Bottoming out* is defined as a distance of less than 1 inch between the surface below the specialized support surface and bony prominences.

Dynamic support surfaces are recommended for patients who are unable to assume a variety of positions, who cannot stay off the ulcer, or who cause a static support surface to bottom out. Having a wound that does not show evidence of healing is another indication for a dynamic support surface. Air-fluidized beds are indicated for patients at high risk for developing pressure ulcers and patients with difficult to manage ulcers. Low-air-loss beds are indicated for moderate risk patients and those with manageable ulcers. Overlay type PRDs are indicated for patients at minimum to moderate risk and ulcers that do not require pressure relief to heal. At the time the AHCPR guidelines were written, panel members could not find any compelling evidence that one support surface for beds performed better under all circumstances.

Kinetic therapy beds were not addressed in the AHCPR guidelines. Older types rock from side-to-side (KCI RotoRest, KCI, San Antonio, TX). Newer specialty beds from KCI, Hill-Rom, and Huntleigh (Eatontown, NJ) accomplish the equivalent of rocking motion by rhythmically inflating and deflating air chambers across the bed from side-to-side. In addition, these newer beds can provide airway clearance by vibrating the support surface. The use of this type of bed, however, does not eliminate the need for a turning schedule.

The AHCPR recommended several considerations specific to sitting. These include an assessment of postural alignment and interventions such as instruction, orthoses, or cushions to provide postural alignment. Positioning should be used to ensure optimal distribution of weight, balance, stability, and continuous pressure relief. Although more favorable from a cardiopulmonary standpoint, sitting even in a well-cushioned chair causes very high interface pressures. Recommendations from the AHCPR guidelines include avoiding sitting if an ulcer develops on a sitting surface such as the sacrum or the ischial tuberosities. Bear in mind, however, that these guidelines were developed prior to the development of newer seating cushions. One type in particular, the Isch-Dish (see Figure 7-6C), takes weight completely off the ischial tuberosities and sacrum and redistributes weight to the posterior thighs. If pressure can be relieved totally, the guidelines recommend that the patient may sit a limited time. As with the bedbound individual, the person should have an individualized written plan. In addition, each person should have an individually prescribed cushion, be repositioned every hour and should shift weight every 15 minutes, if possible.

Medicare Part B Support Surface Guidelines

Medicare Part B Support Surface Guidelines Policies for reimbursement for support surfaces are divided into groups I, II, and III. Criteria for group I devices are either complete immobility or limited mobility or any stage ulcer on the trunk or pelvis and at least one of the following contributing factors: impaired nutritional status, fecal or urinary incontinence, altered sensory perception, and compromised circulatory status. The need for a pressure redistributing device needs to be included in a plan of care established by the patient's physician or home care nurse, documented in the medical records, and including education of the patient or caregiver on prevention or management of pressure ulcers, regular assessment by a healthcare practitioner, appropriate turning and positioning, appropriate wound care, appropriate management of moisture (incontinence), nutritional assessment and intervention consistent with the overall plan of care, and a written order must be provided by the physician. Devices in group I include alternating air pressure mattresses and overlays, gel mattress or overlay, and water pressure mattresses and overlays.

Group II products include low-air-loss beds noted as *powered air flotation bed*. This group includes powered pressure-reducing air mattress, non-powered advanced pressure reducing overlay for mattress, powered air overlay for mattress, and non-powered advanced pressure reducing mattress. Requirements for a group II product include multiple stage II pressure ulcers located on the trunk or pelvis and that the patient has been using a group I support surface as part of a comprehensive treatment program with worsening or no improvement over the past month; or large or multiple stage III or IV pressure ulcers on the trunk or recent myocutaneous flap or skin graft for a pressure ulcer on the trunk or pelvis with surgery within the past 60 days, and the patient has been on a group II or III support surface immediately prior to discharge. Coverage is limited to 60 days for operative repair of ulcers. Again, a written order and a comprehensive plan as described above for group I surfaces are required. Use of the group II surface is allowed until the ulcer is healed

or documentation in the medical record shows that other aspects of the plan of care are being modified to promote healing or that the group II surface is medically necessary for wound management.

Group III only includes air-fluidized beds. Requirements include the presence of a stage III or IV pressure ulcer, the patient is bed- or chairbound due to severely limited mobility, the patient would require institutionalization without the air-fluidized bed, and failure of more conservative treatment. A comprehensive plan of care including the air-fluidized bed is required as described under group I devices. In general, a more conservative plan of care should have been in effect for at least one month prior to use of an air-fluidized bed with failure to improve. Other limitations also need to be addressed. These include presence of coexisting pulmonary disease, lack of a caregiver willing and able to provide care required by a patient on an air-fluidized bed, and inadequate electrical system or structural support for these extremely heavy beds.

Turning Schedules

Any bedbound individual with compromised mobility or other risk factors should be repositioned according to an individualized schedule that should be written, posted, and carried out by the patient's caregivers. Historically, a recommendation of turning on a schedule rotating among prone, sidelying to one side, supine, and sidelying to the other side every 2 hours has been made. Rather than using a directly sidelying position, pillows or wedges should be used to turn the patient 30 degrees to avoid positioning directly on the greater trochanter. Patients should not need to be put completely prone for a similar reason. Skin over a number of bony prominences can be put at risk, such as the frontal bone, patellae, and dorsum of the foot. Rather than complete prone positioning, a wedge or pillows can be used to rotate the patient 30 degrees in either direction. This position may also be found more comfortable for the neck and for breathing. For individuals at high risk, especially those who are emaciated and malnourished, 2 hours in one position may be too long.

Blindly repositioning without regard to neurologic deficits, musculoskeletal injuries, or particular areas of skin at high risk is a disservice to the patient. Moreover, a patient should never be positioned directly over an ulcer if possible, and if not possible, the patient should be on a pressure-redistributing surface. To prevent injury caused by bony prominences contacting each other, pillows, foam wedges, or other devices should be used to keep the knees or ankles apart. Anyone with impaired mobility who is bedbound should have a device that totally relieves pressure on the heels, usually by raising the heels off the bed (floating the heels). This may consist of simply placing pillows under the legs or may include more complex devices

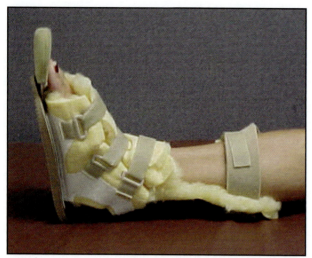

Figure 7-7. Multipodus boot. The heel is protected from the weight of the patient, and the loss of dorsiflexion produced by constant weight of sheets and blankets on the foot is minimized.

such as Multipodus boots (Restorative Care of America, St. Petersburg, FL, Figure 7-7). Donut devices should never be used on anyone at risk for pressure ulcers. These devices are designed only for temporary comfort use in individuals not at risk for pressure ulcers.

In addition to pressure, shear must be minimized. Shear stress increases directly in proportion to the incline of a bed or chair. In the case of reclining, shear is placed on the skin over the sacrum when skin adheres to the support surface as body weight pulls downward. These forces also occur during transfers, turning and bed mobility. To minimize injury due to shear, the clinician should maintain the head of the bed at the lowest degree of elevation consistent with medical conditions and other restrictions such as increased intracranial pressure, pulmonary edema, congestive heart failure, and gastroesophageal reflux. To further decrease shearing, the patient can be placed in the Fowler's position. Raising the foot of the bed puts a patient in hip and knee flexion such that weight is placed on the posterior thigh to stop the patient from sliding downward in bed when in supine. However, prolonged Fowler's position needs to be avoided due to the risk of hip and knee flexion contractures. The use of a trapeze or draw sheets to lift and avoid dragging individuals in bed who cannot assist during transfers and position changes is recommended.

Patient Assessment

Three instruments for assessing risk are described below. These are the Norton scale, the Braden scale, and the Gosnell scale. The Norton scale is a sum of ordinal scale values for overall physical condition, mental condition, activity level, bed mobility and continence. Each item is scored between 1 and 4 and the five item scores are added. Risk is then determined by the sum. The scoring system for the Norton Scale is shown in Table 7-3. The lowest possible score is 5 and the highest is 20. A score of 14 or less indicates risk for developing pressure ulcers and a score of 12 or less indicates high risk. Based on the risk, prevention and intervention strategies may be undertaken. Although some of the items require judgment of the clinician, the reliability of the scale is sufficient for most needs. As with any instrument using ordinal scales, the numerical differences cannot be treated mathematically. For example, a score of 7 does not necessarily represent 30% more risk than a score of 10.

The Braden scale uses some similar indicators of risk. It has 6 items, also on an ordinal scale of 1 to 4. With this scale, risk also increases with a lower score. This scale uses sensory perception rather than mental condition and moisture rather than incontinence. It, similar to the Norton scale, uses mobility and activity level. The Braden scale scores 2 additional items. Risk of friction and shear, which are somewhat related to bed mobility, and nutrition are addressed in this scale, but not in the Norton scale. The Braden scale does not give a score to the clinician's overall impression of physical condition. The scale gives a maximum score of 23; one item (friction and shear) only scores between 1 and 3. Scoring is shown in Table 7-4. For this scale, a person with a score of 16 or below is generally considered to be at risk, although for certain populations a score of 17 to 18 is considered to be at risk for development of pressure ulcers.

The Gosnell scale is an adaptation of the Norton scale. One major difference is the reversal of the scores such that a high number represents a greater risk. With this adaptation, 5 is the lowest possible score, indicating the least risk and a score of 20 represents the greatest risk. Other differences between the Gosnell scale and Norton scale is the replacement of "physical condition" with nutrition. Other items appear on the tool, but are not used in the scoring directly. In addition, very detailed instructions are included on the tool.

Nutritional Assessment

A clear association between malnutrition and new ulcer development has been observed. Particular risk factors cited include low dietary protein and hypoalbuminemia. Nutrition is addressed specifically in Chapter 4. The AHCPR guidelines recommend an evaluation of nutritional status using a nutrition screening manual. Preferably, a clinical dietician would be available to perform a thorough nutritional assessment. The AHCPR also recommends that a reassessment be made every three months. Nutritional risk factors addressed in the guidelines include inability to take food by mouth, a history of involuntary weight loss, immobility, altered mental status, and educational deficit. The guidelines recommend encouraging dietary intake

Table 7-3

Scoring Based on the Norton Scale

	4	3	2	1
Physical condition	good	fair	poor	very bad
Mental condition	alert	apathetic	confused	stupor
Activity	ambulant	walk/help	chairbound	stupor
Mobility	full	slightly limited	very limited	immobile
Incontinent	not	occasional	usually/urine	doubly

Table 7-4

Scoring Based on the Braden Scale

	1	2	3	4
Sensory perception	completely limited	very limited	slightly	no impairment
Moisture	constantly moist	moist	occasionally	rarely
Activity	bedbound	chairbound	walks occasionally	walks frequently
Mobility	completely immobile	very limited	slightly	no limitations
Nutrition	very poor	probably inadequate	adequate	excellent
Friction and shear	problem	potential problem	no apparent problem	

and supplementation of the diet if the person is malnourished, including nutritional support by tube feed or other means if necessary. An intake of 30 to 35 kcal per kilogram of body mass each day with 1.25 to 1.50 g of protein per kg per day is recommended.

Pain Assessment

Pain management is discussed in Chapter 10. For an individual with limited mobility, complaints of pain from a body surface should be treated as a sign of imminent skin injury. A thorough investigation of the cause of the pain, rather than simply treating the pain, needs to be performed. Routine assessment of pain is recommended by the AHCPR, although they also recommended further research into this topic. Specifically addressed is the potential for intensified pain during dressing changes and debridement. They suggest that pain should be managed by eliminating or controlling its source and providing analgesia during painful procedures such as debridement. All patients should be assessed for pain related to the pressure ulcer or its treat-

ment. Controlling the source of pain may include covering wounds, adjusting support surfaces, or repositioning.

Psychosocial Assessment

In many situations, healthcare professionals cannot provide all of the care; the patient or other caregiver must take a major role. Even in the acute care hospital, psychosocial issues may promote or impair the efficacy of provided services. Issues that need to be addressed include whether the patient comprehends the plan of care and if the patient is motivated to adhere to the plan. The clinician needs to understand values, lifestyle, psychosocial needs and goals of not only the patient, but also the family, or if different, the caregiver. The AHCPR guidelines specifically mention mental status, learning ability, depression, social support, polypharmacy or overmedication, alcohol and/or drug abuse, goals, values, and lifestyle, sexuality, culture and ethnicity, and stressors. With these issues in mind, the clinician, patient, family, and other caregivers should set treatment goals collabora-

Table 7-5

Differential Diagnosis of Ulcers Caused by Neuropathy and Arterial Disease

Characteristic	Neuropathic	Ischemic (Arterial Insufficiency)
Appearance	Round or elliptical	Dry surrounding skin Irregular, wet or dry gangrene Atrophy of skin, thickened nails, loss of hair Rubor of dependency
Location	Sites of pressure or shear during weightbearing and ambulation	Distal, especially toes and heels, but may occur anywhere arterial vessels occlude
Pain	None, but may have dysesthesia	Painful
Tests	Sensory testing shows loss of protective sensation, loss of vibration, position sense, reflexes	Low ankle brachial index Low transcutaneous oxygen Claudication during treadmill

tively. In addition, when developing a home plan of care, the clinician needs to determine whether the patient and family have the resources available to be treated at home. These resources are not only financial, but also include the ability to understand and the physical ability and skills to follow through on the treatment plan. Periodic reassessment is also recommended by the AHCPR and follow up should be planned in cooperation with the individual and caregiver.

NEUROPATHY

In Western civilizations, diabetes mellitus represents the major cause of peripheral neuropathy and as such plantar ulcers in people with diabetes mellitus are the emphasis of this section. Other causes of neuropathy include spinal cord injury, tumors, stroke, spina bifida, syringomyelia, other sensory neuropathies, and leprosy (Hansen's disease). Although diabetes is also associated with peripheral arterial disease, the mechanism of neuropathic ulcers is mechanical, not vascular. A person may have both arterial disease and neuropathy due to diabetes and the combination of these two further complicates treatment. However, the wounds caused by these two etiologies are generally easy to distinguish. Wounds caused by peripheral artery disease are painful and occur on the distal part of the foot. The affected extremity has a low

ankle brachial index (ABI), the wound has an irregular shape, and a pale wound base. Neuropathic ulcers occur on areas of weightbearing and shearing, especially under metatarsal heads and sites of bony abnormalities including the dorsal, medial, and lateral surfaces of the foot, including the toes (Figures 7-8 and 7-9). The wounds are round and not painful. Characteristics leading to a differential diagnosis between neuropathic and ischemic ulcers are displayed in Table 7-5.

Although the lack of sensation is commonly believed to be the root cause of plantar ulcers in diabetic feet, this type of ulcer is generally due to neuropathy of three systems and loss of any of the three systems may be more responsible for ulceration than the other two in a given individual. Approximately 15% of all individuals with diabetes mellitus will develop foot ulcers. Moreover, 20% of all hospital admissions of those with diabetes mellitus are due to foot ulcers. People with diabetes mellitus average one hospital admission per year for foot problems after 65 years of age. The most common sites of diabetic foot ulcers include the plantar great toe, 30%; the head of first metatarsal, 22%; the dorsum of digits, 13%; the plantar aspect of other toes, 10%; the fifth metatarsal head, 9%; the second metatarsal head, 6%; the arch, 4%; the third metatarsal head, 2%; the fourth metatarsal head, 2% and the heel, 1%.

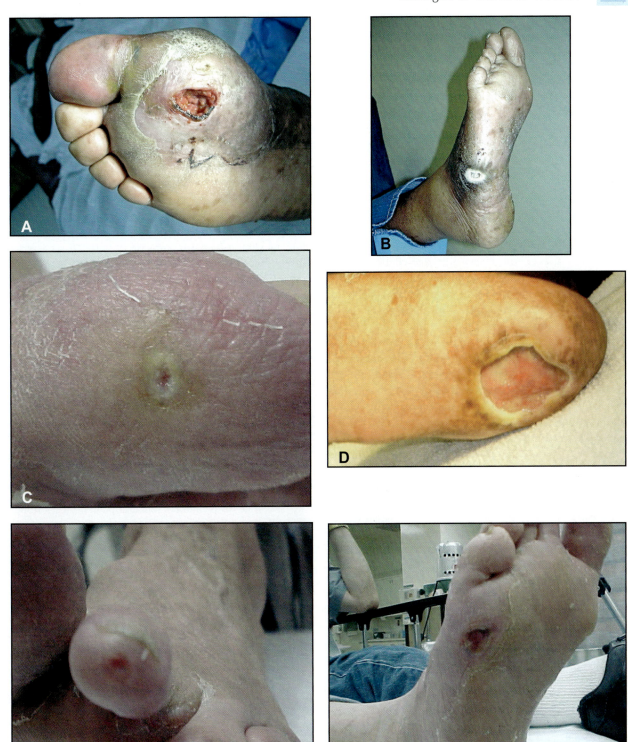

Figure 7-8. Common sites for neuropathic ulcers. (A) Below second metatarsal head, (B) Styloid process of fifth metatarsal, (C) Medial surface of great toe, (D) Heel, (E) Tip of second toe (tip-top-toe syndrome).

Figure 7-9. Shallow ulcer characteristic of Wagner grade 1 ulcer. Note the dryness and callus formation over the entire plantar surface.

Problems Caused by Hyperglycemia

Multiple systems are affected by diabetes mellitus, particularly when glycemic control is poor. Of particular importance for this discussion are neuropathy, retinopathy, glycosylation of proteins, and atherosclerosis, which leads to peripheral arterial disease, ischemic heart disease, stroke, and renal disease. Glycosylation has been suggested to cause reduced elasticity of skin, tendons, and ligaments, contributing to altered biomechanics of the foot.

Diabetic Neuropathy

Neuropathy implies an injury to nerves, which may be more general or specific depending on the disease. In spite of the focus of lay people and even some clinicians on sensory nerves, the neuropathy caused by diabetes mellitus affects sensory, motor, and autonomic nerves. Each of these components of neuropathy contributes to the plantar ulcers associated with diabetes and other distal neuropathies.

The triple threat of neuropathy needs to be carefully addressed by evaluating sensory, motor, and autonomic function. Sensory neuropathy leads to glove and stocking sensory loss, which is characterized by loss of sensation occurring distally and progressing proximally. Glove and stocking sensory loss results from the greater probability of damage to longer neurons and, as the disease progresses, shorter neurons become involved. Therefore, sensory loss is most likely to occur first in the foot and progress centrally. Sensory loss may also progress to the hand, usually about the time that sensory loss occurs near the knee. Damage to sensory neurons is also manifested as the bizarre brief burning sensation termed *dysesthesia* and chronic discomfort of the feet. Treatment of diabetic foot pain is addressed below.

Motor neurons, like sensory neuron, are also affected based on neuron length. The foot muscles most affected are those located within the foot itself (intrinsic) rather than the muscles located in the leg and attached to the foot by long tendons. Frequently, the peripheral neuropathy results in a combination of weak intrinsic flexors and normal extrinsic extensors, which produces foot deformities, contributes to limited joint mobility within the foot, and leads to abnormal biomechanics. These biomechanical abnormalities create pressure and shearing under metatarsal heads, shearing under other bony prominences, and a condition known as tip-top-toe syndrome in which the tips and tops of toes are damaged by friction against the inside of the patient's footwear. Biomechanics are also altered by glycosylation of joints of the foot with loss of foot's ability to dissipate force by relaxation of muscles and splaying of the foot. Inability to dorsiflex, in particular, places the great toes at increased risk of shearing as the foot fails to progress normally from heel strike to toe off.

The results of these biomechanical changes are often obvious from inspection of the patient's shoes.

Autonomic involvement causes loss of sweating, dry skin, and loss of control of blood vessels within the foot. Increased blood flow to the foot has been implicated in resorption of bone leading to the deformity known as Charcot foot (described below). Charcot foot carries with it an increased risk of fracture of osteopenic bone and with it, an increased risk of creating new shear/pressure points on the foot. As a result of triple neuropathy, individuals with poor glycemic control experience a number of health problems, which left unmanaged, are nearly certain to result in a downward spiral of the person's health. These conditions include dry, flaky skin prone to hyperkeratosis and cracking, which can provide a portal for bacterial entry, especially if the patient soaks the feet.

Sensory neuropathy results in the loss of protective sensation. Motor neuropathy produces weakness of intrinsic foot muscles and changes in the shape of the foot with altered biomechanics and risk of injury. Thirdly, autonomic neuropathy causes the loss of sweating to protect the skin against drying. As a result of damage to all three neural systems, altered biomechanics of the foot cause pressure and shear in typical locations, and dry, hyperkeratotic skin and callus increase the damage caused by pressure and shear, and skin damage is allowed to go undetected with the result of round/elliptical wounds occurring under bony prominences.

Factors Leading to Foot Wounds

A single factor is unlikely to cause plantar ulcers alone. Generally, several factors interact to cause the wound and, therefore, several factors must be addressed in the treatment plan. Among these problems are altered biomechanics, an insensate foot, arterial insufficiency, the inability to monitor the feet, competition for time and resources with other pathologies, bad information received from others, and denial. Denial is particularly easy when a person with an insensate foot has more immediate and obvious problems such as end stage renal failure, heart disease, stroke, and diminished ability to inspect the feet due to poor mobility, decreased sensation in the hands, and diminished vision.

Having an insensate foot requires one to more carefully monitor footwear to the point of inspecting the inside for foreign objects. Those with neuropathy must be taught to carefully check their shoes before donning them, including turning them over and feeling with their hands. Foreign objects may compress a foot causing ischemic injury, or cut or puncture a foot without the wearer's realization. Some individuals retain the sensation of deep pressure and may wear shoes substantially smaller than they would otherwise, leading to crowding of the foot and frictional and ischemic injuries. A second common problem is the warming of feet. Either because of concomitant arterial disease or simply due to cold weather, a person with neuropathy may attempt to warm the feet with soaking in hot water, application of a heating pad, or propping feet up near a fireplace. Tremendous thermal injury may result before the person notices. One example of note is a person who wore black rubber boots while cutting grass on a riding mower on a hot, sunny day. The effect of the heat absorbed by the boots and transmitted to the feet was not noticed until the boots were removed and much of the skin under the boots was removed with the boots. Additionally, those without pain in the injured foot are less likely to voluntarily reduce tissue loading on the foot. Whereas a person with normal sensation and an injury to the foot will reduce gait-induced stresses on the foot, the person lacking pain is unlikely to alter the gait pattern.

Deformities of the foot produce abnormal pressure and shear points on the foot manifested initially as callus, erythema, and progressing to hemorrhage under callus. Callus itself is a risk factor for ulceration because callus formation increases load on the tissue by 30%. A simple demonstration of the effect of callus can be performed by having a person with normal sensation walk with a coin taped in the bottom of the shoe. Moreover, wounds developing beneath callus can be hidden from view, leading to extensive infection with tunneling and osteomyelitis. Such a wound may not be detected until tissue erodes in an area of the foot that is in plain sight or when blood or purulence is seen on a sock.

Pathway to Amputation

Diabetes mellitus frequently leads to amputation. The reasons for amputation of diabetic limbs are multiple and many pathways lead to amputation. The usual pathway (72%) consists of minor trauma, cutaneous ulceration, and wound-healing failure (Pecoraro, Reiber, Burgess). This pathway is depicted in Table 7-6. Factors cited as indications for lower extremity amputation are as follows: ischemia, 46%; infection, 59%; neuropathy, 61%; faulty wound healing, 81%; ulceration, 84%; and gangrene, 55%. Initial minor trauma was cited in 81% of cases of lower extremity amputation in persons with diabetes mellitus. Because statistically identifiable and potentially preventable events appear to precede most amputations, the federal government has instituted a program through the National Institutes of Health called the LEAP program. This acronym stands for Lower Extremity Amputation Prevention. It consists of educational material for both individuals with diabetes and the clinicians caring for them. These materials include instructions for screening and proper fitting of footwear. The materials can be obtained from their Web site http://www.hrsa.gov/leap/.

Table 7-6

Causal Pathway to Amputation With Diabetic Neuropathy

Neuropathy
Minor trauma
Ulceration
Faulty Healing
Gangrene
Amputation

Table 7-7

Wagner Grading System of Neuropathic Ulcers

0 = pre-ulcerative lesions, healed ulcers, presence of bony deformity

1 = superficial ulcer without subcutaneous involvement

2 = penetration through the subcutaneous tissue; may expose bone, tendon, ligament or joint capsule

3 = osteitis, abscess, or osteomyelitis

4 = gangrene of digit

5 = gangrene of the foot requiring disarticulation

Wagner Grades

The Wagner scale is used for prognosis and intervention decisions for neuropathic ulcers. The scale does not represent a progression of a given wound, rather it represents degrees of severity of the injury and the invasiveness required for treatment of the wound. As the descriptions detail, neuropathy, infection, and ischemia are all involved. The scale ranges from grade 0 to grade 5. See Table 7-7 for descriptions. A grade 0 ulcer represents damage to the foot, but the skin remains intact. Severe subcutaneous tissue injury may be present and as such, minor trauma to the foot may lead to a serious infection of the necrotic tissue within the foot. Grade 1 is used to describe a partial-thickness or superficial ulcer (see Figure 7-9). A full-thickness wound with subcutaneous involvement is classified as a grade 2 neuropathic ulcer (Figure 7-10). Note that only 2

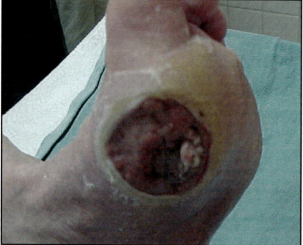

Figure 7-10. Deep ulcer characteristic of a Wagner grade 2 ulcer. Note the thick rim of callus around the wound. Also note the presence of hammer toes, which increase the shearing forces under the metatarsal heads during gait.

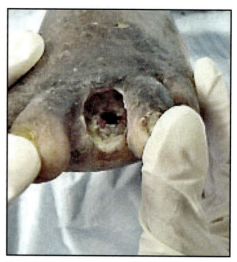

Figure 7-11. Infection with subsequent amputation of the third ray (toe and metatarsal). Infection is characteristic of Wagner grade 3.

Table 7-8

University of Texas Wound Classification System of Diabetic Foot Ulcers

Grades 0-3

0 = pre- or post-ulcerative lesion completely re-epithelialized
1 = superficial wound, not involving tendon, capsule, or bone
2 = wound penetrating to tendon, capsule, or bone
3 = wound penetrating to bone, or a deep abscess

Add Stages A-D as appropriate to number above

A = no infection or ischemia
B = with infection
C = with ischemia
D = with infection and ischemia

grades are used to denote the depth of the ulcer. A wound is classified as a grade 3 ulcer when infection is present, manifested as either an abscess or osteomyelitis (Figure 7-11). Progression to forefoot gangrene is documented as a grade 4 ulcer and grade 5 represents gangrene of most of the foot. Treatment of neuropathic ulcers will be described based on Wagner grade below.

Another useful classification scheme is the University of Texas Wound Classification System (Table 7-8). This system provides more flexibility for wound classification than the Wagner grades. The examiner assigns a number

for the depth of the wound and a letter that describes complications associated with the wound. For example a superficial wound with infection is classified as 2B.

Interventions for neuropathic ulcers include local wound care, periodic foot screening for deformities, callus formation, sensation, reflexes, strength, and range of motion. Decreased range of motion of the articulations of the foot are predictive of future ulceration. Inspection of footwear and either offloading or protecting the foot may become necessary. Of all possible interventions, metabolic control is the most important factor for long-term health.

Patients must be reinforced and rewarded by all members of the healthcare team to maintain blood glucose as close to normal (about 100 mg/dL) as possible. With multiple demands on the patient's life, blood glucose control is often difficult prior to ulceration, but only becomes more difficult with infection. In fact, rising blood glucose is suggestive of infection.

Offloading

To allow healing and prevent recurrence, the mechanical forces causing the wounds must be addressed. Following healing, more definitive measures can also be undertaken to minimize future ulceration. Because the 2 most important aspects of offloading are patient education and adherence to the plan of care, the clinician must evaluate the patient's understanding of the plan of care and willingness to adhere to the plan. Based on this information, the clinician can select the most appropriate offloading techniques. The most appropriate technique will be determined based on a number of factors, including the skill level of the clinician to apply them, the perceived adherence of the patient, and the skill level of the patient or caregiver to follow up at home. Several means are available for protecting the foot. These include bed rest, crutch walking, and specialized footwear. Bed rest is largely impractical due to the potential for severe cardiopulmonary decline and exacerbation of blood glucose control. For many individuals, especially older patients with multiple health problems, crutch walking is also impractical. Diminishing balance due to loss of proprioception and vision creates safety concerns. Moreover, the tremendous prevalence of obesity in type 2 diabetes and the potential for cardiovascular disease with increased energy demands of crutch walking compared with unaided gait may increase the risks associated with ambulation with crutches. Means of offloading discussed below include off-the-shelf shoes, total contact casting, walking splints, the Charcot Restraint Orthotic Walker (CROW), DH Pressure Relief Walker, CAM walkers, healing sandal, and OrthoWedge Healing Shoe.

Off-the-Shelf Shoes

In mild cases before significant changes in the shape of the foot or injury to the skin, a patient may sufficiently benefit from ordinary, but well-constructed off-the-shelf shoes without any special modifications. Attention to construction and fit are important at this phase of neuropathy. Good quality running shoes, walking shoes, or shoes with a crepe sole absorb forces that a stiffened foot would not. Dress shoes with stiff leather soles are to be avoided as they do not adequately dissipate forces to accommodate a person with a stiff foot. Stiff uppers are also a risk factor for injuring the dorsum of the foot. A tracing of the foot should be used to determine proper fit. This tracing is cut out and placed in a prospective shoe. If wrinkling of the foot template occurs, a shoe of a different size or last shape is needed. After a shoe is selected, it must still be checked with the person standing in it for proper fit. Shoes need to be 1 to 2 cm longer the great toe (or second toe if it is longer). The paper template should be drawn sufficiently long to judge this, but a second person should still check this aspect of fit.

Similarly, the width of the shoe should be checked even after using the foot template by having another person pinch the material of the shoe top over the metatarsal heads. If the material is too taut to be pinched, the shoes are too narrow. Excessive width, however, allows excess movement within the shoe, which may also lead to injury. Third, ensure that the distance between the metatarsal heads and heel is correct, allowing the shoe to flex at the metatarsal heads. Flexing of the shoe at a different point can exert force on the end of the toes or on the heel, depending on the flex point. Any new shoes should be worn sparingly until they are broken in. This process can be facilitated by hand if done properly. A common recommendation is a 2-hour limit on wearing new shoes with a gradual increase in wearing time. For this reason, new shoes should be obtained prior to the old shoes becoming so worn that they are no longer safe to wear. This allows one to continue to use the old shoes as the new shoes are broken in.

Feet with deformities that increase the height of the foot, such as hammer toes or claw toes require shoes with increased depth (depth shoes). These shoes, like off-the-shelf shoes do not need to be customized for individuals. Modifications that may be required, however, include a rocker bottom for individuals who cannot perform the normal transition from heel strike to toe off, including lack of dorsiflexion, hallux rigidus, loss of MCP joint motion, and partial foot or toe amputations. Flared heels may be required if the patient shows excessive foot varus. This problem can be identified easily by excessive wear on the outside of the shoe's sole.

Total Contact Casting

Total contact casting is used for diabetes mellitus and other chronic sensory neuropathies, such as Hansen's disease (leprosy). This technique is based on the concept of protecting the foot against repetitive stress on insensate feet. Total contact casting is the preferred method of temporary offloading of the foot for Wagner grades 0, 1, and 2 provided no contraindications exist. Contraindications include Wagner grades 3 to 5, fragile skin, and poor adherence to the care of the total contact cast. Poor adherence and failure to follow up as directed may cost the patient's limb or worse. Total contact casting reduces excessive plantar pressure by redistributing pressure and immobilizing the foot and ankle to correct biomechanical problems and minimize shearing. The cast also controls edema and protects the foot from trauma.

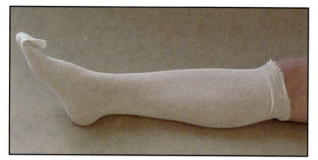

Figure 7-12A. Total contact casting. Stockinette applied from the knee, beyond the toes, and folded onto the dorsal surface.

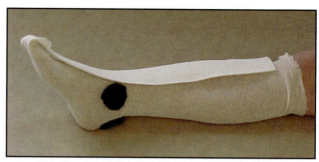

Figure 7-12B. Padding required for total contact cast. A thin layer of felt is placed over the tibial crest, and foam is placed over both malleoli and the insertion of the heel cord.

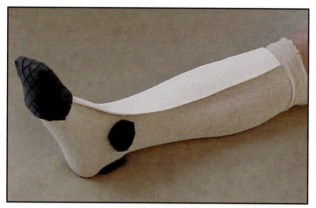

Figure 7-12C. Foam is placed over the toes, including the metatarsals, with beveling of the edge under the metatarsal heads to improve foot biomechanics.

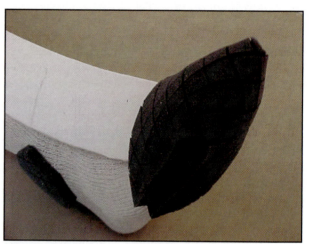

Figure 7-12D. Close-up view of foam over the forefoot.

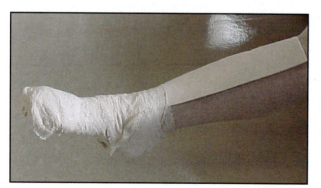

Figure 7-12E. The first plaster bandage is applied. Several turns around the ankle are necessary to maintain rigidity. Ankle must be maintained in neutral as plaster or fiberglass bandages are applied.

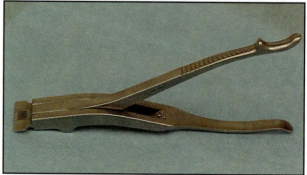

Figure 7-12F. Cast spreaders used to remove a cast.

Statistically, healing occurs in 73% to 100% of the time over 37 to 65 days with an average of 43 days. In addition, those using total contact casts for neuropathic ulcers reported fewer hospitalizations for infection or amputation. However, total contact casting does create some potential problems. Forty-three percent of those using total contact casts reported minor complications. Those listed included abrasions from suboptimal fit and fungal infections treatable topically. Other possible risks include undetected osteomyelitis or deep infection, sepsis, amputation, or death. However, these complications can be minimized by careful application and frequent follow-up.

Total contact casts are constructed of plaster or fiberglass bandages used for other types of orthopedic casts (Figure 7-12). One significant difference is the amount of padding used. In a total contact cast a minimum of padding is used. First, the web spaces are protected by cotton batting or lamb's wool. A length of stockinette is applied to the leg and foot. The distal end of the stockinette is brought to the top of the toes to prevent pressure on the toes caused by a seam in the stockinette. The proximal end of the stockinette should extend to the knee. Padding is placed over the malleoli, around the toes, and along the crest of the tibia. A quick set plaster bandage is applied distally to cover the toes, and applied with overlapping spirals proximally up the leg. Typically 2 to 3 plaster bandages are needed to cover a leg. The surface of the plaster is smoothed with water as the bandages dry. Extra care is needed to reinforce the cast at the ankle. The cast is only allowed to come to about a finger's width below the head of the fibula. A shorter cast is more susceptible to torque and a longer cast will interfere with knee range of motion. A cast that ends close to the head of the fibula may injure the peroneal nerve. The cast may then be reinforced by a layer of fiberglass casting tape. The use of layered plaster allows visualization of drainage from the wound into the cast. Fiberglass improves the durability of the cast, but compromises visualization of drainage. Another option is leaving a window in the cast where the wound can be visualized. The fiberglass roll must be wet with cold water and applied quickly to prevent premature hardening. Various types of bracing mechanisms have been placed in total contact casts in an effort to improve biomechanics and reduce stresses on the foot.

In general, the initial cast will be worn for 1 week, and subsequent casts are worn up to 2 weeks, depending on issues unique to each patient. The clinician must be confident in the patient's ability to follow directions, monitor the fit of the cast, and seek emergency care for the cast when needed. Some individuals place a rubber heel on the cast to allow ambulation. Others fit the patient for a postop sandal to wear on the bottom of the cast to protect the cast. Casts may be worn in the shower if care is taken to protect them from water. A plastic trash bag can be secured over the cast and dry towels using a rubber band. Towels are wrapped over the top of the cast to absorb any leakage into the plastic bag.

Walking Splint

An alternative to total contact casting is the walking splint. It is similar to a cast, but made of more durable materials, and it is cut along both sides (bivalved) to allow it to be put on and taken off. The 2 pieces are secured with Velcro straps or elasticized bandage rolls. Like the total contact cast, the foot and ankle are immobilized, pressure is distributed more evenly on the plantar surface, and edema is prevented. A walking cast has the advantage of frequent inspection of the foot, but the disadvantage that the patient may fail to wear the device and edema control diminishes over time. With this device and the 2 below, offloading of an infected ulcer may be more safely performed.

Charcot Restraint Orthotic Walker

The Charcot Restraint Orthotic Walker (CROW) has features in common with the walking splint. The orthosis is a rigid polypropylene boot walker with a rocker sole. The anterior half of the shell is removable with velcro straps and shares the advantages and disadvantages of the walking splints. The device is custom made and lined with perforated plastazote to provide fit, cushioning, and ventilation. The rocker sole built into the orthosis allows pressure and shearing forces to be minimized. A custom molded insert is used to accommodate the shape of the foot. Because the CROW is custom-made and may require multiple modifications, it can be very expensive.

DH Pressure Relief Walker

Similar to the CROW, the DH Pressure Relief Walker (Royce Medical, Camarillo, CA) is an extended foot ankle orthosis, covering the leg to just below the head of the fibula. It is similar to the boots used for lower extremity fractures and features a rocker sole bottom and customizable insole. The insole consists of an array of hexagonal plugs attached with Velcro. Individual plugs are removed easily and can be reconfigured as needed to determine the optimal pressure relief for the patient's foot. The advantages and disadvantages are similar to the CROW and walking splint, with the exception of edema control. The DH Pressure Relief Walker is not rigid and may allow swelling to occur. The convenience of pressure relief without custom molding may be considered an advantage, but is also a disadvantage because the insole will not conform carefully to the plantar surface of the foot. One published study (Lavery, et al), however, indicates that this orthosis is as effective as total contact casting for reducing forefoot pressure. A much less expensive alternative to the CROW or DH pressure relief walker is a simple CAM walker (controlled ankle motion) used for lower extremity fractures.

The advantage of the total contact cast is enforced compliance. Removable orthoses are worn by 15% of patients at home, and for only 50% of daily activities. Only total contact casting guarantees that the patient will wear the device at all times during ambulation. Even patients with otherwise good compliance in wearing the orthosis will remove an orthosis when retiring for the night and if getting up at night, will ambulate what he or she can rationalize as an insignificant distance. Compliance with wearing these alternatives to total contact casts may be enforced by wrapping them with fiberglass or plaster bandages. The combination of casting material and boot is more readily removed for routine care or during an emergency than a complete total contact cast. Plastic cable ties may be used,

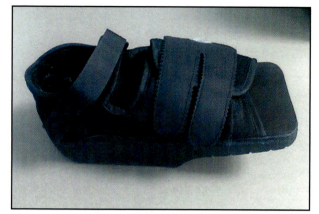

Figure 7-13A. OrthoWedge shoe. Note the dorsiflexion imposed by the shoe and the lack of weightbearing on the forefoot.

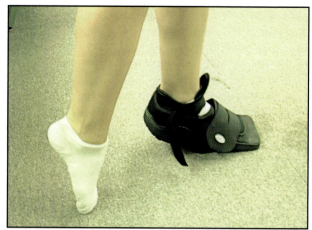

Figure 7-13B. Walking in an OrthoWedge shoe. A patient can place weight on the forefoot without appropriate gait.

but due to their accessibility, they may be simply cut off at home and replaced just before a clinic visit.

OrthoWedge Healing Shoe

The OrthoWedge Healing Shoe (Darco International, Huntington, WV), as the name implies, has a wedge shaped sole that provides 10 degrees of dorsiflexion and suspends the forefoot, as the wedged bottom part of the sole extends only to the metatarsal head. The design limits motion of the ankle and foot similar to the orthoses described above, but removes weightbearing nearly completely from the forefoot. The patient will also ambulate with a shorter stride. Because the device only covers the foot, edema control is not provided. The orthosis is readily removed for inspection of the foot and, of course, can be left off by the patient. An awkward gait may lead to noncompliance by some patients (Figure 7-13).

Healing Sandal

Another device to assist in healing of neuropathic ulcers that is less invasive, but also less effective and therefore recommended for individuals at lower risk of impaired healing, is the healing (cutout) sandal. A piece of thermoplastic is cut to fit a postop sandal and glued inside the sandal. A relief area is then cut into the sandal. The bottom of the foot requiring relief is marked with ink, betadine, benzoin, or other suitable marking substance and the individual is asked to stand on the thermoplastic material or the sandal may be carefully applied to the foot to emulate standing position. The stained thermoplastic is cut out. This process may require several trials to create the proper size and shape. These sandals may, however, cause pressure around the ulcer. Use of this option also necessitates meticulous callus removal. Callus formation on the edges of the cutout may generate unacceptable pressure around the wound. A similar procedure can be performed with either felt or foam padding cut to fit around the ulcer to relieve pressure on the site. Healing sandals may also be used temporarily until appropriate footwear is obtained. Like the walking splint, the healing sandal has the disadvantage that the patient may choose to walk without the device. Other disadvantages are the lack of ankle immobilization and edema control.

Walking Patterns

A number of ambulation strategies have been proposed to reduce peak plantar pressure and shearing. Shortening step length has been shown to reduce pressures, presumably by decreasing push off forces. Mueller has proposed what he terms a *hip strategy* to reduce plantar pressure.[7] Ground reaction forces are reduced by using hip flexion to advance the swinging extremity, rather than plantar flexion and strong toe off of the fixed extremity. The patient is also instructed to shorten step length, but not walking speed. Another proposed strategy is the step-to-gait pattern. By decreasing the length of the step on the uninvolved extremity by stepping to the involved foot, forefoot pressure is reduced by 53%. Many patients naturally adopt these walking strategies when placed in offloading footwear. Just as compliance is an issue with footwear, it is even more critical if gait pattern is the major preventative strategy. In particular, patients may not wish to be seen in public with an unusual gait pattern.

Protection of Surrounding Skin

In addition to glycemic control and offloading the foot, protection of the skin is vitally important. Compromised skin integrity of a foot with diminished immunity and possibly necrotic tissue represents a tremendous risk for infection and movement toward limb amputation. Management of drainage needs to be considered carefully. The presence of moisture on surrounding skin is likely to cause maceration and cracking of the skin, providing a portal for infection. In addition, excessive dryness of skin can cause cracking of the skin. Cracking can be prevented by moisturizing the skin of the foot other than the web spaces. Web spaces tend to accumulate moisture. Use of cotton batting or lamb's wool between toes will wick moisture away from the web spaces to protect this area.

Diabetic Foot Wound Care

Appropriate local wound care consists of debridement, selection and application of appropriate dressings, application of topical agents and modalities, and protection of surrounding skin. The American Diabetes Association recommends aggressive debridement to viable tissue due to the high risk of infection of open wounds with necrotic tissue and frequent immunosuppression. Trimming callus should be done as needed. Callus is formed by abnormal shearing forces on the skin. Even with removal of the abnormal shear, callus often returns and must be debrided by either peeling or by shaving the tissue tangentially with a sharp scalpel. Dry gangrene should never be debrided. As a general rule, necrotic tissue is removed from a wound to allow healing from viable edges of the wound toward the center. In the case of dry gangrene, no healthy tissues exist under the necrotic surface. Debridement exposes necrotic tissue to the outside environment. This, combined with the frequent immunosuppression of individuals with poor glycemic control, creates tremendous risk for a rapidly progressing infection of the extremity. Stated simply, no good comes from debriding dry gangrene, whereas tremendous risk is associated with removal of the covering of the moist necrotic tissue below.

When cleansing a neuropathic ulcer, avoid using a whirlpool or any type of soaking. Soaking increases the risk of maceration and potential for skin cracking, and provides a portal of entry for bacteria. When selecting a dressing, the clinician's foremost consideration must be the high risk of infection. An appropriate dressing allows frequent observation and avoids occlusion. A cavity requires loose filling to promote healing from the center of the wound toward the periphery. Available fillers include alginates and hydrofibers, amorphous gels, and various gauze products such as 4 x 4 gauze sponges. However, gauze promotes inflammation which, in turn, leads to continual use of gauze due to drainage caused by the inflammatory response to gauze. One particular study demonstrated that collagen-alginate filler increases healing compared with gauze, but at a higher cost per dressing change. On the other hand, the ease of dressing removal and comfort of the alginate or hydrofiber dressings produces greater patient satisfaction.

At this time, topical agents shown to be effective for wound healing include platelet-derived growth factor (PDGF) and platelet-rich plasma gel. Regranex (becaplermin, Johnson & Johnson, New Brunswick, NJ) is recombinant PDGF. AutoloGel (formerly Procuren, Cytomedix, Rockville, MD) is available at specific wound care centers where it is prepared from the patient's own blood. Both Regranex and the process for isolating growth factors from a patient's blood are very expensive. PDGF is discussed in more detail in Chapter 14. Topical antiseptics and antibiotics are not recommended due to cytotoxicity. The ADA recommends oral or parenteral antibiotics instead. Chemical debriders are not recommended by the ADA due to the risk of infection in these wounds. Sharp debridement down to healthy tissue is recommended instead.

Wound Management by Wagner Grade

A grade 0 ulcer has intact skin and must be protected by offloading the foot by total contact casting or other methods described above including orthotic or special shoes. The foot needs to be inspected for the presence of subcutaneous necrosis and potential breach of the skin. An analogy to a volcano is often drawn. Subcutaneous necrosis below intact skin frequently produces a greenish hue to a circumscribed region beneath at-risk skin. Management of grade 1 and 2 ulcers includes local wound care as described above, management of edema, protection from maceration, and protection of the foot by total contact casting or another method. Total contact casting both offloads and controls edema. The control of edema, however, presents 2 serious challenges to the clinicians. Resolution of edema may compromise the fit of the total contact cast, causing damage to the skin under the cast. On the other hand, increased swelling within the cast may cause ischemic injury. Patients must be taught to monitor the cast carefully and to seek immediate care if swelling causes vascular compromise within the cast and to return for recasting if the cast becomes too loose. Grade 3 ulcers require referral to an orthopedic surgeon or podiatrist who may perform resection of bone or bony prominence with osteomyelitis and incision and drainage of the abscess. The surgeon may decide that selective removal of foot bones may be required to rid the foot of infection. Oral or parenteral antibiotics, but not topical, are recommended by the ADA. Total contact casting is contraindicated for Wagner grades 3 to 5. Wounds should be cleaned by sharp debridement and selective cleansing such as pulsatile lavage with concurrent suction, rather than whirlpools and wet to dry dressings. Grades 4 and 5 neuropathic feet with dry gangrene require referral to a vascular surgeon with possible revascularization or amputation of the limb.

Charcot Foot

A particularly devastating complication of neuropathy is the complex of sensory, motor, and autonomic changes that lead to structural and vascular changes known as Charcot foot. Charcot foot most commonly occurs with diabetes, but may occur with other diseases. Up to 13% of those seen in high-risk diabetes clinics have this condition. The term *Charcot arthropathy* refers to skeletal damage secondary to neuropathy, and may also be called neuropathic osteoarthropathy. Charcot foot is characterized by progressive, multiple osteoarthropathy with joint dislocation, pathologic fractures, and deformities. The most common deformity is a boat-shaped foot in which the concavity of the arch of the foot is not only lost, but the bottom of the foot becomes convex (Figure 7-14). The toes frequently lose contact with the support surface of the foot and tremendous shear forces are exerted at the metatarsal heads. Pathologic fractures of the diabetic foot and deformities must be considered high-risk factors. Charcot arthropathy was named for a prominent French neurologist and was first described as a consequence of syphilis. It was originally believed to be due to lack of sensation and accumulated trauma, but was later shown to have a neurovascular component. This includes an increased blood flow due to denervation, accompanied by demineralization of the bones of the foot. Osteopenia combined with the loss of sensation leads to fractures of the foot. Moreover, motor denervation and resultant muscle imbalance lead to a very high risk of ulceration of the plantar surface as well as dorsal surfaces of hammer toes.

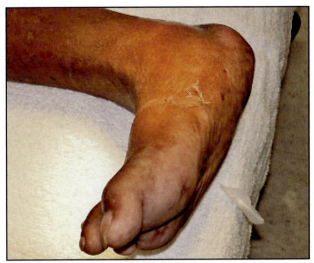

Figure 7-14. Example of a Charcot foot. Note the boat-shape deformity and healed forefoot wound. This foot now has an open wound on the heel (same foot as 7-8D).

Diagnosis of Charcot Foot

Unilateral swelling, elevated temperature, and erythema with no significant radiographic changes may represent the early stage of Charcot foot, requiring careful observation, rest, elevation, immobilization and referral to specialists experienced in treating Charcot foot. These events are associated with the increased blood flow caused by denervation of blood vessels of the lower extremities. Further examination may reveal joint effusion, bone resorption by imaging techniques, an insensate foot, and usually some degree of pain. Approximately 40% of those with Charcot foot have already experienced ulceration. Because of the swelling, heat, erythema, and pain of Charcot arthropathy, this condition may be confused with osteomyelitis. Differential diagnosis can be performed with a bone scan, blood work, especially white count, and bone biopsy.

Charcot foot has been described as having 4 stages for convenience of discussion. The first stage is characterized by a hot, red, swollen, foot with bounding pulses. During stage 1, resorption of bone produces severe osteopenia. For diagnosis, an increase of 2°C is considered necessary. During the second stage, dissolution, fragmentation, and fracture of bone occur as osteopenia weakens bones too much to support the biomechanics of the foot. A patient

is considered to be in stage 3 with development of a rocker bottom foot deformity. Stage 4 consists of plantar ulceration with possible progression to infection, gangrene, and amputation.

Interventions to prevent progression of Charcot foot during stage 1 are nonweightbearing of the affected extremity and, if appropriate, the use of total contact casting until skin temperature is normal. If the disease progresses to stage 3, the patient will need molded shoes or special Charcot shoes with molded inserts and possible surgery to repair deformities to prevent progression to stage 4. Unfortunately, the process may progress to stage 4 and damage to the foot may become so severe as to require amputation.

Another classification of Charcot arthropathy is based on radiographic, thermometric, and clinical signs into either an acute phase or post-acute phase. Although acute Charcot arthropathy may be treated with immobilization and reduction of stress, including decreased weightbearing with crutches, unloading one foot overloads the contralateral foot. With the likelihood of bilateral disease, the other foot is placed at greater risk of fracture. Other options that do not overload the contralateral extremity include using a total contact cast for 5 to 6 months, arthrodesis, and open reduction, internal fixation of the fractures. However, immunosuppression and possible arterial disease increase the risk of infection following internal fixation. Long-term solutions can be instituted during the post-acute phase. The classification of post-acute phase may be given after temperature of the affected foot is within 1°C of the contralateral foot. At this time, the patient may be fitted for orthotic shoes, using a removable cast walker until a custom shoe is ready. In about 25% of cases reconstructive foot surgery is performed.

Table 7-9

Risk Factors for Foot Ulceration and Amputation According to ADA

Diabetes mellitus for more than 10 years
Poor glucose control
Presence of cardiovascular, retinal, or renal complications
Peripheral vascular disease
History of ulcers or amputation
Peripheral neuropathy
Altered biomechanics
Evidence of increased pressure manifested as: callus, erythema, hemorrhage under a callus
Limited joint mobility
Bony deformity
Severe nail pathology

Table 7-10

Elements of Foot Examination for Low-Risk Person With Diabetes Mellitus

Use of Semmes-Weinstein monofilament or vibration to detect loss of protective sensation
Taking a history for claudication or examination for pedal pulses
Examination of skin integrity, especially between toes and under metatarsal heads
Examination for erythema, warmth, callus on soles of feet
Examination for bony deformities of the foot
Evaluation for limited joint mobility
Evaluation of gait and balance

ADA Clinical Practice Recommendations

Every year the ADA publishes clinical practice recommendations in its journal Diabetes Care and also makes this information available on its Web site (www.diabetes. org). According to the ADA, the first step is to identify risk factors for foot ulcers/amputations (see Table 7-9). The most important risk factors include having diabetes mellitus for more than 10 years, being male, poor glucose control, and the presence of cardiovascular, retinal, or renal complications, peripheral vascular disease, and a history of ulcers or amputation. In addition, several direct foot-related risk factors for amputation have also been identified: peripheral neuropathy, altered biomechanics, evidence of increased pressure manifested as callus, erythema, or hemorrhage under a callus, limited joint mobility, bony deformity, or severe nail pathology.

The ADA recommends an annual foot examination for all individuals with diabetes mellitus to identify risk conditions including: assessment of protective sensation, foot structure, biomechanics, vascular status, and skin integrity. Based on the results of the yearly foot examination more attention should be paid to certain individuals. Those identified with one or more risk factors should be evaluated more frequently for development of additional risk factors. Secondly, people with neuropathy are recommended to have visual inspection of their feet at every visit to their regular healthcare providers. Elements of a foot examination of a person with low risk are listed in Table 7-10.

Sensory Testing on the Foot

In addition to other tools used to determine sensory integrity, diabetic foot screening commonly uses Semmes-Weinstein monofilaments to assess risk of plantar ulceration in ambulatory, sensory-impaired individuals. These special monofilaments are designed to bend at a calibrated

Figure 7-15A. Sensory testing of the neuropathic foot using a 10 g monofilament. A typical device is shown.

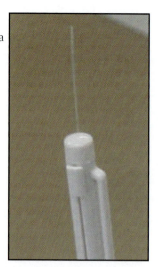

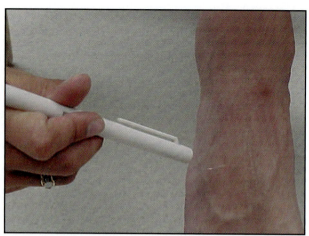

Figure 7-15B. Testing procedure showing bending of the 10 g monofilament on the dorsal foot testing location.

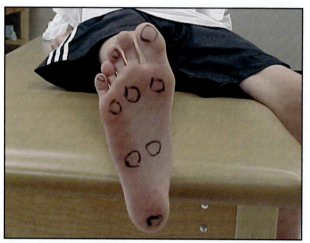

Figure 7-16A. Standard locations for monofilament screening on the plantar surface of the foot.

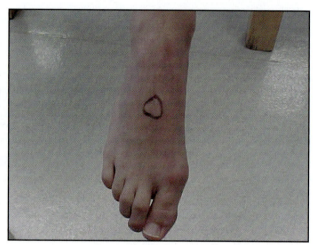

Figure 7-16B. Standard location for monofilament screening on the dorsal surface of the foot.

force. Starting with the thinnest monofilament in the set, each monofilament is touched to skin for total of 1 1/2 seconds: bending for one-half second, left bent for one-half second, and removed for one-half second (Figure 7-15). A person with normal sensation should feel a 10 g monofilament bend. Excessive callus on the foot will, however, decrease the sensitivity of even normal feet. Once a person is able to feel a given monofilament, the clinician stops and records the value. In some cases, a clinician may wish to perform a more thorough test and actually map the entire foot. For a screening procedure, a single 10 g monofilament may be used for a prescribed number of standardized sites (Figure 7-16).

In addition, the clinician should check the foot for deformities and decreased strength, which may alter weightbearing pattern and gait, and visually inspect the skin on each foot. Further sensory testing should be done to distinguish between small and large sensory neuron loss. Reflexes and vibration are carried by large neurons. Loss of these functions indicates a greater degree of neuropathy because loss of neurons generally occurs first in small neurons, progressing to large neurons. Sensations such as temperature and pinprick are carried by smaller, more susceptible neurons. Loss of large neurons is particularly critical. Motor neurons and position sense are carried by large neurons. Loss of the position senses, proprioception, and kinesthesia are likely to exacerbate the problems caused by sensory neuropathy. A typical gait for a person with diminished proprioception includes short, slapping steps and abnormal progression from heel strike to toe off.

Additional testing includes the Michigan Neuropathy Screening Instrument test and vibration perception threshold. Vibration perception threshold is a quantifiable method for testing vibration, instead of a subjective present or absent response. A biothesiometer is applied to the pulp

Patient Version

MICHIGAN NEUROPATHY SCREENING INSTRUMENT

A. History (To be completed by the person with diabetes)

Please take a few minutes to answer the following questions about the feeling in your legs and feet. Check yes or no based on how you usually feel. Thank you.

1. Are your legs and/or feet numb?		Yes	No
2. Do you ever have any burning pain in your legs and/or feet?		Yes	No
3. Are your feet too sensitive to touch?		Yes	No
4. Do you get muscle cramps in your legs and/or feet?		Yes	No
5. Do you ever have any prickling feelings in your legs or feet?		Yes	No
6. Does it hurt when the bed covers touch your skin?		Yes	No
7. When you get into the tub or shower, are you able to tell the hot water from the cold water?		Yes	No
8. Have you ever had an open sore on your foot?		Yes	No
9. Has your doctor ever told you that you have diabetic neuropathy?		Yes	No
10. Do you feel weak all over most of the time?		Yes	No
11. Are your symptoms worse at night?		Yes	No
12. Do your legs hurt when you walk?		Yes	No
13. Are you able to sense your feet when you walk?		Yes	No
14. Is the skin on your feet so dry that it cracks open?		Yes	No
15. Have you ever had an amputation?		Yes	No

Total: _____

How to Use the Michigan Neuropathy Screening Instrument

History

The history questionnaire is self-administered by the patient. Responses are added to obtain the total score. Responses of "yes" to items 1 to 3, 5 to 6, 8 to 9, 11 to 12, 14 to 15 are each counted as 1 point. A "no" response on items 7 and 13 counts as 1 point. Item 4 is a measure of impaired circulation, and item 10 is a measure of general asthenia—they are not included in scoring. To decrease the potential for bias, all scoring information has been eliminated from the patient version.

Physical Assessment

For all assessments, the foot should be warm (>30°C).

Foot Inspection

The feet are inspected for evidence of excessively dry skin, callus formation, fissures, frank ulceration, or deformities. Deformities include flat feet, hammer toes, overlapping toes, hallux valgus, joint subluxation, prominent metatarsal heads, medial convexity (Charcot foot), and amputation.

Vibration Sensation

Vibration sensation should be performed with the great toe unsupported. Vibration sensation will be tested bilaterally using a 128 Hz tuning fork placed over the dorsum of the great toe on the bony prominence of the DIP joint. Patients, whose eyes are closed, will be asked to indicate when they can no longer sense the vibration from the vibrating tuning fork.

In general, the examiner should be able to feel vibration from the hand-held tuning fork for 5 seconds longer on his distal forefinger than a normal subject can at the great toe (eg, examiner's DIP joint of the first finger versus patient's toe). If the examiner feels vibration for 10 or more seconds on his or her finger, then vibration is considered decreased. A trial should be given when the tuning fork is not vibrating to be certain that the patient is responding to vibration and not pressure or some other clue. Vibration is scored as 1) present if the examiner senses the vibration on his or her finger for <10 seconds, 2) reduced if sensed for >10, or 3) absent (no vibration detection).

continued

MICHIGAN NEUROPATHY SCREENING INSTRUMENT

B. Physical Assessment (To be completed by health professional)

1. Appearance of feet	Right a. Normal 0 Yes 1 No b. If no, check all that apply: __Deformities __Dry skin, callus __Infection __Fissure __Other (specify):	Left a. Normal 0 Yes 1 No b. If no, check all that apply: __Deformities __Dry skin, callus __Infection __Fissure __Other specify:

2. Ulceration	Right
	        Absent Present
	           0 1
		Left
		        Absent Present
		           0 1

3. Ankle reflexes	Present Present/Reinforcement Absent
	   0 0.5 1
		Present Present/Reinforcement Absent
		   0 0.5 1

4. Vibration perception at great toe	Present Decreased Absent
	   0 0.5 1
		Present Decreased Absent
		   0 0.5 1

5. Monofilament	Normal Reduced Absent
	   0 0.5 1
		Normal Reduced Absent
		   0 0.5 1

Signature: Total Score: /10 Points

Courtesy of the Michigan Diabetes Research and Training Center, Ann Arbor, MI.

continued

Muscle Stretch Reflexes

The ankle reflexes will be examined using an appropriate reflex hammer (eg, Trommer or Queen square). The ankle reflexes should be elicited in the sitting position with the foot dependent and the patient relaxed. For the reflex, the foot should be passively positioned and the foot dorsiflexed slightly to obtain optimal stretch of the muscle. The Achilles tendon should be percussed directly. If the reflex is obtained, it is graded as present. If the reflex is absent, the patient is asked to perform the Jendrassic maneuver (ie, hooking the fingers together and pulling). Reflexes elicited with the Jendrassic maneuver alone are designated "present with reinforcement." If the reflex is absent, even in the face of the Jendrassic maneuver, the reflex is considered absent.

Monofilament Testing

For this examination, it is important that the patient's foot be supported (ie, allow the sole of the foot to rest on a flat, warm surface). The filament should initially be prestressed (4 to 6 perpendicular applications to the dorsum of the examiner's first finger). The filament is then applied to the dorsum of the great toe midway between the nail fold and the DIP joint. Do not hold the toe directly. The filament is applied perpendicularly and briefly (<1 second), with an even pressure. When the filament bends, the force of 10 grams has been applied. The patient, whose eyes are closed, is asked to respond yes if he or she feels the filament. Eight correct responses out of 10 applications is considered normal, 1 to 7 correct responses indicates reduced sensation, and no correct answers translates into absent sensation.

Courtesy of the Michigan Diabetes Research and Training Center, Ann Arbor, MI.

of toes. The intensity of the stimulus is decreased in stages until it can no longer be detected. The lowest voltage at which the patient can perceive vibration is recorded. Moderate to severe diabetic peripheral neuropathy is defined as a value of 20 to 45 V. The Michigan Neuropathy Screening Instrument consists of a survey instrument consisting of 15 yes/no questions for the patient and 5 areas to be completed by the clinician—foot appearance, presence of ulceration, ankle reflexes, vibration perception at the great toe, and the monofilament test, which have been described as part of a normal physical examination.

Range of Motion

Limited range of motion of the foot and ankle are particularly devastating. A normal foot relaxes and splays as contact is made with the floor to absorb shock. As weight moves from the hind foot to the forefoot, the foot becomes more rigid to allow transfer of force to propel the body forward. Limited range of motion not only causes more energy to enter the plantar surface of the foot as the rigid foot hits the floor, but limited dorsiflexion and first toe extension limit the ability to transfer pressure from the metatarsal head region to the toes. This, in turn, creates a shearing force on the metatarsal heads, especially the first. As a minimum, these biomechanical abnormalities need to be addressed with appropriate footwear from an orthotist or pedorthist.

Shoe Inspection

As discussed with offloading of the foot, part of the evaluation must include inspection of footwear for proper size and construction. Discard any shoes assembled with nails or other sharp objects. Assess the material used for the soles; these should be either rubberized or crepe. Hard leather soles are to be discouraged because of their inability to dissipate mechanical stresses on the foot. As described in the offloading section, draw an outline of the bare foot and stress the importance of using this tracing to compare with any new shoes the patient might wish to purchase. An orthotist or pedorthist can select a shoe with an appropriately shaped last to match the shape of the patient's foot. Individuals with neuropathic feet will frequently purchase shoes that are too small for them. A smaller shoe may create sufficient pressure on the foot to allow perception of the presence of the shoe.

Prevention of high-risk conditions is also recommended. Those at high risk include individuals with distal symmetric polyneuropathy and autonomic neuropathy. Two major recommendations for these individuals are tight control of blood glucose and smoking cessation. In addition, specific recommendations for management include wearing well-cushioned walking or athletic shoes, education on implications of sensory loss and self-monitoring, footwear to distribute pressure if signs of high pressure are evident, debridement of callus to decrease pressure caused

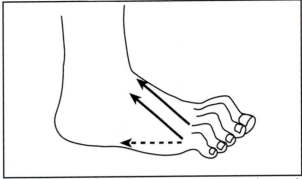

Figure 7-17. Forces producing hammer toes. Normal strength of long extensors of the toes combined with weakness of the intrinsic toe flexors.

by walking on the relatively nondeformable callus, and a vascular evaluation if claudication is determined by history or an exercise test. Extra-wide or depth shoes are recommended if bony deformities such as hammer toes (Figure 7-17) and bunions are present.

Referral to a qualified pedorthist or orthotist for custom-molded shoes should be done if severe deformities, including Charcot foot, are present. Individuals with milder foot deformities may simply need to perform foot tracing before buying shoes to make a comparison of the shape of the foot to the last of the prospective shoe (Figure 7-18). Screening for pressure points on the foot may be performed with a foot imprinter also known as a Harris mat (Figure 7-19). This device consists of an inked mat with a grid system on the underside. Pressure on the imprinter mat causes the inked grid to contact the paper below. The grid system is designed such that low pressures only create a wide grid on the paper, whereas higher pressure creates finer grid lines. Note the high pressures under the first metatarsal head in both examples in Figure 7-19. More sophisticated means of pressure mapping are available, but are quite expensive.

Patient education efforts need to be directed at risk factors and appropriate management, implications of loss of protective sensation, self-monitoring for changes in the foot, foot and nail care, selection of appropriate footwear, and smoking cessation. Learning ability should be assessed individually and the program should be tailored to the patient's preferred learning style. Excellent educational materials are available as part of the Lower Extremity Amputation Prevention (LEAP) program.

American Diabetes Association Position Statement on Foot Care

This position statement addresses management of neuropathic foot ulcers in an attempt to publicize what the ADA believes to be optimal care. Also, the predisposing

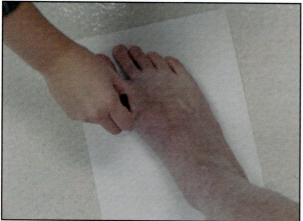

Figure 7-18A. Drawing a template for determining appropriate size and shape of footwear.

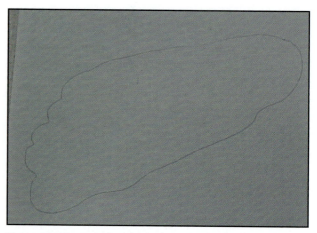

Figure 7-18B. Completed template. This tracing is cut and placed in prospective shoe purchases to determine appropriate fit.

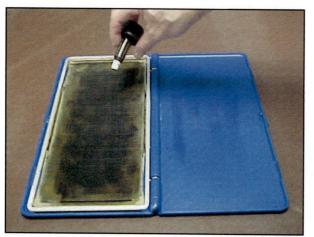

Figure 7-19A. Harris mat foot imprinter is a low-cost screening tool for rapid determination of excess forces on the foot. This figure shows the application of ink to the grid on the underside of the mat.

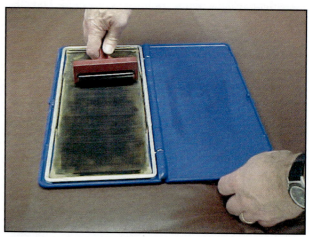

Figure 7-19B. Ink being spread evenly across the grid on the underside of the mat.

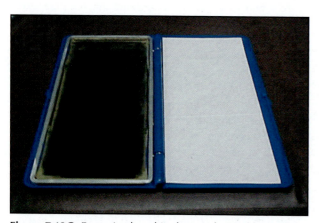

Figure 7-19C. Paper is placed in the tray located beneath the mat.

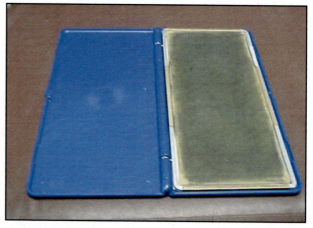

Figure 7-19D. The mat is rotated into its tray with the smooth side up and the inked, grid side down.

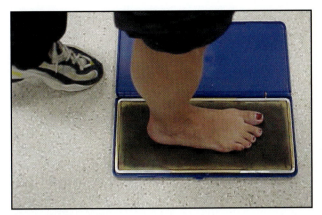

Figure 7-19E. Subject stepping on the mat.

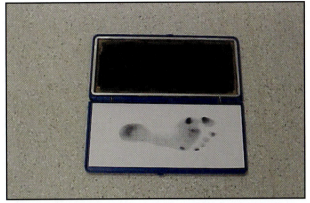

Figure 7-19F. High-pressure areas are indicated by more densely marked portions of paper. Higher pressures are necessary for the progressively closer portions of the grid to come in contact with the paper below it. Note the high pressures on the head of the first metatarsal and proximal, lateral portion of the first toe.

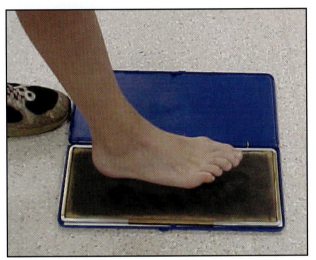

Figure 7-19G. Second subject stepping on mat.

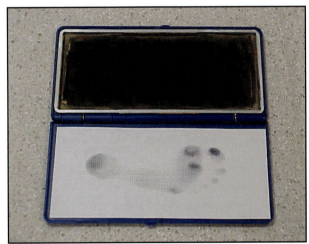

Figure 7-19H. Note the high pressures under the first and second metatarsal heads and first toe.

factors and possible complications relevant to diabetes mellitus should be taken into account rather than simply addressing the open wound. The first priority of the clinician should be determining the ulcer's etiology. Once known, the interventions directed toward cause of the ulcer can be addressed as well as prevention of further ulcers and potential complications that might delay healing. Next the size, depth, and involvement of deep structures should be established. The clinician should examine the wound for purulent exudate, necrosis, sinus tracts, and odor. The surrounding skin should then be assessed for signs of edema, cellulitis, abscess, and fluctuance as well as ruling out systemic infection. The ADA also states that the physical exam should include a vascular exam. The ability to gently probe through the ulcer to bone highly predicts osteomyelitis. A radiologic exam should be done by the physician to exclude subcutaneous gas, presence of foreign body, osteomyelitis, and Charcot's foot. Distinguishing between Charcot foot and osteomyelitis may be difficult in some cases. According to the position

statement, plain radiographs showing periosteal resorption and osteolysis are consistent with, but not diagnostic of osteomyelitis. Rather, a bone scan, WBC imaging, MRI or bone biopsy may be necessary to distinguish osteomyelitis and Charcot foot.

Bacterial cultures and antibiotics are also addressed in the position statement. Because bacterial infections of foot lesions tend to be polymicrobial, broad-spectrum antibiotics should be used immediately, but should be modified based on culture results and patient response to treatment. As discussed more thoroughly in Chapter 9, swab cultures are not sufficient for management decisions. Deep specimens obtained by curettage at the base of wound should be used instead. The ADA states that abscessed infections should be incised and drained with debridement down to viable tissue. The ADA does not specifically endorse the use of topical agents. Rather they state that the use of topical agents is controversial and no adequate evidence exists for their use. Contrary to the popular practice of soaking ulcers, the ADA states specifically that prolonged immersion of feet in water is not recommended.

With regard to mechanical stress, the ADA recommends minimizing weightbearing on ulcers by bed rest or, when ambulatory, by crutches. Also recommended are heel and ankle protection and daily inspection of both lower extremities. Other protection suggested include the use of total-contact casts for protecting healing ulcers, and either shoe inserts or special shoes for those with foot deformities. Candidates for vascular reconstruction include those with slow or inadequate healing, decreased pulses and decreased pressure by Doppler exam, and avoiding vasoconstrictor drugs.

Metabolic control is probably the greatest predictor of long-term health in the person with diabetes mellitus and perhaps even more so in individuals with neuropathic ulcers. Open wounds can make management of blood sugar more complex. Infection and inflammation can cause wide fluctuations in blood sugar. Surgical or medical treatment of the neuropathic ulcer can help control blood sugar. Moreover, poor glucose control hinders healing and overall nutritional status should be monitored by an appropriate clinician. Post-healing management needs to continue to address potential complications. Anyone with neuropathic ulcers is at high risk of future ulceration and requires an education program that emphasizes daily inspection, possible job modification, prescribed footwear, walking or athletic shoes, soft insoles, extra-depth shoes, custom-molded inlays, and custom-molded therapeutic shoes.

Ulcer Recurrence and Failure to Heal

By definition, the term *ulcer recurrence* can apply after 6 months of closure. Recurrence has been shown to happen in 34%, 61%, and 70% of cases after 1, 2, and 3 years. Recurrence after total contact casting has been reported to be between 32% and 57%. Failure to heal is reported to occur in 10% to 22% of cases. Reasons reported for failure to heal include undiagnosed infection and failure of the patient to adhere to the treatment plan. Failure to heal is also reported to be correlated with presence and degree of autonomic neuropathy. Total contact casting is reported to be cost-effective. A typical 8-week course of treatment includes 6 to 8 casts, costing in the range of $810 to $1,050. On the other hand, a short stay in an acute care hospital (3 to 5) days costs more than $2,000, not including physician fees, diagnostic work-ups and procedures, or medications. Other options are less costly than total contact casting and are suitable alternatives for patients who can be trusted to use the orthoses as instructed.

Following complete healing of the wound, definitive treatment to minimize risk of recurrence or new ulcerations is to fit the patient for appropriate shoes. The risk of recurrence of plantar ulcers has been reported to be 26% for those wearing special shoes compared with 83% who wore their own shoes. Either off-the-shelf or custom shoes may be needed for long-term use. Custom-fit shoes designed for the individual require a mold of the foot, analysis of normal and abnormal forces on the foot, and modifications to relieve abnormal pressures. A patient may be referred to an orthotist or pedorthist for proper fitting or molding of custom shoes. In the case of lost range of motion of the foot or fixed deformities, a steel shank rocker bottom can be used to offload the metatarsal heads. Constructed properly, special shoes can offload a foot to nearly normal amounts of pressure and shear. Medicare part B will supply a maximum of one pair of custom shoes per year. The patient must use the shoes prudently. Some have advocated that the patient purchase a new pair every year and rotate through different shoes. If this strategy is undertaken, the clinician must assure that the older shoes are still effectively offloading the foot.

Effects of Diabetic Neuropathy

Diabetic polyneuropathy has a prevalence of 7.5% in newly diagnosed diabetes mellitus, which increases with the duration of the disease. Diabetic polyneuropathy is estimated to be present in 50% of individuals after 25 years of disease with an overall 30% prevalence, which is similar in types 1 and 2. This condition is manifested in multiple ways and a person may have 2 or more types of peripheral neuropathy at once. The types are classified by their anatomic distribution into diffuse neuropathy and focal neuropathy. Diffuse neuropathy may present as distal symmetric sensorimotor polyneuropathy, autonomic neuropathy, or symmetric proximal lower limb motor neuropathy. Focal neuropathy may be superimposed on diffuse neuropathy and present as a complex clinical picture of one or more very specific neurologic deficits with no systematic anatomic basis, autonomic dysfunction, and homogenous distal neurologic deficits.

Derangement of nociceptive neurons frequently leads to neuropathic pain, which may be described as burning, sharp, shooting or deep aching. As the neuropathy advances, signs and symptoms of large neuron involvement become evident. These include the loss of vibratory sensation and proprioception, and absent or reduced deep tendon reflexes, especially the ankle jerk and slow nerve conduction velocity in advanced disease. Numbness, tingling, and a sensation of tightness may also be reported in advanced disease. Autonomic neuropathy is present in 40% of individuals with type 2 diabetes at the time of diagnosis. Typical manifestations of autonomic neuropathy include sexual dysfunction, gastroparesis (diminished motility of the stomach and gastrointestinal tract), diabetic diarrhea, bladder atony, loss of sweating in the feet and cardiovascular abnormalities such as postural hypotension, loss of normal heart rate variability, and arrhythmias leading to sudden death. The pathophysiology of peripheral neuropathy includes damage caused by sorbitol accumulation, ischemia of neurons due to atherosclerosis and diminished expression of nerve growth factor. Excessive blood glucose is converted to sorbitol, which, in turn, accumulates in tissues. Sorbitol accumulation causes decreased production of myoinositol and taurine which leads to decreased Na/K ATPase and slowed nerve conduction velocity. Researchers have attempted to correct nerve injury secondary to sorbitol accumulation with aldose reductase inhibitors, but have yet to be successful in restoring neuronal function.

Pharmacologic Treatment of Neuropathic Pain

Neuropathic pain can be severe and debilitating. It is frequently cited by patients/clients as a reason for not participating in exercise programs. Complaints of sudden burning, shooting pains (dysesthesia), and pins and needles (paresthesia) are common. Patients/clients often also report a greater intensity and frequency of neuropathic pain in affected limbs during weightbearing and exercise. Recently, however, several drugs have been shown to be very effective for reducing neuropathic pain in certain individuals. These include tricyclic antidepressants such as amitriptyline, the anticonvulsant drug gabapentin, which stimulates inhibitory central neurons, and capsaicin, which is used as a topical analgesic for arthritis and musculoskeletal pain. Capsaicin, the active ingredient of chili peppers is believed to work by depletion of substance P, thereby preventing the transmission of pain information to the spinal cord. Doxepin cream has recently been added to the options for treating neuropathic pain. It is a topic tricyclic antidepressant and an antihistamine effective at both H1 and H2 receptors.

Surgical Treatments for Diabetic Neuropathy

Procedures have been described to address altered biomechanics of the foot to decompress peripheral nerves. Surgery may be performed on diabetic feet to correct a painful deformity, reduce risk of ulceration or reulceration due to deformities, or treat infection. Procedures to lengthen the Achilles tendon, tenotomy of toe flexor tendons, and exostomy of bones causing excessive plantar pressure have been described. Midfoot, rear foot, and ankle arthrodeses are described for correction of Charcot foot. Triple and pantalar arthrodeses may be used for extreme cases. Incision and drainage of

abscesses, debridement, and amputations are performed to treat infection.

Decompression of the tibial, deep peroneal, and common peroneal nerves (triple nerve decompression) through ligament release surgery has been reported to reduce risk of plantar foot ulcer incidence. Other studies have shown increased sensation in terms of 2-point discrimination and decreased sway through decompression procedures.

WOUNDS DUE TO CHRONIC VENOUS INSUFFICIENCY

Wounds caused by chronic venous insufficiency (CVI) are very common. Prevalence of varicose veins is estimated at 30% in women and 15% in men. Edema and skin changes (hyperpigmentation and lipodermatosclerosis) occur in about 3% to 11% of the population. Prevalence of ulcers is estimated to be 1% in Western civilization. In addition, healing is generally slow and recurrence is common. Approximately 50% heal within 4 months and 8% remain open after 5 years.

Ulcers caused by CVI have also been called venous stasis ulcers due to a lack of understanding of their pathophysiology; they are not caused by lack of venous flow, but diminished diffusion of nutrients through the interstitial space from capillaries. The root cause of venous insufficiency ulcers is venous hypertension and the consequences of capillary injury by this hypertension. The appearance of involved legs resembles eczema and the term *stasis dermatitis* is often used. *Lipodermatosclerosis* is the preferred term to describe skin with fatty necrosis, and fibrosis of skin and subcutaneous tissue, resulting in induration and hemosiderin accumulation. Through a sequence of events described below, venous hypertension leads to malnutrition of the skin and a limited depth of subcutaneous tissue. In many cases, patients will identify trauma to the affected leg as the cause of the wound. In these cases, however, the patient has simply traumatized necrotic tissue that likely would eventually open into wounds without trauma.

Venous hypertension results in elevated capillary pressure to the extent that capillaries begin to leak fluid, macromolecules, and red blood cells into the interstitial space. As a result, edema of the affected extremity occurs, along with hardening of the skin and the presence of hemosiderin staining. The brawniness of the extremity appears to be due to the leakage of protein into the interstitial space with resultant fibrosis. Leakage of red cells and their breakdown leads to the formation of biliverdin, bilirubin, and hemosiderin (a storage form of iron) in the skin with an obvious brownish-yellow discoloration. The appearance of venous ulcers is shown in Figure 7-20. These wounds are

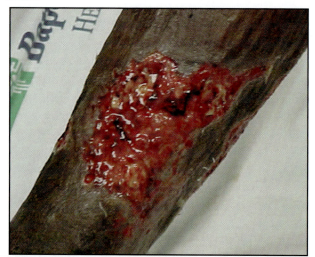

Figure 7-20A. Appearance of leg with wound secondary to chronic venous insufficiency. Note the irregular borders, location, copious drainage, and red granulation tissue.

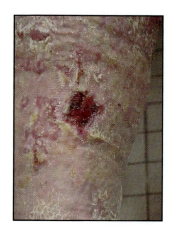

Figure 7-20B. Dermatitis associated with chronic venous insufficiency, frequently termed *stasis dermatitis*. Note deposits of hemosiderin in skin and indentations in skin from compression bandaging.

usually full-thickness with irregular edges, but without subcutaneous involvement. Often the wound bed appears very healthy with a red, shiny appearance due to good arterial inflow. However, many individuals may have peripheral artery disease and venous disease concurrently. This situation complicates treatment and will be discussed specifically below. Many individuals have suffered for years from slow healing and recurrent ulcers because treatment has been directed solely toward the wound without addressing the underlying problem of venous hypertension.

Anatomy of Venous System

Compared with the arterial system, the venous system is highly redundant. This redundancy increases the collective cross-sectional area of veins, allowing venous flow to equal that of the arteries in spite of the much lower pressure present in normal veins. The presence of large numbers of veins also allows the veins to become active components of the thermoregulatory system as warm blood is directed through veins within the skin to dissipate heat. This redundancy also provides additional pathways should a vein become injured or occluded. The venous system of the lower extremities is divided into three components. The veins that accompany arteries and are given the same name as the artery are located subfascially and are termed *deep veins*. Veins that may be seen in the skin are termed *superficial veins*. These veins become more prominent during exercise or with increased core temperature. They are also more prominent in individuals with minimal subcutaneous fat such as body builders. Blood is allowed to drain from superficial veins into deep veins through a system of veins that perforate the fascia. They have been given names such as perforators and communicating veins. Veins have one-way valves that aid flow from distal to

proximal and from superficial to deep veins. The presence of valves in superficial veins of the forearm was critical in the demonstration by Harvey (Scultetus, et al) that blood flows through the body in vessels.

Function of the Venous Pump

This pump, similar to any other pump, requires a force to drive flow, patent conduits, and a one-way valving system. The calf pump uses contraction of leg muscles to pump blood from the dependent lower extremities by taking advantage of one-way valves present in the veins. Without the calf pump, blood pressure in the foot may increase an additional 100 mmHg for an individual approximately six feet in height when moving from supine to standing. To lower venous and capillary pressure to manageable levels, pumping of blood caused by intermittent contraction of leg muscles must be functional. The components of the calf pump are illustrated in Figure 7-21.

Causes of Venous Hypertension

Venous hypertension represents failure of the calf pumping mechanism. In the absence of effective pumping, volume and pressure increases in veins. For blood to move from capillaries into the engorged veins, the outflow pressure of capillaries increases until pressure within capillaries exceeds pressure within the draining veins. This high pressure causes the leakage of water, electrolytes, and other small molecules. As pressure increases, larger constituents of blood including proteins and cells may leak from capillaries. Edema of venous disease results from both high hydrostatic pressure and the high concentration of protein in the interstitial space. As protein leaks from capillaries into interstitial space, the osmotic gradient that normally opposes movement of fluid out of capillaries is decreased, allowing fluid to escape at an even greater rate than it would by the hydrostatic pressure alone.

Normal loss of fluid and plasma proteins can be handled by lymphatic drainage; however, with venous hypertension, proteins leak out faster into the interstitial space than

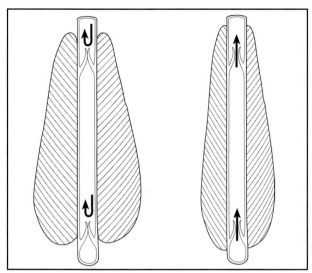

Figure 7-21. Components of the calf pump. Pumping requires the presence of unobstructed vessels, valves to ensure unidirectional flow, and a source of energy (muscle contraction).

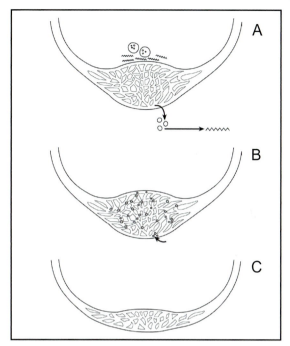

Figure 7-22. Pathophysiology of ulcers due to chronic venous insufficiency. (A) Leakage of proteins from capillaries. (B) Inflammation caused by trapped leukocytes. (C) Rarefaction of capillaries secondary to venous hypertension.

they can be taken up, resulting in accumulation of plasma proteins in the interstitial space. Although edema alone increases the diffusion distance for nutrients, the presence of proteins, particularly fibrinogen has been blamed for tissue injury. Interstitial fibrinogen may be converted to the insoluble protein fibrin, which is the major component of thrombi. Excessive water and protein combined with decreased numbers of capillaries diminish diffusion of oxygen and nutrients required for the health of tissue surrounding the vein. Within the capillaries, hypertension produces dilation, elongation, and tortuosity and frequently thrombosis, similar to the effect hypertension has on superficial veins as they become varicose veins. These changes in capillaries are most pronounced in areas with hyperpigmentation and lipodermatosclerosis. Capillary changes are also most often observed in patients with insufficient perforator and deep veins. Several theories of how venous hypertension results in malnutrition have been proposed. Three particular theories with merit are pericapillary fibrin cuffs, leukocyte trapping, and microangiopathy (see Figure 7-22).

Pericapillary Fibrin Cuffs

The theory of Burnand and Browse is based on the concept of macromolecular leakage due to high capillary hydrostatic pressure. Fibrinogen leaking from capillaries polymerizes into fibrin, creating a diffusion barrier between the capillary and tissues supplied by them. This theory enjoys substantial experimental support, but is inadequate to explain the low tissue PO_2 associated with venous hypertension.

Leukocyte Trapping

The low pressure gradient across capillaries due to venous hypertension is believed to produce sluggish capillary blood flow and enhance the probability of leukocyte adherence to the capillary endothelium, with increased expression of leukocyte adhesion molecules. Leukocyte adhesion then leads to production of chemical mediators of inflammation and tissue injury.

Microangiopathy

Elevated venous pressure due to calf-pump failure causes elevated pressure and dilation of capillaries. Capillary distention can be observed before the tissue injury characteristic of venous hypertension can be observed, and the severity of skin damage and capillary injury are highly correlated. A severe reduction in the number of capillaries can be observed within the ulcer itself and at the edge of the ulcer. A large number of damaged capillaries characterized by dilation, elongation, tortuosity, stasis, and thrombosis can be observed. Thus, avascular areas develop resulting in tissue injury, progressing to tissue death and ulceration of the skin. Wound healing would also be expected to be slow or absent given the lack of nutritive circulation. A correlation between loss of capillaries and transcutaneous oxygen ($TcPO_2$) has been demonstrated in a series of patients with chronic venous insufficiency. During healing, capillary density improved in all cases in both the ulcer and surrounding skin on the ulcer's edge. A greater increase in capillary density was observed in patients with relatively rapid healing compared with patients with relatively slow healing. In addition, $TcPO_2$ increased rapidly in the fast healers and was initially lower in slow healers. Healing was accompanied by an increased $TcPO_2$ in both groups, but was higher in the fast healers. Although healing occurred in these patients, the deranged capillary morphology remained. This, in part, may explain the high recurrence of ulceration in patients simply receiving treatment for ulcerations, but not for venous hypertension.

Risk Factors for Venous Disease

Knowing the parts of the calf pump, possible causes of calf pump failure become easily identified. The causes can be categorized as outflow obstruction, valve insufficiency, or loss of muscle pumping action (Figure 7-23). Venous outflow obstruction may occur from within the venous vessels or be caused by external compression. Typically, internal obstruction results from deep venous thrombosis or clotting. External compression may result from a tumor, such as an enlarged lymph node in the groin, pregnancy, obesity, or inappropriate application of elasticized garments. Insufficient valves may occur in the deep veins running alongside arteries, superficial veins or the communicating veins that allow the superficial veins to drain into the deep veins. Many individuals appear to be genetically predisposed to venous valve weakness. Once venous valves begin to fail, a chain reaction of valve failure results. As a valve fails, pressure rises in the veins until inflow becomes equal to outflow. The lack of outflow results in venous hypertension, dilation, and tortuosity. When dilation and tortuosity of superficial veins are evident, the term *varicose veins* is used. The failure of one segment of a vein predisposes those below it to failure. The inability of leaflets of a venous valve to support the column of blood above it increases the height of the column of blood on the next valve below it. This, in turn, sets in motion propagation of valvular failure, producing a positive feedback of insufficiency and dilation. Loss of muscle pumping action may occur following neuromuscular or musculoskeletal disease or injury or immobilization used to treat a musculoskeletal injury. Potential causes of venous hypertension are listed in Table 7-11.

The greater saphenous vein is particularly susceptible to failure because of its location. Subfascial (deep) veins are readily compressed between bone and muscle during muscle contraction. More superficial veins may still experience pumping due to compression between the skin and muscle. However, the greater saphenous vein primarily runs along the medial surface of the tibia, between bone and skin. This area will not be subjected to as much com-

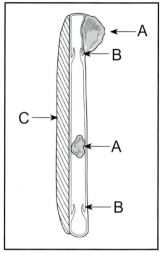

Figure 7-23. Potential causes of calf pump failure. (A) Obstruction of the vein from outside by a mass such as a tumor, and from inside by a blood clot. (B) Incompetent venous valves. (C) Loss of muscle function due to atrophy in this example.

pression as other veins and therefore, is more susceptible to varicosity formation. The greater saphenous vein is also the longest vein in the body, running along the medial thigh and leg. Perforators between the greater saphenous veins and tibial veins located above the medial malleolus are particularly prone to failure and represent a target for surgical treatment for venous disease.

Venous Disease Classification

A classification scheme used for venous disease uses a grading and categorical system to describe the severity, etiology, and the type of vein involved. The CEAP categories are clinical appearance (7 gradations for severity), etiology (congenital, primary, secondary), anatomy (superficial, deep, or perforating), and pathophysiology (obstruction or reflux). For the anatomy and pathophysiology components of this classification scheme, any or all of the terms may be used. Etiology may be congenital (rare) or may be either or both primary and secondary. Primary refers to the cause being attributable to a defect in the vein itself, not secondary to another phenomenon. For example, primary and reflux would be used together to describe a vein with failing valves occurring without any injury to the vein (assumed to be hereditary). The terms *secondary* and *obstruction* are frequently used together because conditions such as compression of veins due to obesity, pregnancy, tumor, or improperly applied elastic bandage or cast is responsible, or clotting within a vein causes the obstruction (the obstruction is secondary to another problem). The definitions for clinical picture are given in Table 7-12.

For example, a case of large tortuous varicose veins caused by valve failure, but no other manifestations of venous disease, the situation is described as $C_2 E_P A_{S,P} P_R$. In the case in which an ulcer is observed, a combination of insufficient valves and compression due to obesity leads

Table 7-11

Causes of Venous Hypertension

Insufficient valves

Insufficient valves of deep veins
Insufficient valves of communicating veins
Insufficient valves of superficial veins (varicose veins)

Obstruction of lower extremity veins

Pregnancy
Obesity
Clotting/thrombosis of veins

Insufficient calf muscle activity

Prolonged standing
Neuromuscular disease affecting the leg muscles
Musculoskeletal injury or disease affecting the leg muscles
Immobilization of the lower extremity

to insufficiency of deep, superficial, and perforating veins, $C_6 E_{P,S} A_{D,S,P} P_{O,R}$ is used.

Differential Diagnosis

The ability to distinguish between arterial and venous disease as causes of ulcers is generally simple with a systematic investigation of the following characteristics: pain, the effect of elevation, the distribution and appearance of the wounds, and special tests described earlier in Chapter 6. Ischemic ulcers can be very painful, increasing with exercise and elevation. Venous ulcers are relatively pain free with some discomfort or bursting sensation, which increases in the dependent position and is relieved with elevation. As discussed above, arterial insufficiency produces ulcers on the most distal areas of the body, especially the toes and heels, whereas venous insufficiency creates wounds almost always on the distal leg superior to the malleoli, with approximately two-thirds occurrence on the medial side and one-third on the lateral side. Arterial insufficiency creates deeper, well demarcated wounds without the presence of granulation tissue. During healing of ischemic ulcers, granulation tissue has more of a pink, rather than the beefy red color of granulation tissue seen in wounds with adequate blood flow.

By the time arterial insufficiency ulcers begin to appear, the patient usually has pain even at rest. Dry gangrene of severe disease is characterized by depressed, punched out, blackened areas. Round or elliptical wounds are generally the result of tissue loading caused by either unrelieved pressure over bony prominences or neuropathy of the foot. Moreover, the skin surrounding the arterial wound displays signs of ischemia such as pallor or mottling of the skin (variegated coloration of the skin).

The appearance of venous ulcers is usually very stereotypical with hemosiderin staining and induration of the surrounding skin, and a granulating wound base that looks ready to heal. However, the edema and induration in severe, longstanding venous disease can produce an appearance similar to that of lymphatic disease. In a minority of cases, some aspects of the appearance of venous ulcers may be overlooked. With a history of varicose veins, or a job requiring a person to stand still throughout the day, then special tests may be necessary to confirm the cause as venous hypertension.

The special tests for the vascular system are described in Chapter 6. These tests include the arterial tests of using a Doppler to determine the presence of distal arterial flow, ABI (indicates occlusion if ankle blood pressure is significantly less than blood pressure in the arm), and pneumoplethysmography waveforms indicating the ratio of blood flow during diastole compared with blood flow during systole. Venous tests include the percussion test, Trendelenburg test, venous filling test, and venous plethysmography (refilling time faster with incompetent valves).

Surgical Treatment of Venous Disease

Several surgical alternatives for correcting venous disease are now available. The type of procedure is

Table 7-12

Descriptions Used for the CEAP System

Clinical Picture

C_0 = No clinical signs
C_1 = Small varicose veins
C_2 = Large varicose veins
C_3 = Edema
C_4 = Skin changes
C_5 = Healed ulcer
C_6 = Active Ulcer

Etiology

Congenital (EC)
Primary (EP)
Secondary (ES)

Anatomy

Superficial (AS)
Deep (AD)
Perforating (AP)

Pathophysiology

Reflux (PR)
Obstruction (PO)

determined by the criteria discussed with the CEAP system. Smaller veins (spider veins) can be managed with sclerotherapy or cosmetic laser. Either procedure results in ablation of small varicosities that are generally more of a cosmetic problem than one leading to skin ulceration. Multiple attempts may be required for some of these veins. Multiple injections of a sclerosing solution are injected into minute varicosities. This technique is being adapted for larger veins as transcatheter foam sclerotherapy with carbon dioxide mixed with the sclerosing agent sodium tetradecyl sulfate.

Most procedures for larger varicosities are directed toward the greater saphenous vein, as this is the most prone to reflux. The old approach of vein stripping is still available for removing superficial veins, but is now done in a way that is less troublesome cosmetically with multiple stab wounds rather than a single, long incision.

A procedure called SEPS (subfascial endoscopic perforating vein surgery) is useful for venous disease caused by perforators. Frequently, both superficial and perforator veins are involved, especially when the condition is more chronic. Other options include radiofrequency ablation and endovenous laser. These two techniques are used to ablate perforators, rather than tying them off. These procedures can provide effective treatment for even severe, prominent, tortuous veins. The endovenous radiofrequency obliteration procedure uses radiofrequency waves to obliterate perforators. It is less invasive and less prone to bruising than laser or SEPS.

Compression Therapy

Definitive treatment for venous ulcers involves compression therapy or surgery to ameliorate the underlying cause of venous hypertension. Gentle cleansing of wounds should be done with each dressing change. Using typical whirlpool therapy creates more problems with venous insufficiency. Typical whirlpool temperatures increasing arterial inflow and the dependent position with the thigh compressed over the edge of the whirlpool tank exacerbate venous insufficiency. Compression may be

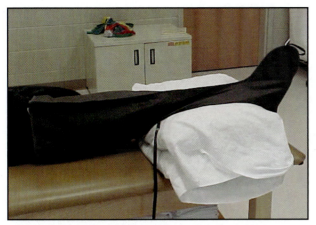

Figure 7-24. Single-cell compression pump. A single air chamber is alternately inflated and deflated. An on-time and off-time must be set as well as the pressure.

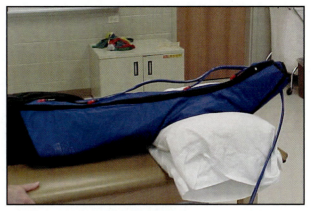

Figure 7-25A. Sequential compression pump. Four air chambers are sequentially inflated in the distal-to-proximal direction. For this model, only the pressure exerted by the pump is adjustable. All 4 chambers are deflated.

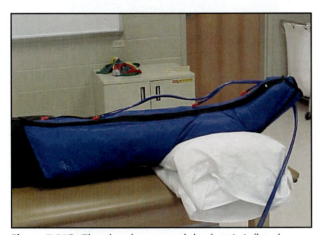

Figure 7-25B. The chamber around the foot is inflated.

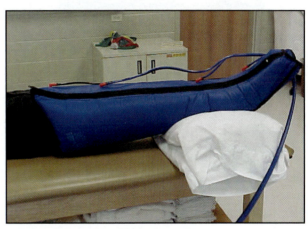

Figure 7-25C. All 4 chambers are inflated.

performed with a clinical or home compression pump. Some older compression pumps are single cell units in which a single sleeve inflates and deflates rhythmically (Figure 7-24). Most newer devices are sequential, multicell pumps in which 3 or 4 cells inflate sequentially from distal (over the foot) toward the knee, then over the thigh. The cells deflate in reverse order and begin inflation distally toward proximally again (Figure 7-25). Any wounds should be covered with an appropriate dressing and a plastic bag to prevent soiling the compression sleeve. The bagged extremity is then placed into the compression sleeve and the affected extremity is elevated slightly. Pumping is done for 1 hour with pressure at 50 mmHg, or less than diastolic pressure. Pressure higher than 50 mmHg is believed to compress lymphatic vessels and pressure less than diastolic ensures some circulation into the extremity for the entire cardiac cycle. If using a single cell sleeve, 90 seconds on, 30 seconds off is commonly used. A sequential pump is simply allowed to run

continuously as described above. If the patient needs to be seen in a clinic, treatment may be done 2 to 3 times per week. A more cost effective strategy is for a rental or a home unit for more frequent treatments up to twice per day.

Compression must be maintained between treatments. Several options are now available in addition to the old standard of the Unna's boot. Unna's boot is messy to apply (Figure 7-26) and regulating the pressure within it is difficult. It is typically only useful in ambulatory patients in whom the semirigid dressing aids the calf pump mechanism. In addition, the Unna's boot loses effectiveness as volume of the leg decreases, the bandage material cannot absorb much drainage and maceration of the periwound skin may occur unless other steps are used to manage drainage from the wound. In many cases, compression is achieved solely with bandaging, rather than use of compression pumps. Multilayer bandaging systems consisting of either 2 (Figure 7-27), 3, or 4 layers

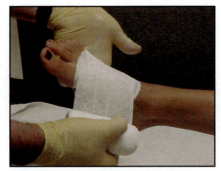

Figure 7-26A. Application of an Unna's boot. Application begins around the metatarsal heads with the bandage applied in a figure 8 fashion proximally.

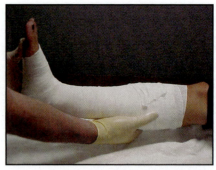

Figure 7-26B. Completed application of the Unna's boot paste bandage.

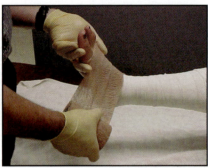

Figure 7-26C. Second layer consists of cohesive bandaging, also applied in a figure 8. This layer prevents soiling of clothing by the material on the Unna's boot bandage and prevents unraveling.

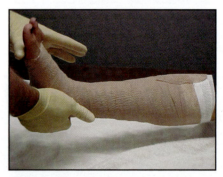

Figure 7-26D. Complete Unna's boot application with paste bandage and cohesive bandage.

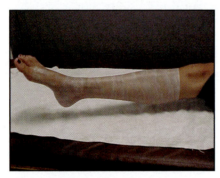

Figure 7-26E. Residue left on patient's leg and foot from the Unna's boot.

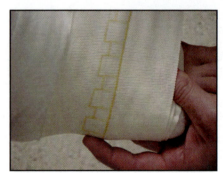

Figure 7-27A. Two-layer bandage application. Markings on the elasticized bandage indicate appropriate tension to produce the desired pressure when applied in half-overlapping spiral technique. Short quadrangles are stretched into squares to produce approximately 30 mmHg pressure in the leg.

Figure 7-27B. Further stretching causes larger quadrangles to form squares and produce approximately 50 mmHg pressure on the leg.

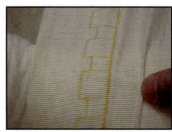

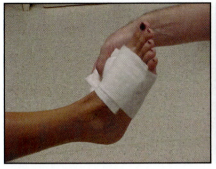

Figure 7-28A. Four-layer compression bandaging. First layer of absorbent batting is applied in half-overlapping spirals with particular attention to filling areas around the malleoli.

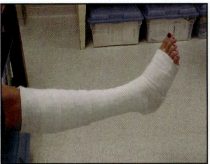

Figure 7-28B. Completion of the first layer.

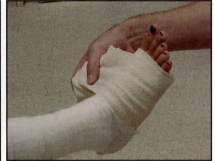

Figure 7-28C. Beginning of half-overlapping spiral technique with the light stretch bandage.

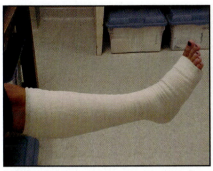

Figure 7-28D. Completion of the second layer.

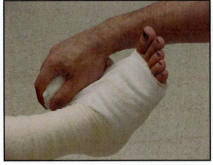

Figure 7-28E. Beginning of third layer, the short-stretch bandage in a figure 8 technique.

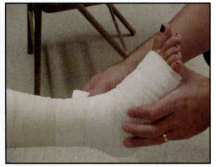

Figure 7-28F. Foot completed; starting up the leg.

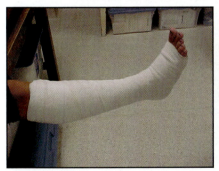

Figure 7-28G. Completion of third layer. Note diamond pattern generated by figure 8 technique.

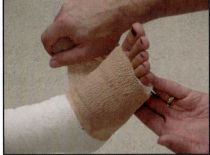

Figure 7-28H. Beginning of fourth layer, the cohesive bandage.

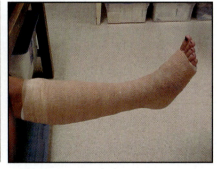

Figure 7-28I. Completion of fourth layer.

(Figure 7-28) can be applied much faster than an Unna's boot, the pressure can be applied easily, the bandages can be removed easily, and the multilayer system creates a more uniform pressure and provides a layer for absorption of drainage. Multilayer bandaging systems utilize short-stretch bandages. These elastic bandages provide compression effectively both at rest and during muscle contraction. Long-stretch bandages, such as ACE wraps, must be pulled with great tension and may provide excessive pressure at rest. During exercise, these bandages give too easily and do not provide useful compression. Regardless of the type of compression system used, the clinician must ensure that the bandaging does not create excessive pressure, and must provide the patient with emergency information of how, and under what conditions, to remove the compression bandaging. A simple test is to check capillary refill (Figure 7-29). Compression pumps and bandages should be used until the clinician is certain that edema has been removed as much as possible. This is determined most objectively

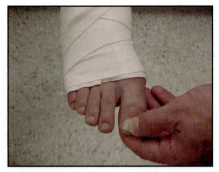

Figure 7-29A. Compressing great toe nail for testing capillary refill.

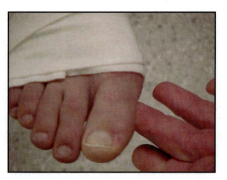

Figure 7-29B. Example of normal capillary refill.

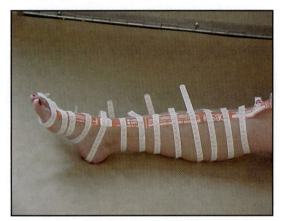

Figure 7-30. Measuring for a custom-fit stocking using device supplied by manufacturer. Note the heel strap, which is used as a reference point in the manufacture of this stocking. Also note the irregular spacing on the foot. This is caused by the requirement to have the second-to-last strap around the metatarsal heads, and the last strap at the base of the toe. On the leg, the straps should be parallel to each other and perpendicular to the spine of the series of straps. Note the fourth strap from the knee is incorrectly applied for the purpose of demonstration.

by serial measurement with a foot volumeter, although multiple girth measurements along the leg or the figure 8 measurement may be used. When volume of the leg is no longer decreasing with compression, the patient should be fitted for custom compression stockings (Figure 7-30). The clinician must check the other leg to determine if venous insufficiency is also present in that extremity.

Multilayer Bandaging

In multilayer bandaging systems, the first layer is generally a layer of absorbent batting. This layer absorbs drainage and fills irregular areas such as those around the malleolus where pressure may be low without appropriate padding. Another layer generally found is a short-stretch bandage. A short-stretch bandage applies adequate pressure with little increase in length, as opposed to long-stretch bandages,

which elongate more for the same increase in pressure. Many of the short-stretch bandages have calibrated markings to indicate the amount of pressure that will be exerted by the bandage at a given length. Typically, rectangles are elongated into squares when the appropriate tension is achieved. An outside layer of cohesive bandage is frequently a component of the multilayer bandage system. Without the outer layer, what may be termed the *folding cup phenomenon* is likely to occur between clinic visits. This phenomenon refers to the propensity for the upper turns of the elastic bandages to become dislodged and slide down the leg, in a manner ascribed to the collapsible camping cup. In a 4-layer system, the second layer, which goes over the absorbent batting, is a moderate stretch bandage, the third layer is a short stretch bandage, and the fourth layer is a cohesive bandage. This type of bandage should be left in place as long as feasible, which typically is about 7 days. Both half-overlapping spirals and figure 8s have been suggested for various layers of the bandaging systems. Half-overlapping spirals are simpler to apply, but unravel more readily and may not control venous hypertension as well. A figure 8 is difficult for the novice (can be performed almost as quickly as a spiral wrap by an experienced clinician) but appears to control venous hypertension more effectively. The absorbent batting layer is generally applied with half-overlapping spirals with extra padding over irregular surfaces. Moderate stretch may be applied with half-overlapping spirals. Short-stretch bandages are expected to be wrapped in a figure 8 and cohesive layers may be applied either way. When using a kit, follow the manufacturer's directions for wrapping each layer. The length of each bandage supplied is based on whether a half-overlapping spiral or figure 8 technique is to be used. A figure 8 technique uses much more bandage length. Using a figure 8 for a layer that the manufacturer instructs using a half-overlapping spiral is likely to result in having insufficient bandage length.

Unna's Boot

Several techniques have been used to apply an Unna's boot. A figure 8 allows some movement between layers and dissipation of excessive pressure. Other options include creating a figure 8 with strips instead of rolling the bandage around the limb. This technique is suggested to allow more give than a figure 8 being rolled. Others simply use half-overlapping spirals and go up, back down, and up again as the length of the bandage allows. Periodic smoothing of the paste should be done as the bandage is applied to provide more even distribution of the paste.

General Wrapping Considerations

Bandaging should produce a greater pressure at the ankle and be progressively decreased as the bandage is wrapped more proximally. This pressure gradient can be automatically developed during the bandaging process by applying equal tension to the bandage as wrapping proceeds. Based on the law of LaPlace, tension equals pressure times radius ($\tau = P \times r$, where τ = tension in the bandage, P = pressure generated by the bandage on the limb, and r = radius of the limb). Therefore, wrapping the bandage with a constant tension as it is advanced from the foot toward the knee results in a greater pressure at the foot where the radius of the turns of the bandage is small and pressure is lower near the knee where the radius of the leg becomes largest.

Using multiple bandages or layers of bandages creates a somewhat more complex situation. An equation used to account for multiple layers and different widths of bandages is given as: $P = NTk/CW$ where N = number of layers, T = tension, k is a constant, C = circumference, and W = width of the bandage. The practical implications of this equation are: 1) more layers create a greater pressure on the limb; 2) with increasing circumference, pressure is reduced; 3) narrower bandages create more pressure; 4) increasing the number of layers increases the circumference, so at some point the effect of adding layers becomes offset by the increase in circumference and the effect of adding layers is lost; 5) if one desires to create less pressure proximally, greater width bandages may be used as one proceeds from distally to proximally. The last implication is the constant in the equation. The actual pressure generated on the limb during simple compression bandaging is not known, but can only be estimated. Experience is needed to ensure that bandaging produces an effective pressure on the limb.

Contraindications for Compression Therapy

The most important aspect of treating venous insufficiency is to first rule out arterial insufficiency. Although a clear diagnosis of venous insufficiency may be made, arterial insufficiency must be ruled out thoroughly because some people may have both. Compression therapy will exacerbate arterial insufficiency and may threaten the limb. Various experts suggest that an ABI of below 0.8 to 0.7 is a contraindication. As a practical rule, do not apply compression when a patient has an ABI value between 0.7 and 0.8 unless you are certain that the patient will be attentive to any problems that might occur with the compression. If the ability of the patient or caregiver to recognize and act upon an emergency situation is questionable, compression should be reserved for a limb with an ABI of 0.8 or greater. Other absolute contraindications include phlebitis and suspected deep venous thrombosis. Relative contraindications include conditions in which mobilization of fluid would occur from the lower extremities to a central circulation that cannot handle the extra fluid (congestive heart failure and pulmonary edema). Diminished sensation is considered a relative contraindication because of the possibilities of malfunction of the pump or foreign objects in the compression sleeve that could injure the patient if undetectable by the patient.

WOUNDS ASSOCIATED WITH LYMPHATIC DISEASE

Although wounds are usually not the primary problem with lymphedema, a number of individuals, especially with severe lower extremity lymphedema, will develop ulcers. A brief description of the lymphatic system and lymphedema and its treatment as it relates to ulcers follows.

Lymphatic Anatomy

The lymphatic system consists of small blind-end lymphatic capillaries that tend to follow small arterioles, venules, and blood capillaries. The ends of the lymphatic capillaries consist of flap-like structures that close off the vessel when interstitial fluid volume is low and open as fluid accumulates. The presence of valves within lymphatic vessels allows forward movement of lymph to occur with the intrinsic contractility of lymphatic vessels, external compression of lymphatic vessels by muscle contraction or other forces, and with negative pressure in the thorax during inspiration. Even the pulsation of the descending aorta is believed to be a factor in moving lymph proximally.

From lymphatic capillaries, lymph moves proximally through progressively larger lymphatic vessels. These larger vessels enter lymph nodes in a number of characteristic locations where lymph is exposed to elements of the immune system. Under normal conditions, pathogens are destroyed, but in some cases the persistence of bacteria or other pathogens stimulates proliferation of immune cells in the nodes and the swelling termed *lymphadenitis*. Should lymphatic defenses be overwhelmed, erosion of the lymph node and overlying skin may occur. Infection spreading along lymphatic vessels produces the red streaks in the skin known as lymphangitis. Failure of the lymphatics to clear pathogens allows them to enter the blood stream and produce septicemia.

Lymphatic drainage from the right upper quadrant of the body drains into the right lymphatic duct. The remainder of the drainage enters the thoracic duct. These ducts drain directly into the right and left subclavian veins, respectively. Lymphatic drainage is increased with increased interstitial volume and may increase by a factor of approximately 10-fold. Other factors are muscle contraction and deep breathing. Creating a strong negative pressure within the thorax creates a pressure gradient driving lymph flow proximally.

Lymphatic Terminology

An area of the body with common lymphatic drainage is called a watershed, analogous to an area of land that drains into a specific body of water. Watersheds have been mapped out through the body and one can obtain a chart demonstrating the watersheds. Obstruction of lymphatic vessels within a watershed produces lymphedema in characteristic locations. One of the theories of lymphedema treatment is that lymphatic drainage can be redistributed to different watersheds that are not obstructed. A segment of lymphatic vessel between valves is termed a *lymphangion*.

Lymphatic Pathophysiology

In many places in the world, lymphedema is usually caused by a worm passed through mosquitoes. *Wuchereria bancrofti* infests the lymphatic system causing obstruction. In Western civilization, most lymphedema is due to injury or resection of lymph nodes and vessels from surgery and radiation therapy for cancer. Breast cancer and uterine cancer treatment are common causes of upper and lower extremity lymphedema, respectively. Because these types of lymphedema are caused by another disorder, they are termed *secondary lymphedema*. A small number of cases of lymphedema are primary. In primary lymphedema, the lymphatic system does not develop normally compromising the ability to return fluid and protein from the interstitial space. Primary lymphedema may be present at birth (congenital lymphedema, 10% of primary lymphedema). A specific type of congenital lymphedema called Milroy's disease accounts for 2% of primary lymphedema. In Milroy's disease lymphatic vessels fail to develop normally due to a genetic defect (autosomal dominant) in a specific type of VEGF. Lymphedema may be delayed until later in childhood or young adulthood in the disorder called lymphedema praecox. By definition, lymphedema praecox, the most common primary lymphedema, is not apparent at birth, but develops before the age of 35. Lymphedema developing after the age of 35 represents 10% of primary lymphedema. It is termed *lymphedema tarda* or *Meige disease*. In all forms of primary lymphedema, lymphatic vessels fail to develop normally.

Characteristics of Skin Injury Secondary to Lymphatic Disease

Skin appearance with lymphedema is generally more severe than with the edema of venous disease, although wounds may not develop until severe skin injury is evident. In the most severe cases, skin eventually becomes thick, redundant, and wrinkled, similar to the skin of elephants, leading to the term *elephantiasis*. The greater loss of protein into the interstitial space produces much of the appearance of the skin. Along with retention of fluid, excessive protein in the interstitial space causes fibrosis and puckering of the skin in a pattern known as peau d'orange (orange peel-like). Hemosiderin staining and bacterial and fungal infections of the skin are also common. Maintaining dry, clean skin may become impossible with severe lymphedema, leading to fungal infection and bacterial superinfection. A common diagnostic test is the Stemmer sign. The edema secondary to lymphatic disease frequently prevents the lifting of the skin distal to the MCP joints. A positive Stemmer sign results when one cannot grasp the skin on the dorsum of the second toe or finger distal to its MCP joint or grasping the skin is difficult compared with grasping the same area on an uninvolved side. By definition, only the second digit is used for the Stemmer sign. A positive Stemmer sign is virtually predictive of lymphedema. However, a negative Stemmer sign (one is able to grasp the skin) does not rule out early or mild lymphedema.

Stages of Lymphatic Disease

For the purposes of diagnosis and treatment, lymphedema is categorized into 4 stages. Stage 0 represents a preclinical presentation, and stage 3 is the most advanced form. A person in stage 0 has a diminished lymphatic transport capacity, but the diminished functional reserve has not yet been challenged to allow manifestations of lymphatic disease to become evident. For example, consider a patient who received surgical and radiologic intervention for uterine cancer many years ago. For all of this time, she has had a diminished capacity to transport lymph from the right lower extremity. However, the need to transport lymph (lymphatic load) had not exceeded its reserve. At this point, she would be said to be in the latency substage of stage 0. Patients in this stage must be counseled about risk factors that could allow them to exceed their lymphatic drainage capacity. After many years, however, many in this stage may begin to ignore this counseling. As a consequence, a stressful event may tip the balance of lymphatic load to a point exceeding reserve. For example, the woman described above needs to mow her lawn after many consecutive rainy days. The grass becomes progressively longer and does not dry sufficiently. The weather is also hot and humid. The heat combined with the physical effort of pushing a lawn mower through long, wet grass results in much greater lymphatic load than she has experienced since her uterine cancer treatment. After more than 10 years of no consequences of subclinical lymphatic disease, she finally exceeds lymphatic transport and lymphedema becomes clinically evident.

Stage 1 is also termed the *reversible stage*. Simple elevation allows the edema to resolve. Pitting edema occurs, but tissue properties are unaltered. No changes in skin color or texture have occurred. Appropriate therapy at this stage is expected to result in return to normal limb volume. Lack of appropriate therapy may allow the disease to progress to stage 2. Another term for stage 2 is spontaneously irreversible lymphedema. The name implies that simple elevation is no longer sufficient to return the limb to its premorbid volume. At this stage, a positive Stemmer sign is expected. Tissue fibrosis and cellulitis are also expected at this stage. Often, lymphedema stabilizes at stage 2. Therapy may be effective in reducing limb volume, but lack of appropriate therapy and development of chronic cellulitis may allow progression to stage 3 lymphedema. Stage 3 is known as lymphostatic elephantiasis. Skin becomes hardened to the extent that pitting becomes difficult or no longer occurs and the Stemmer sign becomes more evident. Skin creases become very deep and pronounced to the point of disfigurement. Hyperkeratosis, fungal infections, and darkening of the skin are common. Papillomas and cysts frequently appear as well as open wounds in the forms of ulcers and fistulas. Treatment at this stage is possible, but restoring limb volume will require more extensive treatment than if it had been initiated during stages 1 or 2.

Treatment of Lymphatic Disease

Many therapies have been developed for lymphatic disease. Like venous disease, successful treatment involves an intensive period of compression therapy followed by lifetime maintenance of compression. A systematic treatment program called complete decongestive therapy (CDT) and several synonymous terms are described at the end of this section. Below, specific elements of compression are described. Although many of the specifics of treatment are different, the general treatment principles described for venous disease apply to lymphedema and some of the specific lymphedema treatments can be used for edema of venous hypertension.

Compression Pumping

Practitioners of CDT discourage the use of compression pumps due to the risk of rare cases of genital edema. The effectiveness of compression pump and its potential for unwanted effects are likely to change with the stage of lymphedema.

Compression Bandaging

Compression bandaging commonly used for lymphedema is somewhat different in terms of the materials than those used for venous disease. Foam sheets are frequently used in the place of absorbent batting material with the hope of breaking up fibrosis. Short stretch bandages of different widths are used depending on the girth of the limb.

Exercise

Exercise of the affected extremities is encouraged with compression bandaging in place. Practitioners of CDT have specific exercises, but any exercise that generates a muscle pumping action without unduly increasing arterial inflow and capillary leakage of fluid may be used.

Manual Lymphatic Drainage

Manual lymphatic drainage (MLD) is touted as the major component of CDT. It uses specific massage-like skin strokes with light pressure to encourage the movement of lymph and the development of alternate pathways around obstructed vessels. MLD is begun at the neck to clear the appropriate duct (right or thoracic), to encourage movement of lymph through both sides. MLD is progressed distally as vessels ahead of the obstruction are "cleared." MLD must be immediately followed by compression bandaging that needs to be left in place between MLD treatments to be effective.

Complete Decongestive Therapy

CDT is an involved program requiring extensive and expensive training. Programs require several weeks and may be divided into specific course levels. The CDT treatment regimen consists of MLD, compression bandaging, remedial exercises, and patient education on skin care.

Medical Treatment

Drugs used include antibiotics to treat cellulitis. In some countries, patients may take drugs called benzopyrones (coumarin and flavonoids) in an effort to minimize fibrosis of the interstitial space. Diuretics and steroids are discouraged. Diuretics will remove water preferentially from other areas of the body that have lower protein concentration. In areas of lymphedema, diuretics will cause the concentration of interstitial protein to increase and create a more fibrotic edema. Steroids are discouraged because of the immunosuppressive effect and fluid retention they would cause when used chronically.

Surgical Treatment

Two types of surgical intervention are used with lymphedema. A debulking procedure may be used to remove excessive tissue and decrease weight of a limb to improve function, but this procedure does not correct the lymphedema. Debulking can be done as staged excision or by liposuction. Procedures are being developed to bypass occlusions in the lymphatic system or to transplant lymphatic vessels.

WOUNDS ASSOCIATED WITH PERIPHERAL ARTERIAL DISEASE

Ischemic ulcers are the result of tissue necrosis secondary to arterial insufficiency of a limb, usually due to atherosclerosis. In addition to tissue necrosis, arterial disease also slows the healing of wounds of other etiologies. In particular, the combination of neuropathy and foot ischemia increases the risk of developing foot ulcers that heal very slowly or not at all requiring amputation. Other causes of ischemic ulcers include sickle cell disease, Buerger's disease (thromboangiitis obliterans), Raynaud's disease, Raynaud's phenomenon secondary to scleroderma and other autoimmune diseases, and primary forms of vasculitis. Types of primary vasculitis include Wegener's granulomatosis, microscopic polyangiitis, Henoch-Schönlein purpura, polyarteritis nodosa, Kawasaki disease, giant cell arteritis, Takayasu's arteritis, and Behçet's disease.

Because the most common form of arterial disease encountered is atherosclerotic, measurement of ankle brachial index should be performed to assess the severity of arterial disease. A value below 0.8 to 0.7 is indicative of arterial disease. In a patient with ABI below 0.45, healing is unlikely. Claudication is likely to occur before ABI becomes this low in physically active individuals, but many with arterial disease do not exert themselves enough physically to experience claudication until ABI falls below 0.5. Segmental blood pressure measurements along the extremity may isolate the area of occlusion noninvasively. A time-consuming, but functional test is transcutaneous PO_2 ($TcPO_2$). This test should be available in a vascular lab to determine the point along the extremity at which oxygen delivery to tissues is compromised. Imaging studies including duplex ultrasound and angiography, which may be required for surgical planning.

In the most common case of atherosclerosis of the lower extremity, tissues at greatest risk of necrosis are the most distal structures. Normally, blood pressure dissipates little along blood vessels of the lower extremity. However, with the obstruction of arterial vessels characteristic of atherosclerotic plaque and thrombosis, necrosis occurs in tissues distal to obstruction, usually on the foot, especially the toes. These wounds tend to be deep wounds with irregular borders outlining the arterial distribution involved. The outward appearance of advanced arterial disease is blackened, dry gangrene on the toes and sometimes more proximal structures.

A number of authorities recommend that dry gangrene not be debrided because it acts as dressing to protect the tissue beneath it. Debridement of dry gangrene is discouraged because debridement exposes necrotic tissue that can quickly support pathogenic organisms and allow disseminated infection. Severe ischemia may require surgical amputation. In some cases, autoamputation occurs in which the necrotic tissue, often a toe, withers and falls off the limb.

Conservative treatment for arterial disease consists of local wound care, but dry gangrene should not be debrided as discussed earlier. Reduction of risk factors such as smoking, elevated blood glucose, hypertension, hyperlipidemia, and limb protection can be offered to the patient. Seemingly trivial mechanical trauma may produce ulcers. Padding, lotions, absorption of excess moisture, and the use of assistive and adaptive devices may help protect limbs at risk for developing infection or injury.

Pharmacologic treatment for arterial insufficiency includes thrombolytic drugs, anticoagulants, vasodilators, and pentoxifylline. Surgical treatment provided by vascular surgeons or interventional radiologists includes bypass surgery, endarterectomy, and percutaneous transluminal angioplasty.

TRAUMATIC, SURGICAL, AND OTHER ACUTE WOUNDS

Traumatic, surgical, and other acute wounds are typically managed initially in the emergency department or by the surgeon creating the wound. Under some circumstances, acute wounds may be seen in other settings for debridement and possibly other interventions due to the nature of the wound. Some acute wounds also carry a high risk of complications requiring prolonged intervention. Acute wounds may be referred to other clinicians in the cases of gross contamination requiring cleansing of the wound before closure, a blistered wound such as a second degree burn over large area, a third degree burn over a small area, infection of an acute or surgical wound, the presence of unhealthy tissue within the wound such that primary closure is not feasible, compromised immune system, dehiscence (defined below), and any other reason for tertiary/delayed primary closure.

Lacerations

Lacerations are among the most common wounds seen in emergency departments. As occurs with any acute wound, lacerations typically have a high risk of contamination. Frequently, however, they can be cleansed sufficiently to allow primary closure with sutures, glue, staples or tape. They are caused by 3 basic mechanisms: shearing, tension, and compression (Figure 7-31). A shearing injury is created by a small amount of energy focused on a small area, basically a sharp edge such as a knife or

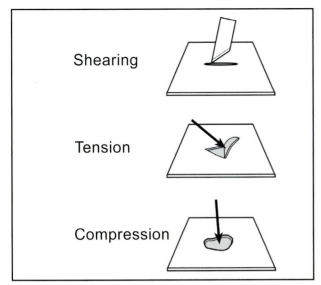

Figure 7-31. Mechanisms of lacerations.

broken glass. The tissue is divided, but minimal cell injury occurs beyond the sharp edge. These wounds can be cleansed and repaired with primary intention with a thin scar and little risk of infection. Striking the body with a blunt object at an angle with high energy creates a tension injury. A triangular flap is created (partial avulsion). The tissue flap is at risk of ischemic necrosis with the loss of blood supply from the free edges, especially if the flap base is distal rather than proximal. The risk of infection is greater due to the potential for ischemia and greater tissue destruction compared with a shearing force. A compression injury is caused by a high force striking straight on, especially over superficial bone. The wound will have jagged and even shredded edges, with much greater cell injury than the other 2 types. The injury may extend to subcutaneous tissue, including the bone. These wounds are at much greater risk of infection, requiring extensive cleansing, irrigation, and debridement. Primary repair is very extensive and may result in a cosmetically poor scar. In many cases, primary repair is not achievable because of the extent of cell injury.

Incisional Wounds

Wounds caused by sharp objects such as scalpels or scissors during surgery are called incisions. Incisions produced with sharp objects by accident or by attack may be categorized with lacerations (above); knives and broken glass are frequent culprits. A deep wound caused by a sharp, narrow object such as an ice pick, nail, or bites by some animals is classified as a puncture wound and is discussed further below. Incision wounds are managed in much the same way as lacerations caused by shearing injuries.

Skin Tears

Due to weakness of skin, minor trauma causes the skin of the elderly to tear easily. Often this occurs due to removal of tape used to keep intravenous lines in place. Skin this fragile is typically thin, almost transparent, and demonstrates multiple ecchymoses and purpura. Prevention of skin tears requires avoiding or minimizing adhesive use on the skin of the elderly as much as possible and meticulous removal of tape to avoid pulling. Younger people are accustomed to pulling tape off the skin without any injury to the skin. Unfortunately, such hasty tape removal is prone to tear the skin of the elderly. Prevention also requires protecting vulnerable areas of skin from trauma. Various means of protection are available, including tubular bandages and bandage rolls. Rather trivial trauma such as striking the dorsal hand and distal forearm on furniture, drawers, cabinets, and so forth when reaching for objects may produce skin tears.

Skin Tear Categories

Category I describes a skin tear without any tissue loss. Frequently this occurs from blunt trauma creating a triangular epidermal flap as described for a tension-type of laceration. Often the flap can be replaced and covered with an appropriate dressing to protect the wound during re-epithelialization. Partial loss of epidermis with the skin tear is a category II. This type of injury is frequently due to removal of adhesives. The adhesion between tape and epidermis may be stronger than the cohesion of the epidermis and adherence to the dermis. Category II may also be caused by a combination of tension and compression. Category III is complete loss of the epidermal flap, either by adhesive removal or blunt trauma to the skin. Category II and III are also treated with dressings that protect the dermis as re-epithelialization occurs. Steri-strips and similar adhesive materials may be used to secure any of the flap that can be salvaged.

Abrasions

Abrasions are also common injuries. Their prevalence is difficult to determine because many are self-treated. These wounds are caused by friction and tangential shearing of skin along a rough surface (see Figure 7-32). Because abrasions commonly occur along the road surface during cycling or motorcycle accidents, and to ejected unrestrained passengers or pedestrians in motor vehicle accidents, the term road rash is often used to describe this injury. Abrasions are superficial wounds and usually only need cleaning and protection. Thorough cleansing is important to remove contaminants for 2 reasons—microbes must be removed to prevent infection, and contaminants that are not removed may remain permanently in the skin causing discoloration,

Figure 7-32. Road rash on the left shoulder from falling off a motorcycle. Note the lack of pigmentation of the abraded skin and the darkening of the burned edges of epidermis. The wound is deeper over the acromion process than the surrounding tissue that is able to deform during the injury.

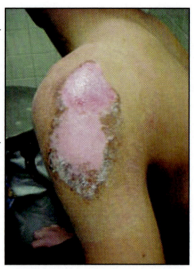

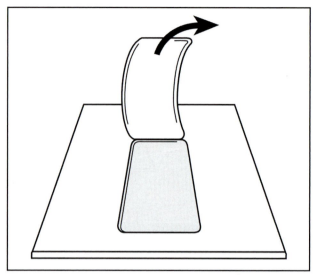

Figure 7-33. Mechanism of degloving (avulsion).

called tattooing. Deeper injuries are produced if abrasion occurs over bony prominences.

Degloving (Avulsion)

A more serious injury in which the skin is pulled from the body is called degloving. This term is particularly descriptive for the upper extremity. It is similar to a tension laceration, but no flap remains; the base of what would be a flap is torn. This type of injury is sometimes also called an avulsion. Degloving occurs during motor vehicle or industrial accidents in which skin catches on a sharp edge while the body is moving away from the object (Figure 7-33). This occurs in motor vehicle accidents in which the skin of a driver or passenger becomes caught on torn metal as the person is ejected from the vehicle. The skin is then torn and pulled away from body. Skin will tear down to an area in which the skin is attached firmly beneath. For the upper extremity, degloving tends to occur distally to the wrist. Depending on the body part, this injury is covered by either a partial or full-thickness graft.

Extravasation and Compartment Syndrome

Extravasation implies that fluid intended to be infused into a blood vessel is instead allowed to accumulate in or below the skin. Enormous quantities may be misdirected, creating pressure below the skin and necrosis. Intravenous catheters may either miss or go through a vein into interstitial space and fill it with fluid. Substantial fluid volume may also be pumped into the skin during hemodialysis intended for a rubber tube shunt placed in the arm. Extravasation may produce injuries similar to those created by compartment syndrome.

Compartment syndrome is typically produced by trauma. The injury may be chronic, for example, run-

ning on hard surfaces, or acutely from a musculoskeletal injury causing swelling of a compartment. Frequently the musculoskeletal injury is a fracture, but severe sprains are capable of causing compartment syndrome. Injury produced by compartment syndrome produces further swelling as cell contents are released into the interstitial space. Permanent injury to peripheral nerves, ischemia within and downstream of the compartment, myonecrosis, and skin necrosis may result. Pressure must be relieved as early as possible by fasciotomy, treatment of inflammation, and if possible, removal of any causes of edema within the compartment.

Puncture Wounds

Long pointed objects such as ice picks, knives, and animal teeth can produce puncture wounds. The feet may also be punctured by nails and other fasteners by stepping on them. The seriousness of puncture wounds is primarily due to the risk of contamination deep into the body, particularly into bone. To assess the risk of a puncture wound and to guide treatment, a puncture wound scoring system has been developed. The scale consists of 4 areas of 1 to 3 points and one with 0 to 9 points. The items consist of age of the wound, shape of the wound, depth of the wound, footwear at time of puncture (if in the foot), and radiographic evaluation. The scoring system is given in Table 7-13.

A score of 1 to 4 indicates need for local cleansing; 5 to 8 indicates local cleansing, irrigation and debridement (I&D), exploration, and placement of a drain. Any score greater than 9 indicates the need for lavage, IV antibiotics, and hospitalization.

Puncture Wound Scoring System

Category	0	1	2	3	9
Age		< 6 hours	6 to 24 hours	> 24 hours	
Classification		Small, sharp, clean edges; superficial	Ragged, irregular margins; moderate depth	Irregular edges, necrotic tissue, foreign body and drainage	
Depth		Only epidermis and dermis	Through dermis with no structural involvement	Through dermis with structural involvement	
Footwear		None	Stockings	Stockings and shoes	
Radiographic exam	No evidence of osseous involvement				Osseous involvement

For presence of concomitant disease, add 1 additional point.

Gunshot Wounds

Pistols, rifles, and shotguns have the potential for transfer of enormous energy injuring the body. Wide ranges of projectile velocity and mass exist, ranging from B-B guns, to large-caliber handguns and high-powered rifles. In addition to the soft tissue wounds along the trajectory of the projectile, gunshot wounds have the potential to cause multiple wounds due to their interaction with tissues. In many cases injuries are immediately lethal, or lethal in a short time, due to direct and indirect injury to the brain (herniation) and tearing of major blood vessels. Gunshot wounds may also cause limb amputation.

Bullets may be arbitrarily divided into low and high velocity. A low-velocity bullet fired from a typical .22 caliber pistol may travel at a rate of less than 1,000 feet per second, whereas a high-powered rifle may propel a bullet more than 3,000 feet per second. In addition, the size of the bullet, the distance from which the gun is fired, and the characteristics of the tissue struck determine the wound produced. With the exception of special handguns, pistols produce low-velocity wounds and most rifles produce high-muzzle velocities. The velocity and mass are determined by characteristics of the bullet. A smaller, more aerodynamic projectile maintains its velocity during flight, whereas large, round shot pellets lose velocity rapidly. As the equation for kinetic energy suggests ($1/2\ mv^2$), velocity is more important than mass. For example, the smaller bullet from a .223 caliber M16 rifle produces approximately 3 times the kinetic energy of a larger bullet of a .45 caliber handgun due to the difference in velocity.

Deformation of a bullet as it passes through tissue causes greater loss of energy and therefore, more transfer of energy to tissues and tissue damage. When a bullet strikes the more dense medium of tissue, its flight becomes unstable; the more unstable it becomes, the more energy it transfers into the tissue. The instability can manifest itself as a tumbling or yawing motion, which increases the surface area of the bullet striking the tissue and transfer of energy into the tissue. Moreover, the irregular movement increases the probability that the bullet may deform or even fragment.

Depending on the depth of the tissue struck relative to the velocity of the bullet, different outcomes are possible. Low-velocity bullets and shot may lodge in tissue with an entry wound only, whereas high-velocity bullets produce both an entry and a larger exit wound. High velocity bullets can also produce devastating cavitation (Figure 7-34). Cavitation is the result of high velocity producing waves of pressure through the tissue. The cyclic expansion and collapse of the track tears tissue; therefore, more cavitation is produced in thicker tissue. A bullet can pass through a relatively thin area of tissue with little cavitation. Very soft tissues, such as internal organs suffer greater cavitation than hard tissues, with skeletal muscle having an intermediate susceptibility to cavitation.

The simplest outcome of a gunshot wound is a small linear wound with an entry wound and a small or possibly

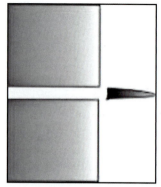

Figure 7-34A. Types of wounds created by gunshots. A high-velocity bullet through a thin target produces a small entry and exit wound and a narrow tract.

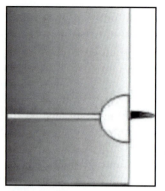

Figure 7-34B. Typical wound created by a high-velocity bullet going through an intermediate thickness target. Cavitation produces a large exit wound.

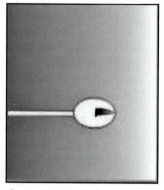

Figure 7-34C. High-velocity bullet entering a thick target producing cavitation, but no exit due to dissipation of kinetic energy within the tissue.

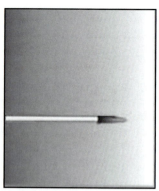

Figure 7-34D. Low-velocity bullet lodged in thick tissue with narrow entry wound and tract.

no exit wound with a narrow tract of tissue damage. This would occur if a high velocity bullet passes rapidly through a narrow path. In the case of a thicker area of tissue, the bullet may produce enormous tissue damage by cavitation with an exit wound. The exit wound may become very large if cavitation occurs maximally at the exit. In addition to the damage caused by the tract of the bullet through tissue, secondary missiles may be produced by fragmentation of either the bullet itself or bone struck by the bullet. On occasion, the bullet may enter a vein and produce a bullet embolism, typically lodging in the right ventricle.

Shot gun shells are available in different sizes and velocity of shot. Shells are classified by the diameter of the shell and the number of shot pellets in the shell. Typical shot guns use either 12 or 20 gauge shells with shell diameters of .729 and .614 inch in diameter, respectively. The pellets within the shell are given numerical sizes as well, typically ranging from .08 to .11 inches in diameter.

Damage is inflicted by the deceleration of a large number of small lead spheres striking tissue. At the muzzle, pellets generally have a velocity of 1,000 to 1,500 feet per second. However, these small, spherical pellets have poor aerodynamic properties and lose kinetic energy traveling through the air before striking tissue. For this reason, the distance of the body from the shot gun is the chief determinant of the damage inflicted. At very close range the individual pellets behave as a large single missile. As the pellets diverge, they become singular missiles.

Depending on the characteristics of different shells, the damage inflicted at different ranges will vary. At a close range (1 to 2 yards) a large single ragged entrance wound is produced, and depending on the depth of tissue, an exit wound may or may not occur. At greater distances, the size of the entrance wound increases and multiple single shot wounds will surround the central wound. As distance increases to about 20 yards, the spray pattern becomes large (1 to 3 feet across), and wounds become singular. At this distance and farther, fewer shot pellets will strike the body and will do so with low kinetic energy. At greater than 50 yards, the probability of damage diminishes rapidly except for the eye.

Although these missiles achieve great kinetic energy and create tremendous heat on striking tissue, bullets and pellets of shot should be considered contaminated. At one time, bullets were considered to be sterilized by the heat generated. However, pieces of material from the body surface are carried into the body and several studies have indicated that microbes can be carried into the body by bullets. Gunshot wounds require careful exploration due to the unpredictable path of tissue destruction. They are generally not closed and require thorough irrigation and filling of the tracts with nonocclusive materials such as packing strip, or if large enough, with a bandage roll. Substantial necrosis of tissue surrounding the tracts is expected and irrigation and debridement may need to be carried out for several days. The material used to fill the tracts is frequently soaked in topical antibiotic solution. Psychosocial issues are common with gunshot wounds. The ability of the clinician to handle these issues may influence the patient's adherence to the plan of care.

Fractures

Fractures represent 2 sets of potential problems related to wound management—wounds created by open fractures and surgical wounds to repair the fracture. The exception would be a closed fracture managed with closed reduction and immobilization. Wounds are created by bone fragments in open fractures, and by surgeons for either open reduction or for external fixation. Open fractures are frequently accompanied by skin loss in the area, although some of these lacerations can be repaired surgically. In other cases, severe avulsion or degloving injuries can cause large areas of skin to be torn from the limb. Open reduction wounds will typically be closed surgically and several incisions may be created, depending on the procedure used. In certain types of injuries, fracture blisters may form and cause severe wounds, often associated with infection. Within this section, care for pins used for skeletal traction following a fracture and external fixation used for management of complex fractures or limb-lengthening will be addressed, and fracture blisters will also be discussed.

Open Fractures

An open fracture, formerly known as a compound fracture, causes tearing of the soft tissues against the sharp edge of the fractured bone. The risk of open fracture depends on several factors, including the mechanism of the injury, the type and amount of soft tissue surrounding the bone, and the pliability of the bone. Open fractures are more likely to occur with injuries caused by high energy mechanisms such as car and motorcycle wrecks, and falls from great heights. Twisting injuries or blows perpendicular to long bones are also more likely to cause open fractures. A bone stabilized by thick pliable tissues such as the femur of an athlete is less likely to tear through soft tissue than a superficial bone with little support such as the distal tibia. Brittle bones of the elderly are more likely to tear soft tissue than the highly pliable bones of very young children.

Open fractures present several serious problems. Bone and soft tissue are exposed to the external environment and, depending on the circumstances, the contamination can be very extensive, eg, a farm implement accident. Contamination of bone with bacteria increases the risk of osteomyelitis, which can be very difficult to clear. Large amounts of necrotic tissue may be present in the wound due to injury from the sharp bone edges. In addition, the border between necrotic and healthy tissue may be difficult to determine early. Failure to remove necrotic tissue from the wound increases the risk of infection. Open fracture wounds need to be probed carefully to find any dead space below the wound surface created by open fractures. Allowing re-epithelialization to occur over an area where dead space has failed to fill with granulation may lead to hematoma and abscess formation in the future.

Neurovascular compromise is always a threat with an open fracture, especially the radial nerve with mid-shaft humerus fractures and the peroneal nerve with tibial/fibular fractures, although any peripheral nerve is at risk. Nerve injuries caused by open fractures and, in some cases, even closed fractures or severe sprains, can lead to complex regional pain syndromes (CRPS), a condition of persistent pain and autonomic dysfunction requiring protracted physical therapy to manage. CRPS is a term that encompasses the variety of dysfunctions formerly known as reflex sympathetic dystrophy, shoulder-hand syndrome, minor causalgia, major causalgia, and others. These conditions are characterized by mechanical allodynia, in which normal mechanical stimulation is perceived as pain, and is accompanied by swelling and atrophy of the skin and bone. Sensory re-education and desensitization are performed in physical therapy. Autonomic blockade of sympathetic ganglia with local anesthetic is sometimes used but is not successful for many individuals with CRPS.

Pin Care

Pin care addresses 3 issues: compromised circulation, pin reaction, and infection. Compromised circulation is caused by excessive skin tension by the pin leading to necrosis of skin around the pin. Pin reaction is described as inflammation due to tissue reaction to the presence of the pin. Signs of inflammation (redness, swelling, tenderness, and discharge) must be present for more than 72 hours to be considered a reaction and clear drainage alone is not considered to be pin reaction. Excessive movement of the pin and blockage of drainage increase the risk of pin reaction. Minor pin reaction refers to a situation in which redness, swelling, tenderness, or clear drainage is present and improves with lancing of the skin. A major pin reaction or infection is defined as a condition that does not improve with lancing and results in the need to remove pins due to the risk of osteomyelitis and the difficulty of managing osteomyelitis. Problems include excessive motion and presence of necrotic tissue around the pin promoting infection and increasing the risk of abscess development around the pin.

Six issues related to pin care include the frequency of pin care, cleansing solutions, use of ointments at the pin-skin interface, management of crusts on the pins, when to use sterile technique, and the use of dressings. Many experts suggest that keeping pins clean and allowing a slow drainage from the tissue onto the pins is the best strategy for avoiding infection. Thus, recommendations given are aimed at promoting free flow of drainage, avoidance of disturbance of the normal balance of skin flora, and avoidance of skin and subcutaneous tissue irritation. Frequency of pin care needs to be individualized. Too frequent pin care causes inflammation, whereas infrequent observation can lead to serious problems. A simple guideline is for pin site care every 8 hours in the presence of drainage and daily with no drainage. Although many individuals commonly use hydrogen peroxide and/or povidone iodine, recommendations are for the use of normal saline only. Normal saline dilutes the bacteria present on the pins, whereas disinfectants have been associated with a higher, not lower, rate of infection. The recommendation is to clean only the pin with alcohol, whereas skin cleansing should only be done as needed and with normal saline. Cleansing also needs to be performed by sweeping away from the skin, and avoiding moving contaminants toward the open wound. Ointment use is discouraged, as they can occlude the pin hole and allow infection to occur. For the same reason, the recommendation is to remove crusts from the pin-skin interface to allow drainage to occur. Some authors have suggested that crust removal is not necessary for pins used for skeletal traction placed in areas with little soft tissue, but crusts should be removed with external fixators. Gauze dressings are recommended for covering the pin sites to reduce surface contamination and to absorb drainage. Dressings should not hold moisture against the skin, nor should they be cut before placing them over the wounds, as frayed ends may irritate the wound. Sterile technique is only recommended during hospitalization due to the presence of multiply-resistant organisms in hospitals.

Fracture Blisters

These wounds occur in a small percentage of fractures in general, but are much more likely to occur in areas of superficial bone with tight skin (5% in these areas). They may also occur in other injuries that do not produce fractures, such as severe ankle sprains. These areas include the ankle, elbow, foot, and distal tibia. In these areas, tissue injury can cause edema between the dermal and epidermal layers of skin.

Because of the proximity of the involved bone or ligaments and the lack of skin mobility in these areas, separation of the epidermis from the dermis with subsequent necrosis of the epidermis results. Fracture blisters are 4 times more likely to occur if surgical stabilization is delayed more than 24 hours. Wound infections, delayed fracture treatment, fracture nonunion, increased hospital stay, and increased costs of care may result from these blisters.

The presence of a fracture blister causes surgical incisions to be placed in areas that may not be optimal for the surgical procedure due to the risk of spreading infection from the blister. Compression may not be useful for prevention of fracture blisters because veins are more superficial in the areas where blisters tend to occur and compression is likely to impede venous flow, whereas compression tends to aid deeper venous return. Prevention efforts include early immobilization, elevation, and surgical repair of twisting injuries of the foot, ankle, elbow, and distal tibia. Rupture of the blister is not recommended, but a dry, absorbent dressing to protect the blister is recommended. Occlusive dressings such as hydrocolloids are recommended once the blister ruptures, if the wound is clean. Topical antibiotics are not recommended unless the wound is infected and not healing. Systemic antibiotics are recommended if infection occurs. In this case, occlu-

sive dressings should not be used. Re-epithelialization of fracture blisters is expected in 4 to 21 days depending on individual factors.

Bites

Several vertebrates may inflict humans with bite injuries, ranging from armadillos to zebras as well as humans. Bite wounds typically contain multiple microorganisms. These may include aerobes, anaerobes, and fungi, and may originate from oral flora of the biting animal or the person's skin. Bites may be complicated by infection, lymphadenitis, lymphangitis, osteomyelitis, septic arthritis, and, particularly when the hand is involved, tenosynovitis. Infections with severe morbidity and possible mortality are possible. Examples include rabies from dogs and wild mammals, tularemia from cats hunting wild rabbits, Herpes B from monkeys, leptospirosis from rodents and dogs, rat bite fever (*Streptobacillus moniliformis*), and cat scratch fever (*Bartonella henselae*). Rat bite fever causes polyarthritis, rash, fever, and headache. It can be fatal due to endocarditis, meningoencephalitis, or septic shock. Cat scratch fever produces pronounced regional lymphadenopathy and signs of system inflammation. Tularemia is also known as rabbit fever, but affects rodents as well. It is acquired by tick bite or handling of the infected animal. The bacterium can also be inhaled or ingested.

The majority of human bites result from striking another with a clenched fist. True occlusional bites represent about 40% of these injuries. Clenched fist injuries are particularly problematic because of involvement of finger tendons from striking another person's teeth. Human bites are likely to lead to infection if untreated and may lead to infection of tendon, joints, and bone with possible loss of tendon function in extreme cases. Hepatitis B, C, and HIV may also be transmitted.

Although several animals commonly bite humans—cats, squirrels, mice, rats, guinea pigs, hamsters, and rabbits—dog bites are particularly likely to cause severe injury. Other animals may be involved depending on occupational or recreational exposure, such as horses, pigs, fish, monkeys, and so on. Most dog bites occur on the lower extremities. In children, however, wounds may also occur on the head, neck, face, and upper extremities. Wound infections are estimated to occur in 5% to 10% of dog bites. Multiple organisms are likely to be obtained; however, intravenous antibiotics are not typically used unless a patient is at high risk for infection. Tetanus shots, however, are given as they would for puncture wounds in general. Several breeds of dogs can create extensive damage during a bite, causing crush injuries in addition to the lacerations and punctures. Crush injuries are more likely to cause tissue necrosis and hematomas that increase the risk of wound infection. Multiple bites during an attack may require thorough debridement of the affected area and grafting. Cat bites are more likely to become infected than dog bites because these injuries are more likely to cause puncture, rather than crushing or laceration. Inoculation with bacteria from the cat's mouth can reach deeply in or through the skin. Small rodents kept as pets are more likely to cause thin lacerations with lower risk of infection than cat or dog bites. Bites from marine animals may transmit *Vibrio vulnificus*, a cause of necrotizing fasciitis, which is discussed below.

Arthropod Bites

Ulcerations caused by chemicals injected by arthropod bites are categorized as toxic ulcerations. Notable among these, in specific areas of the country, is the venom of the brown recluse spider. The venom spreads rapidly through fatty tissue and can produce ulcers several centimeters wide and deep. One of this author's first wound care experiences was a brown recluse injury that created an ulcer 10 x 8 x 7 cm deep in the buttock of a woman bitten while sitting on a wooden outhouse seat. These wounds can be cleaned and healed, but it may take several weeks or months, depending on the size of the wound. As with any wound, the potential for infection exists if the wound is not debrided. With appropriate debridement and dressings, these wounds should heal without complication. Spider bites appear to be extremely overdiagnosed. Skin abscesses due to folliculitis with methicillin-resistant *Staphylococcus aureus* (MRSA) are commonly blamed on spiders without any evidence of the presence of brown recluse spiders in that geographical region.

SKIN DISEASES

Blistering diseases, in particular, may produce acute wounds. Blisters may be formed either by the separation of the epidermis from the dermis or dermis from the basement membrane. In either case the disease results in the loss of the barrier to infection and fluid loss. Epidermolysis bullosa is a genetic disease characterized by defective desmosomes. Pemphigus is an autoimmune disease affecting desmosomes, allowing separation within the dermis, and is life-threatening. Pemphigoid is a disease that superficially resembles pemphigus, but the separation occurs between the epidermal and dermal layers. Blistering may also be toxin-mediated. Staphylococcal scalded skin syndrome (SSSS) is caused in neonates by an epidermolytic toxin of a particular strain of *Staphylococcus aureus*. The skin may come off in sheets and patients must be handled very delicately to prevent further damage. Hypersensitivity reactions may also cause blistering. In particular, Stevens-Johnson syndrome produces blistering of the skin and mucosa. A number of pharmaceuticals, especially antibiotics and sulfonamides in particular, have been linked to this syndrome. Treatment generally consists of protecting the

skin with silver sulfadiazine ointment, although this compound has also been linked to Stevens-Johnson syndrome. Once the skin is at low risk for infection, daily application of sterile hydrogel sheets can be performed. They are soothing, retain fluid and heat, and do not adhere to the wound, making dressing changes less painful for the patient. The patient can also avoid the discomfort of the agitation necessary to remove silver sulfadiazine.

TREATMENT OF ACUTE WOUNDS

The viability of tissue surrounding the wound must also be assessed to determine whether to close a wound. Lacerations, in particular, produce flaps of skin that may lose their blood supply. If this is the case, that part of the wound will need to be left open for 2 important reasons. First, sutures will not hold in devitalized tissue and second, any devitalized tissue is likely to become infected. The amount of tissue loss in a wound needs to be determined to develop a plan for closure. Some areas of a wound can be sutured and other areas left to heal by secondary intention or to receive a graft where tissue loss occurs. Determining the amount of tissue loss can be difficult where tissue is elastic and taut. Plastic surgeons can often develop a plan to close a wound entirely even in the presence of some degree of tissue loss. The depth of injury also affects the plan of care. A small wound can be allowed to re-epithelialize regardless of the depth of the wound, whereas a large wound with full-thickness injury will need to be grafted. Acute wounds must be cleaned before closure. The surrounding skin is carefully prepped, usually with an iodophor such as povidone-iodine, and the wound itself is irrigated and debrided.

Simple lacerations with minimal tissue injury usually require only irrigation. The more complex the wound is and the more extensive the tissue necrosis is, the more extensive the irrigation and debridement need to be. Systemic antibiotics are considered to be of little value in the treatment of acute wounds unless a therapeutic level can be obtained within 4 hours of wounding, and the use of systemic antibiotics after this time may, in some cases, increase infection rate. Systemic antibiotics may be used, however, in the case of spreading cellulitis without purulent drainage.

The cause of the wound will also determine how extensive the irrigation and debridement need to be. An untidy wound such as an industrial accident, farming accident, or bite will need more extensive care. Heavily contaminated wounds can be cleaned with pulsatile lavage or a syringe with an attached catheter. With cleaning of the wound, any embedded material is removed, and a decision of whether debridement is necessary is made. Foreign materials left in the wound will produce inflammation and infection. Long-term consequences include excessive scarring and tattooing. If necrotic tissue or unremovable embedded material remains in the wound, debridement becomes necessary. Debridement needs to be done judiciously to minimize the amount of tissue removed from the wound so that the wound can be closed with a minimum of scarring. Local anesthesia for closure is dependent on the extent of the repair. For simple repairs either 1% or 2% lidocaine is sufficient. For repairs that may require more than 1 hour, a longer acting local anesthetic is needed. Bupivacaine may be used, but it takes longer to achieve anesthesia than lidocaine. Most wounds will be infiltrated with epinephrine in combination with lidocaine. Epinephrine acts as a vasoconstrictor, which decreases bleeding during repairs, and decreases the vascular washout of lidocaine from the tissue, increasing lidocaine's duration of action.

A variety of suture materials are available, with specific advantages for different situations. Suture material may be either absorbable or nonabsorbable, and either monofilament or braided. Absorbable sutures are used subcutaneously or for special conditions in which suture removal is not desired. Polyglycolic acid sutures are braided and degrade by autolytic action rather than phagocytosis, so the risk of tissue reaction is decreased. Nonabsorbable sutures are used for the skin and may be braided or monofilament. The spaces within the braid are a concern for producing tissue reactions or for harboring bacteria. Monofilament sutures, however, are more difficult to tie. Sutures come in different sizes; 6-0 is preferred by many experts for more meticulous work such as the face, whereas 4-0 works well on other parts of the body. Wounds may also be approximated with staples, especially skin grafts. Surgical adhesives are also available, and wounds may also be approximated with tape. Taping reduces the time required for wound closure and the need for local anesthesia, but may not produce as precise a closure as suturing.

Suturing techniques are critical for a good outcome. Poor technique can lead to excessive scarring or dehiscence (the opening of a closed surgical wound). Deep layer approximation becomes necessary when an injury involves subcutaneous tissue. Failure to provide deep layer approximation increases tension on the outer sutures and will leave subcutaneous dead space. Therefore, deep layer approximation reduces the risk of fluid accumulation and infection below the skin. Suturing the skin can be done in a number of ways. The critical component is to gain closure of the wound with minimal tension. Following closure, swelling will increase the tension on the sutures. Excessive tension produces circulatory compromise of the edges of the wound and can lead to infection, dehiscence or both. Sutures can generally be removed in 5 days on the face and 7 days on the trunk. Extremity sutures may be allowed to remain longer than 7 days. Formerly, surgeons were concerned about leaving sutures in too long because of inflammation caused by reaction to the suture material.

Newer synthetic materials allow a longer time to assure adequate wound strength. In some cases, application of skin tape is performed following suture removal to reduce tension on the immature scar to prevent scar widening or dehiscence. The tape strips are allowed to remain for several days until they loosen and detach on their own.

INFECTION

Any defect in the skin places an individual at risk of infection, and even in the presence of intact skin, exposure to some microbes can cause infection. Whether infection occurs with exposure will be determined by the combination of which microbes are present, the wound environment, and the immune status of the patient. Careful skin preparation before surgery, thorough cleansing/irrigation, and debridement reduce bacterial counts in and around the wound. These procedures minimize, but do not eliminate, the risk of infection—even for a person with normal immunity. Even with optimal conditions of a clean wound with minimal necrotic tissue, a person with diminished immunity has a much higher risk of infection than a person with normal immunity who has a contaminated wound.

Risk Factors for Infection

Wound infection is indicated by either localized purulent drainage or surrounding cellulitis and excessive inflammation. Common risk factors for infection are the cleanliness of the wound, the mechanism of injury, age of the wound (how much time has passed since the injury), the extent of the injury, local blood supply, and the presence of necrotic tissue, foreign bodies, hematoma, and dead space.

Several terms have been used to describe the cleanliness of a wound. The terms tidy and untidy indicate a degree of contamination with foreign materials. Clean, clean-contaminated, and contaminated, have also been used to describe the cleanliness of surgical wounds. A clean or tidy wound has little, if any, foreign material and a low level of bacterial contamination. How clean the wound is can often be inferred from the mechanism of the injury. A wound from farming equipment or a bite is likely to have a much greater degree of contamination than one from a piece of glass or kitchen knife. A kitchen accident with broken glass or a knife would be considered to be tidy or clean, although some bacteria will be introduced. An untidy wound or contaminated wound has foreign materials that are likely to produce inflammation and is likely to carry large numbers of viable bacteria and spores. Clean, as it is used in surgical terminology, implies that proper sterile technique was maintained, and no trauma or inflammation that might contaminate the site is present. Clean-contaminated refers to surgical or diagnostic procedures on the gastrointestinal, respiratory, or genitourinary tracts in which no significant contamination occurs, ie, spills from the tracts do not occur. These tracts are exposed to the outside environment and are likely to be contaminated with bacteria. Contaminated is used to describe a situation in which either spillage from a tract or a significant break in sterile technique occurs. Dirty implies the presence of frank purulence, inflammation, or necrotic tissue in the surgical site.

The possibility of embedded materials and amount of tissue necrosis of the wound can be deduced from the mechanism of injury. The age of a wound is important in deciding whether closure or healing by second intention is preferable. The longer a wound is left untreated, the greater the risk of infection. However, the local blood supply also is a factor in the decision whether to close a wound. A greater blood supply provides a better immune response. Facial injuries are commonly sutured even after 12 hours. In the past, the concept of a *golden period* dictated that closure must be accomplished within 6 to 12 hours, or the wound should be left open to heal by secondary intention. Modern practice with better debridement and antibiotic coverage allows greater latitude on how long a wound may be left open before surgical closure.

Surgical Site Infection

Surgical wounds present the least potential for complications associated with wounds in general. The skin is prepared with an antiseptic such as povidone-iodine and the wound is created under sterile conditions. In addition, areas surrounding the sterile field are draped to avoid contamination. Although surgical site infection (SSI) has a low probability (2%), given the large number of surgical procedures, approximately 600,000 SSIs are expected annually with a mortality of 20,000 per year. In response to this problem the Center for Disease Control has issued SSI guidelines. Several of the recommendations to be discussed include avoiding shaving the surgical site, applying antiseptic to an area large enough for any possible incision during the procedure in concentric circles moving peripherally, adequate oxygenation of the patient, smoking cessation, glucose control, and appropriate sterile technique.

Adequate preparation of the skin is critical to prevent surface flora from being carried into the wound. For this reason, shaving of hair is discouraged. Instead, hair should be trimmed sufficiently to prevent loose hairs from entering the sterile field or hairs becoming entangled in the sutures. Shaving is likely to abrade the skin and may transmit surface bacteria into the skin. Preparation of the skin is then done after hairs are trimmed from the area of interest. Circular biopsy punches of the skin may be approximated with sutures to decrease the size of the scar. Alternatively, these wounds could be covered with an occlusive dressing and allowed to heal by secondary intention.

Complications may result from contamination released by surgery on the gastrointestinal tract or undetected bleeding forming a hematoma. The other major complications are related to suturing technique and excessive tension placed on wounds by movement, coughing, and other maneuvers that increase abdominal pressure leading to dehiscence. Although the vast majority of surgical wounds heal without complications, a number of these wounds will experience complications of infection, dehiscence or both. Several risk factors for infection have already been discussed earlier in this chapter and will be discussed further in Chapter 9.

Surgically closed wounds with purulence, peripheral cellulitis, and induration require incision, irrigation, and drainage. Once bacterial burden is below 100,000 per gram, delayed closure has a 96% success rate. Excessive tension placed on sutures can cause necrosis of the wound margins leading to infection or dehiscence of the wound. Dehiscence is discussed in greater detail below. In addition, poor nutrition, corticosteroid use, diabetes mellitus, and smoking are among the potential causes of delayed healing and may prevent healing or lead to necrosis of the wound margins or infection.

Only two-thirds of SSI are due to the incision; one-third are due to infection of the space or organ involved in the procedure. Both hematoma and dead space present the problem of allowing bacteria to accumulate under intact skin. Dead space can occur in several ways. During surgery, subcutaneous tissues must be approximated before the skin is closed. Failure to achieve subcutaneous tissue approximation leaves a space for bacterial growth to occur. In chronic wounds, dead space occurs when the base of the wound fails to completely granulate before re-epithelialization occurs bridging the dead space. Hematomas may form postoperatively if adequate hemostasis is not attained before surgical closure. Blood may accumulate gradually and go unnoticed until sufficient tension on the suture line allows blood or pus to escape. Hematomas may also result from trauma that injures subcutaneous structures and causes bleeding under intact skin. Generally, these are musculoskeletal injuries, especially muscle tears. Hematomas create an additional risk factor beyond dead space by providing nutrients to bacteria possibly accelerating their growth beyond the capacity of the immune system to destroy them.

Dehiscence

The opening of a surgical wound is termed dehiscence. This type of wound is caused by the failure of sutures or staples to maintain primary closure of a surgical wound. A wound dehisces when the sutures, staples, tape, adhesive, or the skin itself is overcome by pressure or shear. Common causes include excess or improper lifting, necrosis of the wound edges due to vascular compromise or infection, or weakness of the skin caused by corticosteroids or other causes.

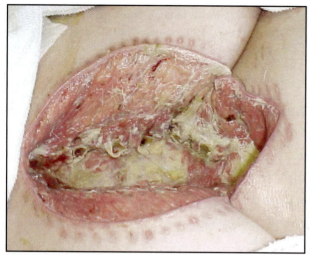

Figure 7-35A. Dehiscent sternotomy wound. Note the degree of gapping and the inflammation of the suture wounds.

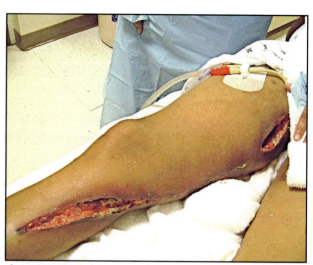

Figure 7-35B. Dehiscent saphenous vein harvesting sites.

Sternotomy wounds caused by open heart surgery and other procedures are frequently dehisced by patients who ignore lifting restrictions, or are not taught proper transfers and other precautions to reduce sternal stress. These precautions include avoidance of shoulder extension, bilateral abduction, and pushing up in bed from long sitting. Instead, the patient needs to be taught to roll into sidelying and drop the legs off the bed as a counterweight to come to sitting. Some patients may prefer to scoot in prone until the legs are cleared from the bed. Patients need to be taught to avoid low furniture with soft cushions and to avoid pushing up through the hands to come to standing from sitting. A typical example of ignoring lifting restriction is one particular person who lifted his bass boat into the water from his trailer. Abdominal surgical wounds may dehisce due to lifting, but also due to intra-abdominal pressure or bloating.

Infection can cause a wound on any part of the body to become dehiscent. In many cases the dehiscent wound becomes so contaminated or the potential for tissue loss or necrosis is so great that primary closure is not attempted again. In this case, the typical approach is lavage, antibiotics, and delayed primary closure when the wound is clean and stable and sufficient granulation tissue formation has occurred to relieve strain on the apposed edges of delayed primary closure. In other cases, secondary closure is allowed to continue to completion, which may take months for some large abdominal wounds. Infection may cause dehiscence or be a result of dehiscence. Dehiscence may occur due to the pressure caused by accumulation of purulence beneath the skin. Alternatively, dehiscence may be caused by poor healing of a surgical incision site allowing microbes access to subcutaneous tissue and infec-

tion. Wounds may be closed by gradual third intention in which sutures are placed across the wound and tied as the wound becomes clean and sufficiently filled with granulation tissue to minimize tension on the sutures. A dehiscent sternal wound is shown in Figure 7-35.

Managing Risk of Dehiscence

Patients at risk for dehiscence should be identified and given particular attention to avoid events that might lead to dehiscence. The patient's history gives some risk factors: smoking, diabetes, obesity, and use of corticosteroids. Additional risk factors include disorders associated with coughing and large pendulous breasts for sternal wounds and constipation or other conditions associated with the Valsalva maneuver for abdominal wounds. The patient's nutrition and glucose need to be carefully monitored and corrected. Body mechanics during transfers from bed to sitting and from sitting to standing should be taught, monitored, and corrected as needed. Trapeze bars should be removed from beds and use of bed rails or other pulling techniques during transfers must be discouraged.

Inspection of the wound needs to be done regularly. Visual inspection should show epithelialization bridging the incision. The absence of epithelialization, increased separation of the sides of the incision, and continued signs of inflammation or evidence of infection are signs of potential dehiscence. Erythema, edema, pain, and warmth should be decreasing. Increasing signs of inflammation with the addition of induration and purulence place the wound at high risk of dehiscence. Within 5 days, a definite healing ridge should be palpable. Absence of a healing ridge from postop days 5 through 9 represents delayed healing and risk of dehiscence.

Complications of Specific Types of Surgical Wounds

Certain types of surgical wounds are more prone to complications such as infection and dehiscence. Sternotomy, lower extremity incisions for harvesting of veins for coronary artery bypass grafting (CABG), incisions for bypass surgery of the lower extremities, fasciotomy, tumor excision, joint replacement surgery, abdominal surgery, panniculectomy, and pilonidal cysts are discussed below.

Median Sternotomy

Median sternotomy is the typical access site for open heart surgery. Perioperative complications occur in a small percentage of cases, including hematoma, infection, and wound dehiscence. Any of these 3 factors may lead to the others. Lack of adequate hemostasis leading to hematoma provides a suitable environment for rapid proliferation of bacteria. Inadequate primary closure of the soft tissue overlying the sternum can lead to dehiscence. However, dehiscence may occur in the presence of technically adequate wound closure, presumably due to excessive forces placed on the sternum and overlying tissue particularly in patients who are overweight, have large pendulous breasts, and diseases that stimulate frequent coughing. Large mechanical stresses are commonly believed to be a risk factor for dehiscence and subsequent infection. Infection of the soft tissue overlying the sternum may then predispose the patient to osteomyelitis of the sternum and to mediastinitis, which is associated with a high (~40%) mortality. Osteomyelitis generally requires sternectomy, debridement of necrotic soft tissue and plastic surgery to close the wound.

Lower Extremity Incisions for Bypass Surgery and Fasciotomy

Other common sites of postop infection include lower extremity incisions used to harvest the saphenous vein for CABG. Depending on the quality of vein harvested, multiple incisions may be necessary to retrieve sufficient length of usable vein. Many patients receiving CABG have other ischemic disease, including the lower extremities, putting the incisional wounds at risk for infection and dehiscence. Incisional wounds created for bypass surgery of arteries of the lower extremities may have a similar fate. Likewise flaps and grafts used to cover wounds may fail for the same reasons that the wounds would not close without plastic surgery.

Fasciotomy wounds are similar to bypass graft donor sites, except the wounds are deeper. These wounds are at risk due to the injury that required the fasciotomy. An additional problem is the potential for premature closure of the skin without complete granulation, leaving a dead space that in the future may lead to abscess formation.

Tumor Excision

Tumor excision wounds may be relatively simple in the cases of squamous cell or basal cell carcinoma of the skin, but excision of melanoma is more complex. The risk of metastasis of melanoma is related to depth of skin involved. Therefore, the excisional wound may be full-thickness and removal of regional lymph nodes may be performed for diagnostic and therapeutic reasons.

Arthroplasty

Joint replacement surgery is very common and a small fraction of these surgical wounds will be complicated by infection. Removal of the prosthesis and implantation of antibiotic releasing material is frequently performed to allow for future implantation of a new prosthesis.

Abdominal Surgery

Abdominal wounds, especially those created for intestinal surgery are at risk for infection. Bacteria from the inside of the bowel may contaminate the surgical site and incision in spite of copious irrigation. Edema, pain, induration, and expression of purulence are obvious signs of infection. Complete reopening of the entire wound is usually not necessary for drainage. Frequently an abscess will be limited to one or more small areas beneath the incision. Careful probing of the wound is necessary to discover any tracking of the wound. Subcutaneous connections between openings are common, requiring irrigation through the tracts and packing to prevent the openings from closing before the tunnels are granulated.

Panniculectomy

Panniculectomy is the surgical removal of redundant abdominal skin and subcutaneous tissue following extreme weight loss. The panniculus (pannus, "apron") may substantially overlap tissue producing intertrigo, a condition of maceration, inflammation, and fissuring of the skin. Intertrigo complications include fungal infection, bacterial superinfection and skin breakdown. Insurance coverage for panniculectomy remains controversial as some payers see this procedure as strictly cosmetic rather than recognizing it as a risk factor for tissue injury and infection.

Pilonidal Cyst

Abscess formation within pilonidal cysts is a common problem. The term pilonidal means *nest of hair*. Those with pilonidal cysts have a dimple and increased hair growth in the sacrococcygeal area, just superior to the gluteal cleft. Cysts most often become problematic in late teen and early adult years. Although abscesses within these cysts are frequently treated with incision and drainage, they do not heal well and these infections are notoriously recurrent even after wound closure. Alternatives to incision and drainage are excision of the cyst with primary closure or

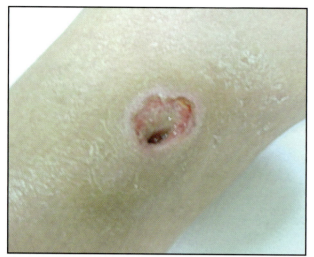

Figure 7-36. Wound over the fibular head caused by ill-fitting prosthesis.

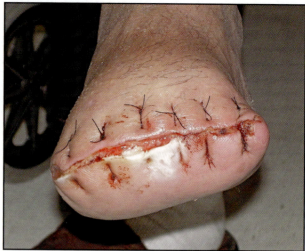

Figure 7-37A. The beginning of infection and dehiscence of an amputation wound. This amputation was subsequently revised and healed.

plastic surgery and excision with healing by secondary intention. Statistically, excision with secondary intention has the best outcome, and incision and drainage has the highest rate of complications and recurrence. Abscessed pilonidal cysts have a great propensity for sinus tract formation, including multiple and long tracts that may extend along the fascia of the posterior thigh. Because of the long tracts, they also have the tendency to close on the surface even as they are still expressing purulence. If allowed to close over purulent dead space, recurrence is very likely. These wounds need to be irrigated frequently and packed to stay open until all tracts have granulated and the wound bed fills.

Amputation Sites

Depending on the cause and site, amputation wounds may need to be closed in different ways. In general, a suture line is not desired on a weightbearing surface. To create a suture line on the anterior surface of a residual limb, sufficient viable skin must be left on the posterior surface of the extremity to be brought over the weightbearing surface and sutured or stapled to the anterior surface. If this condition cannot be met because of excessive loss of functional limb length, equal amounts of skin from the posterior and anterior surface of the limb can be approximated across the weightbearing surface. This approach, however, risks damage and possible dehiscence with early weightbearing, preventing a common goal of post-amputation rehabilitation. Sufficient soft-tissue is needed between the skin and the residual bone to prevent injury to the skin making contact with a prosthesis (see Figure 7-36).

Complications of amputation sites may occur shortly after the procedure or years afterwards. Acute wounds

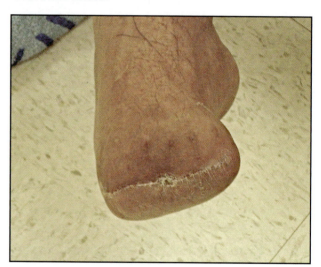

Figure 7-37B. The same foot after revision and healing of the amputation site.

are generally caused by infection of the surgical site. The wound site may open due to pressure caused by the volume of purulence, but wounds may become infected because the surgical wound opens up due to poor healing (see Figure 7-37). In either case, dehiscence of an amputation wound requires intervention. Because large pus-filled tracts may occur, careful examination of the wound must be performed as described in the next chapter. Wounds may be caused years after the amputation due to excessive wear of the prosthesis, or an ill-fitting prosthesis. If the patient still has postop swelling of the residual limb during a prosthetic fitting, the socket may become too large, causing movement inside the socket and damage to the skin of the residual limb.

Skin and Soft Tissue Infections

This type of wound is increasing in prevalence and may be the most common type of wound seen in some practices. The causative agent is frequently MRSA. Increased incidence is likely due to the development of community-acquired MRSA, whereas in the past MRSA was generally a nosocomial infection. Excessive use of antibiotics and failure of patients to finish courses of antibiotics have been blamed for the increased incidence of MRSA. According to the AHRQ, 5% of the 368,600 patients hospitalized in 2005 for MRSA died. Most of these were either elderly or had a low income. Hospitalization for MRSA infections is related to insurance coverage. AHRQ statistics show 332 Medicare patients per 100,000 were hospitalized for MRSA, 184 per 100,000 for Medicaid patients, 29 per 100,000 for patients with private insurance, and 43 per 100,000 for those without health insurance. These numbers do not necessarily indicate differences in the incidence of MRSA infection among these groupings, but could reflect differences in comorbidity and access to outpatient or ambulatory care services. Regional differences also exist in hospitalization, which may be due to regional practice patterns or incidence of MRSA infections. Hospitalization was greatest in the South (113 admissions per 100,000), followed by the West (96 admissions per 100,000), and lowest in the Northeast and Midwest (89 admissions per 100,000 population).

Skin and soft tissue infections (SSTI) typically occur in the forms of folliculitis and skin abscesses, either as furuncles or carbuncles. A furuncle is a skin abscess with a limited area, generally surrounding a hair follicle or other opening in the skin. A carbuncle is a coalesced mass of furuncles that typically occur within a fascial plane. Areas of loose skin to fascia attachment such as the nape of the neck are particularly prone to carbuncle development. Most skin abscesses tend to occur on the back and between the waist and knee, although they may appear anywhere on the body. Some individuals are prone to recurrent SSTIs. They may develop abscesses on a buttock, then several months later, one on the thigh, then one on the back, or they may develop in similar or the same areas. A severe form of SSTI is necrotizing fasciitis.

Hidradenitis Suppurativa

Infection of the apocrine sweat glands, located in the axilla, groin, perineum, perianal area, buttocks, scrotum, and submammary region is termed hidradenitis suppurativa. The process is similar to folliculitis in general, in which keratin comedones occlude the apocrine ducts, promoting inflammation and infection. Rapid proliferation of bacteria leads to abscess formation, chronic infection, and spread of infection through the glandular mass. As the process is allowed to continue induration and tract formation may occur, allowing infection to spread through the area's apocrine glands. This disease is divided into 3 stages. Stage 1 is characterized by single to multiple abscesses, but no sinus tracts or scarring. In stage 2, the patient has recurrent abscess formation, tracts, and scarring. Diffuse involvement with multiple interconnected tracts and abscesses throughout the region of glands is observed in stage 3. Patients may require a large number of small incisions to allow purulence to drain. Due to its recurrent nature, excision of the apocrine sweat gland masses in these areas may become necessary.

Necrotizing Fasciitis

Necrotizing fasciitis has been dubbed *flesh-eating bacteria*. It may be linked to traumatic or surgical wounds, but frequently occurs idiopathically. The typical patient is a middle-aged man with a secondary immunodeficiency, especially a combination of poorly controlled diabetes and alcoholism. The typical case (type 1) is produced by mixtures of aerobic gram-negative and anaerobic bacteria that act synergistically, eroding fascial planes and necrotizing subcutaneous tissue seemingly overnight. Accumulation of subcutaneous gas usually occurs due to anaerobic, gas-producing microorganisms.

Three categories of necrotizing fasciitis have been described based on the bacteria involved. Type 1 necrotizing fasciitis is a mixture of aerobes and anaerobes. Typical organisms for this type are group A beta-hemolytic *Strep*, *S. aureus*, *E. coli*, *Clostridium* species, and *Bacteroides*. Unusual components are group B, C, and G *Strep*, *Hemophilus b*, *Pseudomonas aeruginosa*, and *Vibrio vulnificus*. A combination of group A beta-hemolytic *Strep* and *S. aureus* exists in type 2 necrotizing fasciitis. Type 3 is caused by *Vibrio vulnificus*. This type is frequently caused by entry directly into a wound from contaminated seawater (bay or river mouth) or indirectly through a bite from fish or insects. An example of type 3 necrotizing fasciitis due to entering contaminated seawater with an open neuropathic ulcer is shown in Figure 7-38.

Overlying skin must commonly be excised to adequately halt progress of tissue necrosis. Frequently a combination of excision and incision and drainage must be performed, leaving pockets that benefit from daily irrigation and packing pockets and tracts with topical antibiotic in addition to systemic antibiotics. Because of the different mixtures of flora in different individuals, the clinical course may vary tremendously. The mortality of necrotizing fasciitis remains high, partly because of compromised immunity that preceded the infection such as poorly controlled diabetes, cancer, peripheral arterial disease, organ transplants, HIV, neutropenia, and alcoholism.

Necrotizing fasciitis occurs in hypoxic areas due to the effect of hypoxia on neutrophils that allows aerobic bacteria to proliferate. Consumption of oxygen by the aerobes

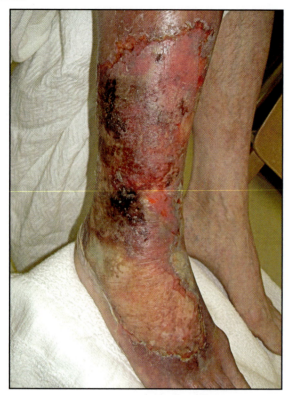

Figure 7-38. Example of type 3 necrotizing fasciitis (*Vibrio vulnificus*) caused by going into seawater barefoot with an open neuropathic ulcer.

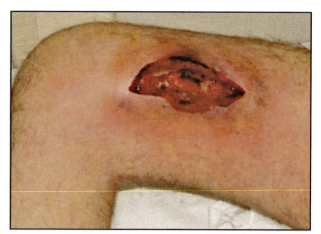

Figure 7-39. Incision and drainage wound due to skin abscess with MRSA. The wound requires packing to allow drainage to continue.

then allows anaerobes to proliferate as well. Patients generally require supplemental oxygen, one or more surgical excisions, and multiple antibiotics to cover the variety of possible bacteria. Hyperbaric oxygen has been shown in multiple studies to tremendously decrease the mortality. Usually group A hemolytic *Strep* or *S. aureus* is the initiator of the process, followed by any of a number of anaerobes. The combination of bacterial toxins can disable multiple parts of the immune system and digest tissue allowing fascial spread. The patient usually presents with a painful, edematous, and erythematous area with crepitus that progresses to anesthetic and dusky. The spread is dependent on the thickness of subcutaneous tissue. Spread is particularly rapid through the scrotum and penis due to their lack of subcutaneous fat.

Fournier's Gangrene

The term Fournier's gangrene is used specifically for necrotizing fasciitis of the perineum/scrotum and often the penis of adults. The scrotum may become several times its normal size. Early diagnosis may allow treatment with incision and drainage, but excision of some or all of the scrotal skin and, on occasion, that of the penis and perineum may become necessary depending on the spread of the infection. Plastic surgery to rebuild the scrotum or creation of pockets in the thigh to implant the testes is necessary in severe cases. The term Fournier's gangrene has been applied to women and children by some sources if necrotizing fasciitis of the perineum is present.

Diagnosis of SSTI

SSTI is generally easily diagnosed. Commonly, patients report a sudden onset of swelling and pain in the area of the SSTI. Purulence may be expressed spontaneously, or from the patient squeezing or picking at the abscess. The volume of purulence can be disturbing to the patient as a great deal of space within a fascial plane may fill seemingly overnight. Palpation of the area demonstrates warmth and induration in addition to the observation of erythema and the complaint of pain from the patient.

Treatment for SSTI

The standard treatment is incision and drainage (I&D) in conjunction with systemic antibiotics such as clindamycin, vancomycin, or the combination drug, trimethoprim and sulfamethoxazole (bactrim). One or more incisions are placed in the abscesses and purulence is expressed. The open wound created is irrigated and allowed to drain as the wound closes by secondary intention. Patients may be treated by a physician as an outpatient and given oral antibiotics or the patient may be admitted to a hospital and placed on intravenous antibiotics. Patients may require more than one I&D procedure (Figure 7-39). The wound is usually filled with packing strip—either plain or iodoform to allow the purulence to drain. An alternative to packing strip is a Penrose drain. This is a length of flat rubber tubing that prevents premature closure of the incision and allows drainage to continue as long as it is deemed necessary. Other types of drains using vacuum bulbs, such as Jackson-Pratt, may be used in some cases. Packing strip is changed daily or more often and will generally be coated with thick yellow drainage early for a variable number of days. In some cases, purulence may persist as the wound granulates in and preventing re-epithelialization may become difficult, but critically important.

SSTI occurs frequently in diabetic feet. When deep infection is suspected, I&D is generally indicated. This procedure is also used for infected surgical wounds, osteomyelitis, puncture wounds, tunneling, or sinus tracts. Deeper wounds may require the placement of a drain in addition to packing. In select cases, delayed primary closure may be used rather than secondary intention. Packing of larger wound may be done with saline-moistened gauze sponges or bandage rolls to prevent the wound from filling with granulation tissue if delayed primary closure is desired.

Pulsatile lavage is suitable for this type of wound to remove bacteria and necrotic tissue. Patients who are admitted to a hospital will generally need to continue therapy as outpatients. With the placement of peripherally-inserted central lines (PIC lines), patients can continue with intravenous antibiotics either at home or at an outpatient IV service if oral antibiotics are not appropriate. When the wound is clean and stable, closure may be performed with sutures, staples, or plastic surgery techniques discussed below. Readmissions occur occasionally. Some patients may be seen cyclically as an inpatient, outpatient, and inpatient again over a period of months to years.

Peritonitis

A life-threatening infection of the abdominal cavity, peritonitis most commonly develops from perforation of the bowels (including the appendix) with release of bacteria into the peritoneum. The esophagus and stomach may also be the source. Spillage of gastric acid due to a perforated ulcer, bile acids from a perforated gall bladder or lacerated liver, and digestive enzymes from an inflamed pancreas are also potential causes. Infected fallopian tubes or ruptured ovarian cysts are potential causes in women. Disease may be manifested as either generalized inflammation (peritonitis) or intra-abdominal abscess. Like necrotizing fasciitis, peritonitis can spread rapidly. Peritonitis may be divided into primary, secondary, and tertiary. Primary occurs spontaneously (does not involve perforation), whereas secondary peritonitis exists if the cause is either a disease process or iatrogenic. Tertiary peritonitis refers to recurrent disease. Mortality is low if the disease is uncomplicated and treated promptly (5% to 10%), but may reach 70% in cases of massive infection and organ damage.

Primary peritonitis is most commonly caused by chronic liver disease. A percentage of patients with cirrhosis and ascites (~30%) will develop spontaneous bacterial peritonitis. This form is usually due to a single bacterial species, usually gram-negative, and most commonly *E. coli.*

Common causes of secondary peritonitis are appendix rupture, perforated gastric and duodenal ulcers, strangulation of the small bowel, and perforated sigmoid colon secondary to diverticulitis or cancer. This type of peritonitis is usually due to anaerobes that do not cause problems within the gastrointestinal tract, but are allowed to proliferate within the peritoneum. Massive fibrosis or abscess formation may occur within the peritoneum, sequestering bacteria and impairing an immune response.

A patient with peritonitis will present with typical signs of systemic inflammation, complaints of abdominal pain and tenderness on palpation and will have abdominal wall muscle rigidity. The onset ranges from acute to insidious and the clinical presentation may range from limited, mild disease to systemic disease with septic shock. Treatment includes appropriate antibiotics and either percutaneous or open abdominal drainage. Dehiscence of surgical wounds for open drainage of peritonitis is 3 times as likely as abdominal surgery in general.

Another complication of peritonitis is abdominal compartment syndrome (ACS). This syndrome is characterized by intra-abdominal hypertension and multiple organ dysfunction. Excessive intra-abdominal pressure can affect multiple systems, notably pulmonary, cardiovascular, renal, and splanchnic. It may also damage skin and musculoskeletal structures. ACS is most commonly associated with massive hemorrhage, the need for extensive fluid resuscitation, prolonged surgical procedures, and coagulopathies. ACS may develop insidiously or acutely. In either case the abdominal compartment will eventually lose extensibility and pressure will rise steeply.

Similar to compartment syndromes of the extremities, ACS results in compression and then injury to whatever is located in the compartment. Hollow organs collapse, ischemia and metabolic acidosis occur in the abdominal organs, and release of bacteria, histamine, and serotonin into the peritoneum increase fluid accumulation in the peritoneum, furthering ischemia of abdominal organs, and impairing the kidneys, central circulation, ventilation, and cerebral perfusion. ACS is increasingly being suspected for acute decompensation in critically injured patients.

ACS is suspected in those with a predisposing injury and with a distended abdomen, and difficulty breathing with wheezes, crackles, and cyanosis. The patient will appear ill (wan appearance), pale, listless, weary. Surgical drainage and supportive care are required, but mortality is very high. Untreated ACS is considered to have 100% mortality; overall the mortality of documented cases of ACS is approximately 70%.

Burns: Thermal, Chemical, Electrical, Radiological

Etiology of skin injury due to different types of burns are described below. These include thermal, electrical, chemical, and radiological. In addition to injury to the skin, burns are associated with high morbidity and mortality. Loss of skin's barrier function allows body heat and water to escape and allows microorganisms access to injured tissue. Even with recovery, loss of sensation, sweating, sebum secretion, and skin elasticity occur. Mortality may occur rapidly due to airway injury. Massive quantities of fluid may be lost into the injured tissue due to the osmotic effect of particles released from tissue necrosis. Failure to rapidly replace multiple liters of fluid lost to the injured tissue will lead to hypovolemic shock. Infection may cause mortality rapidly or weeks after the injury. Rehabilitation for thermal injuries is more specifically addressed in Chapter 15.

Risk Factors and Populations

Burn injuries are very common; nearly everyone experiences them on occasion. Fortunately, most of these are inconsequential with a short period of discomfort. Although most are self-treated and are not reported, an estimated 2.5 million burn injuries per year require some degree of medical attention with 70,000 of these requiring hospitalization. A disproportionate number—approximately 35%—of serious burn injuries involve children. Many serious burn injuries occur either on the job or in motor vehicle and other crash injuries; however, 75% to 85% occur in the home, particularly in the kitchen and bathroom, with hot foods and liquids spilled in the kitchen being the largest single source of burns to children. As described in the section on neuropathy, individuals with peripheral neuropathy secondary to diabetes mellitus are also at great risk due to lack of sensation and may experience scalds from not being able to adequately determine the temperature of bath water or injuries from placing feet too close to a fireplace. Wet heat as in a scald from fluid or steam transfers more heat to the body than hot gas as in a flame. Contact injuries, particularly with very hot metallic objects such as mufflers, will transfer tremendous heat to the skin and may produce deep injuries even with brief contact due to their high conductivity.

The 2 primary age groups at risk for death from burn injury are very young children up to 5 years old and adults older than age 65 who lack the ability to escape life-threatening situations and are less able to tolerate the physical stress of the post-burn injury period. Up to the age of approximately 5 years old, burns consist mainly of scald injury with an estimated 70% of these scald injuries being preventable. These injuries include kitchen injuries from cooking, unattended hot food, liquids, and appliances; bathroom injuries from hot water, chemicals, and in older homes electric grooming appliances in the absence of ground-fault interrupter circuits. Other areas of concern in the home include lamps with dangling cords, radiators and space heaters, and hot mist vaporizers. Unattended matches and lighters in the hands of small children of this age are also a major concern. In the older child (5 to 12 years old) experimentation with heat-producing products, power lines, and above ground transformers become major sources of risk of burn injury. In teenage years with greater involvement in household and working experience, preparing food, gasoline, car repairs, occupational accidents, and sun become more prominent as causes of burn injury. In adults, gasoline, smoking, electric accidents, and occupational accidents become more common causes of injury. Finally, in the adult older than age 65, falling asleep while smoking, scalds, burning yard waste, ignition of clothing, tripping and falling on hot pipes, heaters, and radiators become important causes.

Evaluation of Burn Injuries

To explain evaluation of thermal injuries of the skin, a review of several aspects of skin anatomy is necessary. The epidermis is the avascular layer of the skin with 4 strata (5 on the palms and soles). The deepest stratum, the stratum basale, is the regenerative layer. The interface of the dermis and epidermis forms an undulating, wavelike surface; the area of the dermis that extends up into these waves is the papillary dermis and the thicker region of the dermis beneath this is the reticular dermis. Melanocytes are present in the stratum basale and necrosis down to this layer carries the risk of pigment loss from the skin. Of the sensory receptors located in the dermis, the Pacinian corpuscle is located most deeply. Hair follicles and other appendages of the epidermis dive deeply into surrounding reticular dermis. Knowledge of these points is necessary to perform an examination to reveal the depth of injury.

Two systems for communicating depth of injury are commonly used. The lay terminology of first-, second-, and third-degree burns continues to be used even in healthcare facilities. The newer system to identify the depth of injury uses the terms superficial, superficial partial-thickness, deep partial-thickness, and full-thickness. A subdermal burn injury is usually created by contact with a very high voltage source. This type may be termed a fourth-degree burn injury.

Most burn injuries other than superficial thickness will be combinations of depths. Progressing away from the area exposed to the greatest amount of heat, a less severe depth of injury is observed from the site of injury. Definite determination of the stage of injury may require 3 to 4 days due to evolution of the wound and presence of eschar. A concept frequently used to explain this phenomenon is to classify areas of the injury into 3 zones: the zone of coagulation, the zone of stasis, and the zone of hyperemia. The zone of coagulation represents the area that received the most severe injury producing irreversible cell injury. The zone of stasis represents an area of less severe insult with reversible cell injury characterized by sluggish blood flow. This region surrounds the zone of coagulation and cell death may occur in this zone in the presence of further insult. Surrounding the zone of stasis is the zone of hyperemia. This area is inflamed, but is expected to recover completely, even without further care. A deep partial-thickness wound is an example of a wound with a zone of coagulation that extends to the reticular dermis. The remainder of the reticular dermis would likely be in the zone of stasis. Further injury to the reticular dermis would convert the deep partial-thickness injury into a full-thickness injury. Additionally, areas of the body have different skin thicknesses and skin thickness changes with age. Areas of very thin skin or the skin of infants and elderly will receive greater depths of injury as classified below for the same amount of heat transferred to the skin.

Superficial/First Degree

An injury limited to the epidermis will not directly damage blood vessels or living cells. However, injury to the epidermis frequently leads to erythema and tenderness due to inflammation of the vascular layer below. Over the next few days, itching may become problematic. Eventual exfoliation (peeling) of the injured epidermis occurs over the next several days as new epidermal cells replace the injured cells without scarring. Usual causes include sunburn and brief contact with small quantities of hot liquid or mildly hot objects. Unless an injury of this depth of covers an extensive percentage of body surface area, no treatment is necessary.

Superficial Partial-Thickness/Second Degree

A greater intensity of insult creates reversible injury to the papillary dermis in addition to the loss of epidermis. In this depth of injury, generally no more than one-third of the dermis receives irreversible injury. The greater depth of injury causes more severe inflammation with leakage of fluid from the capillaries of the papillary dermis into the space between the dermis and epidermis. In areas of greater intensity of injury, massive quantities of serous fluid can accumulate, breaking desmosomes between the layers. Blistering, erythema, and pain are characteristic of this level of injury. Blistering may range from less than 1 cm to several centimeters in diameter and height above the surrounding skin. Because of the presence of intact sensory receptors, exquisite pain will result. An example is shown in Figure 7-40.

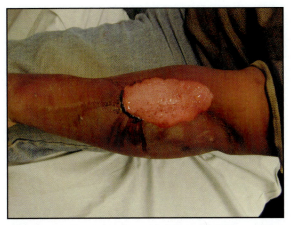

Figure 7-40. Example of superficial partial-thickness burn injury. Courtesy of Arkansas Children's Hospital, Little Rock, AR.

The decision to deliberately rupture blisters remains controversial. The intact, but nonviable and stretched epidermal layer prevents contamination of the dermis below and loss of water vapor from the wound. However, these blisters may rupture spontaneously and become contaminated under uncontrolled conditions. Molecules related to the inflammatory process are present within the blister fluid, slowing healing of the wound. Blisters may be debrided with surrounding necrotic tissue and covered with a broad spectrum antibiotic such as silver sulfadiazine, or polymixin and bacitracin, which is often used on the face. As the inflammatory process proceeds, blisters may continue to evolve within the injured area over 3 to 5 days with new blister formation and increasing size of blisters. One should assume that any erythematous and painful area will develop blisters and treat these areas as if blisters will form. Superficial partial-thickness injuries are typically caused by scalds, brief contact with hot objects, and brief contact with flame. If the blisters rupture, the wound will appear moist and red. Healing occurs spontaneously within 2 weeks without scarring. Pigmentation of the injured area will require several days to weeks and some alteration of normal skin pigmentation may occur.

Deep Partial-Thickness

This depth of injury does not have a term in the first-, second-, third-degree system, but a term for this depth is important to communicate that the prognosis of this depth of injury is different from a full-thickness injury. Deep partial-thickness burns (Figure 7-41) are the most difficult to distinguish, especially early on. They may be a variety of colors, ranging from tan to white and red. Severe injury to the papillary dermis that extends partially into the reticular dermis coagulates blood vessels in the papillary dermis, but leaves the deepest parts of hair follicles and other appendages that produce epidermal cells intact. Blisters

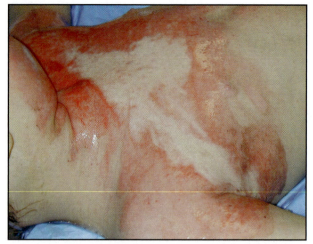

Figure 7-41. Example of deep partial-thickness burn injury. Courtesy of Arkansas Children's Hospital, Little Rock, AR.

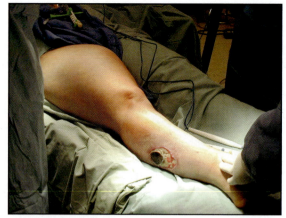

Figure 7-42A. Example of full-thickness injury prior to debridement. Courtesy of Arkansas Children's Hospital, Little Rock, AR.

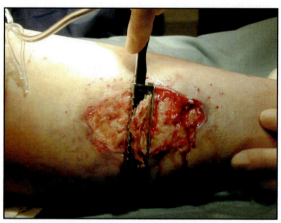

Figure 7-42B. Same leg as Figure 7-42A during debridement. Courtesy of Arkansas Children's Hospital, Little Rock, AR.

will not be evident even in the presence of severe edema due to the thickness of injured tissue and the adherence of injured tissue.

In this depth of injury, blood vessels in the deeper reticular dermis remain viable, but slow capillary refill will be present compared with more superficial injuries. Sensory testing will reveal preservation of pressure sensation to a pin prick, but not a normal sharp sensation. Because of the depth of the hair follicle within the skin, hair follicles are still viable in deep partial-thickness injuries. Therefore, one may be able to distinguish deep partial-thickness injuries from full-thickness by pulling on available hairs. If the injury is caused by flames, however, hairs may not be available for evaluation of the depth.

With this depth of injury, the skin can re-epithelialize and regain nearly normal appearance and function over the course of weeks to months of remodeling of the injured dermis. However, necrosis of more superficial tissue with loss of its barrier function places the reversibly injured deep dermis at risk of irreversible injury and necrosis due to infection, trauma, and other stresses.

Full-Thickness/Third Degree

In a full-thickness injury (Figure 7-42), cell death through the reticular dermis causes anesthesia and coagulation of the blood vessels throughout the skin. Blood may be trapped in coagulated vessels visible from the surface of the skin, but the skin will not blanch and refill. A wound that does not extend through the entire reticular dermis will allow blanching and refill of the skin. In addition, if the deep reticular dermis remains viable, vibration and pressure sensations will be intact from the Pacinian corpuscles located deep in the dermis. This depth of injury destroys all cells capable of regenerating dermis and the sources of epidermal cells from within the wounded

area. In full-thickness wounds, hairs slide out easily, in contrast to the resistance to pull that occurs with deep partial-thickness injury. Full-thickness burns are caused by prolonged contact with hot objects, scalding with very hot liquid, and particularly by ignition of clothing.

Full-thickness injuries require generation of granulation tissue, epidermal cell migration across the surface from surrounding epidermis, and will contract unless extensive scar management is provided (covered in Chapter 13). Although some smaller wounds may close due to granulation tissue and epithelialization from the edges, wound contraction associated with healing by secondary intention of full-thickness wounds more than a few centimeters across is likely to cause functional impairments; therefore grafting is generally done on all full-thickness burn injuries. However, skin grafts may also contract without appropriate intervention. In addition, very deep partial-thickness injuries may not close with enough dermal depth for satisfactory healing to occur and may also

Classification System of Burn Injuries*

Degree	Cause	Appearance	Pain level	Healing time
First/superficial	Sunburn, scald, flash flame	Dry, no blisters	Painful	2 to 5 days with peeling, no scarring
Second/superficial partial-thickness	Brief contact with hot liquids or solids, flash flame, chemical	Pink to cherry red; moist blisters	Painful	5 to 21 days, no grafting
Deep partial-thickness	Similar to above and below with corresponding greater or lesser intensity	Mixed white, waxy, pearly, or deep khaki; blanches with pressure; dry, leathery; hairs (if any) resist tugging	Some pain	If no infection, then 21 to 35 days; if infected, converts to full-thickness
Third/full-thickness	Contact with hot liquids or solids, flame, chemical, or electrical	Mixed white, waxy, pearly, deep khaki, mahogany, or charred; dry, leathery	No pain in this area, but painful in surrounding areas of partial and superficial thickness	Large areas may need months with skin grafting; small areas need weeks with or without grafting

*Table adapted from Burn Awareness Kit. Burn Awareness Coalition, Box 17840, Encino, CA 91416.

require grafting. Table 7-14 summarizes characteristics of the different classes of burns.

In all types of injury, new epithelial cells will be thinly layered and dry, and therefore easily damaged. Regenerating skin must be protected from mechanical trauma, elevated temperature, and sun exposure. In deep partial-thickness and full-thickness injuries moisturizers are needed to prevent excess drying secondary to damage to sebaceous glands. Coagulated tissue may form eschar with tremendous swelling and, as in compartment syndrome, possible vascular and neural compromise can occur. Therefore, capillary refill of distal tissues must be checked. In the case of circumferential eschar with swelling in deep partial-thickness and full-thickness burns, an incision through eschar to relieve pressure on subcutaneous tissues, called an escharotomy, will need to be performed (Figure 7-43). Depending on the location, an escharotomy may be needed even if the wound is not circumferential due to pressure within a limb compartment.

Subdermal burns are unusual and require tremendous transfer of heat. They may occur when a person is exposed to prolonged heat such as being trapped in a fire, but most often are associated with high voltage electrical injury.

These wounds are very extensive and will frequently require more than a simple skin graft such as a flap containing subcutaneous tissue to cover the defect. These wounds will likely not experience much swelling, but they are associated with a high risk of death from cardiac and respiratory arrest and internal injuries. Particularly severe exit wounds may occur if high-voltage power lines are touched while standing on metal ladders. Electrical injuries are discussed further below.

Body Surface Area

Two methods of computing extent of burned body surface are in common use. Both are used to quantify extent in terms of percentage of body surface area. The Lund and Browder method uses charts with percentages of body surface area assigned to certain body parts based on careful research of typical body proportions. Diagrams for adults and children are in shown in Figure 7-44. The adult chart may be used for children 7 years of age to adult. The child's version is used for newborns up to age 7. Certain body parts are not assigned a number directly, but a letter. A legend below the chart corresponding to the letters assigns values for the head and lower extremities on both the adult and child ver-

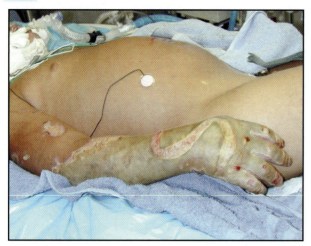

Figure 7-43. Escharotomy to relieve pressure with the forearm and hand. Courtesy of Arkansas Children's Hospital, Little Rock, AR.

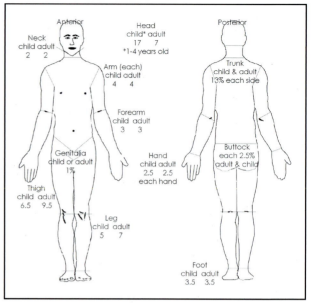

Figure 7-44. Computation of body surface area by the Lund and Browder method for adult and child.

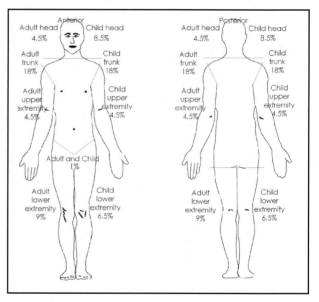

Figure 7-45. Rule of nines chart for determining percentage of body surface area for adult and child.

sion. Although this method is fairly accurate and takes into account changes in body proportions with age, the Lund and Browder method takes some time to compute.

The rule of nines (Figure 7-45) was developed to estimate percentage of body surface area involved rapidly for triage purposes. Areas of the body are divided into segments with 9% of body surface area, except for the trunk (18% for the front and 18% for the back) and the perineum is assigned 1% to make 100%. Each upper extremity is given 9% (4.5% for the anterior surface and the posterior surface). The anterior surface of each lower extremity is given 9%, as is the posterior surface, the front of the head and back of the head are each given 4.5% for a total of 9%. The head is 9%, each upper extremity is 9%, each lower extremity is 18%, the trunk is 36%, and adding 1% for the perineum yields 100%. This system is not as accurate, but is rapidly computable. An additional shortcoming is that this system does not account for changing body proportions with age as well as the Lund and Browder system. Only a child's and an adult's rule of nines chart is available and the simplicity of adding nines is also lost for the child. The need for this system is not as important as it once was due to decreasing mortality with improved treatment of burn injury.

Because the percentage of burned surface area alone is not a sufficient predictor of need for medical attention, the burn index was developed. The burn index takes into account both body surface area (BSA) involved and severity of burns. Burn index (BI) is computed as: BI = (% BSA with partial-thickness burn x 1/2 point) + (% BSA with full-thickness x 1 point). For example if 30% of the BSA has superficial or deep partial-thickness burns and 10% has full-thickness: BI = 30 x 1/2 + 10 = 25. A second example is a situation in which 10% has partial-thickness and 15%

has full-thickness. Burn index in this case is: BI = 10 x 1/2 + 15 = 20). Burn index is used to compute risk of mortality, but does not take into account the person's preexisting medical condition. Prognosis must also take the patient's age and general state of health into account. A frequently used rule of thumb is to subtract the patient's age and the percentage of body surface area burned from 100 to determine the probability of survival.

Frostbite

Prolonged exposure to subfreezing temperatures produces necrosis that may be similar in appearance to that caused by heat. These injuries typically occur due to a person being stranded outdoors in cold weather (homeless or outdoor sports-related) or due to excessive occupational exposure in a freezer. Mountain frostbite may occur in mountain-climbers due to the additive effects of cold and hypoxia. Risk of frostbite is increased by peripheral artery disease, Raynaud's disease or phenomenon, diabetes mellitus and other peripheral neuropathies, smoking, use of beta blockers, and alcohol consumption. Apical areas of the body are most susceptible to frostbite due to their large surface area relative to mass. The nose, ears, fingers, and toes are most likely to be injured. Amputation of affected areas may be required. Sophisticated plastic surgery techniques are available to reconstruct noses and ears.

The injury of frostbite is complex, involving ice crystal formation leading to loss of cellular water and damage to proteins, DNA synthesis, and cell membranes. Freezing of blood injures capillaries in the affected area. Further injury occurs during rewarming, particularly to blood vessels. Necrosis can be furthered by reperfusion injury. Thawing and refreezing is particularly damaging. The depth of injury is categorized in the same way as burns due to heat.

Frostbite injury may initially appear pale, and feel indurated and cold. The affected area is anesthetic with possible deep, aching pain. As the area warms, however, it may show extreme erythema and the patient may experience intense pain. If skin freezes, however, the tissue becomes white, no sensation returns, and necrosis occurs. Skin becomes darker, blisters, then demonstrates wet gangrene with possible injury to deeper structures including bone. In addition to these injuries, a person is likely to experience hypothermia with risk of injury to internal organs and arrhythmia.

Care includes fluid resuscitation, rapid rewarming with water at 40°C to 42°C for approximately 20 to 40 minutes until flushing of the affected area is noted. Debridement of clear, fluid-filled blisters is recommended, but not hemorrhagic blisters due to risk of infection.

Electrical Injuries

Electrical injuries include thermal injury to the skin and the effect of electrical current on subcutaneous structures and blood. The amount of heat dissipated in tissues is determined by I^2R (current squared times resistance) and the time of the exposure. Dry skin has a higher resistance than moist skin, therefore more energy is dissipated in the skin. Dry skin, therefore, increases the risk of skin injury, but decreases the risk of internal injury. With wet skin, burns of the skin are minimized, but internal injury could become severe. Mucous membranes also have a low resistance and subcutaneous injury is more likely to result. The size of the injury is also related to the body surface area (current density). A given current limited to a small area is more likely to cause injury, eg, biting into an electrical cord.

Household current of 120 V is unlikely to cause injury to intact skin. The 220 V current used in appliances such as ranges, electrical dryers, and air conditioning units is more likely to damage skin. This voltage is also used for household current in most of the world outside North America and the Caribbean. High voltage lines of 500 V and greater are very likely to cause skin injuries. Depending on the path of high voltage current, severe edema and thrombosis of blood vessels in the damaged area can occur. Edema, compartment syndrome, and thrombosis compound the injury caused by the electrical exposure by adding a component of ischemic injury. Internal organs and skeletal muscle may be severely injured. In the case of touching a high voltage line while standing on a conductive surface such as a metal ladder, shattering of bone and open fractures may result. Cardiorespiratory arrest is possible due to ventricular fibrillation and damage to the brain stem.

Chemical Injury

A wide variety of chemicals are capable of injuring skin. Exposure to acidic, alkaline, or other injurious chemicals may rapidly produce skin necrosis similar to that of a thermal injury. Other chemicals produce erythema, blistering, and more gradual necrosis. Chemical injuries are usually the result of industrial accidents due to inadvertent release of caustic substances from their containers. The extent of injury is related to the concentration of the substance and the time of exposure. For this reason, chemicals must be flushed from the skin as quickly as possible including removal of clothing and contact lenses. Treatment of this type of injury is also discussed in Chapter 15.

Radiation Burns

Either naturally occurring radioactive substances or artificially generated radiation may be encountered. Release of radioactive materials into the environment has occurred with disasters such as the Chernobyl accident in Ukraine in 1986 and explosion of nuclear weapons. Some cases of occupational exposure to radiation may also occur, but radiation injury is most commonly due to the treatment of neoplastic disease. Sources of ionizing radiation include x-rays, alpha particles, beta particles, and gamma rays. Alpha particles are helium nuclei (2 protons and 2 neutrons) that can produce tremendous damage, but because of their mass, they do not penetrate tissue. However, alpha particles can be released in the lungs due to the inhalation of radon gas and cause lung cancer. Beta particles are essentially electrons emitted from particular radioactive species with high energy. Beta particles have much less mass than alpha particles and can penetrate a limited depth of tissue. Beta-particle emitters may be used to treat a superficial form of cancer, mycosis fungoides.

Because gamma rays and x-rays have no mass they can travel long distances and penetrate tissues. The emission of these can be controlled and used either diagnostically or therapeutically. X-rays are generally useful for diagnostic imaging. Gamma rays may be used therapeutically to irradiate tumors and may also be used diagnostically for imaging, generally by placing a gamma-emitting substance into the body to localize its distribution within the body. Gamma radiation may be controlled precisely in a device called a gamma knife to reach otherwise inoperable tumors. A form of radiation therapy called brachiotherapy uses seeds of radioactive materials implanted in specific areas of the body to locally damage cancer cells.

Although the application of radiation therapy is designed to minimize injury to skin and subcutaneous tissue while producing irreversible injury to neoplastic tissue, beams of radiation from sources such as Cobalt-60 are capable of inflicting tremendous genetic injury to healthy tissue between the source of radiation and the tumor. Therefore, multiple beams are aimed from different directions toward the neoplasm to enhance the injury to the tumor and minimize damage to other tissues. However, the accumulation of injury may still result. Short-term complications of radiation therapy are estimated at 5% to 15%. Longer range complications may be seen in patients irradiated many years ago, but the true rate is not known due to death of patients before long-term complications can be observed. Patients with fistulas, osteonecrosis, sclerosis of skin and skeletal structures may be seen in a typical clinic due to remote radiation therapy.

Acute radiation injury is primarily due to direct damage to DNA. Indirect injury may also occur due to the generation of free radicals by ionizing radiation. Cell death may occur immediately, or cells may not be able to replicate following exposure. Additionally, blood vessel injury may produce ischemic injury to additional tissue. Long-term effects are mainly fibrosis of tissue in the path of the ionizing radiation. Skin loses its rete pegs, elastic fibers are damaged, and abnormal fibroblast activity is induced by the injury. Because of genetic damage induced by radiation, other malignancies and nonhealing wounds may develop over time. The loss of fibroblasts and dysfunction of remaining fibroblasts may require wide excision of the injured tissue and either grafting or a flap to cover the wound.

Radiation injury may be classified as acute, subacute, or chronic. Acute injuries are generally the result of acci-

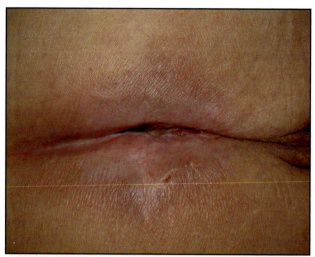

Figure 7-46. Example of injury incurred from radiation therapy for colon cancer. Note erythema and induration.

dental exposure. This type of injury requires a dose in the range of 5,000 to 10,000 rads, producing skin injury with an appearance similar to a thermal burn. Patients may experience a range of effects from severe erythema, edema, pain, and itching, to desquamation of the skin, to a depth of tissue necrosis, including blood vessels and other subcutaneous structures. Desquamation and tissue necrosis greatly increase the risk of infection. Very high doses of ionizing radiation impair the ability to produce blood cells.

Subacute injury is more likely to be seen clinically as a result of cancer radiation therapy. Recurrent exposure to low doses of radiation produces erythema, edema, and severe induration (see Figure 7-46). Mild cases may have transient erythema only. Greater damage may cause dry desquamation with erythema, itching, and epidermal peeling. With wet desquamation, erythema and blistering of the skin occur. These conditions can progress to tissue necrosis with sloughing. Damage to blood vessels, fibroblasts, and epidermal cells may lead to delayed or nonwound healing.

Chronic injury is due to long-term, repeated, and usually occupational exposure to radiation. Damage may eventually become similar or worse than that observed with subacute injury. Blood vessels are generally damaged more severely in chronic than subacute injury, leading to additional ischemic tissue injury.

OPERATIVE REPAIR OF WOUNDS

Operative repair of ulcers represents surgical management and, as such, is performed only by a qualified and licensed surgeon. Possible techniques for operative repair include direct closure with sutures, staples, or adhesives. In certain cases, healing by first, second, or third intent is not adequate for wound closure. Alternatives include skin grafting and flaps. Living skin equivalents may be used in the same manner as grafts. Skin grafts are commonly used for full-thickness burns. A piece of skin is removed completely from the body and transplanted to another site, where it is revascularized by the recipient site. Another approach is the flap in which the transplanted tissue is transferred with its own blood supply. In some cases, the transplanted tissue is not completely excised and may have a number of different tissue types within them.

Operative repair is addressed in AHCPR pressure ulcer treatment guidelines. At the time of publication, the recommendation was for operative repair for clean stage III or IV pressure ulcers not responding to optimal care, although the panel stated that more research was needed to identify criteria clearly. Operative repair should not be undertaken until a wound is clean, stable, and free of necrotic tissue. In the case of large wounds, conventional treatment including debridement and dressing changes may be carried out for several weeks before grafting is feasible. Operative repair is recommended only for patients who are medically stable, adequately nourished, and otherwise able to tolerate surgery. In some cases, especially terminal illness, wound closure is not a feasible goal; simple protection of the wound may be sufficient.

For the operative repair candidate, a number of factors may improve operative outcome. Preoperatively, the clinician should address smoking cessation, treatment for spasticity, wound colonization, urinary and fecal incontinence, and urinary tract infection. Common procedures include direct closure (third or delayed primary intent), skin grafting, skin flaps, musculocutaneous flaps, and free flaps. Types of flaps are described in Chapter 2. Postoperative follow-up care for operative repair of ulcers includes using an appropriate support surface. An air-fluidized bed or low-air-loss bed is recommended for up to 2 weeks post-op, depending on multiple factors, especially the patient's ability to remain off the operative surface and the risk for development of new ulcers. Tissue viability in the operative site should be monitored carefully with a slow increase in the time that the patient is positioned on the flap or graft. Monitoring flaps or grafts for pallor or redness that persist after 10 min of pressure is recommended. In addition, shear forces, including excessive stretching of the operative site should be avoided.

SUMMARY

The purpose of this chapter is to understand the mechanisms of these wounds and what may lead to the referral to clinicians reading this material. Pressure ulcers are caused by a number of factors, including pressure, shear, friction, excess moisture, heat or skin dryness, and lack of nutrition. Both time and pressure on a body surface must be considered in assessing risk of skin injury. Staging of pressure ulcers is based on the tissue involved and, therefore, reverse staging cannot be done logically. Positioning must account for pressure, the patient's body composition, mental status, and support surface. Guidelines for appropriate support surfaces are discussed as is the need for adequate nutritional and psychosocial assessment. Methods to enhance healing of pressure ulcers are discussed in subsequent chapters.

Neuropathic ulcers are formed by the chain of events including loss of sensory, motor, and autonomic innervation of the foot, leading to loss of protective sensation, altered biomechanics of the foot, and dryness of the foot. Foot screening is performed at regular intervals and more frequently in patients with established high risk. The Wagner scale is a series of progressively worse conditions, rather than a continuum of wound severity. The Wagner scale begins with pre-ulceration, then ulceration of the foot, infection, then ischemic ulcers of the forefoot and entire foot. A noninfected foot without arterial insufficiency needs to be protected from further injury by offloading, including total contact casting. Total contact casting may not be appropriate for all individuals. Infection (stage 3) needs to be cleared before casting. Stages 4 and 5 require referral and further evaluation by a vascular surgeon. Other options for offloading may be less effective, but allow better inspection of the affected foot.

Arterial, venous, and lymphatic disease can create ulcers requiring skilled assessment and therapy. A thorough differential diagnosis is critical. Arterial disease can create an emergent surgical problem and the treatment for chronic venous insufficiency is contraindicated in the presence of arterial insufficiency. Arterial insufficiency may occur anywhere, but is most common where vessels are the most distal, on the toes and heels. Venous ulcers are located most commonly just proximal to the medial malleolus, sometimes proximal to the lateral malleolus and rarely elsewhere. Arterial insufficiency can be painful at rest, increasing with elevation and the wounds tend to be pink rather than red. Venous insufficiency may cause an uncomfortable pressure in the leg, which is relieved by elevation, and the wounds tend to be red and very wet with hemosiderin staining of the skin surrounding the ulcer. Failure to treat the underlying venous hypertension is a frequent cause of failure to heal or recurrence of the leg ulcers. Compression therapy includes compression bandaging, pumping, and fitting for custom stockings when edema is removed.

Traumatic wounds are typically managed in the emergency room or operating room, but complications may involve other clinicians. Complications include infection and dehiscence due to a number of factors unique to each patient. Common causes of acute wounds include burns, dehiscence of surgical wounds, amputation wounds, lacerations, incisions, gunshot wounds, and open fractures. A brief discussion of operative repair is also included in this chapter.

QUESTIONS

1. Why is body composition important in the risk for developing pressure ulcers?

2. Why are the occiput and lateral condyles of the elbows at such high risk for skin breakdown?

3. Why is reclining such an important risk factor in sacral ulcers?

4. List reasons that a person might require a specialty bed.

5. What options are available for reducing risk of pressure ulcers in a person during sitting?

6. Why are psychosocial factors important in preventing pressure ulcers?

7. Trace the sequence of events leading to lower extremity amputation.

8. Distinguish between diabetic ulcers caused by arterial disease and by mechanical forces on the foot.

9. Discuss the roles of motor and autonomic neuropathy in causing neuropathic ulcers.

10. What is the basis for the Wagner scale? Does it represent increased severity of a given condition?

11. What is the value of testing for pain, vibration, reflexes, and muscle strength in the diabetic foot?

12. Why is bed rest frequently a poor option for offloading a diabetic foot?

13. Describe indications for different types of offloading devices for aiding neuropathic ulcer healing.

14. Which type of vascular ulcer tends to be dry? To be wet?

15. What is the physiological basis for the moisture of venous wounds?

16. Who is more likely to develop venous insufficiency, a tall person or a short person? A person who moves or one who stands all day?

17. Contrast arterial and venous ulcers in terms of how malnutrition of tissue occurs.

18. Why is compression contraindicated in the presence of arterial insufficiency? What simple test can be used to screen for arterial disease?

19. Why is compression therapy contraindicated in the presence of congestive heart failure?

20. Why is a gunshot wound likely to become infected even if the bullet reaches a high temperature?

21. What are the advantages and disadvantages of placing the amputation wound at the distal end of the residual limb?

22. What are the relative risks of poor outcomes from the three basic types of lacerations? Which is generally better, a triangular flap with its apex distal or proximal?

23. What are the potential problems created by an open fracture and the use of external fixation?

24. How does radiation therapy affect wound healing?

25. Why is a clean wound, free of infection, required for operative repair?

REFERENCE

1. NPUAP. *Pressure Ulcer Stages Revised by NPUAP.* Available at http://www.npuap.org/pr2.htm. Accessed September 9, 2009.

BIBLIOGRAPHY

AHCPR Supported Clinical Practice Guidelines. Available at: http://www.ncbi.nlm.nih.gov/books/bv.fcgi?rid=hstat2.section.4521. Accessed September 9, 2009.

American Diabetes Association 2009 Clinical Practice Recommendations. Available at http://care.diabetesjournals.org/content/32/Supplement_1. Accessed September 9, 2009.

American Diabetes Association: Consensus development conference on diabetic foot wound care (consensus statement). *Diabetes Care.* 1999;22:1354-1360.

Backonja M, Beydoun A, Edwards KR, et al. Gabapentin for the symptomatic treatment of painful neuropathy in patients with diabetes mellitus: a randomized controlled trial. *JAMA.* 1998;280(21):1831-1836.

Barczak CA, Barnett RI, Childs EJ, Bosley LM. Fourth national pressure ulcer prevalence study. *Adv Wound Care.* 1997;10:18-26.

Blair SD, Wright DD, Backhouse CM, Riddle E, McCollum CN. Sustained compression and healing of chronic venous ulcers. *BMJ.* 1988;297:1159-1161.

Bone RC, Balk RA, Cerra FB, et al. Definitions for sepsis and organ failure and guidelines for the use of innovative therapies in sepsis. The ACCP/SCCM Consensus Conference Committee. American College of Chest Physicians/Society of Critical Care Medicine. *Chest.* 1992;101(6):1644-1655.

Brienza DM, Geyer MJ. Understanding support surface technologies. *Adv Skin Wound Care.* 2000;13:237-244.

Brienza DM, Karg PE. Seat cushion optimization: a comparison of interface pressure and tissue stiffness characteristics for spinal cord injured and elderly patients. *Arch Phys Med Rehabil.* 1998;79:388-394.

Brown HE, Mueller MJ. A step to gait pattern decreases pressures on the forefoot. *J Ortho Sports Phys Ther.* 1998;28:139-145.

Burnand KG, Browse NL. The cause of venous ulceration. *Lancet.* 1982;31:243.

Butler ED, Gant TD. Electrical injuries, with special reference to the upper extremities. A review of 182 cases. *Am J Surg.* 1977;134(1):95-101.

Calianno C. Assessing and preventing pressure ulcers. *Adv Skin Wound Care.* 2000;13:244-246.

Cancio LC, Jimenez-Reyna JF, Barillo DJ, Walker SC, McManus AT, Vaughan GM. One hundred ninety-five cases of high-voltage electric injury. *J Burn Care Rehabil.* 2005;26(4):331-340.

Catanzariti AR, Haverstock BD, Grossman JP, Mendicino RW. Off loading techniques in the treatment of diabetic plantar neuropathic foot ulceration. *Adv Wound Care.* 1999;12:452-458.

Chase CW, Franklin JD, Guest DP, Barker DE. Internal fixation of the sternum in median sternotomy dehiscence. *Plast Reconstr Surg.* 1999;103(6):1667-1673.

Coleridge Smith PD, Thomas P, Scurr JH, Dormandy JA. Causes of venous ulceration: a new hypothesis. *Br Med J.* 1988;296:1726-1727.

Dellon AL. Treatment of symptomatic diabetic neuropathy by surgical decompression of multiple peripheral nerves. *Plast Reconstr Surg.* 1992;89(4):689-697.

Dietzek AM. Endovenous radiofrequency ablation for the treatment of varicose veins. *Vascular.* 2007;15(5):255-261.

Doughty DB. Prevention and managing surgical wound dehiscence. *Adv Skin Wound Care.* 2005;18:319-322.

Driscoll JA. Integumentary management of the patient with multiple traumatic injuries. *Acute Care Perspectives.* 1999;7(2):1-18.

Ducic I, Taylor NS, Dellon AL. Relatioinship between peripheral nerve decompression and gain of pedal sensibility and balance in patients with peripheral neuropathy. *Ann Plast Surg.* 2006;56(2):145-150.

Edberg EL, Cerny K, Stauffer ES. Prevention and treatment of pressure sores. *Phys Ther.* 1973;53(3):246-252.

Edmonds ME, Blundell MP, Morris ME, Thomas EM, Cotton LT, Watkins PJ. Improved survival of the diabetic foot: the role of a specialized foot clinic. *Q J Med.* 1986;60(232):763-771.

Evans RJ, Little K. Fracture due to shock from domestic electricity supply. *Injury.* 1991;22(3):231-232.

Exton-Smith AN, Sherwin RW. The prevention of pressure sores. Significance of spontaneous bodily movements. *Lancet.* 1961;2(7212):1124-1126.

Finley JM, McConnell RY. *Emergency Wound Repair.* Baltimore, MD: University Park Press; 1984.

Goldstein B, Giroir B, Randolph A. International pediatric sepsis consensus conference: definitions for sepsis and organ dysfunction in pediatrics. *Pediatr Crit Care Med.* 2005;6(1):2–8.

Heggers JP, Robson MC, Manavalen K, et al. Experimental and clinical observations on frostbite. *Ann Emerg Med.* 1987;16(9):1056-1062.

Helm PA, Walker SC, Pulliam GF. Recurrence of neuropathic ulceration following healing in a total contact cast. *Arch Phys Med Rehab.* 1991;72:967-970.

Hess CT. Management of the patient with a venous ulcer. *Adv Skin Wound Care.* 2000;13:79-83.

Irion GL, Boyer S, McGinnis T, Thomason M, Trippe A. Effect of upper extremity movement on sternal skin stress. *Acute Care Perspectives.* 2006;15(3):1-6.

Irion GL, Boyte B, Ingram J, Kirchem C, Weathers J. Sternal skin stress produced by functional upper extremity movements. *Acute Care Perspectives.* 2007;16(3):1-5.

Kaplan EN, Hentz VR. *Emergency Management of Skin and Soft Tissue Wounds. An Illustrated Guide.* Boston, MA: Little, Brown, and Company; 1984.

Kravitz SR, McGuire JB, Sharma S. The treatment of diabetic foot ulcers: reviewing the literature and a surgical algorithm. *Adv Skin Wound Care.* 2007;20:227-237.

Kuo J, Butchart EG. Sternal wound dehiscence. *Care of the Critically Ill.* 1995;11:244-248.

Landis EM. Microinjection studies of capillary blood pressure in human skin. *Heart.* 1930;15:209-228.

Lavery L, Vela SA, Lavery DC, Quebedeaux TL. Reducing dynamic foot pressure in high risk diabetic subjects with foot ulcerations. *Diabetes Care.* 1996;19:818-821.

Levy MM, Fink MP, Marshall JC, et al. 2001 SCCM/ESICM/ACCP/ATS/SIS International Sepsis Definitions Conference. *Crit Care Med.* 2003;31(4):1250-1256.

Lopez A, Phillips T. Venous ulcers. *Wounds.* 1998;10:149-157.

Lower Extremity Amputation Prevention. Available at http://www.hrsa.gov/leap/brochure.htm. Accessed September 9, 2009.

Lund CC, Browder NC. The estimation of areas of injury. *Surg Gynecol Obstet.* 1944;79:352-358.

Max MB, Culnane M, Schafer SC, et al. Amitriptyline relieves diabetic neuropthy pain in patients with normal or depressed mood. *Neurology.* 1987;37(4):589-596.

McCallum I, King PM, Bruce J. Healing by primary versus secondary intention after surgical treatment for pilonidal sinus. *Cochrane Database Syst Rev.* 2007;(4):CD006213.

McCleane G. Topical application of doxepin hydrochloride, capsaicin and a combination of both produces analgesia in chronic human neuropathic pain: a randomized, double-blind, placebo-controlled study. *Br J Clin Pharmacol.* 2000;49(6):574-579.

McGuckin M, Stineman M, Goin J, et al. *Venous Leg Ulcer Guideline.* University of Pennsylvania; Philadelphia, PA; 1997.

McKenzie LL. In search of a standard for pin site care. *Orthopaedic Nursing.* 1999;18:73-78.

Mueller MJ. Off loading techniques for neuropathic plantar wounds. *Adv Wound Care.* 1999;12:270-271.

Nelson RG, Gohdes DM, Everhart JE, et al. Lower extremity amputations in NIDDM: 12-year follow-up study in Pima Indians. *Diabetes Care.* 1988;11:8-16.

Nicholaides AN. Investigation of chronic venous insufficiency. *Circulation.* 2000;102:e126-163.

O'Sullivan B, Levin W. Late radiation-related fibrosis: pathogenesis, manifestations, and current management. *Semin Radiat Oncol.* 2003;13(3):274-289.

Panel on the Prediction and Prevention of Pressure Ulcers in Adults. Pressure Ulcers in Adults: Prediction and Prevention. Clinical Practice Guideline, No. 3 AHCPR Publication No. 92-0047. Rockville, MD: Agency for Health Care Policy and Research; May 1992.

Peacock EE. *Wound Repair.* Philadelphia, PA: W.B. Saunders; 1984.

Pecoraro RE, Reiber GE, Burgess EM. Pathways to diabetic limb amputation. Basis for prevention. *Diabetes Care.* 1990;13:513-521.

Petrone P. Surgical management and strategies in the treatment of hypothermia and cold injury. *Emerg Med Clin North Am.* 2003;21(4):1165-1178.

Proebstle TM, Vago B, Alm J, Göckeritz O, Lebard C, Pichot O. Treatment of the incompetent great saphenous vein by endovenous radiofrequency powered segmental thermal ablation: first clinical experience. *J Vasc Surg.* 2008;47(1):151-156.

Puggioni A, Kalra M, Gloviczki P. Superficial vein surgery and SEPS for chronic venous insufficiency. *Semin Vasc Surg.* 2005;18(1):41-48.

Quintavalle PR, Lyder CH, Mertz PJ, Phillips-Jones C, Dyson M. Use of high-resolution, high-frequency diagnostic ultrasound to investigate the pathogenesis of pressure ulcer development. *Adv Skin Wound Care.* 2006;19(9):498-505.

Rains C, Bryson HM. Topical capsaicin. A review of its pharmacological properties and therapeutic potential in post-herpetic neuralgia, diabetic neuropathy, and osteoarthritis. *Drugs Aging.* 1995;7(4)317-328.

Robson MC. Wound infection. A failure of wound healing caused by an imbalance of bacteria. *Surg Clin North Am.* 1997;77:637-650.

Robson MC, Shaw RC, Heggers JP. The reclosure of postoperative incisional abscesses based on bacterial quantification of the wound. *Ann Surg.* 1970;171:279-282.

Rudolph DM. Pathophysiology and management of venous ulcers. *J Wound Ostomy Cont Nurs.* 1998;25:248-255.

Rudolph R, Arganese T, Woodward M. The ultrastructure and etiology of chronic radiotherapy damage in human skin. *Ann Plast Surg.* 1982;9(4):282-92.

Scultetus AH, Villavicencio JL, Rich NM. Facts and fiction surrounding the discovery of the venous valves. *J Vasc Surg.* 2001;33(2):435-441.

Siemionow M, Alghoul M, Molski M, Agaoglu G. Clinical outcome of peripheral nerve decompression in diabetic and nondiabetic peripheral neuropathy. *Ann Plast Surg.* 2006;57(4):385-390.

Sims DS, Cavanaugh PR, Ulbrecht JS. Risk factors in the diabetic foot. Recognition and management. *Phys Ther.* 1988;68:1887-1902.

Sinacore DR. Total contact casting for diabetic neuropathic ulcers. *Phys Ther.* 1996;76:296-301.

Steins A, Junger M, Zuder D, Rassner G. Microcirculation in venous leg ulcers during healing: prognostic impact. *Wounds.* 1999;11:6-12.

Stone NC, Daniels TR. Midfooot and hindfoot arthrodeses in diabetic Charcot arthropathy. *Can J Surg.* 2000;43(6):449-455.

Swan KG, Swan RC. *Gunshot Wounds. Pathophysiology and Management.* Chicago, IL: Year Book Medical Publishers; 1989.

Ulrich AS. Hypothermia and localized cold injuries. *Emerg Med Clin North Am.* 2004;22(2):281-298.

Varela CD, Vaughan TK, Carr JB, Slemmons BK. Fracture blisters: clinical and pathological aspects. *J Orthop Trauma.* 1993;7:417-427.

Veal J, Sellars BB. Reduce sternal dehiscence and infections. *Cardiovasc Dis Manage.* 2002;8(11):6.

Ward P. Care of skeletal pins: a literature review. *Nurs Stand.* 1998;12:34-38.

Wells JA, Karr D. Interface pressure, wound healing and satisfaction in the evaluation of a non- powered fluid mattress. *Ostomy Wound Manage.* 1998;44:38-42.

Wu SC, Armstrong DG. The role of activity, adherence, and off-loading on the healing of diabetic foot wounds. *Plast Reconstr Surg.* 2006;177(7 Suppl):248S-253S.

Young MJ, Cavanaugh PR, Thomas G, et al. The effect of callus removal on dynamic plantar foot pressures in diabetic patients. *Diabetes Med.* 1992;9:55-57.

Zeitani J, Bertolodo F, Bassano C, et al. Superficial wound dehiscence after median sternotomy: surgical treatment versus secondary wound healing. *Ann Thorac Surg.* 2004; 77(2): 672-675.

Assessing Wounds

OBJECTIVES

- List observations necessary for assessing wounds.
- Describe appropriate methods for documentation of the following and discuss the potential implications associated with:
  - » Color of wounds
  - » Odor
  - » Drainage
  - » Extent
  - » Surrounding skin.
- Identify tissue types within a wound.
- Document undermining, pocketing, tunneling, and sinus tracts.
- Describe and distinguish signs of infection and inflammation both locally and systemically.
- Perform differential diagnosis of wounds of different etiology.
- Provide a prognosis for different wounds; list factors that may alter the anticipated number of visits or time for reaching goals.
- Conduct a complete wound examination/evaluation.
- Recognize the need for and utilize the results of various diagnostic imaging procedures.

Previous chapters have been directed toward assessing patients and the etiology of wounds. However, given 2 wounds with identical characteristics, patients with different cultural, work, family backgrounds, and comorbid conditions may have different goals or prognoses for that wound. A thorough examination must be performed on the initial visit with periodic re-examination appropriate for the setting. Every visit is an opportunity for re-examination, including an update on history, home, and work activities. The depth and breadth of each re-examination will be determined by a number of factors: the severity of the wound, the progress of the wound, and any signs of deterioration, such as development or worsening of odor or drainage. The purpose of this chapter is to develop a systematic method of wound examination and testing so one can develop a differential diagnosis and a prognosis for reaching appropriate goals based on the individual needs of the patient. Development of a plan of care will be discussed in Chapter 18.

Irion G.
Comprehensive Wound Management, 2nd ed. (pp 149-160)
© 2010 SLACK Incorporated

WOUND CHARACTERISTICS

The 5 critical aspects of wound characteristics are color, odor, drainage, extent, and surrounding skin (CODES). The mnemonic CODES will be used to develop a systematic examination of the wound. Methods for observing the CODES and the measurements of wounds are discussed along with interpretation of findings. The tools for an examination can be relatively simple such as cotton-tipped applicators and paper rulers; however, a thorough examination requires adequate lighting to visualize the details of the wound and surrounding skin. A dedicated exam light is useful because it can be used during debridement as well. A pocket flashlight and magnifying glass are tremendously useful to see detail, particularly deep into a wound where an exam light might be difficult to aim. Otherwise, injury through different layers of tissue could be missed. The ability to determine which tissue layers are involved in wounds, and to observe the colors deep within the wound can facilitate the diagnostic process greatly.

Color

This item refers to the color within the wound. The color of surrounding skin is discussed below. Three basic colors may be observed in a wound: black, yellow, and red. Black tissue within a wound represents desiccated necrotic tissue. With certain exceptions, black tissue should be debrided to allow migration of new cells to fill the defect and resurface it with epithelial cells. An exception to debriding blackened tissue is the presence of dry gangrene, usually on the foot, caused by severe ischemia. Such advanced arterial disease often requires amputation, and autoamputation of toes may occur. Debridement in the case of dry gangrene is unlikely to assist in healing due to the lack of delivery of nutrients necessary for healing, rather it exposes necrotic tissue to the risk of infection.

Yellow may represent one of 3 possibilities. Pus (purulent exudate) within a wound has a thick texture, usually has an odor, and may have a color ranging from a greenish tint to a darker yellow. Purulence is a clear sign of infection with pyogenic (pus-producing) organisms, which may require the temporary use of topical antimicrobials or systemic antibiotic drugs along with more aggressive debridement of the wound. A second yellow substance is fibrin. Fibrinogen leaks from vessels during inflammation and is converted to fibrin. Fibrin is the end product of the blood coagulation cascade, forming an insoluble fiber that, along with platelets, creates thrombi. Fibrin forms a difficult to remove hardened sheet on wound beds, which may require debridement with specific chemicals or sharp instruments. The third material is termed *slough* (pronounced sluff). This is partially solubilized necrotic tissue. It ranges from a grayish to brownish-yellow color depending on how well autolytic debridement (breakdown of necrotic tissue by enzymes produced by cells in the wound) is proceeding. Autolytic debridement is also associated with soupy brownish drainage and stringy tissue. It should not be confused with purulence.

A beefy red color is observed in a clean, granulating wound. A wound with this color needs to be protected from both environmental factors and from harsh handling by the clinician or caregiver. Appropriate dressings for clean, granulating wounds are discussed in Chapter 12. Redness of tissue is due to the presence of hemoglobin of red blood cells circulating through tissue. As blood flow declines with arterial disease, granulation tissue becomes less red, becoming pink instead. A lighter pink color indicates poor arterial circulation. A dusky red is an indication of impending necrosis suggesting infection of the granulation tissue.

Odor

Although words may fail to describe odors well, a few words are commonly used to describe them. Healthy wounds generally have no odor, but the absence of odor does not ensure the absence of infection. Foul is used for wounds with that have an unpleasant odor that generally induces a withdrawal reaction from those not accustomed to infected wounds. Putrid is reserved for a very strong, foul odor associated with decaying meat. A putrid odor may be present in a wound, such as a pressure ulcer, that has had a large amount of necrotic tissue for an extended time. A fruity/sweet odor is characteristic of infection with *Pseudomonas aeruginosa*. *Pseudomonas* is also characterized by bluish-green color on the wound surface and greenish drainage. Treatment for *Pseudomonas* infection is frequently topical application of acetic acid, the active ingredient of vinegar, which also has a characteristic odor. Proteus produces a characteristic ammonia odor. A foul-smelling wound is usually, but not always infected. A wound with a strong foul odor from a distance or with the dressing still in place, however, is very likely to be infected. Large quantities of slough as discussed above may have an odor, and a clinician must be prepared to distinguish the odor of an occluded wound from infection. Slough left under an occlusive dressing (a dressing holding fluid under it) for a number of days may have an odor, but this odor is typically milder than that associated with infection and will be lost when the wound is cleansed, whereas an infected wound will continue to have a foul odor after the wound is cleansed.

Drainage

Drainage should be described both in terms of amount and quality of the drainage. Terms used to describe the quantity are rather subjective. A continuum of desiccated, minimum, moderate, and maximum (or copious) is used. The terms *desiccated* and *maximum* are easily identified. A wound bed that is dry needs intervention to increase its moisture to a level compatible with healing. The term *maximum* or *copious drainage* may be used when the primary dressing (dressing directly in contact with the wound) and secondary dressings are soaked with drainage. A small area of moisture on the primary dressing may be described as minimum. Moderate drainage may be appropriate when the primary dressing is nearly full but not saturated with drainage. However, judgment of quantity may be difficult when the time that the dressing has been in place is not constant. For example, a dressing may be changed overnight or during early morning rounds with no indication of how long the dressing has been accumulating drainage. Copious drainage needs to be managed by selecting an appropriate dressing or combination of dressings to absorb drainage and protect the surrounding skin from excessive moisture. Optimizing healing is often a balancing act of maintaining wound moisture without maceration of surrounding skin and requires good clinical judgment.

The color and consistency of drainage are also important. Clear drainage is caused by leakage of fluid from blood vessels during inflammation. By definition, a clear fluid consisting of water and small particles such as electrolytes is a transudate, whereas exudate contains larger elements such as cells and proteins. If the equivalent of serum (the fluid part of blood with removal of proteins) is present, the adjective serous is used. Because serum and transudate represent the same type of fluid, the term *serous exudate* should not be used. Moreover, distinction between exudate and transudate cannot always be made visually. On the other hand, *purulent exudate* is acceptable terminology. This fluid obviously has cells and proteins in it. The safest term to use is *drainage* if the clinician is unsure whether the fluid is transudate or exudate. Soupy brownish drainage is associated with autolytic debridement (breakdown of necrotic tissue using enzymes produced by macrophages and other cells). An example of copious bluish green sanguinopurulent drainage (bloody/purulent) due to *Pseudomonas aeruginosa* infection is depicted in Figure 8-1. Copious serous drainage indicates either venous insufficiency or inflammation and a need to reduce handling of the wound and to provide adequate absorption to prevent maceration. A desiccated wound indicates the need to use a dressing to retain fluid within the wound and to add moisture to a wound using dressings described in Chapter 12.

Extent

The extent of a wound may be assessed in many ways. The 2 basic methods are to measure representative distances or to measure volume. Within the wound, an

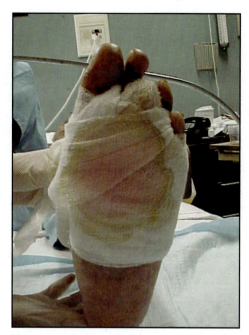

Figure 8-1. Red and green sanguinopurulent drainage of a diabetic foot infected with *Pseudomonas aeruginosa*.

estimated percentage of the wound bed of different tissue types or colors should be documented. One may use the terms: 1) *granulation tissue* vs *necrotic tissue*, 2) *granulation tissue, slough,* and *eschar,* or 3) *red, yellow,* and *black,* and give percentages adding up to 100%. Examples of these ways of reporting include: 1) 40% granulation tissue and 60% necrotic tissue, 2) 40% granulation tissue, 30% slough, and 30% eschar, or 3) 40% red, 30% yellow, and 30% black (see examples in Figure 8-2). The shape of the wound, if not drawn, should also be described. A round or elliptical wound is a reliable sign that the wound was caused by tissue loading such as pressure or shear. Vascular wounds tend to have irregular shapes. Arterial insufficiency produces a dry depression due to the loss of moisture from the necrotic tissue.

Measuring Wounds

Determining the size of a wound is a necessary part of the wound evaluation. Many individuals involved with wound care place great importance on wound measurements and much research has been performed on the best practice and reliability of different techniques. However, a few important points need to be considered. In general, patients with wounds will be referred to physical therapy because of the quality of the wound, rather than the quantity of the wound. Secondly, measurements may vary tremendously due to patient positioning. For measurements to be reliable, a patient will need to be positioned in the same manner each time a measurement is performed. Because of infection control considerations,

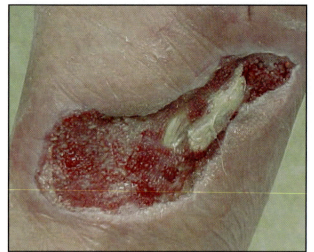

Figure 8-2A. Examples of tissue types within wound beds. This dorsal foot wound has 100% granulation tissue. Note that much of the granulation tissue has a pink color, indicative of diminished arterial blood flow. Also note the presence of tendons within the wound bed. Tendons and ligaments must not be confused with necrotic tissue.

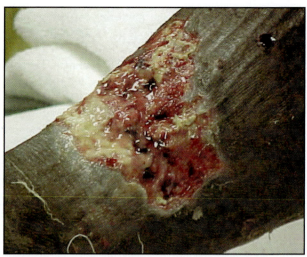

Figure 8-2B. In this example, the wound bed consists of 10% black necrotic tissue, 40% yellow necrotic tissue, and 50% red granulation tissue. Note the healthier appearing granulation tissue in this wound compared with the wound in 8-2A.

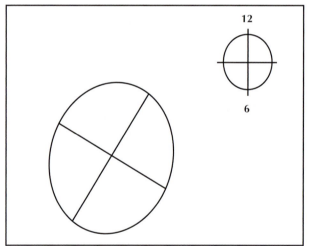

Figure 8-3A. Measuring the surface dimensions of a wound. In this example, the longest dimension is measured and the width perpendicular is also measured.

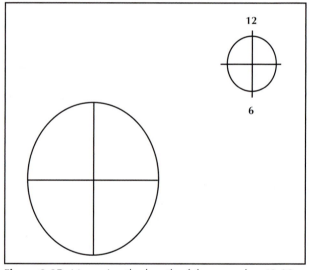

Figure 8-3B. Measuring the length of the wound as 12:00 to 6:00, and the width as 9:00 to 3:00.

precise measurements may not be practical. Methods for measurements are discussed below. One needs to be aware that an error in measurement is likely to be greater than any real day-to-day changes in wound size. Wound size will usually change little until the wound is relatively clear of infection. When wound size begins to decrease rapidly, patients may need to be discharged from the outpatient setting.

Surface Area

Measurement of only the surface area of a wound is suitable in the absence of subcutaneous tissue involvement (Figure 8-3).

Clock Notation

A means of establishing consistent directions for the measurement is clock notation. Using clock notation, we indicate the cephalic direction on the trunk and proximal direction on a limb as 12:00 and the caudal direction on the trunk or distal direction on a limb as 6:00. Using this notation, the term *length* refers to the distance from 12:00 to 6:00 and width is measured from 9:00 to 3:00. Three generally accepted means of measuring across a wound are in common use. One method is to measure the greatest width and greatest length regardless of the shape of the wound. A second method is to measure width and length regardless of size. In this method, length is defined as the distance across the wound from 12:00 to 6:00 and width is defined from 3:00 to 9:00. The preferred means currently is measuring the greatest dimension across the wound and the distance perpendicular to this measurement. Using any of these methods, the two measurements may be multiplied to determine a crude number to describe the cross-sectional area of the wound. Multiplying length times width overestimates the true surface area. The error is small for a wound with a shape approaching that of a rectangle, but error increases as the wound deviates from a rectangular shape and is maximal when a wound is perfectly round. In the case of a highly irregularly shaped wound, measurements may need to be taken at multiple locations. In such cases, a map of the wound should be drawn in the medical record with representative distances marked clearly on the map.

Tools for measuring the distance across the wound include sterile cotton-tipped applicators, transparent grids and plastic materials such as sandwich bags. Sterile cotton-tipped applicators offer the advantage of low cost. The wooden end is held to one edge of the wound as the thumb of a gloved hand is slid to the opposite side of the wound. The cotton-tipped applicator is then held close to a ruler to measure distance in centimeters. If the wound is less than 1 cm across, the distance may be reported in millimeters instead. An alternative is the use of a clear plastic template designed for wound measurements. Some of these are found sterile in dressing packages; these may be placed directly on the wound for measurement. Otherwise, clean plastic templates may be held over a wound, but not in direct contact, to measure it. These devices have a centimeter scale along one edge and a calibrated system in the middle. Many of these systems are a series of concentric circles or ellipses. Care must be taken to determine whether the numbers printed on the wound template refer to the radius or the diameter of the concentric circles or ellipses. Wound templates placed over the wound allow both length and width to be read rapidly, but if held away from the wound, greater risk of error is incurred. An exact system is to use a plastic sheet material such as plastic wrap or a sandwich bag to trace a wound for a permanent record. The wound tracing can be digitized on a computer or a planimeter and may be used to compute surface area accurately. The problem using a single sheet of plastic is the potential for contamination. A sandwich bag or a doubled-over piece of plastic wrap allows the top layer to be kept and the surface in contact with the wound to be discarded. Wound tracings may be photocopied or scanned to be placed in a paper or electronic record permanently.

Depth

Depth of a wound should be determined for wounds with significant subcutaneous involvement such as stage IV pressure ulcers. The volume of shallow wounds such as

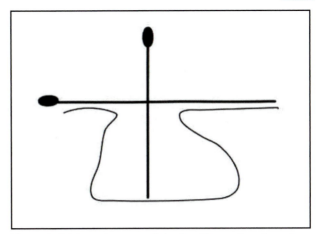

Figure 8-4. Measuring wound depth with a cotton-tipped applicator. A second cotton-tipped applicator is placed across the wound to estimate the reference point of the intact skin, rather than estimating it by eye.

burns without subcutaneous involvement, stage II or stage III pressure ulcers, arterial ulcers or venous ulcers is generally not practical as the depth is not much greater than the error in measurement.

The simplest means of providing an index of volume is to measure wound depth with a cotton-tipped applicator in a way that is similar to measurement of cross-sectional area (see Figure 8-4). To reduce error in means of localizing the skin surface, one cotton-tipped applicator is placed across the wound and another is placed in the wound with the wooden stick end into the wound next to the cotton-tipped applicator lying across the wound. The point at which depth is measured depends on the configuration of the wound. Generally, one should use the deepest spot. If a wound has multiple depths such that one number could not accurately describe the wound, a map of the wound may need to be drawn with depths indicated on the map.

Obtaining measurements of length, width and depth allows only a crude approximation of wound volume to be made. More precise means of volume determination can be performed by filling the wound with a suitable material. Sterile saline from a premeasured syringe may be used. Volume of the syringe is recorded before and after the wound is filled from the syringe. Volume is simply calculated by subtracting the final volume of the syringe from its initial volume. This method is only effective if the patient can be positioned in such a way that the surface of the wound is parallel to the floor. If this position is not practical, hydrogel, a more viscous material may be infused instead. A more involved procedure is the use of dental impression gel, such as Jeltrate (Dentsply International, York, PA). An equal volume of warm water is added to the powder from the canister and mixed. Before the material hardens, it can be placed into the wound and allowed to become firm. Jeltrate is biocompatible and is easily removed from a wound after it hardens. The impression of the wound can be placed in a graduated cylinder to determine wound volume. The volume of the impression gel must be measured before it dries completely and loses volume from evaporation.

Tunnels, Tracts, Fistulas

Linear erosion extending from a wound may be termed *tunneling* or called a *tract*. These form most readily along fascial planes. The term *sinus tract* is commonly used when erosion of subcutaneous tissue from an abscess occurs (sinus refers the space created by the abscess). A fistula is an abnormal opening between 2 structures. Fistulas can form between the esophagus and trachea, colon and bladder, skin and intestines, and other locations. For example, fecal material may be discovered in the depths of an opened abdominal abscess from an enterocutaneous fistula. Probing needs to be done meticulously to determine whether an opening in the wound is a simple sinus tract or a fistula. Fistula management is more complex due to the openings on both ends and may require months to close.

The locations of tunnels and sinus tracts are documented using clock notation, and the distance a cotton-tipped applicator can be inserted beneath intact skin is noted. An example of appropriate notation is a 5 cm tunnel at 11:00. However, in many cases, one cannot be certain that the end of tunnel can be reached. This may also occur in cases in which 2 wounds communicate subcutaneously. One may not be able to move a cotton-tipped applicator from one wound to the other, but fluid may be observed coming out of one wound while pulsed lavage is being applied to the other. In such cases, one may note that probing completely between the 2 wounds could not be accomplished, but the 2 wounds appear to be connected beneath intact skin.

Undermining/Pocketing

Undermining can be visualized as a cliff caused by necrosis of tissue more susceptible to hypoxia than skin is. It is commonly associated with pressure ulcers produced by shearing. This phenomenon is depicted in Figure 8-5. Undermined areas tend to have a maximal distance at a certain point and symmetrically decrease in an arc of the wound's perimeter. To document undermining, a broken line is drawn to indicate the distance of undermining and to denote the arc involved. If not drawn, one may use clock notation to indicate the location and extent of undermining. For example, in Figure 8-5 undermining is present from 1:00 to 6:00. The term *pocket* may be used to describe a type of subcutaneous defect that extends under intact skin, but does not have a cliff-like appearance. These are generally the remnants of abscesses that may be found incidentally when drainage is found emanating from the pocket, but should be found during the initial and sub-

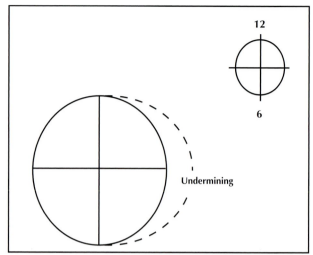

Figure 8-5. Documenting undermining. The arc typical of an undermined wound such as a pressure ulcer is noted with a dashed line. Numbers representative of the distance that undermining occurs may be written on a diagram or as text in a note. The arc is given in clock notation as 1:00 to 5:00.

sequent wound assessment by checking for whether the edges of the wound are adherent.

Surrounding Skin

Due to total focus on the wound itself, the surrounding skin is often neglected to the detriment of wound healing. Surrounding skin is the primary source of new epithelial cells to resurface wounds. Unhealthy surrounding skin will slow healing tremendously, even if the wound fills with granulation tissue. Moreover, potential problems with wound healing frequently show in surrounding skin first. Concerns include maceration, inflammation, hydration, nutrition, callus or hyperkeratosis, and induration. The color of skin may also provide important information.

Skin Color

White indicates lack of blood flow or arterial insufficiency. Blue coloration (cyanosis) is a sign of severe lack of oxygen in the tissue due to arterial insufficiency, heart failure, or respiratory disease. A blackened area surrounding a wound represents necrosis, probably due to severe arterial disease. A yellowish-brown, variegated coloration, especially when it is located on the lower part of a leg near the medial malleolus is indicative of venous insufficiency as described in Chapter 7. Redness is described separately below.

Nutrition

A combination of dry, thin skin is indicative of a lack of nutrition to the skin producing skin atrophy. Skin nutrition is specifically addressed in Chapter 6.

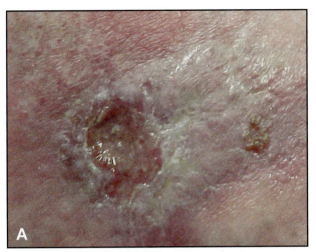 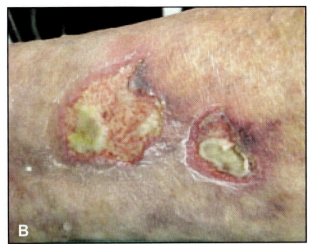

Figure 8-6. Features of wounds. (A) Note the maceration. (B) Note yellow slough, and the mottling and atrophy of the skin.

Inflammation and Infection

Signs of inflammation of surrounding skin are expected for infected wounds. The wound will be surrounded by an area of erythema, the skin will be thickened by edema and fibrosis, resulting in induration, a hardening of the skin. The surrounding skin must, therefore, be examined not only visually, but also by palpation. Along with induration, increased warmth may be detected. Harsh handling of a wound may also cause inflammation. A small area of inflammation of a few millimeters may exist in the absence of infection. A large area of inflammation may represent infection of the surrounding skin, termed *peripheral cellulitis.* Further spread of infection may reveal increased size and firmness of lymph nodes draining the area (lymphadenitis) and red streaks in the skin (lymphangitis).

Skin Hydration

Skin hydration and turgor are examined together. With normal aging, both hydration and turgor may be lost. Normally hydrated skin conforms to the surface below and resists compression. This is tested by pinching a fold of skin. Dehydrated skin without turgor folds into a tent shape and remains tented. In certain areas of the body, notably the neck, tenting is present in elderly individuals without pinching the skin. Elderly skin is at high risk for damage due to trauma, in particular the use of tape and indiscriminate removal of the tape as described in Chapter 7 under skin tears.

Maceration

Maceration is a result of excessive hydration of skin (see Figure 8-6). It can be seen in normal skin following long exposure to moisture, such as long baths or swimming. The macerated skin becomes swollen and lighter in color in addition to an appearance of fissuring. Surrounding skin becomes macerated from using dressings that cannot keep drainage off the surrounding skin, not changing dressings frequently enough, or failure to use moisture barriers or skin sealants to protect the skin from moisture. Maceration may also be caused by rough handling of the wound or placing cotton gauze in direct contact with the wound leading to chronic inflammation of the wound bed.

Excessive Dryness of Skin

A range of normal skin hydration may be found across individuals. The term for excessively dry skin is *xerosis.* The skin of those from Subsaharan African descent has greater propensity for xerosis, often described as being "ashy." Additionally, diabetes and arterial disease lead to skin dryness. A combination of all 3 of these factors is common and can result in fissuring of the skin, a risk for infection. Xerosis can also be the result of systemic disease, especially if found in atypical areas in a person who does not have a history of ashy skin.

Scale

Scaling may be the result of a number of disease processes that may be local or systemic. Scale represents abnormal keratinization and may be accompanied by signs of inflammation. The color of the scale may also be indicative of a specific disease. Psoriasis produces silvery scaling and may produce papules and plaques. Scaling on sun-exposed skin, especially in older individuals may represent actinic keratosis, a precursor of squamous cell carcinoma. Eczema is generally associated with both scaling and inflammation with weeping and crusted lesions.

Chronic Injury to Surrounding Skin

Skin surrounding and near the wound should be inspected for signs of chronic injury. The presence of healed scars may suggest an ongoing or intermittent underlying problem causing wounds to occur in an area of the body. For example, multiple scarred areas may be found near the medial malleolus and other areas on the legs of a person with venous disease. Scars from old wounds near the lateral malleolus and elsewhere may be the result of sickle cell disease. Scarring is also likely to be found on problem areas in diabetic neuropathy and arterial disease.

The insult responsible for creating a wound may also produce a milder, reversible injury to the skin around the wound. Bleeding into the skin may be caused by excessive shearing, or pressure exerted on the skin, or by venous hypertension. Red blood cells break down in the tissue releasing hemoglobin. As hemoglobin is degraded into first biliverdin and then bilirubin, the tissue takes on a greenish, then yellow appearance from these pigments. After bilirubin is removed, iron from the hemoglobin remains in the storage form of hemosiderin. Hemosiderin is cleared slowly by macrophages. The color of the surrounding skin may, therefore, help reveal whether the injury is mild, new, continuous, or old. Measures to correct chronic injury to the skin may be taken by offloading the area or addressing venous hypertension.

Chronic shearing, when accompanied by stiffness of the skeletal structures of the foot and dryness of the skin in diabetes produces callus on shearing points such as metatarsal heads and heels. However, callus may cover the entire plantar surface of the foot and extend along the medial and lateral sides of the foot toward the dorsal side. The dorsal surfaces of toes at the interphalangeal joints may also be callused due to shearing between the skin and the tops of shoes. Callus creates increased pressure on the skin below it during ambulation and must be debrided.

Callus is considered a form of hyperkeratosis, but hyperkeratosis may occur without external shear forces. Dry skin over extensor surfaces may become thickened by the excess accumulation of material of the stratum corneum. Normally, the stratum corneum is shed as quickly as new keratinocytes reach this layer from below. Some skin diseases are also characterized by hyperkeratosis.

Wound Edges

The edges of a wound are one of the two fronts for wound healing. As the base of the wound granulates, a wound that is full-thickness or deeper epithelializes only from the edges. Partial-thickness wound epithelialize from hair follicles and other accessory structures that are lined with epithelial cells. Whereas the wound bed needs to be moist, the intact epidermis around the wound must maintain normal hydration for epidermal cell migration onto the edge of the wound. Wound edges must be inspected for hydration status, signs of ongoing injury, and adherence of the edge to the wound bed. Hydration status and signs of injury are described above for surrounding skin in general. Adherence of edges is inspected both visually and by palpation. Epiboly, as described in Chapter 3, prevents migration of epidermal cells. Lack of

adherence indicates subcutaneous injury. This can take the form of tunneling/tracts, undermining, and pocketing. Although patients may experience discomfort from probing, discovery of tunnels and pockets is critical. These subcutaneous defects may close prematurely, walling off bacteria and increasing the risk of abscess formation. Patients may return for a new episode of wound care due to subcutaneous cavities left along a fascial plane. Even if infection does not occur immediately, patients have developed abscesses months or years later due to introduction of bacteria into these cavities.

Wound-Related Pain

Wound pain serves an important diagnostic role and can have a major impact on patient function, including home interventions. A sudden increase in pain, especially if accompanied by increased odor and drainage is indicative of infection. Even in the absence of infection, excessive pain may cause a patient to avoid cleansing or dressing changes at home. Pain may also impair a person's ability to return to work with devastating economic impact. Chapter 10 addresses pain management specifically.

TESTS AND MEASURES

Appropriate tests and measures to assist in diagnosis and prognosis include temperature, ABI, culture (addressed in Chapter 9), and tests described in Chapter 6 for sensation, mobility, strength, range of motion, gait, and need and use of assistive devices. Temperature may be assessed simply by palpation and comparison to other parts of the body. A more reliable indication of temperature, however, is use of either a thermistor or radiometer to measure temperature. These devices are very accurate, precise, and reliable. A thermistor measures temperature using a probe that varies in resistance to the current applied to it with temperature. Radiometers measure infrared radiation to determine temperature. Thermistor systems are relatively cheap if used on a large number of persons. The thermistors can be cleaned and disinfected between patients. The advantage of a radiometer is its ability to measure temperature without coming in direct contact with a wound. These devices, however, are very expensive.

DIAGNOSIS

Diagnosis encompasses several aspects of the wound and the patient. Examination of the patient was covered in Chapters 5 and 6. Many times the diagnosis in terms of the ICD-9 code is given with the referral. However, a diagnosis includes more information than the simple description of the ICD-9 code. Many times the code provides the actual etiology and in other cases the code given will only address the body part. In addition, the stage of wound healing should be described. On occasion, the referring diagnosis may not be correct. Etiology was discussed in the previous chapter. Even if the correct etiology is known, additional information necessary to guide a plan of care must often be obtained by examining the wound and interviewing the patient or caregivers. Elements that need to be addressed include the percentage of the wound bed that is red, yellow, and black; the drainage type (color, consistency, and presence of purulence); the quality of the tissue in and around the wound; signs of infection; presence of anatomic structures; and phase of healing, including chronicity in a given phase. Color of the wound bed and drainage were addressed above.

Quality of Wound Bed

Issues with the wound bed include the relative health and turgor of the wound. A healthy wound bed is red, firm, and does not bleed with trivial trauma. Unhealthy wound beds may result from infection or critical colonization, ischemia, and lack of moisture. Pink tissue is indicative of diminished blood flow to the wound bed. Dusky, bleeding, stringy, weak tissue without turgor (friable tissue) indicates injury most likely caused by infection or critical colonization. Brown, darkened areas within the wound bed are caused by tissue necrosis, frequently due to infection. Boggy tissue within the wound indicates deep necrosis and edema. Such a wound requires further exploration. Hardness results from either desiccation or the presence of hardened fibrin on the wound surface.

The percentages of red, yellow, and black and the quality and quantity of drainage are factors in determining the plan of care, regardless of the etiology. Type of debridement, dressings used, and frequency of visits are among issues that will depend on the quality of the wound bed.

Infection and Critical Colonization

Determining the level of bioburden is generally important in developing a plan of care. All chronic wounds are assumed to be colonized by a number of bacterial species. Contamination refers to the introduction of material from outside the wound. In general, contamination is to be avoided because of the risk of a new pathogen or excessive numbers of a particular pathogen. Contamination does not guarantee infection and theoretically could be beneficial by altering the composition of the flora in such a way that no one pathogen will flourish in the wound. Infection control will be addressed more specifically in Chapter 9. Both infection and critical colonization will slow or halt wound healing. Critical colonization refers to a level of colonization that impedes wound healing through competition for resources, through toxins, or by maintaining chronic inflammation. Infection, beyond slowing healing, may cause wound deterioration and spread either locally or systemically.

Signs of infection have been described by the mnemonic IFEE, which stands for induration, fever, erythema, and edema as described in Chapter 2. These are also signs of inflammation, although the presence of induration is more suggestive of infection, especially when associated with injury beneath intact skin. Copious or maximal drainage exceeding the expected amount for the size and location of the wound is also suggestive, whereas the presence of purulence is considered sufficient to diagnose infection. In wounds with large subcutaneous components, purulence may be missed. During palpation of the wound and surrounding skin, one should gently attempt to express drainage to determine whether purulence is present. Purulence may also be initially detected within tracts and pockets during probing with a cotton-tipped applicator. Many patients may indicate exquisite pain during the first few treatments due to inflammation, but this pain should resolve with removal of bacteria and necrotic tissue during these initial visits. A return or increase in odor that persists after wound irrigation and increased pain in the wound should make the clinician suspicious of infection or reinfection.

Infection may take one or more of several forms beyond purulence within a wound bed and subcutaneous defects. Infection may spread to bone (osteomyelitis), particularly in wounds that can be probed to a bone's surface. As discussed above, cellulitis is the spread of infection through the interstitial space producing erythema, warmth, and pain. Lymphadenitis and lymphangitis may also be present. Erysipelas is a specific type of cellulitis that is most commonly caused by group A *Strep*. This type of infection is more common when venous or lymphatic drainage of the area is compromised. Facial (cheek and bridge of nose) and leg erysipelas account for almost all cases. In addition to localized heat, pain, and erythema, systemic effects (fever, chills, decreased appetite, and somnolence) are commonly present at diagnosis. Spread of infection through the blood is given the general terms *sepsis* or *septicemia*, although the more specific terms of *bacteremia*, *viremia*, and *fungemia* may be used. Although sepsis and septicemia may be used interchangeably, sepsis may also be used to indicate local infection. Septicemia may be considered a more specific type of sepsis to indicate an infection spread to the blood.

Although swab cultures are still done commonly, they may not detect the true culprit, but only surface contaminants. If a swab culture is performed, the wound should be irrigated initially or fluid deep in the wound should be used. Biopsy of wound tissue is more likely to detect infection and allow sensitivity testing to correctly identify appropriate antibiotics. Biopsy is also the preferred means

Table 8-1

Systemic Inflammatory Response Syndrome Criteria for Sepsis

Heart rate greater than 90 bpm (tachycardia)

Either hypothermia or fever

- Core temperature less than 36°C (96.8°F)
- Core temperature greater than 38°C (100.4°F)

Increased respiration as either tachypnea or hypocapnia/hyperventilation

- Respiratory rate greater than 20 breaths per minute (tachypnea)
- $PaCO_2$ less than 32 mmHg (hypocapnia/hyperventilation)

White blood cell count shows elevation, depression, or increased bands (immature neutrophils)

- WBC count greater than 12,000 per mm^3 (leukocytosis)
- WBC count less than 4,000 per mm^3 (leukopenia)
- Bands greater than 10% (bandemia)

of determining osteomyelitis. Because biopsy is invasive and could potentially introduce contaminants from soft tissue into bone, imaging is likely to be performed and biopsy be reserved for more difficult cases. Plain film x-ray can be used to detect osteomyelitis if osteonecrosis including deformity can be visualized. Ultrasound and MRI imaging may also be performed if necessary.

Indicators of systemic infection include increased blood glucose, including wide fluctuations of blood glucose from hypoglycemia to values of 400 mg/dL or greater, elevated WBC count, increased sedimentation rate, and elevated C-reactive protein. Clinical signs of sepsis are produced by the patient's immune response to the infection. The collection of signs accompanying sepsis are called the systemic inflammatory response syndrome (SIRS). Criteria for sepsis based on SIRS are listed in Table 8-1.

Sepsis is present if an infection is either present, or highly suspected, and 2 or more of the criteria exist. Fever and leukocytosis are part of the acute phase reaction along with anorexia and somnolence. Tachycardia and tachypnea indicate cardiovascular and metabolic disturbances. For children, heart rate (HR), respiratory rate (RR), and WBC must be compared with norms for the age.

Criteria for HR and RR are greater than 2 SD above mean. The criterion for hypothermia is the same as adult, but the criterion for fever is 38.5°C. Bandemia is also 10%.

Etiology

Generally, acute wounds do not present difficulty in determining etiology. Certain types of chronic wounds,

however, need to be identified by etiology to determine the proper plan of care to address the underlying cause. Mechanical causes may include open fracture, degloving, laceration, incision, and abrasion (road rash). Thermal injuries include burn, scald, and frostbite. In addition, the cause of the burn, whether by contact, flash, or ignition of clothing, should be noted. Chemical and radiation burns, and dehiscence of a surgical wound, can also be determined from history, as well as toxic ulcerations, eg, those caused by brown recluse bites.

Differential diagnosis is particularly important in determining whether the patient has a pressure ulcer, a neuropathic ulcer, or if the ulcer is caused by venous insufficiency or arterial insufficiency. The history, physical examination, and special tests should be sufficiently rigorous to determine the cause. However, diabetes can predispose an individual to arterial, pressure, and neuropathic ulcers and, because venous insufficiency is so common, a person can have a combination of conditions.

Pressure ulcers should be classified according to NPUAP definitions as stage I, II, III, IV, deep tissue injury, or unstageable based on the depth of structures involved as described in Chapter 7. Before a stage is determined, however, the base of the wound should be visible. Several days of debridement may be required before an accurate staging can be performed.

The Wagner grading system is commonly used for neuropathic ulcers (see Chapter 7). However, the system does not grade the severity of the wound, but the severity of the injury to the foot. It combines aspects of neuropathy, arterial insufficiency, and infection. By definition, a Wagner grade 0 indicates intact skin, although deeper skin may be poised to break down. Grade 1 represents a superficial ulcer, grade 2 represents a deep ulcer, and grade 3 includes infection as indicated by abscess or osteomyelitis. Gangrene of the forefoot is documented as grade 4, and grade 5 represents gangrene of most of the foot.

Burns should be classified by the depth of tissue injury. Older terminology of *first-*, *second-*, and *third-degree burn* continues in common use today, however. Injury limited to damage to the epidermis with inflammation of the dermis is documented as a superficial or first-degree burn, which is equivalent to sunburn. Injury to the superficial dermis causes sufficient inflammation for fluid to accumulate between the dermis and epidermis, thereby producing the blisters characteristic of superficial partial-thickness or second-degree burns. The 2 other classes of burns are more difficult to distinguish from each other. Both may have a charred, pearly or khaki, hardened appearance. The difference between a deep partial-thickness and a full-thickness burn is observable if preservation of hair follicles and blood vessels can be determined. In a deep partial-thickness burn, hair follicles and blood vessels in the deep dermis are still viable. Tugging on a hair also can be used to distinguish the two. However, in certain types of burn injuries, especially those involving flames, hairs may be singed and not available for testing. In a full-thickness burn, a tugged hair slides easily from the follicle. Resistance to tugging indicates a deep partial-thickness injury. Blanching with pressure indicates the presence of viable blood vessels and therefore a deep partial-thickness burn, whereas a wound with a full-thickness injury is not blanchable.

Other types of wounds should be classified by the depth of injury into superficial, partial-thickness, full-thickness, or full-thickness with subcutaneous involvement. Many individuals, however, incorrectly attempt to use the NPUAP definitions for wounds with causes other than pressure. A superficial wound exhibits damage to the epidermis only and may display some erythema. No treatment other than protection is usually needed. These wounds are usually caused by mild abrasion of the skin. Partial-thickness wounds have evidence of damage through the epidermis and into the dermis. These injuries include skin tears, deeper abrasions, blisters, partial-thickness graft donor sites, and others. Full-thickness wounds injure the skin through the entirety of the dermis. Causes of full-thickness injuries include full-thickness skin graft donor sites, venous insufficiency ulcers, surgical wounds, neuropathic wounds, and degloving or avulsion injuries. Full-thickness wounds with subcutaneous involvement injure tissues below the skin, including subcutaneous fat, muscle, tendon, ligament, and bone. Surgical wounds, arterial insufficiency, pressure, and open fractures are common causes of this type of wound.

Next, the clinician must determine the current phase of healing and whether a wound is failing to progress from one phase to the other, or becomes chronic in a given stage of wound healing. A nonhealing wound may be chronically in the inflammatory, proliferative, epithelializing, or remodeling stage. The wound may also fail in one of these steps: inflammation, proliferation, epithelialization, or remodeling.

Critical decision-making points are whether the wound is infected, whether the wound requires debridement, requires filling of depth, undermining, tunnels, or sinus tracts, and the degree of drainage. Many of these points are addressed together; however, in some cases the clinician may need to work with competing goals to optimize wound healing. For example, sharp debridement accomplishes the goals of treating infection and the presence of large quantities of necrotic tissue. On the other hand, use of autolytic debridement and preventing maceration of surrounding skin may be difficult. The assessment for wound infection has been described frequently by the mnemonic IFEE. An infected wound often has the characteristics of induration, fever, erythema and edema. The odor and color of drainage from the wound can aid in this determination. The presence of dusky or brownish patches within the wound is also very suggestive of wound infection.

Debridement can be a difficult decision process and is discussed extensively in Chapter 11. Filling or packing a wound is discussed in Chapter 12 and is dependent on the presence of undermining, tunneling, sinus tracts, and the risk of abscess formation. Deciding on a dressing based on the drainage of a wound and choice of using skin sealants and moisture barriers will be described in Chapter 12 also.

A diagnosis and prognosis based on the *Guide to Physical Therapist Practice* can be made. These patterns are straightforward, except when other systems are also affected, as in a case of multiple trauma. Pattern A, primary prevention, should be applied to individuals at risk for neuropathic ulcers, pressure ulcers, and venous insufficiency ulcers. Prevention of ischemic ulcers may be limited to detection of arterial insufficiency and referral to a vascular surgeon. Pattern B is applied to those with superficial skin involvement and may be limited to patient education. Pattern C describes partial-thickness wounds and may involve multiple interventions including a brief course of direct intervention, and patient education. Full-thickness injuries are described by pattern D, and pattern E includes involvement of fascia, bone, or muscle. Both patterns D and E require substantial direct intervention including debridement, dressing changes, possible adjunctive therapies, work or lifestyle modifications, and patient education.

Prognosis is the predicted optimal level of improvement in function and amount of time to reach that level based on the information available. Goals refer to remediation of impairments and may address characteristics of the wound and specific deficits in related areas, eg, limited mobility. The prognosis is based on multiple factors and is not limited to the wound itself. For example, a person who remains on his feet all day will have more difficulty in healing a venous insufficiency or neuropathic ulcer. Home resources and the ability to learn how to handle the wound at home are also important prognostic indicators. An example of a prognosis is that the wound will be clean and stable and ready for grafting in 10 visits and the patient will return to all previous roles in 6 weeks. The goal of the clinician's intervention also needs to be considered. In many cases, involvement may simply be limited to providing a clean, stable wound ready for grafting or delayed primary closure. Another common goal is to have the wound stable enough for the patient and any caregivers to manage at home with or without home health assistance. In longer-term healthcare settings, complete healing may be the goal of therapy. Goals may include prevention of pressure ulcers, protection of a wound, prevention of contamination or infection, management of drainage, management of edema, complete healing (more reasonable for long-term care rather than in an acute care facility), clean and stable wound (typical for acute care) with self-care, follow-up with home health, or long-term facility, clean and stable wound ready for surgical closure, or a clean and stable wound ready for grafting. Outcomes should be addressed relative to history, such as return to family, work, and social roles, or may include the need for modified assistance using equipment, continued care in a different type of facility, or the need for assistance at home. These may include minimizing limitation of function, optimizing health status, preventing disability, and optimizing patient satisfaction.

Interventions are discussed in the plan of care (see Chapter 18). Within the assessment, the clinician may need to note that debridement of necrotic tissue may initially increase the size of the wound. An argument should also be developed for the plan of care in terms of frequency of treatment, particular type of dressing, method of cleansing wound, and type of debridement.

Summary

Assessment of the wound requires clinical judgment based on objective tests, history provided by the patient or caregiver, and direct observation by the clinician.

Whereas acute wounds usually present no problem with determining the cause, many chronic wounds may not present an obvious cause. In addition, the clinician needs to determine why the wound failed to heal and why any previous treatment failed. Observation of the wound can be based on the CODES system described above. Measurement of surface area is sufficient for superficial or full-thickness wounds. For wounds with substantial subcutaneous involvement, either wound volume or depth characteristic of the wound need to be documented. A discussion of the systems for characterizing wounds of different types is provided.

Questions

1. Why is the color of the wound important in the diagnosis and prognosis for a wound?
2. What is the importance of the condition of the surrounding skin of a wound?
3. What types of wounds require measurement of the volume or depth?
4. What influence does the history have on diagnosis of a chronic wound?
5. Why must social and work history need to be considered to develop a prognosis?

Bibliography

American Physical Therapy Association. Guide to physical therapist practice. *Phys Ther.* 1997;77:1177-1619.

Armstrong DG, Holtz-Neiderer K, Wendel C, Mohler MJ, Kimbriel HR, Lavery LA. Skin temperature monitoring reduces the risk for diabetic foot ulceration in high-risk patients. *Am J Med.* 2007;120(12):1042-1046.

Armstrong DG, Lavery LA, Liswood PJ, Todd WF, Tredwell JA. Infrared dermal thermometry for the high-risk diabetic foot. *Phys Ther.* 1997;77(2):169-175.

Flanagan M. Improving accuracy of wound measurement in clinical practice. *Ostomy Wound Manage.* 2003;49(10):28-40.

Harlin SL, Willard LA, Rush KJ, Ghisletta LC, Meyers WC. Chronic wounds of the lower extremity: a preliminary performance measure set. *Plast Reconstr Surg.* 2008;121(1):142-174.

Jessup RL. What is the best method for assessing the rate of wound healing? A comparison of 3 mathematical formulas. *Adv Skin Wound Care.* 2006;19(3):138-147.

van Rijswijk L. The fundamentals of wound assessment. *Ostomy Wound Manage.* 1996;42(7):40-46.

Interventions

Having taken a history, performed a physical examination, and evaluated the wound, the clinician is prepared to make decisions appropriate for the given wound and the given patient. These decisions are elaborated in the plan of care. Although many combinations of interventions are possible, and any number may be appropriate for a given wound, an understanding of the patient's situation will limit the possibilities. Moreover, the clinician should anticipate a progression of interventions, including contingency plans, foreseeing possible outcomes of the interventions, and determining appropriate referral to other healthcare providers and type of patient education.

Different interventions and a description of appropriate indications for them are presented in the chapters of this unit. The issue of informed consent, as well as other ethical issues, needs to be addressed for all interventions. The 4 basic ethical principles are beneficence, nonmaleficence, utility and autonomy. Beneficence is the cornerstone of the patient/clinician relationship. The patient trusts the clinician to provide services solely for the benefit of the patient. With this in mind, we are ethically bound to provide the optimum plan of care for each patient as an individual. Nonmaleficence implies that the patient can trust the clinician to not intentionally injure the patient. Utility is based on the principle of risk/benefit ratio. Based on this principle, the clinician designs a plan of care that provides the greatest benefit relative to the risk. Although utility is a greater issue in prescribing medicine or performing surgery, the clinician involved in wound management needs to explore the risk and benefits of the plan of care and understand the patient's willingness to incur more or less risk to increase the chances of benefit. The fourth principle, autonomy is the basis of informed consent. As described for utility, certain risks and benefits may be derived from interventions and education provided by the clinician. The patient has a reasonable expectation to be informed sufficiently of the risks and benefits to consent to any interventions. Included in informed consent are the risks associated with the procedure, benefits expected to be derived from the procedure and the risk of choosing to forego the proposed intervention. The level of informed consent is likely to vary tremendously from facility-to-facility and for different procedures. A minimum of an oral informed consent should be obtained for each procedure, whereas some facilities may desire a written and signed informed consent form for each procedure. In particular, surgery or procedures that may be perceived as surgery, such as sharp debridement may require a written, signed informed consent and a time out period before the procedure is started to ensure that the correct procedure is performed.

Infection Control

9

OBJECTIVES

- Discuss the need for infection control and use infection control measures.
- Discuss the issues involved with latex sensitivity for both the patient and the healthcare professional.
- Describe the microbiology of wounds, including common bacteria responsible for wound infection.
- Describe risk factors for wound infection and means of preventing surgical site infection.
- Discuss the indications for culturing wounds and the limitations of culturing.
- Contrast the use of wound biopsy and culture.
- Contrast the processes of sterilization and disinfection.
- Contrast aseptic and sterile techniques.
- Discuss appropriate use of sterile and clean techniques for acute and chronic wounds.
- Discuss indications for systemic medicines for wound infection.
- Discuss indications for topical antimicrobial agents.
- Describe appropriate OSHA regulations for handling potentially infectious material.
- Discuss relevant CDC recommendations for isolation precautions in hospitals, including the evolution of isolation practices.
- List the types of precautions and patients requiring various isolation precautions.

The susceptibility of individuals to infection is determined by a number of factors. Factors include host defense mechanisms, pathogenic properties of microbes, the presence of predisposing factors to infection, and sources of organisms in wounds. Below, common organisms found in wound infections, and control of both endogenous and exogenous organisms are discussed.

HOST DEFENSE MECHANISMS

Both passive and active mechanisms reduce the opportunity for infection, particularly the intact skin. The mechanical barrier provided by skin due to waterproofing is effective for the vast majority of organisms. In addition, growth is diminished by the acidity of skin, the presence of molecular defense molecules called defensins and col-

Irion G.
Comprehensive Wound Management, 2nd ed. (pp 163-190)
© 2010 SLACK Incorporated

Table 9-1

Host Defense Mechanisms

Cell Mediated	*Humoral*	*Molecular*
• T-cell	• Antibodies, especially IgA	• Defensins
• Neutrophils		• Collectins
• Macrophage		

lectins, and competition with other microbes. Mucosal surfaces are protected additionally by antibodies. If intact skin is breeched by injury, elements of the immune system including neutrophils, macrophages, T cells, and antibodies are usually able to prevent infection. Unfortunately, a number of circumstances can lead to infection in different individuals in different ways. First of all, each person's immune system is somewhat different due the inheritance of unique combinations of cellular and humoral immunity genes from each parent. Secondly, a large number of local and systemic factors may compromise the effectiveness of the immune system. Types of host defense mechanisms are categorized in Table 9-1.

Defensins are 15 to 20 amino acid polypeptides effective against bacteria, fungi, and enveloped viruses. Alpha defensins are found in neutrophils, macrophages, and specific cells in the intestines, whereas beta defensins are secreted by epithelial cells and leukocytes. In addition to the ability to create pores in microbes, defensins have multiple roles related to their immune function. Production of human beta defensin-2 occurs in keratinocytes and increases during infection and inflammatory disease of the skin, especially psoriasis. Human beta defensin-2 specifically destroys gram-negatives. In addition it stimulates chemotaxis of memory T cells, production of cytokines, and stimulates wound repair through its effects on keratinocyte migration and proliferation.

Collectins are often the first line of attack of the immune system. Eight types of collectins have been described. Collectins bind selectively to specific carbohydrate components of microbes through a part of their molecules termed the *carbohydrate recognition domain. Collectins*, as the name implies, cause aggregation (collecting) of microbes, which also results in opsonization to increase phagocytosis of the bound microbes. Additionally, production of cytokines and free radicals used in phagocytosis are stimulated. Some collectins also activate the complement system.

Complement is a family of serum proteins that serves to complement the cellular components of the immune system. Similar to what collectins perform on surfaces, complement molecules opsonize bacteria and stimulate cytokine production. A major stimulus of complement is the binding of antibodies to antigens.

Neutrophils are nonspecific cellular components that respond innately to abnormal cells and microbes. They arrive early at the scene of a tissue injury. They produce some cell killing by secretion of proteolytic enzymes. Macrophages may be resident in certain tissues (varies by type of tissue) or may be carried as monocytes through the circulation to the site of injury. Macrophages phagocytize microbes as the name implies and stimulate repair to the site of injury. Macrophages also innately respond to microbes without any specific activation.

Lymphocytes are divided into 2 major groups of B cells and T cells. Both types of lymphocytes are considered adaptive. In the face of an immune challenge, particular types of B and T cells are recruited against specific nonself antigens. During development, a wide array of B and T cells are generated against different types of potential antigens. Those that would respond to self-antigen are removed from the lymphocyte pools. B cells release antibodies, whereas T cells are selected by macrophages that remove antigen from microbes and present the antigen to T cells, which directly destroy microbes bearing the antigen presented to them. Both B and T cells proliferate rapidly in response to the appropriate antigen and stimulation by complement, helper T cells and other components of the immune system. Following eradication of the antigen, memory B and T cells are made available for a rapid future response against the antigen (memory cells).

Thus, B and T cells are considered to be adaptive, cell-mediated components of the immune system. Antibodies are an adaptive part of the immune system and because they are carried within the blood and body fluids, they are considered to be adaptive and humoral components. Neutrophils, macrophages, defensins, collectins, and complement naturally respond to broad categories of antigens and are considered to be innate. Neutrophils and macrophages are cell-mediated innate components and defensins, collectins, and complement are humoral, innate components.

PATHOGENIC PROPERTIES OF MICROBES

A number of bacteria are capable of penetrating the mechanical barrier of the skin and mucosa, in particular those causing sexually transmitted disease. Specific properties conferring virulence are seen in certain bacteria that allow them to escape detection or killing by the immune system. Capsule-forming bacteria such as *Streptococcus pneumoniae* and *Hemophilus influenzae* are common culprits in infections of the throat, middle ears, and upper airways. Leukocidins are chemicals produced by *Staphylococcus aureus* and *Clostridium perfringens* that are toxic to white cells. *Pseudomonas aeruginosa* and *Staphylococcus aureus* produce molecules that interfere with lysosomal function. Molecules produced by some bacteria allow rapid spread, especially through fascial planes, due to their proteolytic properties. Streptokinase is produced in laboratories to be used as a thrombolytic agent.

Injury-causing molecules on the surface of bacteria are called endotoxin. Certain endotoxins are very dangerous, especially those found on the surface of gram-negative bacteria. Bacteremia with gram-negative organisms may produce septic shock and death. Other molecules called exotoxins are released from bacteria and may interfere with metabolic processes causing cell injury. The presence of bacteria and their chemical products can have a profound effect on healing. At low bacterial levels, certain aspects of wound healing may occur at a faster rate, but high levels of bacteria inhibit healing. Even at some distance, the presence of an abscess can delay healing of a wound elsewhere on a patient.

A definitive diagnosis of infection requires the presence of purulent drainage or inflammation spreading beyond what is expected of normal healing (cellulitis). Quantitatively, a culture obtained by tissue biopsy demonstrating greater than 100,000 organisms per gram or the presence of ß-hemolytic streptococci in even lower concentration is strongly suggestive of infection. A commonly used rule of thumb is that a wound that heals primarily without discharge is uninfected but is infected if purulent discharge occurs. In such cases, bacteria may not be detected in culture if the purulent drainage consists only of dead bacteria, neutrophils and tissue debris. However, biopsy of the wound itself, rather than swabs of the drainage, are likely to truly demonstrate infection if it exists; therefore, swab cultures (see below) are discouraged. Purulent drainage confined to a suture site (stitch abscess) is not considered infected if healing occurs and the suture sites clear within 72 hours.

PREDISPOSING FACTORS TO INFECTION

Immunodeficiency is a general term for reduced effectiveness of the immune system. A related term is *immunosuppression*, which implies that something has suppressed the immune system, making it deficient. Based on the underlying cause, immunodeficiency can be divided into two basic categories. Primary immunodeficiency is caused by genetic defects in the immune system, resulting in a lack of specific or more general components of the immune system. Specific deficiencies include the lack of antibodies, X-linked agammaglobinemia (Bruton's disease), and thymic dysplasia (DiGeorge syndrome) in which the thymus and other specific embryologic structures, including the heart, fail to develop normally. A number of more global deficiencies also occur.

Far more common are immunodeficiencies with underlying causes other than genetic, termed *secondary immunodeficiencies*. In the context of wound care, the most important is diabetes mellitus. In particular, neutrophil function is depressed in poorly controlled diabetes mellitus. Other common forms of secondary immunodeficiency include kidney disease, burns, malnutrition, alcohol and drug abuse, cancer in general, and certain types of cancer of the immune system in particular. All surgery carries some risk of infection. A recent study (Greif, et al), however, indicated that supplemental oxygen during surgery drastically reduces the risk of operative infection. Other secondary immunodeficiencies include AIDS and administration of immunosuppressive drugs to treat autoimmune diseases (rheumatoid arthritis, lupus, scleroderma and others) or to prevent transplant rejection. Other terminologies that may be used with causes of secondary immunodeficiency are *immunosuppression* or *compromised immunity*.

Infections that occur because of a deficient immune system are called opportunistic infections. The organisms and viruses that cause opportunistic infection typically do not lead to illness in someone with a normal immune system. Many opportunistic infections are caused by fungi. Only a small number of fungal species are pathogenic in those with normal immunity.

Another mechanism for infection is alteration of the microenvironment where microbes exist, promoting proliferation of particular types of organisms. Infections that occur under these altered conditions are called *facultative infection*. This term implies that the infection would not have occurred without the environment being facilitated for the organism. This facilitation may occur for a number of reasons. Use of antibiotics that reduce competition for the local microenvironment may allow resistant organisms to proliferate. A classic example is the vaginal yeast infection that occurs frequently after an antibacterial drug is administered for an upper respiratory or urogenital bacterial infection. In addition, altered pH, temperature, or humidity may promote the growth of particular organisms. An important facultative infection is *Clostridium difficile*, which can produce diarrhea when competition with other organisms in the gastrointestinal tract is reduced by the use of antibiotics.

Postoperative infections are believed to be due to factors other than simple presence of airborne bacteria. An estimated 30,000 to 60,000 airborne bacteria fall within a 3 to 4 m² operating room per hour; however, postoperative infection rate is not highly correlated with the quantity of bacteria present in the air or even those present in the wound at the time of surgery. The strongest factor seems to be the duration of the surgical procedure, ranging from 3.6% for procedures of less than 30 minutes to 16.4% for procedures lasting more than 5 hours. Another factor, infection in another area of the body, increases the risk of infection during surgery by 3-fold. In the case of traumatic wounds, time also plays an important role. The number of organisms recovered from traumatic wounds increases rapidly with time. The average time since injury for wounds with fewer than 100 organisms per gram is 2.2 hours compared with 3 hours for wounds with 100 to 100,000. The average time for wounds with greater than 100,000 organisms per gram was 5.17 hours and only the wounds with greater than 100,000 per gram developed clinical infection in the emergency room series described by Robson, Duke, et al.

SOURCES OF ORGANISMS

A number of normal flora colonizing the skin, sweat glands, hair follicles, and mucosa (resident microbes) can proliferate and become virulent when introduced into body tissues. Approximately 1,000 organisms per gram of tissue reside in sweat glands and hair follicles. Common resident microbes colonizing the skin include *Staphylococcus epidermidis*, *Pseudomonas aeruginosa*, and *Staphylococcus aureus*. Transient microbes are introduced by contact with objects or other persons, or animals. Intestinal flora may be introduced to wounds by fecal incontinence, poor hygiene, or by accidental puncture during surgical procedures. Notable examples of transient microbes include various *Enterococci*, *Escherichia coli*, *Proteus*, *Klebsiella*, and *Lactobacillus* species. Multiple organisms colonizing the mouth and pharynx may be introduced due to poor hygiene or human bites. A tremendous number of bacteria from the environment may contaminate wounds, especially the *Clostridium* species. Bacteria may also enter wounds by direct contact with others, including healthcare workers, due to improper handwashing (skin-to-skin contact) or by aerosol inhalation. Ingestion of contaminated food or drink, particularly by the fecal-oral route due to improper

hygiene or sanitation is another important means of transmitting bacteria. Some infections may also be caused by arthropod or vertebrate bites.

Indirect contact or secondary contamination is caused by contact with contaminated bedding, clothing, instruments, or equipment. Inanimate objects that transfer microbes are called fomites. Hospital (or other facility) acquired infections are termed *nosocomial infections*. The most common nosocomial infections are caused by *Staphylococcus aureus*, *Escherichia coli*, and *Pseudomonas aeruginosa*. Overall, the most common organism involved in wound infection is *Staphylococcus aureus*. Wounds may also be infected by facultative gram negative bacteria such as *E coli*, *Proteus*, *Enterobacter*, and *Klebsiella* due to fecal contamination of wounds. Deep wounds are frequently infected by anaerobes such as *Bacteroides*, *Actinomyces*, and *Clostridium* species.

COLONIZATION, CONTAMINATION, AND INFECTION

The ability to control wound infection depends on a thorough understanding of the differences between colonization, contamination, and infection. All wounds—whether acute or chronic—are exposed to microbes. Our ability to reduce the risk of infection is determined by the characteristics of the bacteria and the environment in which the bacteria live. Three factors that determine whether infection occurs are the number of organisms, the virulence of the organism, and the patient's immunity to the organism. *Virulence* is a term that expresses how likely an organism is to cause an infection for a given number of them. For example, the virulence of ß-hemolytic strep is about 10 times that of most bacteria. The risk of infection is increased by the number of organisms, the virulence of the organism, and decreased by the patient's immunity to it. Some have suggested expressing this as a mathematical equation: Risk of infection = number x virulence/immunity. This is an obvious oversimplification, but it is a useful tool for understanding the factors involved in infection. For example, a large number of organisms are very likely to cause infection in anybody; a person with suppressed immunity is likely to develop an infection when exposed to only a small number of bacteria, and a virulent organism such as ß-hemolytic strep is more likely to cause an infection for a given number of bacteria and a given immunity.

Colonization simply represents a stable population of resident bacteria in low numbers on a surface. As long as the environment remains stable, the surface does not become overrun and microbes do not invade tissues surrounding the surface. Contamination refers to the introduction of transient microbes to a surface. If a colonized

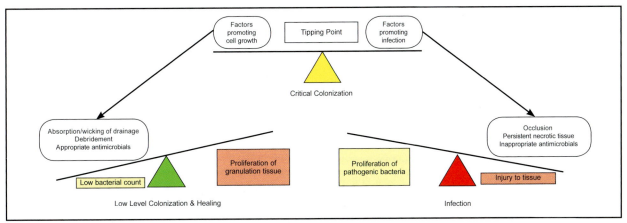

Figure 9-1. Relationship between cells of the wound bed and bacteria that define colonization, critical colonization, and infection. This diagram illustrates the principle of a tipping point in which conditions become favorable for granulation tissue formation at the expense of bacterial growth, or conditions become favorable for bacterial growth at the expense of the cells of the wound producing infection. An area near the tipping point represents critical colonization. Granulation cannot take place rapidly due to competition for resources between the cells of the wound and bacteria.

surface such as an open wound experiences contamination, 3 outcomes are possible. Microbes contaminating the wound may be particularly virulent or suited to the environment and the risk of infection is increased. A second possibility is that the microbe has weak virulence or the environment is unsuitable resulting in no change in the wound's status. A third possibility is that the new microbe introduced to the wound competes for resources or alters the environment of the wound in such a way that actually improves the wound's status. Such a strategy is used for treatment of fungal infection of the mouth (thrush). Introduction of specific bacteria diminish the proliferation of fungus, which clears thrush. However, contamination of a wound is generally to be avoided as we cannot predict the outcome of contamination.

A level of bacterial involvement intermediate between colonization and infection is critical contamination. This term implies that the quantity of bacteria becomes a drain on local resources, impairing wound healing ability. Low-level production of toxins may also be responsible for impaired healing. The terms *colonization, critical colonization,* and *infection* need to be viewed as a continuum in which either granulation tissue or bacteria are "winning." In colonization, a small number of bacteria are able to survive and wound healing is able to progress. In critical colonization, the host's tissues are able to survive, but not proliferate and produce healing. Infection implies that bacteria are prospering at the expense of tissue of the wound. At this point on the continuum, the wound does not stagnate, but deteriorates. Infection occurs when tissue is invaded by bacteria that proliferate and harm the tissue in the wound instead of remaining as a stable population. Operationally, infection is defined as 100,000 (10^5) organisms per gram. In a deteriorating wound, necrosis is observable as a dete-

rioration of the wound or darkened dusky or brown areas developing on the wound surface. As discussed above, the presence of purulence and spreading cellulitis are indicators of infection.

The relative prosperity of the host and the microbe and the terms associated with them are depicted in Figure 9-1. This figure also suggests how the concept of tipping point can be applied to a wound's health. At a point near critical colonization, changes in the wound's environment can cause the balance of prosperity to tip in either direction. Interventions are directed at making the wound move from infection and then tip toward the health of granulation tissue. Many things might happen to a given individual to allow a wound to tip toward infection. Moving away from infection toward critical colonization gives the immune system the opportunity to restore tissue health and allow healing. If conditions allow proliferation of bacteria in tissue to occur faster than the immune system can destroy them, the wound goes past the tipping point toward infection. Systemic or topical antimicrobials are a way to move past the tipping point toward healing. Other means of tipping toward healing involve improving the environment of the wound.

A moist, warm environment with necrotic tissue such as an occluded wound is conducive to bacterial overgrowth. The risk of infection is great in an acute wound with large amounts of necrotic tissue available for nourishment of microbes. In particular, burned tissue and hematomas serve as a tremendous growth medium for bacteria, likely to tip the wound toward infection. Cavities within the body such as sinuses created by allowing abscesses to close over, subcutaneous spaces created by surgery and not adequately approximated afterward, spaces along prostheses, and foreign materials left in the body after surgery are particularly likely to promote bacterial growth. Partial-thickness wounds that might have healed without scarring and loss of skin elasticity can easily degenerate into full-thickness injuries with compromised skin function because bacteria were able to proliferate and cause necrosis through the remaining depth of dermis at the base of a burn injury.

Large, contaminated acute wounds, especially those with substantial injuries and tissue necrosis, should be allowed to heal by granulation, allowing the base and sides of the wounds to push outward, rather than closing such a wound. Suturing and other forms of primary closure of this type of wound produce cavities that provide an ideal environment for bacterial overgrowth and no opportunity exists to observe the wound. Exposure to air, irrigation, and filling the wound with absorbent, nonocclusive material such as gauze to wick drainage out of a wound can decrease bacterial count, tipping the wound toward healing. However, an open wound may dry out and slow healing. Occlusive dressings, on the other hand, promote a moist wound environment, but provide conditions suitable for bacterial overgrowth. Choice of dressing and means of debridement of wounds are clinical decisions that must be made based on individual characteristics of the wound and the patient. Thorough sharp debridement can reduce the bacterial count of a wound rapidly. Moreover, once sharp debridement is completed, bacterial counts will remain low (<100 per gram) in almost all cases.

CULTURING WOUNDS

The goals of culturing wounds would seem to be identification of any microorganisms that might impede wound healing, finding an appropriate antibiotic to eradicate that microorganism, and restoring normal healing trajectory. Unfortunately, indiscriminate use of antibiotics has instead resulted in the development of antibiotic-resistant bacteria. Culturing has a place in wound care, but may cause more harm than good if used inappropriately.

Types of Cultures

The 2 basic reasons for culturing wounds are to determine the bioburden of the wound (quantity of microbes present) and to identify which microorganisms are present. A quantitative culture is used to determine the microbial burden. A qualitative culture is used to identify which microbes are present and may be followed by sensitivity testing to determine the optimal antimicrobial drug to treat the infection. Identification of the microbe will allow the virulence of the microbe to be taken into account as well.

Another classification of culturing is aerobic vs anaerobic. Aerobic culturing is straightforward and is performed simply as described below. An anaerobic culture must be obtained with a special culturette and handled in such a way that the anaerobes are not excessively exposed to air and killed before a culture is plated.

Issues Associated With Culturing Wounds

Although performing routine cultures would seem to have great value in directing wound management efforts, routine swab culture of chronic wounds is not recommended by AHCPR for several reasons and may actually lead to poorer wound management. Two important mistakes may result from indiscriminate use of cultures. An appropriate antibiotic may not be given or an antibiotic may be prescribed when it is not needed. In the first case, infection may be allowed to spread. The second case might seem to be benign, but antibiotics are not harmless; administration of antibiotics carries some risk of injury to the patient. Therefore, the risk/benefit ratio of antibiotic treatment may become inappropriate.

The concept that infection interferes with acute wound healing can be illogically extrapolated to chronic wounds. The presumption of infection as the cause of a slow healing wound leads to the use of routine cultures and indiscriminate application of topical or systemic antibiotic agents, rather than thoroughly investigating the causes of slow healing. Topical agents then further slow wound healing, leading to even harsher handling of the wound and further courses of antibiotics. Chronic wounds are expected to be colonized; therefore, cultures will grow resident microbes that are unlikely to be the cause of any problems with wound healing. The harm of systemic antibiotics can be many. In addition to harm done to the wound bed, patients may develop allergic, anaphylactic, or other immune system injuries. Penicillins and cephalosporins, in particular, have been linked to anaphylaxis. Less severe allergic responses may also be seen with these and other drugs. Antibiotics can produce the immune injuries called Stevens-Johnson syndrome (described in Chapter 7) and serum sickness. In serum sickness, deposit of antigen-antibody complexes in tissues leads to extreme pain. This syndrome was initially described in patients who were exposed to horse serum as a source of immunoglobulins.

Some antibiotics may be selectively toxic to certain tissues. In particular, a number of nephrotoxic and ototoxic drugs are well known. These include penicillins, cephalosporins, ciprofloxacin, vancomycin, streptomycin, kanamycin, neomycin, gentamicin, tobramycin, amikacin, netilmicin, erythromycin, clarithromycin, and azithromycin. Because gut bacteria are sources of biologically important substances such as vitamins K and B12, vitamin deficiencies may result.

Antibiotics may also cause facultative infections. The loss of bacteria from the gastrointestinal tract and its mucosal surface may lead to thrush, a fungal infection of the mouth, and vaginal yeast infection. Finally, the gut may be overrun with *Clostridium difficile* due to the use of antibiotics either singly or in combination. Diarrhea during antibiotic therapy is frequently due to *C difficile*. The patient may need to cease that specific antibiotic therapy and use other antibiotics to eradicate the *C difficile*.

Another issue is the incorrect identification of pathogenic organisms. Swabbing the surface of a wound may miss organisms growing beneath the surface, which are our major concern. Two very serious consequences may then result. A swab culture of a wound with copious purulent drainage may grow little if anything in the lab, because the offending organism was not accessible during a swab. Secondly, incorrectly identifying the source of infection can lead to the use of antimicrobial agents that may further slow healing of the wound and may have adverse effects for the patient either locally or systemically. The wrong antimicrobial may worsen an infection if sensitivity tests are conducted on the wrong microorganisms. By eliminating competing microorganisms the true culprit may be allowed to flourish.

All chronic wounds, including stage II-IV ulcers, are considered to be colonized; therefore, culturing a wound that does not appear to be infected provides no useful information. Instead of treating a colonized wound with antimicrobials, the risk of colonization progressing through critical colonization and infection will be minimized through cleansing and debridement of wounds. If purulence or foul odor develops, more frequent cleansing or debridement should be done. As discussed, healing of even chronic wounds may be delayed if greater than 100,000 organisms per gram or osteomyelitis exist. The AHCPR has taken the position that swab cultures should not be done routinely for determining whether a wound is infected. Instead, the Centers for Disease Control (CDC) recommends either drawing wound fluid through needle aspiration or taking a tissue biopsy. Because infection is largely dependent on the presence of necrotic tissue, adequate cleansing and debridement will prevent infection in most cases. The AHCPR guidelines recommend a 2-week trial of topical antibiotics if a clean ulcer is not healing or if exudate continues despite optimal care for 2 to 4 weeks and to evaluate bone for osteomyelitis.

Culturing Techniques

Culturing may be done by any of a number of personnel, including physicians, nurses, medical technicians, and physical and occupational therapists. When unsure of the preferred technique of a facility, the best option is to ask the medical technician who will be performing the cultures exactly how the swabbing and transport of the culturette should be done. Aerobic and anaerobic culturettes are handled somewhat differently and instructions given with the culturette need to be followed carefully. Some general rules for performing the culture include avoiding swabbing over eschar, which will likely have different microbes present than the wound itself due to the vastly different microenvironment. The tip needs to be rotated to cover as much of the swab tip as possible. While swabbing, cover from one edge to the other in a zigzag pattern such that 10 points (5 on each side) are covered from one end of the wound to the other. A newer technique, the Levine technique may be performed to allow swab culturettes to capture bacteria in the wound fluid. In this technique, a wound bed is cleaned thoroughly then the culturette is pressed into the wound bed sufficiently to cause fluid to be expressed from the wound bed and absorbed onto the culturette as it is rotated over a 1 cm^2 area.

Antimicrobial Methods

Several important definitions must be understood to practice good infection control. These terms include *sterilization*, *disinfection*, and *antisepsis*. Sterilization refers to total destruction of all microbial life, including spores and viruses. Antisepsis is a reduction in the number of organisms present on skin or tissues. A related term, *disinfection*, is defined as a reduction of the number of organisms present on inanimate objects.

Antimicrobial methods may be divided into physical and chemical methods. Certain types are more appropriate for sterilization, others for antisepsis or disinfection. Factors to be considered for any method include how long the process is applied, the temperature and pressure at which the process is applied, the quantity or concentration of heat or chemical, the nature of the item receiving the process, the type and quantity of microbe, including spores, and whether the items are contaminated with body fluids that may act as a protective layer for the microbe.

Physical methods include heat—both dry and moist, pressure combined with heat, cold, desiccation, radiation, ultrasound, filtration, and hypertonicity. In general, physical methods are useful for sterilization, whereas chemicals are frequently used for antisepsis and disinfection. However, a combination of physical and chemical methods may be used for any of the 3 types of antimicrobial methods.

Sterilization

Heat can be used for either sterilization or disinfection. However, heat is not suitable for many items and certainly not for antisepsis. To achieve sterilization, a combination of time and temperature is necessary. The heat required for sterilization is increased if items are contaminated with any body fluids that might form an insulating coat on the microbes. If instruments are contaminated with body fluids, thorough cleaning and chemical disinfection may be required prior to sterilization with heat. Dry heat is less effective on some types of microbes, especially on items contaminated with body fluids. Moist heat delivered as either steam or boiling is more effective at removing proteinaceous material from instruments. Of particular concern is destruction of viruses that may withstand boiling. The combination of pressure and heat used in an autoclave is effective at destroying spores and viruses that may survive heat alone. Safe guidelines promoted in the literature include autoclaving for 20 minutes at 250°C and 15 psi, boiling for 30 minutes (longer at higher elevations) or dry heat (baking) for 1 hour at 356°C. Appropriate packaging, including pressure sensitive tape, should be used for autoclaving. Due to the heat and pressure of the autoclave, no sealed containers should be used. Items that cannot tolerate normal autoclave temperatures may be treated at a lower temperature for a longer time, or may require chemical disinfection. Another approach for heat-sensitive items such as catheters is gas sterilization. Ethylene oxide is a chemical oxidizing agent, which is highly effective, but is also difficult to use. Radiation is another method used to sterilize items. X-rays or gamma rays (ionizing radiation) induce sufficient genetic damage to sterilize instruments as well as foods and drugs. Ultrasound is highly effective at removing adherent materials from the surface of metal. The cleansed materials may then be further disinfected and sterilized.

Disinfection

Three levels of disinfection are commonly described. High level disinfection destroys all microorganisms and viruses. Intermediate level disinfection destroys all microbes except spore-forming, and some nonlipid and small viruses. The third type, low level disinfection, provides little action against spore-forming bacteria, mycobacteria, and some fungi and small viruses. Some items such as laundry can be disinfected sufficiently by using very hot water. The effectiveness of chemical disinfection can be altered by the interaction of disinfectants and microbes. The concentration of the chemical, the pH, and presence of any body fluids on the items to be disinfected determine the effectiveness of chemical disinfectants; therefore, instructions need to be followed carefully. As discussed with sterilization, instruments and other items should be washed thoroughly before disinfection to remove proteinaceous material that may protect microbes from the disinfectant. High level disinfection needs to be used when concern exists regarding spore-forming bacteria or viruses.

Although disinfection is useful for treating items that come in contact with intact skin, instruments used for debridement must be sterilized. For routine wound care clean exam gloves are sufficient. No differences have been found in infection rates between clean examination gloves and sterile gloves used for closing wounds in emergency departments. Although clean gloves may be used on chronic wounds of individuals with relatively normal immunity, exam gloves, dressings, or anything else that might touch the wound should not be left in the open for extended periods where they may accumulate unnecessary surface contamination. Materials used in wound management should be kept in their original sealed packaging inside cabinets or drawers to protect them from airborne contamination or splashing until they are needed. Sterile gloves should be considered for any patients with significantly depressed immunity.

Chemicals chosen for disinfection should be chosen for the particular situation. A large number of high level disinfectants are available commercially. Their effectiveness is determined by the factors described previously, in particular, concentration, temperature, and the presence of body fluids. Surfaces should be scrubbed with detergent to remove body fluids. Surfactant and chelating agents in the detergent increase their effectiveness in removing proteinaceous contaminants. In addition, the disinfectant should be left on the surface for the prescribed time to be effective.

Disinfectants include several types of agents including soaps/detergents, alcohols, heavy metals, oxidants, chlorine and iodine compounds, and other agents. Phenolics are used commercially in home disinfectants, eg, Lysol (Reckitt Benckiser, Wayne, NJ). Phenolics include carbolic acid, phenol, xylenols, cresol, and orthophenylphenol. Similar to alcohols, these agents are effective tuberculocides and sporicides. In particular, chlorine compounds are used in hydrotherapy. Sodium hypochlorite, the active ingredient of laundry bleach, has a short half-life and is inactivated readily by organic material. Sustained release forms of chlorine, such as Chlorazene (Ferno-Washington, Inc., Wilmington, OH), are frequently used to disinfect water used for hydrotherapy in a whirlpool tank. Although they are indicated for skin preparation prior to surgery and for hand scrubbing prior to surgery, sustained release forms of iodine, such as povidone iodine, have also been used to disinfect water used for hydrotherapy.

Antisepsis

Like disinfection, chemical antimicrobial methods are the mainstay of antisepsis. Chemicals used for antisepsis are called antiseptics. Physical means are generally not suitable for antisepsis due to the potential damage to skin or body tissues. Moreover, many chemicals that are highly effective for disinfection are too toxic to be used as antiseptics. Although antiseptics reduce the number of microbes on the body surface, microbes may still be harbored in hair follicles and the ostia of sweat and sebaceous glands. A reduction of approximately 95% is expected with good technique. Soaps and detergents act as antiseptics by removing surface microbes. In addition, they damage cell membranes by dissolving phospholipids. Many soaps and detergents have antimicrobial agents added, such as acetic acid and benzoic acid, for handwashing. As with disinfection, some degree of scrubbing is necessary to remove residues that could harbor bacteria beneath them.

Chlorhexidine gluconate (Hibiclens, Mölnlycke Health Care US, LLC, Norcross, GA) and hexachlorophene (Phisohex, Sanofi-aventis US, Bridgewater, NJ) are commonly used as antiseptics for handwashing or topical bacterial infections. Both of these should be rinsed thoroughly from the skin. Hexachlorophene is neurotoxic if it is absorbed through the skin. These agents are used occasionally as whirlpool disinfectants, although they have questionable value at the dilutions used and may be ineffective against a number of organisms at their full strengths.

Ethyl and isopropyl alcohol in 70% solutions are effective disinfectants for bacteria and are tuberculocidal and sporicidal. Aerosolized ethyl alcohol foams and isopropyl alcohol gels are available for handwashing to rapidly reduce the counts of transient bacteria. Because these formulations appear to be more effective antiseptics than soap and water, some organizations have suggested these be used either in place of, or in addition to, handwashing with soap and water.

Iodine can be formulated as a slow release polymer such as Betadine (Purdue Pharma L.P., Stamford, CT) to produce continual release of iodine on the skin surface or combined with alcohol (tincture of iodine). Alcohol and iodine solutions are used for antiseptic scrubs to further reduce microbial counts. Even with surgical scrubbing, microbial counts are still unacceptably high, requiring the use of sterile gloves. Iodine compounds are approved by the Food and Drug Administration (FDA) for surface antisepsis as either a skin scrub or surgical prep, but are not approved for use in open wounds. Iodine compounds have been shown clearly to interfere with the processes of wound healing. In addition, high concentrations of iodine can cause iodine burns and absorption of antiseptics can lead to systemic iodine toxicity, manifested as neuropathy, cardiovascular, renal, and hepatic toxicity.

Acids such as acetic acid and boric acid are effective against a number of common bacteria. Acetic acid is commonly used for treating wounds infected by *Pseudomonas aeruginosa*, and Dakin's solution is used to destroy *Staphylococcus* and *Streptococcus* species. Antiseptics are also used in sprays as air fresheners containing ingredients such as alcohol, triethylene glycol, and benzethonium chloride.

Hydrogen peroxide is a commonly used, commercially available agent proposed to work as an oxidizing agent, particularly for anaerobes, and produces effervescence due to the reaction with tissue catalase, providing a mild debriding function.

Heavy metals, halogens, iodine, and bromine are bactericidal, virucidal, tuberculocidal, and sporicidal. Salts of heavy metals are available commercially as antiseptics. Mercury chloride is commonly used for first aid on acute wounds (Merthiolate, Mercurochrome) and silver nitrate has been used as an ophthalmic antiseptic for neonates. Silver nitrate left on skin or open wounds is highly toxic. It causes severe drying and necrosis of tissue and is not recommended for use on open wounds.

In addition to chemical means of antisepsis, ultraviolet lamps have been approved. Like x-rays and gamma rays, ultraviolet produces severe genetic damage. The dose necessary for antisepsis is relatively small, requiring exposure for several seconds with minimal risk to growing tissue in the wound when used appropriately.

As discussed with iodine compounds, the use of antiseptics as topical agents for wounds is discouraged. No research has shown that use of antiseptics on wounds reduce bacterial counts within them. Some antiseptics can be absorbed and cause toxicity as noted above for iodine and hexachlorophene. Excessive use of antiseptics (and disinfectants) may lead to development of resistant microbes. Other limitations on antiseptics are their ineffectiveness with high bacterial counts and the inactivation of antiseptics by excessive organic material, especially purulence.

Physical Methods of Infection Control

Paper and gauze may be used to filter substances to decrease contamination with microbes. Paper is frequently used for face masks and gauze is frequently placed as a covering over wounds. Paper and gauze need to be kept dry to be effective as filters. Wet gauze, in particular, can transmit microbes into a wound. Moist dressings are usually covered by a dry gauze or paper material to prevent transmission of microbes from the air into the wounds. Additionally, high-efficiency particulate air (HEPA) filters are used to decrease microbes, as well as allergens from the air. Ionizers may also be used to remove particulate material from the air; however, the ionized particles settle on surfaces and require dusting, vacuuming, or mopping to remove them.

Cold is primarily bacteriostatic, rather than bactericidal. Cold reduces the rate of growth of microbes. Allowing temperature to increase to room temperature causes bacterial growth to resume and spores to germinate. Refreezing will simply slow the growth of a larger number of bacteria. Desiccation (drying) is frequently used in the preparation of foods and drugs. Desiccation combined with vacuum is called *lyophilization*. Unfortunately, desiccation can also preserve microbes, especially spores. These microbes encased within desiccated body fluids may be found in a patient's environment, particularly on floors, dressings, clothing, and other items. Disturbing these may result in airborne dust that can be carried into wounds where a warm, moist, and frequently occluded environment may aid in the proliferation of the microbe. Hypertonicity is generally used for preserving food rather than wound management.

CONTROL OF ENDOGENOUS ORGANISMS

Endogenous organisms refer to those already present on the person. Several means are available to control endogenous organisms. A common means of preventing bacterial access to wounds is skin preparation with chlorhexidine/alcohol or iodine/alcohol. Cleansing wounds with mechanical irrigation such as pulsatile lavage with concurrent suction is useful for traumatic wounds with gross contamination. Generally, if given the choice of topical and systemic antimicrobial drugs, systemic drugs are preferred. The depth of penetration of topical agents is often insufficient. The concern with bacteria in the wound is not surface colonization, but invasion of tissue below the wound surface where topical agents are unlikely to reach. Protecting wounds on the sacrum and ischial tuberosities from feces is another important aspect of managing colonization and preventing infection. Placing patients in full body whirlpools creates the opportunity for fecal material and organisms colonizing other parts of the body to be carried into wounds. Patients also need to be discouraged from placing an untreated leg in a whirlpool with the leg being treated as the quantity of organisms in the tank will be increased and the species of organisms may be different.

CONTROL OF EXOGENOUS ORGANISMS

Microbes present on a surface other than the body are termed exogenous organisms. Control is usually achieved by sterilization of invasive instruments and disinfection of equipment such as hydrotherapy tanks and turbines. Although we tend to focus on transient microbes, resident microbes—while not generally pathogenic—can cause infection in immunocompromised individuals, or when deposited into a patient's tissue. Moreover, microbes may also be transmitted from patients to clinicians.

Although not completely effective in removing microbes from the skin, care needs to be taken during

handwashing to minimize what is left on the skin of the clinician. Handwashing or application of approved hand sanitizer (alcohol preparations discussed above) is to be done before and after each patient. One must distinguish between handwashing, which is done to minimize the number of transient organisms on the hands, and scrubbing, which is done to minimize both transient and resident organisms present on the hands. Handwashing is a vigorous and brief rubbing of hand surfaces together with lathered hands, followed by rinsing with flowing water. Scrubbing is a specific sequence lasting up to 10 minutes, using antiseptics, before surgery is performed in an operating room. A surgical cap, mask, shoe covers, and sterile gown are also required. Handwashing involves soap or detergent, sometimes combined with mild antimicrobial agents. Scrubbing is done with a combination of iodine and alcohol or other harsh antimicrobial agents.

For handwashing, disposable soap containers are preferred to refillable containers; bar soap should not be used due to potential contamination from other users. During handwashing, nothing should touch the hands and forearms other than soap, running water, and one's own hands and forearms. Because the average person only washes hands when they are obviously contaminated, the sink, its controls, and soap dispensers are generally heavily contaminated and should not be touched directly with the hands. One must also avoid being splashed at the sink due to the possibility of microbes being transmitted from the sink. Water controls and nonrefillable soap dispensers that use knee or foot controls are preferable to controls that require the use of hands. Care must be taken during handwashing to prevent contamination with *Pseudomonas* and other microbes from contact with the sink, handles, and faucet, or from using solutions diluted with nonsterile water. If hands-free controls are not available, use clean paper towels to touch faucet controls. A scrub cannot be performed without knee or foot controls. A scrub must be followed by drying with a sterile towel, whereas clean paper towels are sufficient for handwashing. In obtaining paper towels, contact with the outside of the towel dispenser must be avoided. The steps of proper handwashing are listed in Table 9-2. Proper handwashing techniques are depicted in Figure 9-2.

TOPICAL ANTIMICROBIAL AGENTS

A large number of antimicrobial agents have been used on open wounds. Most of these, however, are designed for preparation of the skin preoperatively and for immediate use on acute wounds. These are not designed, indicated, or approved for use on chronic wounds. These agents are frequently misused or overused. Although they may be useful temporarily, they must be used prudently with the specific goal of preventing or treating infection. Because infection

Table 9-2

Handwashing Technique

- Turn on the faucet with foot or knee control, or a clean paper towel
- Operate soap control with foot control or use a clean paper towel
- Wash thoroughly for 30 seconds
- Rinse thoroughly under flowing water, but do not make contact with the faucet or sink; do not allow splashing from the bottom of the sink
- If contact or splashing occurs, handwashing must be restarted
- Allow water to run toward elbows; do not allow water from arm to run down to hands
- Dry with clean paper towels and then turn off water with paper towels
- Use of automatic paper towel dispenser is preferred; avoid using crank type dispenser
- Disposable soap containers are preferred to refillable containers; bar soap should not be used

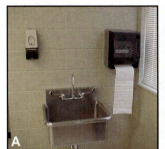
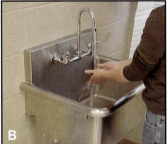
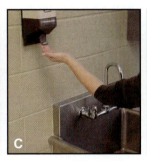
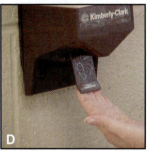

Figure 9-2. Hand washing. (A) Soap dispenser, sink, and paper towel dispenser, (B) Wetting hands, (C) Obtaining soap, (D) Close-up of nonrefillable soap dispenser.

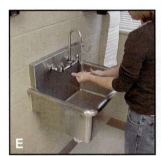
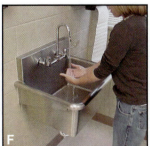
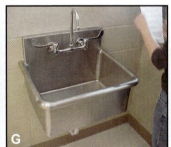
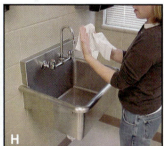

Figure 9-2. (E) Lathering, (F) Rinsing, (G) Obtaining paper towel, (H) Drying hands.

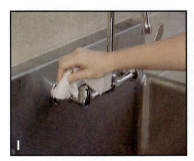
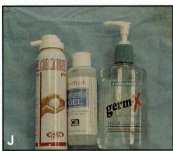

Figure 9-2. (I) Turning off faucet handles with paper towel, (J) Isopropyl alcohol based hand sanitizers.

and eschar slow healing, these agents are used often in an illogical attempt to speed healing. Considering that these agents are toxic to bacteria, fungi, protozoa, and even many viruses, the clinician should also consider what these agents do to fibroblasts and epithelial cells. If the immediate goal is to rid the wound of unacceptable numbers of microbes, then a limited course may be prudent. One must keep in mind, however, that the concern is for organisms that have achieved a true tissue level, not simply bacteria colonizing the surface of a wound. Moreover, many topical agents lack the penetration necessary to be effective when applied topically. Of the commonly used topical agents, silver sulfadiazine is sufficiently water soluble to be effective. Once a wound is debrided, clean and stable, these topical antiseptic agents will only retard wound healing. AHCPR recommends a 2-week trial of topical antibiotics for clean ulcers that are not healing or are continuing to produce exudate after 2 to 4 weeks of optimal care. If an antibiotic is selected for topical use, the AHCPR recommends using an agent that is effective against gram-negative, gram-positive and anaerobic organisms. Triple antibiotic and silver sulfadiazine are mentioned specifically.

The AHCPR guidelines recommend against use of topical antiseptics such as povidone iodine, iodophor, sodium hypochlorite, Dakin's solution, hydrogen peroxide, and acetic acid in wound tissue. In these guidelines, systemic, rather than topical, antibiotic therapy is suggested for patients with bacteremia, sepsis, advancing cellulitis, or osteomyelitis. These guidelines also indicate that systemic antibiotics are not required for pressure ulcers with only clinical signs of local infection. The ADA recommends against the use of any topical antiseptics or antibiotics and recommends aggressive sharp debridement and systemic antibiotics. As discussed above, povidone-iodine is a compound designed to produce sustained release of iodine. It is very beneficial in reducing risk of infection as a surgical preparation and temporary use on acute wounds. However, it is not recommended for use in chronic wounds. It may be used to prevent cross-contamination of hydrotherapy equipment. At a concentration of 0.001% it is noncytotoxic for fibroblasts. However, it is often used on gauze packed wounds in concentrations much higher than this and has never received approval to be used in wounds, but only for prepping skin for surgery or as a surgical hand scrub solution. Hypochlorite (household bleach) and the less cytotoxic chloramine (Chlorazene) are used routinely to prevent cross-contamination of hydrotherapy equipment. Unless a patient has more than one wound in a whirlpool tank or other container, the use of these chlorine compounds is questionable.

Triple antibiotic is a solution of 3 antimicrobials: neomycin, polymyxin B, and gramicidin. It is useful topically on a temporary basis for either a deep acute wound,

such as a gunshot wound, or as a short topical course for a nonhealing chronic wound suspected to be infected. Silver sulfadiazine inhibits DNA synthesis of microbes and is a broad spectrum antimicrobial with a cream formulation for topical application. It is especially useful for burns, has a soothing effect, and prevents gauze bandages from adhering to wounds. Although it may have adverse effects on fibroblasts and keratinocytes, it is highly effective in reestablishing bacterial balance. Therefore, it should be discontinued once bacterial balance is achieved. Silver sulfadiazine has also been implicated in Stevens-Johnson syndrome, an immune reaction that results in epidermal and mucosal blistering. This condition is potentially, but rarely, lethal. Stevens-Johnson syndrome has also been linked to a number of other antibiotics in addition to silver sulfadiazine. An alternative to silver sulfadiazine is Sulfamylon (UDL Laboratories, Rockford, IL). Sulfamylon may be preferred for full-thickness burn injuries as it penetrates eschar better. However, silver sulfadiazine may be preferred with large percent body surface area wounds. Sulfamylon may cause electrolyte problems when applied to large surface area wounds. Patients need to be monitored and instructed to look for local reactions or more widespread allergic/anaphylactic reactions.

Cadexomer iodine is available in multiple forms—an ointment, sheet, or powder. It has been used in a variety of wounds, both acute and chronic, including venous, arterial, pressure ulcers, and purulent wounds. It releases iodine gradually as the material absorbs exudates, and manufacturers claim that the release rate of iodine is not cytotoxic. In addition to absorption, it reduces odor and prevents maceration that might otherwise occur due to leakage of drainage onto surrounding skin. Although it may be applied to cover the wound bed, it requires a secondary dressing over it. When the material changes color from brown to a yellow or gray color, it should be replaced. However, the nature of the ointment and its color also obscures visibility of the wound bed and interferes with assessment of drainage quantity and quality.

Mercurochrome has useful antimicrobial action on small, partially healed, superficial wounds, or for a small number of applications to minor acute wounds. Neosporin is a combination of 3 antibacterial drugs (neomycin, polymyxin B, and bacitracin) and is highly effective against most gram-negative and gram-positive bacteria found on skin, and is indicated for most minor acute wounds. Moreover, its petrolatum base allows moisture retention to prevent scab formation. Polysporin only contains 2 of the 3 antimicrobials present in Neosporin (missing neomycin). Sensitivity to neomycin is common. Because Polysporin does not contain neomycin, it is a good alternative to neosporin. It also has a petrolatum base and it is commonly used on facial wounds, including burns.

Polysporin is also available in a powder, which can be poured into open wounds.

Hydrogen peroxide is a tremendously overrated antimicrobial agent. Although it is a household staple for treatment of minor acute wounds, it has little antimicrobial action compared with other available agents. It is sometimes used for its mechanical effect of effervescence. The enzyme catalase in blood converts H_2O_2 to H_2O and O_2, but this provides minor debridement value, which could be performed in other ways. Hydrogen peroxide has mostly entertainment value. Silver nitrate is very effective against gram negative bacteria, especially in a single application following contamination, but it is more useful as a hemostatic agent. It is very caustic and will discolor the skin (black). Its caustic nature allows the skilled clinician to use it to burn off excessive granulation tissue or to open curled over wound margins (epiboly).

Dakin's solution is a combination of sodium hypochlorite and boric acid that is effective against *Staphylococcus* and *Streptococcus* species. It was an important development in treating acute wound infections and likely prevented a number of wartime amputations. However, it is frequently prescribed for use on chronic wounds that are not infected. It is highly cytotoxic unless diluted and the AHCPR guidelines state explicitly that Dakin's solution should not be used on chronic wounds. Acetic acid, the active ingredient of vinegar, in a 0.25% solution is highly effective against *Pseudomonas*, but is caustic and damages healthy tissue. The AHCPR guidelines also make specific mention of acetic acid in terms of harming healing tissue. Acetic acid may be useful for a short course of several days in wounds infected by *Pseudomonas aeruginosa*.

SYSTEMIC ANTIMICROBIAL AGENTS

Many systemic antimicrobial drugs are available to treat infection. Entire texts are written to describe them. For chronic wounds, antibiotics are often not useful because systemic antibiotics do not reach therapeutic levels in chronic granulation tissue. However, these drugs become important in cases of acute wounds with advancing cellulitis. The purpose of this section of the chapter is to provide some background information for the clinician working with a patient for whom these drugs have been prescribed by a physician. As with any type of drug, antimicrobial agents have a therapeutic index that must be considered. Therapeutic index (TI) is the ratio of the median toxic concentration (TD_{50}) to the median effective concentration (ED_{50}); $TI = TD_{50}/ED_{50}$. Ideally, all antimicrobial drugs would have selective toxicity that would only harm bacteria (or protozoa or fungi), rather than the patient. Another consideration physicians have in prescribing antibiotics is that some antibacterial drugs are bacteriostatic, whereas others are bactericidal. Under most conditions,

simply rendering bacterial replication difficult (bacteriostatic agents) is sufficient to allow the immune system to tip the wound away from infection and toward healing. However, certain conditions dictate using drugs that kill existing bacteria (bactericidal agents).

Antibiotic strategies commonly used include inhibition of cell wall synthesis, damaging bacterial cell membranes, inhibition of bacterial protein synthesis, inhibition of bacterial DNA/RNA function, and modification of energy metabolism. As research continues on bacterial genomes, we should expect to have newer and more specific strategies available in the future. The earliest and still important category is the cell wall active agents (Beta lactams). These drugs prevent synthesis of cell walls around bacteria, but are not effective on mycoplasma, which lack a cell wall. Drugs in this category include penicillins (amoxicillin, oxacillin, methicillin, ampicillin, piperacillin, nafcillin, etc), cephalosporins, vancomycin, bacitracin, monobactams, and carbapenems. Polymyxin acts at the cell membrane, rather than the cell wall and, along with bacitracin, is more suitable for topical use than systemic use due to toxicity. Penicillins were the first antibiotics. These drugs were initially isolated from Penicillium molds that contaminated bacterial cultures and inhibited the culture's growth. Unfortunately, some bacteria have an enzyme called beta-lactamase that alters the structure of the active part of the penicillin molecule and confers resistance. One drug developed to overcome the problem is Augmentin (GlaxoSmithKline, Research Triangle Park, NC), a combination of the penicillin amoxicillin and a beta-lactamase inhibitor (clavulanate). Allergies to penicillins are common and can be severe.

Cephalosporins have an action similar to penicillins and may be used as an alternative drug if penicillin is ineffective or contraindicated due to allergy. These drugs are classified as first, second, third generations with an increasingly broader spectrum. Unfortunately, these drugs have also been linked to allergic reactions similar to penicillins. Like the penicillins, these drugs are easily identified by their names. Cephalosporins usually have ceph-, cef-, or kef- in the name, with the exception of some of the trade names such as Ceclor, Suprax, and Fortaz.

Vancomycin also inhibits the synthesis of cell wall and is frequently reserved as a "last resort" for resistant species or given empirically until sensitivity testing is completed in the lab. Vancomycin, as well as several other -mycin antibiotics, is nephrotoxic and ototoxic. Clindamycin also interferes with synthesis of cell walls.

Bacterial protein synthesis inhibitors include aminoglycosides, macrolides, and tetracyclines. Aminoglycosides are broad spectrum aerobic gram-negative antibiotics. They bind to bacterial ribosomes to disrupt protein synthesis. Like vancomycin, they are ototoxic and nephrotoxic. Several are in common use and have names that end in -mycin. Some antimicrobials with -mycin in the name are not aminoglycosides. These exceptions include vancomycin, clindamycin (above) and macrolides listed below. Popular examples include gentamycin, streptomycin, neomycin (used topically as discussed above), and tobramycin, which is also available in a form that can be inhaled for infections commonly seen in cystic fibrosis.

Macrolides interfere with enzyme systems responsible for bacterial protein synthesis. Unfortunately these also may interfere with the breakdown of certain other drugs. Available types include the erythromycins, azithromycin (Zithromax, Pfizer, New York, NY), clarithromycin (Biaxin, Abbott Laboratories, Abbott Park, IL). Tetracyclines interfere with ribosomal function and are broad spectrum agents. They are commonly used for chlamydial and rickettsial diseases (typhus, Rocky Mountain spotted fever, Q fever), and for Lyme disease. However, serious adverse effects limit its use—the drug interacts with calcium, discolors teeth in children and pregnant women, and impairs growth and development of teeth and bones.

Antibacterials that inhibit DNA/RNA include quinolones such as Ciprofloxacin (Cipro, Bayer Pharmaceuticals, Wayne, NJ), which inhibit coiling of DNA, and sulfonamides, which disrupt folic acid synthesis. These drugs are sometimes combined with trimethoprim (Bactrim, Hoffmann-La Roche Inc., Nutley, NJ; Septra, Monarch Pharmaceuticals Inc., Bristol, TN). However, these drugs are also associated with allergic reactions, including Stevens-Johnson syndrome, and some severe hematologic disorders.

Metronidazole (Flagyl, Pfizer, New York, NY) is frequently used for anaerobic infections with penetrating injury and rupture of the GI tract, but is associated with peripheral neuropathy, seizures, and leukopenia. The same drug is also used for certain protozoal infections and is used topically as a gel for rosacea. Fungal infections are unusual in wounds. In general, fungal infections are usually either facultative or opportunistic. Several agents are available for treating either systemic or surface fungal infections.

RESISTANT ORGANISMS

Methicillin resistant *Staphylococcus aureus* (MRSA) is now a common problem. Prior to the use of penicillin, *Staphylococcus aureus* bacteremia had a mortality of greater than 80%. Methicillin was developed to overcome the mechanism of penicillin resistance of strains of *Staphylococcus aureus*. MRSA was reported in 1961 and now represents a large proportion of isolated *Staphylococcus aureus*. Vancomycin has been the major antibiotic used against penicillin resistant *S. aureus* since the 1950s. The proportion of *Staphylococcus aureus* strains varies tremendously among locations. Once primarily nosocomial, com-

munity-acquired MRSA is now among the most common causes of skin and soft tissue infections. MRSA may be a resident microbe on the skin and inside the nose. Patients may develop recurrent skin abscesses and spread MRSA to others. Methicillin resistant *Staphylococcus epidermidis* (MRSE) is considered to be less of a problem than MRSA, but it may become important in those with reduced immunity and implanted devices, including catheters.

Another important resistant organism is vancomycin-resistant *Enterococcus* (VRE). These bacteria (*Enterococcus faecalis* and other species) are spread easily by contact between healthcare providers and patients due to breakdown in standard precautions. VRE may be present in fecal matter and inadvertently spread to a patient's skin where it may then be transmitted to a person or object coming in contact with the contaminated area.

Vancomycin resistant *S. aureus* (VRSA) was reported in 2002, presumably due to the transfer of genes from VRE to *S. aureus*. Although it is somewhat resistant to vancomycin, it is still treatable by trimethoprim/sulfamethoxazole (Bactrim, Septra) and other antibiotics. The term *Vancomycin intermediate resistant S. aureus* (VISA) is used for strains that require lower concentrations of vancomycin to inhibit growth than VRSA requires. By definition, the concentration of vancomycin needed to inhibit growth of VRSA is 2 to 4 times that needed for VISA.

Multi-drug resistant tuberculosis (MDR TB), while not directly involved in skin and soft tissue infections has become an increasing problem. MDR TB may, however, be transmitted between patient and clinician. By definition, MDR TB is resistant to at least 2 of the primary antituberculosis drugs, particularly isoniazid and rifampicin. Extensively drug resistant tuberculosis (XDR TB) is resistant to isoniazid, rifampicin, fluoroquinolones, and at least one of the drugs used for cases resistant to these three. For those with compromised immunity, especially those with HIV infection, mortality is very high.

PERSONAL PROTECTIVE EQUIPMENT

In the course of wound management, the clinician must be protected from accidental exposure to pathogens. In addition to pathogens involved in wounds, clinicians must be protected against transmission of blood-borne pathogens such as hepatitis B virus (HBV), hepatitis C virus (HCV), and human immunodeficiency virus (HIV). Additionally, patients must be protected against the transmission of pathogens from the clinician. Pathogenic organisms can be transmitted easily from one patient to a clinician's clothing to another patient. OSHA (Occupational Safety and Health Administration) requires protection of all workers from biohazards. Specific OSHA requirements are discussed at the end of this chapter. Personal protective equipment (PPE) consists of gloves, devices to protect mucous membranes such as masks and eye shields, and coverings for clothing and shoes. Personal protective equipment is shown in Figure 9-3.

Gloving

As a minimum, clean examination gloves should be worn both to protect the clinician from the patient's body fluids and to protect the patient's body fluid from contaminants on the clinician's hands not removed by handwashing. Donning sterile gloves requires special techniques, which are sometimes obvious from following package instructions, but not all manufacturers include instructions. Technique for donning sterile gloves is derived from 2 basic rules: 1) the inside of gloves is considered unsterile and 2) the outside of the gloves is considered sterile. Therefore, the hands may only make contact with the inside of the gloves and only the outside of a glove is allowed to touch another glove. Furthermore, the inside of the package is sterile until touched by hands. Based on these rules, the clinician peels the package open and makes certain that all other needed packages are open before gloving and that the clinician's hands will not need to go outside of sterile field.

The glove package is oriented so the words "right" and "left" or "R" and "L" are upright. The inside package is folded so the part of the package that becomes the outside of the wrapper can be grasped without touching the inside of the package. The inside package can then be pulled open using this folded-over part of the wrapper in the center. Avoid touching the inner surface of this wrapper and pull hard enough to keep the wrapper open. The wrapper will re-close if not pulled far enough. The following sequence is based on the concepts discussed above.

Reaching carefully, place the fingers of the nondominant hand into the glove in a scooping manner. With the dominant hand, pull on the inside surface of the glove until the fingers are in, but do not try to pull the first glove all of the way on. Next, using the gloved nondominant hand, scoop underneath the fold in the cuff of the glove for the dominant hand so that the glove on the nondominant hand only makes contact with the outside of the glove on the dominant hand. The partially gloved nondominant hand is used to pull the glove fully onto the dominant hand, but only touching the outside of the 2 gloves to each other. At this point, the dominant hand is completely gloved and the nondominant hand is partially gloved. To finish gloving the nondominant hand, place the fingers of the gloved dominant hand inside the folded cuff of the other glove, and pull the glove all of the way onto the nondominant hand, only touching outside of the glove.

When gloves are removed, the outsides of the gloves should only touch the outside of the other glove, not the skin; carefully pull gloves off inside-out so that hands only

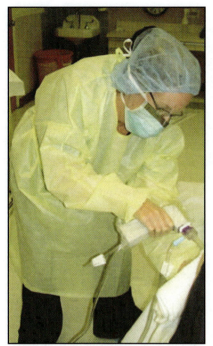

Figure 9-3. Personal protective equipment: surgical cap, face shield, gown, and gloves.

contact the inside surface of the gloves. Wash your hands as soon as possible after gloves are removed. Do not write notes, restock supplies, or anything else before doing so to avoid secondary contamination from the gloves onto other objects. Techniques for donning and doffing sterile gloves are demonstrated in Figure 9-4. Gloves should be removed first when removing PPE.

Latex Sensitivity

Latex is a major concern in wound management. Both the clinician and patient need to be considered. Due to the institution of universal precautions, a large number of both patients and clinicians have been exposed and sensitized to latex. Latex allergy is potentially fatal and must be taken seriously. An irritant dermatitis (type IV immune injury) is much more common than a type I allergic/anaphylactic reaction. About 7% to 12% of healthcare workers who are exposed to latex on a regular basis have positive skin tests to proteins present in latex gloves. All patients with spina bifida are automatically treated as if they are latex-sensitive, although the actual percentage is believed to be between 28% and 67%. Moreover, clinicians must be familiar with objects other than gloves containing latex that may contaminate surfaces that contact the latex-sensitive person. For this reason, latex and nonlatex exam gloves should be kept apart and hands should be washed after using latex gloves to avoid contaminating others with latex proteins. Powder-free gloves are less likely to expose

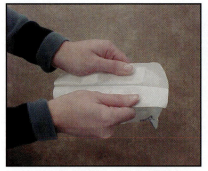

Figure 9-4A. Opening any sterile package should be done in this manner to avoid touching inside the package.

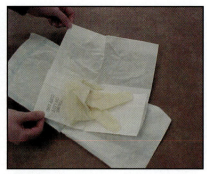

Figure 9-4B. Opening package to reveal the first glove.

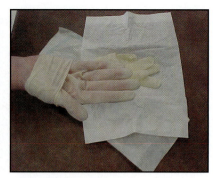

Figure 9-4C. Donning first glove to leave cuff turned over.

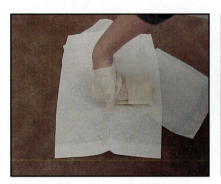

Figure 9-4D. Scooping second glove, touching on the outside of the second glove with the outside of the first glove.

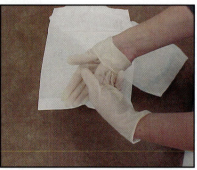

Figure 9-4E. Pulling down the cuff of the first glove with the second glove, touching only the outside of the first glove.

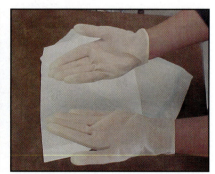

Figure 9-4F. Completed gloving.

individuals to latex proteins by minimizing airborne latex exposure. Other PPE may contain latex in elastic bands and other parts. Latex free equivalents for these may be necessary. Employers are required to provide latex-free PPE to employees. Clinicians should also keep fingernails trimmed and remove jewelry to avoid accumulation of latex molecules beneath them. Non-water-based skin care products should not be used under latex gloves as these may degrade the gloves. The CDC recommends using these skin care products only at the end of patient care for the day.

Face Protection

The mucus membranes of the eyes, nose, and mouth are potential sites for pathogen transmission. Aerosolization of fluid under pressure used to irrigate wounds, splashing of body fluids from open wounds and spurting blood may result in contamination of mucus membranes. When any of these situations might occur, the clinician is expected to use protective eyewear, masks, gloves, and in some cases protective gowns and caps. A combination face mask with an attached anti-fog eye shield provides better

protection than separate eyewear and mask. Splashes may bounce off the face, under eyewear, and strike the eye. A full face shield provides even greater protection, but can become uncomfortable and impede visibility due to fogging. Although almost all clinicians will never experience a facial splash, one cannot predict with complete confidence that fluid from any given wound will never splash. The cost of disposable masks and reusable goggles is small compared with the possible outcome of infectious material contacting the eyes, nose, or mouth.

SEQUENCE OF DONNING AND DOFFING PPE

Surgical or bouffant caps are the first item for donning, followed by a face mask, unless the design of the face protection dictates an opposite sequence. Shoe covers are donned after face protection, and hands are then washed or scrubbed as appropriate. Gowns follow handwashing and drying. Gloves are the last part of PPE donned. After use, gloves are removed first, taking care not to touch the outside. Gowns are pulled off from the inside and the mask, cap, and shoe covers are removed from the back. Hands are then washed again.

The logic of the donning and doffing sequence is related to the likelihood of contacting body fluids and the cleanliness of the part of the body being covered. Gloves are the most likely item to touch a patient, followed by the gown. These are donned last to avoid any contact with the face or shoe protection. Any contamination from the head is unlikely to affect the clinician's shoes, whereas contaminating the hands while donning shoe covers is highly likely. Therefore, shoe covers follow face protection in the donning sequence. Handwashing, as well as scrubbing, takes place with shoe covers and face protection in place. When doffing PPE, gloves must be discarded first to avoid contamination and gowns follow. Removal of face protection precedes removal of shoe covers to minimize any contamination from shoes onto the head. When doffing, only the inside or the back of the PPE is touched with the hands as any body fluids present on the PPE will only be on the front and outside.

INFECTION CONTROL

Two classifications of problem solving for infection control are work practice controls and engineering controls. Work practice controls refer to how a task is performed, including the physical layout and work flow. Engineering controls refer to the creation of devices or processes to minimize risk of infection.

Engineering Controls

Examples of engineering controls include the development of sharps containers, suction canisters, powders to solidify fluid within suction canisters, hands-free sinks and soap and paper towel dispensers. As people learn how to defeat previous engineering controls, for example, pushing needles down into a sharps container, better engineering controls must be developed.

Practice Controls

As much as possible, any equipment or supplies not essential to the task should be protected from any contamination by splash or aerosolization. Supplies must be kept in closed drawers or cabinets. Sinks, soap dispensers, and paper towel dispenser must be present. Dispensers for hand sanitizers should also be conveniently located within the room where the procedure is performed. This room must have solid walls and a door that can be closed fully. A sign should be placed on the door to indicate that a procedure is occurring to prevent unwanted traffic. A curtain between treatment areas is not considered sufficient for infection control. Any PPE should be donned and doffed within the room and not worn outside the room.

To prevent unnecessary traffic outside a treatment room, determine whether all equipment and supplies are present and working before donning PPE. Only under extreme circumstances should a clinician leave a room before the procedure is complete. Access to assistance by intercom, telephone, or call button should be present to minimize the need to leave the room.

The room should be designed and equipment and supplies arranged to minimize movement through the treatment area. The process of setting up a treatment room may seem trivial initially, but through the course of treating patients, unforeseen circumstances may dictate rearrangement of the room. Waste containers including sharps containers should be kept within the clinician's reach to avoid spilling body fluids on the floor, dropping objects, or accidentally contacting self or others when carrying objects. Laundry may become rather wet during procedures such as pulsatile lavage. Soiled linen hampers should be brought as close as possible to the laundry rather carrying wet or contaminated linens across the floor. If body fluids are spilled or splashed onto the floor, the floor must be disinfected as soon as a reasonable opportunity occurs, and anything dropped on the floor must be disinfected or put in a waste container as appropriate. To minimize contamination by splashes, spills, or aerosolization, packaged supplies and PPE should be closed within drawers or cabinets until they are about to be used. Handles or knobs for cabinets and drawers should be disinfected between patients. Sinks and soap and hand sanitizer dispensers must be placed within the enclosed room in such a way that they can be used before leaving the room and so the clinician can avoid encountering anything such as waste and laundry containers or spills on the floor on the way to the sink. Generally, this can be accomplished by locating waste and laundry containers on the side of the patient farthest from the door. Supply and linen cabinets are located between the patient and the sink. The sink and dispensers for soap, paper towels, and hand sanitizer are located as close to the door as possible. An uncluttered path must be maintained among all of these areas.

Body Substance Isolation Precautions

In addition to the use of PPE, the manner of performing tasks is part of the policies and procedures known as body substance isolation precautions. These procedures are termed *universal precautions*, implying that they are applied under all situations. All procedures involving patients with the potential for body substance exposure are to be done as if pathogens might be transmitted between any patient and clinician. The term *standard precautions* contains additional behaviors to be used during patient care. If standard precautions are executed properly, clinicians will not perform procedures any differently when a patient is known to have a blood-borne pathogen.

Table 9-3

AHCPR Recommendations for Body Substance Isolation Precautions

- Use clean gloves for each patient
- When treating multiple ulcers on the same patient, attend to the most contaminated ulcer last (change gloves if **any** fear of cross-contamination)
- Use sterile instruments for debridement
- Use clean dressings
- Follow local regulations for disposal of contaminated dressings
- Additional barriers such as gowns, plastic aprons, masks, or goggles must be worn when moist body substances (secretions, blood, or body fluids) are likely to soil the clothing or the skin or splash in the face.

Universal Precautions

Universal precautions include wearing gloves for anticipated contact with blood, secretions, mucous membranes, nonintact skin, and moist body substances for all patients. Handwashing between patients is essential and gloves must be changed before treating another patient. With any type of patient contact, the hands should be washed for 10 seconds with soap and friction to remove transient microbial flora, and then rinsed with running water. Application of alcohol foam or gel is now considered an acceptable alternative to handwashing because these destroy 99.9% of pathogens on the skin compared with 95% for the best handwashing practices. Periodic handwashing, however, is recommended to remove residues from the skin. Each institution should have policies and procedures in place related to infection control, and each clinician is responsible for following body substance isolation (BSI) precautions. Body substance isolation precautions suggested by the AHCPR are listed in Table 9-3.

Standard Precautions

These precautions apply to all patients. They do not differ with diagnosis or infection status. Standard precautions are applied to all body fluids, including blood, secretions, and excretions with the exception of sweat; the presence of visible blood within fluids is irrelevant. These precautions also apply to nonintact skin and mucous membranes. As with universal precautions, PPE (gloves, gowns, face, and eye protection) are to be used and handwashing guidelines are to be followed—ie, handwashing or application of approved hand sanitizer is to be done before and after patient contact. Use of gloves does not substitute for handwashing. To avoid trapping pathogens beneath them, jewelry is not worn, nails are kept short, and artificial nails are not used. Sharps are placed in approved containers as soon as feasible and are not recapped. No drinking, eating, application of makeup, lip balm, or contact lenses is permitted in patient care areas. Direct touching of mucous membranes is not allowed. Linens are placed as soon as feasible in approved laundry bags or hamper. Wastes are placed in appropriate containers as soon as feasible.

Anyone exposed to body fluids covered by standard precautions is to seek immediate assistance and submit an incident report. OSHA defines exposure incident as "a specific eye, mouth, other mucous membrane, nonintact skin, or parenteral contact with blood or other potentially infectious materials that results from the performance of an employee's duties."[1] Reporting exposure is meant to protect employees, and not to punish them if consequences of body fluid contact occur. Without appropriate reporting, health claims remote from the exposure may not be considered a workplace incident affecting workman's compensation and other legal matters.

Isolation

Procedures related to isolation have been simplified in an effort to enforce them. Three categories of isolation are now designated by the CDC. Basically, previous categories have been collapsed into these categories with the understanding that isolation procedures that addressed all of the issues with the previous categories will be more easily enforced. The new categories are contact, droplet, and airborne precautions. Optimally, patients under isolation are placed in private rooms specific to the reason for isolation or minimally a patient will share a room with another individual with the same reason for isolation. Rather than depending on individual healthcare providers to remember the details of each category, precautions are posted plainly on doors, bed, and charts with specific instructions posted at the patient's door for each type of precautions.

Most of this chapter has dealt with microbes that fall into the category of contact precautions. Contact precautions primarily enforce standard precautions, incorporating contact, enteric, and drainage and secretion precautions. Gloves must be used in the patient's room. Gowns are worn if contact with the patient or any surfaces within the room might occur. Other standard precautions are used as needed, for example shoe covers, eye and face protection during pulsatile lavage in an isolation room. Upon leaving the isolation room, hands must be washed with an approved soap or hand sanitizer must be used. Gloves should be changed when material with a known high concentration of microbes is touched and regloving performed. Care must be taken to avoid inadvertently touching any surfaces with hands or clothing while in the room. As much as practical, dedicated equipment is to be used. Stethoscopes, blood pressure cuffs, pulse oximeters, thermometers, and walkers are left in the room. Suction pumps and other equipment needed for procedures should also be left in the room and thoroughly disinfected when no longer needed or when the patient is discharged. Any equipment that must otherwise be removed from the patient's room must be placed in a clearly marked biohazard bag or other appropriate container. Contact precautions are used commonly for patients with MRSA or VRE. Other reasons for contact precautions include surface infections such as impetigo, other antibiotic resistant organisms, *C. difficile*, and other causes of diarrhea, and exoparasites such as lice and scabies.

Airborne precautions are primarily those used for tuberculosis. Other diseases transmitted this way include paramyxoviruses (measles) and varicella zoster virus (chicken pox, shingles). Airborne pathogens are capable of traveling longer distances through the air than those involved in droplet precautions. These precautions are designed to protect people from droplet nuclei containing particles 5 μm or smaller, contents of evaporated droplets that remain suspended in air for long periods, and dust particles that can carry microbes. Air currents may carry these materials throughout a room and may be inhaled. Special rooms with negative airflow are required. Doors must be kept closed whenever possible. Air within the room is drawn out by vacuum and outside air is brought in. A specialized type of mask is required that meets standards for preventing airborne pathogens from being inhaled around the edges of the mask. These masks meet NIOSH N95 (National Institute for Occupational Safety and Health) standards and a fitting session with employees is required. Patients must wear masks when they must be removed from the room and transport should be limited as much as possible. Although gloves and gowns are not required, standard precautions must be followed. For varicella zoster virus, both airborne and contact isolation are enforced. If possible, anyone who might be susceptible to measles or varicella should not enter the room. Those who are known to be immune are not required to wear respiratory protection.

Droplet precautions are used when infection could be passed by inspiring aerosolized respiratory secretions or saliva containing infectious material and transmitted to conjunctivae and mucous membranes of others. Droplets may be produced by coughing, sneezing, or even talking. Suctioning and bronchoscopy may also produce droplets. Aerosolized droplets may travel some distance across a room. In addition to standard precautions, a mask is mandatory when working within 3 feet (1 meter) from the patient as these particles are larger than 5 μm. Diseases transmitted this way include mumps and *Neisseria meningitidis*. Preferably, a mask is worn anytime the room is entered. Likewise, if a patient is removed from a room, the patient is required to wear a mask; however, transport of patients from their rooms should be minimized as much as possible. Good quality, well-fitting masks that do not directly touch mucous membranes are preferable to cheaper masks with simple ear loops that easily contact the mouth and may become wet, transmitting bacteria across them. Duckbill or other types with a rigid material keeping space in front of the mouth and nose should be used if possible. With droplet precautions, a private room is required and handwashing is required when entering and leaving the room. Specialized ventilation is not required for droplet precautions.

CLEAN AND STERILE TECHNIQUES

Absolute sterile technique is not justifiable for all patients. Even for surgical procedures, varying levels of sterile techniques are practiced. In particular, much greater precautions are taken for orthopedic surgery than for other types. For most wound care, clean technique and universal precautions are sufficient. Clean technique dictates that during treatment of multiple ulcers on the same patient, the clinician should attend to the most contaminated ulcer last (eg, the perianal region). In contrast, with normal sterile technique, the clinician would change sterilized gloves for each wound on the patient.

Clean dressings, rather than sterile ones, may be used on pressure ulcers and other chronic wounds, as long as dressing procedures comply with institutional infection-control guidelines. Clean dressings may also be used in the home setting. Disposal of contaminated dressings in the home should be done in a manner consistent with local regulations. In some areas, this may allow the disposal of all items in the regular trash or may require the use of biohazard containers. Clean techniques are listed in Table 9-3 as part of body substance isolation precautions.

Sterile Techniques

No matter how well done, no technique can be completely sterile. We can strive for conditions that are as close as reasonably possible, but even in an operating room, we cannot guarantee sterility. With the presence of

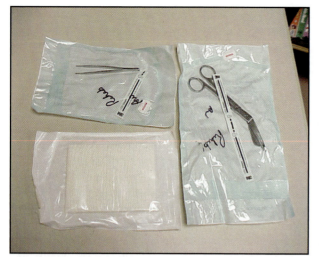

Figure 9-5A. Variety of sterile packages: sterilized forceps, scissors, and disposable towel.

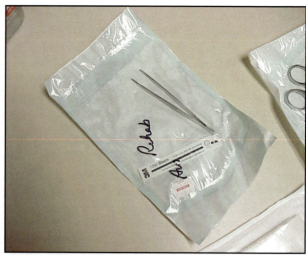

Figure 9-5B. Sterile packages. Note the indicator strip in the packages to insure sterilization has occurred.

any air movement, nonsterile clothing, and any particulate matter in the room, deposition of a small number of microbes onto what we would consider sterile is virtually assured. However, the cleaner our procedures are, the lower the risk of infection becomes.

Sterile refers to the complete absence of viable microbes, often in conditions such as surgery. A sterile field is an area in which no viable microbes exist. In contrast, unsterile can refer to a condition that may result from a number of causes. An item is considered unsterile if it has not been appropriately sterilized, if it has come in contact with an item that is no longer considered sterile, has entered a field that is not sterile, or if it has exceeded its shelf-life. Shelf-life is the length of time that an item that has been sterilized and packaged is considered to still be sterile if the package is unopened. Some packages of materials have expiration dates on them; however, exceeding shelf-life is highly unlikely given the rate at which supplies are used in most facilities. Packages of sterilized equipment typical of those obtained from a central sterile supply are shown in Figure 9-5.

Contamination is the process in which an item, surface, or field has come in contact with anything that is not sterile. Some general rules may be followed to prevent contamination and maintain a field as close to sterile as possible. First, only sterile materials should be used in a sterile field. Care should be taken to avoid leaning over, or passing an upper extremity or other object over a sterile field. Packages containing sterile materials to be placed on the sterile field should not be shaken excessively over the sterile field. Preferably, sterile objects are tossed from inside their packages onto a sterile field. A sterile towel (Figure 9-6) may be used to create a sterile field, but only one side of a sterile towel will be sterile and because the

corner of the sterile towel is handled to create the sterile field, a 1-inch border around the towel is considered to be unsterile. When a sterile towel is used to dry a patient from a sterile whirlpool, the sterile side is used; the other side may be touched with clean, unsterile hands, although gloved hands would be preferable. Any wet surface will be contaminated as water carries contaminants through to the sterile side of the towel.

Packages placed on a clean surface are considered to be contaminated on the outside, but the inside of the sterilized package may be used as a sterile field (Figure 9-7). However, wet paper packages used for circumstances such as wet-to-dry dressings are not sterile fields, but are usually acceptable for a short time, usually within the range of less than 1 minute before water soaks through and allows contamination to be carried from below the towel (Figure 9-8).

Sterile gowns are used infrequently outside the operating room or burn unit. These gowns are considered sterile only down to the waist in the front; the forearms (up to the elbow) are considered sterile, but anywhere between the elbow and shoulder is not considered sterile. The logic behind the declaration of sterile and nonsterile areas along the upper extremity is due to the inability to see behind and the possibility of bumping an object. For these same reasons, one should never face the back of another person working with a sterile field; being back-to-back or front-to-front is acceptable. Communication with the other individuals, however, is the best way to prevent contamination of others. Also, using the same simple rules, sterile gloved hands must be kept within prescribed sterile areas of the gown and not allowed to hang below the waist. When using sterile materials on a sterile, draped table, similar rules apply. Tables draped with a sterile field are considered sterile only on the top surface; sides are not.

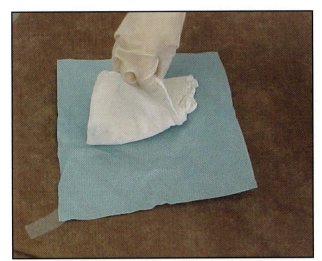

Figure 9-6A. Sterile towel. Removal of package by its corner.

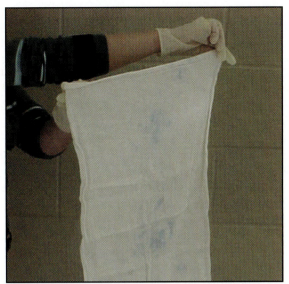

Figure 9-6B. Handling of sterile towel by 2 corners. By convention, none of the corners or edges within 1 inch are considered sterile.

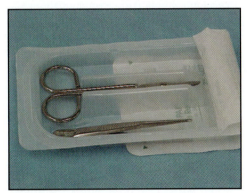

Figure 9-7A. Proper use of a package as a sterile field. Inside of the package is considered sterile and may be used as a sterile field.

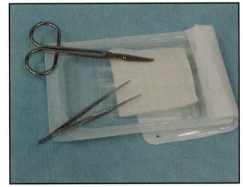

Figure 9-7B. Placing items on the edges of packages contaminates them.

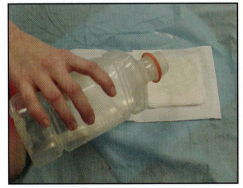

Figure 9-8. Excessive wetting of a sterile 4 x 4 leads to contamination due to soaking through the package.

Several rules regarding containers must be enforced. For the most part, these rules follow common sense as we consider the potential for secondary contamination vs the potential for airborne contamination. The foremost rule is that the edges of any container are unsterile unless the container has been sterilized and has just been opened from a package. Following this rule, cap edges and tops are considered to be unsterile. Caps must not be removed with sterile or clean gloves that have been, or will be, in contact with the wound or regloving must be done. When removing caps from containers, the cap is laid inside-up, but not within the sterile field. We are generally willing to accept some degree of airborne contamination, but not surface contamination that results if the cap is laid inside-down. Tubes from which contents are squeezed require either a second person to squeeze the tube as the contents are needed or the contents must be squeezed onto a sterile surface such as a 4 x 4 gauze sponge or sterile tongue depressor before gloving. We need to assume that the outside of the tube is unsterile. If a second person is squeezing the tube onto the clinician's gloved finger to apply to the wound or surrounding skin, the clinician must be careful to avoid touching any part of the tube.

The inside of any sterile package can be considered sterile if peeled open properly. Opening the package completely to avoid reaching over an unsterile area of the package is a safer approach in one sense, but, on the other hand, the longer a package is open to the atmosphere, the greater is the risk of airborne contamination. Using this approach, tools such as scissors and forceps may be placed back in the package or on a sterile towel. When using this technique, one must avoid allowing the instrument to contact the edges of the packages where they were opened. Laying an instrument over the edge of a package to improve the ease of picking up the instrument is very tempting; however, doing so contaminates the handles of instruments.

When working under either sterile or clean conditions, the clinician must cover all hair including facial hair, as well as removing all dangling earrings, bracelets, and necklaces. Although many individuals seem comfortable in covering rings and wristwatches with gloves, jewelry traps material underneath, which cannot be effectively removed by handwashing or hand antiseptic. All jewelry should be removed before patients are seen and hands should be washed. Jewelry should remain off until the clinician is finished seeing patients for the day and hands are washed. Following the rules of sterile fields can be difficult, but these rules are important for minimizing risks to both the patient and clinician. One of the simplest means to facilitate good practice is to have nonsterile personnel available for help as needed to avoid breaking a sterile field or having to reglove.

WHIRLPOOL

Equipment used for whirlpool therapy requires specialized care for infection control. The tank and turbine might be used for multiple patients on a daily basis. Pathogens potentially could be transmitted from one patient into the whirlpool tank or into the turbine and then to another patient. Areas of particular concern are the drain, the uppermost part of the tank, and the inside of the turbine where disinfection may prove difficult. A further concern is the possibility of aerosolization due to the agitation created by the turbine. Bacteria and other microbes present in the wound will be randomly distributed throughout the tank. Although this may remove pathogens from the wound, their distribution on the tank, within the tank and onto any parts of the patient's body can become problematic. Pathogens from multiple wounds, intact skin, and the perineal area will be deposited in the tank, turbine, and elsewhere on the body, including the open wound. Therefore, the potential for a wound to become more contaminated instead of less exists. The movement of pathogens from one area on a patient to another is termed *cross-contamination*.

High level disinfectants need to be rinsed thoroughly to avoid injury to the patient. Surfaces of whirlpool tubs usually receive high level disinfection, but they are left open to airborne contamination and contaminants may be present in tap water used to fill the whirlpool tub. When hydrotherapy is used, the ability of water to be aerosolized carrying microbes onto other surfaces must be taken into account. In addition to keeping equipment and supplies covered, all horizontal surfaces in the treatment room must be disinfected between patients. After a patient is removed from a whirlpool, the submersed body part should be rinsed to remove contaminants, including disinfectants/antiseptics that were in the tank. Although sterile normal saline has been used routinely for irrigation, infection rate is actually lower when wounds are irrigated with tap water than with normal saline provided a comparable decrease in bacterial count occurs.

Strategies for minimizing contamination and cross-contamination consist of the addition of iodine or chlorine releasing molecules such as povidone iodine (betadine) and chloramine T (Chlorazene). Whirlpool liners decrease the risk of contamination from patient to tank and tank to patient, but they do not address contamination between the inside of the turbine and the patient, nor do they address cross-contamination. Between patients, the tank and turbine must be cleaned and disinfected. A cleansing agent that removes proteinaceous residue must be used first to allow the disinfectant to reach the tank's surface. During this cleansing and disinfecting procedure, care must be taken to reach all surface areas that may contact the patient or the water that will be placed in the tank for the next patient. Difficult to reach areas include the drain, the rim, along the contours of the turbine, and a thermometer if it is present. Overlooked areas that may be missed include the upper part of the tank, the rim, and over the outside of the tank. Although the floor may become wet from doing so, these areas should be cleaned and disinfected. In addition to disinfection of the whirlpool tub, the inside and outside of the turbine must be disinfected. Running the turbine inside a bucket of appropriate disinfectant for 10 minutes is usually recommended by manufacturers. Following cleaning and before the next patient use of the tank, high-level disinfectants must be rinsed from the tank thoroughly to avoid injury to the patient.

Spills onto the floor must be promptly cleaned and the floor disinfected. Patients at risk for respiratory infection may require a mask. Aerosolization and splashing may also occur during irrigation, especially pulsatile lavage. Masks should be worn by both the clinician and patient and splashing contained by a plastic sheet or a towel. In addition to keeping equipment and supplies covered, surfaces must be disinfected between patients.

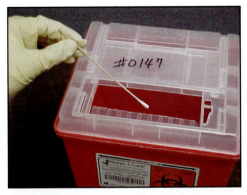

Figure 9-9A. Cotton-tipped applicators are placed in a sharps container due to the possibility of breaking and creating a sharp edge that could puncture a bag.

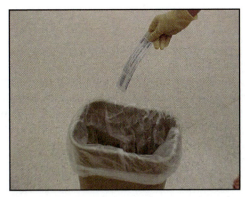

Figure 9-9B. Items not grossly contaminated with body fluids are placed in a regular trash can.

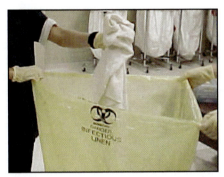

Figure 9-9C. Typical contaminated laundry bag.

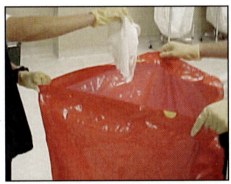

Figure 9-9D. Typical biohazard disposal bag.

WASTE DISPOSAL

Waste disposal is generally the last item that occurs following patient care, although some waste disposal may be necessary during procedures. In many facilities, clinicians may be observed disposing of all waste in red biohazard containers. Noncontaminated waste placed in biohazard containers costs each facility thousands of dollars each year needlessly for special disposal. Careful consideration allows the clinician to be selective in disposal of materials. The quantity of outer packages that are grossly contaminated during procedures can be minimized by handling only the contents or through the judicious use of sterile fields. Certainly, any grossly contaminated items and sharp instruments must be placed in appropriate biohazard containers, whereas packages that do not contact body fluids directly should be placed in regular waste containers. Contaminated dressings, gauze, gloves, and similar items should be placed in a red, marked biohazard bag. Waste containers are depicted in Figure 9-9. Personnel should never attempt to retrieve items that have been placed accidently or deliberately in any waste containers, whether regular, biohazard, or sharps. In addition to trash, soiled reusable articles and linen should be placed in containers that are securely sealed to prevent leaking. Double bagging is not necessary unless the outside of the bag is visibly soiled.

Sharp instruments such as needles, scalpel blades, forceps, and scissors that could puncture a biohazard bag should also be placed in puncture-resistant, rigid sharps containers (Figure 9-10). Cotton-tipped applicators should also be placed in a sharps container. If they break after being placed in a plastic bag, a jagged edge that can pierce a plastic bag and injure another person may result.

Regulations exist for both reusable and disposable sharps. For reusable sharps, the regulations call for them to be placed immediately, or as soon as possible after use, in appropriate containers until properly reprocessed. By OSHA regulations, a container is considered to be appropriate if it is puncture resistant, it is labeled or color-coded, and leakproof on the sides and bottom. Single use contaminated sharps are to be discarded immediately or as soon as feasible in closable, puncture-resistant, leakproof (sides and bottom), and labeled or color-coded containers. OSHA calls for placement of containers such that during use containers are easily accessible and located as close as is feasible to the immediate area where sharps are used.

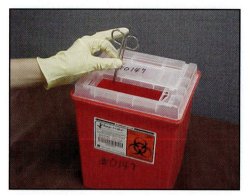

Figure 9-10. Disposable scissors being placed in an approved sharps container.

The containers are to be kept upright throughout use, replaced routinely and are not allowed to be overfilled. Sharps containers must be closed immediately prior to removal or replacement to prevent spillage or protrusion of contents during handling, storage, or transport and placed in a secondary container that is closable and made to contain all contents and prevent leakage if leakage is possible. Secondary containers must also be labeled or color-coded according to OSHA standards. Reusable containers, typically used for reusable sharps, are not to be opened, emptied, or cleaned manually or in any other manner which would expose employees to the risk of percutaneous injury. Note that the requirement for sharps containers are for containers that are puncture resistant. Protrusion of the contents through the walls of puncture resistant containers will not occur under normal use. However, mishandling of these containers could result in puncture. Also note that the primary container is to be leakproof on the bottom and sides. These containers can leak if moved from an upright orientation or if overfilled. Personnel using or handling these containers should be trained to avoid spilling or puncturing the containers.

ADDITIONAL OSHA REGULATIONS

Facilities are obligated to examine engineering controls periodically and maintain or replace them on a regular schedule. Important work practice controls dictated by OSHA include a specific statement that all procedures involving blood or other potentially infectious materials are to be done to minimize splashing or spraying. OSHA also requires certain work practice controls. Eating, drinking, smoking, applying cosmetics or lip balm, and handling contact lenses are prohibited in work areas where exposure is likely to occur. Food and drink are not allowed to be kept in refrigerators, shelves, and other areas where blood or other potentially infectious materials are present. For conditions that engineering and work practice controls cannot completely eliminate or minimize exposure, PPE is required by the OSHA regulations. For such conditions, employers are obligated to provide PPE at no cost to employees. According to OSHA, appropriate PPE may consist of gloves, gowns, laboratory coats, face shields or masks and eye protection, and mouthpieces, resuscitation bags, pocket masks, or other ventilation devices. OSHA defines appropriate in such a way that the PPE does not permit blood or other potentially infectious materials to pass through to or reach the employee's work clothes, street clothes, undergarments, skin, eyes, mouth, or other mucous membranes. This is qualified by stating that blood and other potentially infectious material does not pass through the PPE under normal conditions of use and for the duration of time during which PPE is used. Employers are responsible for ensuring that employees use appropriate PPE with the exception of extraordinary circumstances in which the PPE, in the opinion of the employee, might cause more harm than benefit. Under these circumstances an analysis of the circumstances is to be undertaken to determine whether policy or procedure changes are necessary to prevent such problems from recurring. Employers are responsible for having PPE appropriate for any personnel requiring it, including any necessary sizes or accommodating allergies, eg, providing hypoallergenic gloves. Employers are also responsible for cleaning, laundering, disposal, repair, or replacement of PPE as needed to maintain its effectiveness, at no cost to the employee. To prevent spread of pathogens contaminating the PPE, all PPE must be removed and left within the work area. Facilities will typically place disposal containers within the appropriate work area rather than in common areas such as gyms or hallways, and durable PPE is left in a designated area within the work area and not carried out into common areas. OSHA states that after use, all PPE is to be placed in an appropriately designated area or container for storage, washing, decontamination, or disposal.

Employers are responsible for ensuring that worksites are maintained in a clean and sanitary condition. Because of variation in the type of activities and patient populations, appropriate written schedules for cleaning and methods of decontamination are to be determined and implemented based upon characteristics of the worksite, type of surface to be cleaned, type of soil present, and tasks or procedures being performed in the area. Regardless of the cleaning schedule, however, all equipment and environmental and working surfaces are to be cleaned and decontaminated after contact with blood or other potentially infectious materials. Contaminated work surfaces are to be decontaminated with an appropriate disinfectant after completion of procedures. Decontamination is to be done immediately or as soon as feasible if surfaces are overtly contaminated, or after any spill of blood or other potentially infectious materials.

Table 9-4

OSHA Requirements for Employee Training

- Where the regulations can be accessed and an explanation of the regulations
- The epidemiology and symptoms of blood-borne diseases
- The modes of transmission of blood-borne pathogens
- The employer's exposure control plan
- Tasks and other activities that may involve exposure to blood and other potentially infectious materials
- Use and limitations of methods to prevent or reduce exposure including appropriate engineering controls, work practices, and personal protective equipment
- Types, proper use, location, removal, handling, decontamination, and disposal of personal protective equipment
- The basis for selection of personal protective equipment
- Information on the hepatitis B vaccine and the appropriate actions to take and persons to contact in an emergency involving blood or other potentially infectious materials
- Methods for reporting any incident involving blood-borne pathogens and the medical follow-up that will be made available
- Information on the post-exposure evaluation and follow-up that is required of the employer
- Signs, labels, and any color coding required for biohazardous materials
- An opportunity for interaction with the person conducting the training session

OSHA regulations state that handling of contaminated laundry should be minimized and bagged or containerized at the location where it was used. To minimize handling, contaminated laundry is not to be sorted or rinsed in the location of use. Contaminated laundry is to be placed and transported in bags or containers labeled or color-coded appropriately. In cases in which universal precautions are used in the handling of all soiled laundry, any labeling or color-coding that permits recognition by all employees is acceptable. As discussed with sharps containers and any other biohazard container, any time that soak-through or leakage from the bag or container is likely, laundry is to be placed and transported in leak-proof bags or containers. Employers are also responsible to ensure that employees who have contact with contaminated laundry wear protective gloves and other appropriate PPE.

Employers are obligated to offer the hepatitis B vaccine and vaccination series to all employees who have occupational exposure. Employers are also responsible for postexposure evaluation and follow-up to all employees who have had an exposure incident. Evaluations are to be made available at no cost to the employee, available at a reasonable time and place, and performed by or under the supervision of a licensed physician or by or under the supervision of another licensed healthcare professional, and provided according to recommendations of the US Public Health Service, and all laboratory tests are to be conducted by an accredited laboratory at no cost to the employee.

Contaminated waste is placed in containers that are readily recognized by any employees. Labels are to be fluorescent orange or orange-red, or predominantly so, with lettering and symbols in a contrasting color and affixed as close as feasible to the container by string, wire, adhesive, or other method that prevents their loss or unintentional removal. Red bags or red containers may be substituted for labels.

OSHA regulations require that employers provide and ensure participation by all employees with occupational exposure in a training program provided at no cost to the employee and during working hours. Training is to be provided at the time of initial assignment to tasks where occupational exposure may take place, and at least annually thereafter. Employers are also to provide additional training as needed if changes in tasks or how tasks are performed affect the employee's occupational exposure. The training program must, at the minimum, address the elements shown in Table 9-4.

SUMMARY

Working with wounds creates the opportunity for wounds to be contaminated, and for wounds to contaminate clinicians and others working in the facility, including those who empty waste containers or transport or clean laundry. Control of infection in wounds requires an understanding of the terms *colonization, infection* and *contami-*

nation, resident microbes, and *transient microbes.* Acute wounds contaminated with any microbes are at risk for infection and, therefore, are treated harshly with aggressive debridement, irrigation, application of topical antibiotics, and on occasion, systemic antibiotics. Chronic wounds are colonized by a number of species of microbes in a limited number. Contamination of an open wound presents the opportunity for a new microbe to grow out of control, causing infection. The terms sterilization, antisepsis, and disinfection were introduced. Sterilization removes all microbes and is necessary whenever invasive procedures or sharp debridement are performed. Routine wound care requires clean technique, but following general principles of sterile technique reduces the risk of contamination. Individuals with compromised immune systems require greater care to minimize the introduction of new microbes to the wound. OSHA standards require both work practice and engineering controls to minimize risk of exposure to blood-borne pathogens and use of PPE when these controls cannot eliminate the risk. PPE includes protection of the eyes, nose, and mouth with goggles, glasses, face masks, or face shields as appropriate, gloves at any time of exposure to body fluids, and gowns, caps, and shoe covers when appropriate. Universal precautions dictate assuming that any body fluids contain blood-borne pathogens. Both the employer and employee are obligated to follow OSHA regulations. Annual review of OSHA regulations is required.

QUESTIONS

1. What is the difference between colonization and infection?

2. What role does contamination play in the risk of infection?

3. List common causes of immunosuppression.

4. How is management of these patients different?

5. Describe the differences between sterilization, disinfection, and antisepsis.

6. When is the use of antiseptic agents in wounds appropriate?

7. During what aspects of wound management is the use of gloves required? Of gowns? Of shoe covers? Of caps?

8. Under what type of wound care must sterile instruments be used?

9. What types of items should be disposed of in a red or biohazard-labeled bag?

10. What items should be placed in a biohazard-labeled puncture-resistant container?

11. What items should go in the regular trash?

REFERENCE

1. OSHA Regulations (Standards - 29 CFR) Bloodborne Pathogens.- 1910.1030. http://www.osha.gov/pls/oshaweb/owadisp.show_ document?p_table=STANDARDS&p_id=10051. Accessed July 28, 2009.

BIBLIOGRAPHY

Ad Hoc Committee of the Committee on Trauma, Division of Medical Sciences, National Research Council: Report: Postoperative wound infections; the influence of ultraviolet radiation of the operating room and the influence of other factors. *Ann Surg.* 1964;160(suppl 1).

AHCPR Supported Clinical Practice Guidelines. Available at: http://www.ncbi.nlm.nih.gov/books/bv.fcgi?rid=hstat2.section.4521. Accessed September 9, 2009.

American Diabetes Association 2009 Clinical Practice Recommendations. Available at http://care.diabetesjournals.org/content/32/Supplement_1. Accessed September 9, 2009.

Bill TJ, Ratliff CR, Donovan AM, Knox LK, Morgan RF, Rodeheaver GT. Quantitative swab culture versus tissue biopsy: a comparison in chronic wounds. *Ostomy Wound Manage.* 2001;47(1):34-37.

Bochner BS, Lichtenstein LM. Anaphylaxis. *N Engl J Med.* 1991;324(25):1785-1790.

Bohannon RW. Whirlpool versus whirlpool rinse for removal of bacteria from a venous stasis ulcer. *Phys Ther.* 1982;62(3):304-308.

Bucknall TE. The effect of local infection upon wound healing: an experimental study. *Br J Surg.* 1980;67(12):851-855.

Burton GRW, Engelkirk PG. *Microbiology for the Health Sciences.* 5th ed. Philadelphia, PA: Lippincott-Raven Publishers; 1996.

Centers for Disease Control and Prevention (CDC). Guidelines for infection control in dental health-care settings, 2003. MMWR 2003; 52 (RR17): 1-68. http://www.cdc.gov/mmwr/preview/mmwrhtml/rr5217a1.htm. Accessed July 28, 2009.

Cooper ML, Laxer JA, Hansbrough JF. The cytotoxic effects of commonly used topical antimicrobial agents on human fibroblasts and keratinocytes. *J Trauma.*1991;31(6):775-782.

Cutting KF, White RJ. Criteria for identifying wound infection—revisited. *Ostomy Wound Manage.* 2005;51(1):28-34.

Gardner SE, Frantz RA, Doebbeling BN. The validity of the clinical signs and symptoms used to identify localized chronic wound infection. *Wound Repair Regen.* 2001;9(3):178-186.

Grayson ML, Gibbons GW, Balogh K, Levin E, Karchmer AW. Probing to bone in infected pedal ulcers. A clinical sign of underlying osteomyelitis in diabetic patients. *JAMA.* 1995;273(9):721-723.

Greif R, Akca O, Horn E-P. Kurz A, Sessler DI. Supplemental perioperative oxygen to reduce the incidence of surgical-wound infection. *New Engl J Med.* 2000;342:161-167.

Guideline for the Prevention of Surgical Site Infection. http://www.cdc.gov/ncidod/dhqp/gl_surgicalsite.html. Accessed August 25, 2009.

Guideline for Isolation Precautions in Hospitals. http://www.cdc.gov/ncidod/dhqp/gl_isolation.html. Accessed August 25, 2009.

Hospital Infection Control Practices Advisory Committee. Guidelines for Isolation Precautions in Hospitals. Hospital Infection Control Advisory Committee Publication date: 01/01/1996 http://wonder.cdc.gov/wonder/prevguid/p0000419/P0000419.asp. Accessed August 25, 2009.

Levine NS, Lindberg RB, Mason AD, Pruitt BA. The quantitative swab culture and smear: A quick, simple method for determining the number of viable aerobic bacteria on open wounds. *J Trauma.* 1976;16(2):89-94.

Lineaweaver W, Howard R, Soucy D, et al. Topical antimicrobial toxicity. *Arch Surg.* 1985;120(3):267-270.

Mertz PM, Oliveira-Gandia MF, Davis SC. The evaluation of a cadexomer iodine wound dressing on methicillin resistant Staphylococcus aureus (MRSA) in acute wounds. *Dermatol Surg.* 1999;25(2):89-93.

Moscati RM, Mayrose J, Reardon RF, Janicke DM, Jehle DV. A multi-center comparison of tap water versus sterile saline for wound irrigation. *Acad Emerg Med.* 2007;14(5):404-409.

Moscati RM, Reardon RF, Lerner EB, Mayrose J. Wound irrigation with tap water. *Acad Emerg Med.* 1998;5(11):1076-1080.

Niederhuber SS, Stribley RF, Koepke GH. Reduction of skin bacterial load with use of the therapeutic whirlpool. *Phys Ther.* 1975;55(5):482-486.

OSHA Regulations (Standards - 29 CFR) Bloodborne Pathogens.-1910.1030. http://www.osha.gov/pls/oshaweb/owadisp.show_document?p_table=STANDARDS&p_id=10051. Accessed July 28, 2009.

Robson MC. Wound infection. A failure of wound healing caused by an imbalance of bacteria. *Surg Clin North Am.* 1997;77:637-650.

Robson MC, Duke WF, Krizek TJ. Rapid bacterial screening in the treatment of civilian wounds. *J Surg Res.* 1973;14:426-430.

Robson MC, Stenberg BD, Heggers JP. Wound healing alterations caused by infection. *Clin Plast Surg.* 1990;17(3):485-492.

Shankowsky HA, Callioux LS, Tredget EE. North American survey of hydrotherapy in modern burn care. *J Burn Care Rehabil.* 1994;15(2):143-146.

Sussman GL, Beezhold DH. Allergy to latex rubber. *Ann Intern Med.* 1995;122:43-46.

Sussman GL, Liss GM, Deal K, et al. Incidence of latex sensitization among latex glove wearers. *J Allergy Clin Immunol.* 1998;101:171-178.

White RJ, Cutting KF. Critical colonization—the concept under scrutiny. *Ostomy Wound Manage.* 2006;52(11):50-56.

Zamora JL, Price MF, Chuang P, Gentry LO. Inhibition of povidone-iodine's bactericidal activity by common organic substances: an experimental study. *Surgery.* 1985;98(1):25-29.

Zhou LH, Nahm WK, Badiavas E, Yufit T, Falanga V. Slow release iodine preparation and wound healing: in vitro effects consistent with lack of in vivo toxicity in human chronic wounds. *Br J Dermatol.* 2002;146(3):365-374.

Pain Control

10

OBJECTIVES

- Discuss options available for medical management of pain and how individual characteristics must be evaluated based on the characteristics of the patient and any medications.
- Describe electrical modalities available for management of wound-related pain including contraindications.
- Discuss the use of topical agents used by providers other than physicians for management of pain associated with wound management.
- Implement wound-related pain interventions.

In the management of wounds, the focus on healing can easily obscure the need for management of pain associated with the wound. Although pain management is very specifically addressed in the AHCPR guidelines, it has not yet seemed to reach the consciousness of healthcare providers. Too often, pain is considered an inevitable consequence of dressing changes and debridement. Moreover, the responsibility for pain management is delegated to the physician and nurse, leaving everyone else to ask, "Has the patient received his pain meds?"

Pain is a complex biopsychosocial phenomenon. Some have insisted on considering pain as a fifth vital sign along with heart rate, blood pressure, temperature, and respiratory rate. The perception of pain results from physical stimuli, complex neurologic connections among the periphery, spinal cord, and multiple areas of the brain—the biologic part of the biopsychosocial model. The person's psychological state also has a strong influence on the perception of pain, as well as pain perception having a profound impact on a patient's psychological status. Social influences are multiple and may determine a patient's perception of pain, but may also determine the degree to which a patient is willing to express pain. Awareness of the patient's pain is not simply a matter of reducing suffering experienced by the patient, but pain slows wound healing and may be a sign of infection.

Itching (pruritus) is a related problem. Although it may not cause as much suffering as intense pain, pruritus can be more than a nuisance. Chronic pruritus can be debilitating and lead to scratching and injury to the skin. Itching is related to release of histamine and frequently accompanies the rapid granulation of a wound as it heals. Pruritus may have causes other than the wound. It is associated with chronic renal failure, especially ure-

Irion G.
Comprehensive Wound Management, 2nd ed. (pp 191-202)
© 2010 SLACK Incorporated

mia, cirrhosis, lymphoma, exoparasites such as lice and scabies, or simply dry skin. Patients may get relief from patting rather than scratching. Pruritus associated with wounds that becomes a significant problem can be treated topically with 5% doxepin cream, or with oral medications including gabapentin (anticonvulsant), ondansetron (serotonin blocker used to treat nausea), and diphenhydramine (histamine blocker).

The management of pain, therefore, must take on all 3 components of the biopsychosocial model of pain. Emphasis on the biologic aspect is understandable, given the wide selection of pharmacologic approaches available; however, pain management is more likely to be effective when psychological and social influences are appreciated and exploited to minimize the negative impact associated with painful stimuli.

Three types of pain management are addressed specifically in this chapter: medical management, electrotherapy, and topical medications. In addition, we have the responsibility to assess the causes of pain and take reasonable steps to eliminate or minimize pain through means such as positioning and selection of dressings in addition to the types of interventions described below. The assessment of pain can also aid in diagnosis of wound etiology.

Pain Assessment

In many cases, wound etiology is known, but in other cases, assessment of pain may help in the diagnosis of wound etiology. Some conditions, such as sickle cell ulcers or wounds secondary to skin abscesses, can be exceedingly painful. Wounds associated with venous disease may be mildly uncomfortable or very painful depending on the patient's position, and some patients will have no pain associated with their wounds, especially those with neuropathic ulcers of the foot. In some cases, patients with diabetic neuropathy may not have normal pain sensation, but may still complain of neuropathic pain caused by nerve injury. Pains associated with neuropathy may include shooting or burning pains, or the perception of brief electric shocks, called dysesthesia. Arterial disease can cause severe pain and increases with positions that decrease blood flow further such as elevation, or placing a leg or thigh over an edge. Regardless of the etiology, pain should be assessed for all patients, even if the patient has no pain.

Just as pain interventions must account for all 3 biopsychosocial aspects, the assessment of pain must also. Key elements for the biological piece include patient history of both the intensity and character of the pain, a neurologic screening, and referral for further diagnostic testing if the cause is not identified. Identifying whether the pain is somatic, visceral, referred, or emotional is a major part of the assessment, and different treatments and referrals to other healthcare providers may become necessary. To make this assessment, the history must discover factors that worsen or alleviate the pain, whether pain changes over the course of the day, whether it wakes the patient at night, and whether it is independent of movement or positioning of the area of the body where pain is localized by the patient. Additional information from the physical examination and history needed to assess pain should include local and body temperature (fever), malaise, anorexia, somnolence (sleepiness), odor from the wound or elsewhere, and any cellulitis or induration surrounding the wounds. Although pain might be expected due to the presence of a wound, pain may be caused by something other than the wound and dismissing the patient's pain may allow another patient condition to go undiagnosed.

A large number of pain assessment tools are available for use. Simple forms include verbal report, visual analog scale, and the facial scale (FACES). Visual analog scales are very simple to use. The left end of the line represents no pain and the right end represents the worst possible pain the patient could imagine experiencing. The patient marks the line at a distance between the ends of the line that represents the fraction between the two ends of the pain perceived. FACES was developed initially for the pediatric population based on pictures drawn by children in an effort to allow them to express their levels of pain. The final version of the images on the scale was designed to avoid bias based on gender, age, and race. This tool has also been used to communicate pain intensity by non-English speaking patients. Instructions in different languages are available from the Wong on Web site. Figure 10-1A demonstrates a visual analog scale and the Wong-Baker FACES pain scale is shown in Figure 10-1B.

More complex and time-consuming tools may be appropriate for certain situations. An intermediate level tool is the short form of the McGill Pain Questionnaire. It consists of 4 parts, including a list of terms that might be used to describe the quality of the pain. The terms are *throbbing, shooting, stabbing, sharp, cramping, gnawing, hot-burning, aching, heavy, tender, splitting, tiring-exhausting, sickening, fearful,* and *cruel-punishing.* The first 11 of the 15 terms are considered sensory; the last 4 are considered affective. Three columns are provided for choosing the intensity of the pain (mild, moderate, and severe). None is implied by failing to mark a column for a given term. The scoring for each of the 15 terms is 0, 1, 2, or 3. A visual analog scale is scored from 0 to 10 with 10 as maximum pain. The patient is also presented with a pain diagram to mark where on the body pain is perceived. A total is generated from the sensory, affective, and visual analog scale scores. Sensory is scored with a maximum of 33, affective is scored with a maximum of 12, and the visual analog scale has a maximum of 10. This questionnaire has been adapted for a number of specific uses. A third part, an evaluative overall

No pain ━━━━━━━━━━━━━━━━━━━━━━━━━━━ Worst pain imaginable

Directions: Indicate your pain in relation to the two extremes. Make a mark at the distance across that you think your pain is. A mark made in the middle of the line means your pain is half of the worst possible pain you could experience.

Figure 10-1A. Visual analog scale used for patients to indicate the intensity of pain.

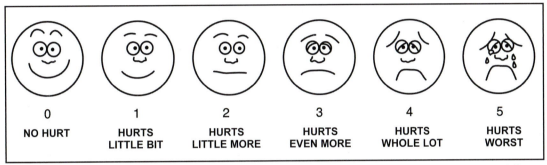

0	1	2	3	4	5
NO HURT	**HURTS LITTLE BIT**	**HURTS LITTLE MORE**	**HURTS EVEN MORE**	**HURTS WHOLE LOT**	**HURTS WORST**

Figure 10-1B. Wong-Baker FACES pain rating scale. Originally designed for children, but can be used for individuals who cannot use a visual analog scale. Instructions are also available in a number of other languages on the Wong on Web site. From Hockenberry MJ, Wilson D. *Wong's Essentials of Pediatric Nursing.* 8th ed. St. Louis, MO: Mosby; 2009. Used with permission. Copyright Mosby.

intensity of pain may be included as part of this tool. This part is scored from 0 to 5, using the words, no pain, mild, discomforting, horrible, and excruciating. The short form of the McGill Questionnaire is shown in Figure 10-2.

MEDICAL MANAGEMENT

Although this text is directed toward a broad audience, the majority of individuals reading this text will not be in a position to prescribe drugs to manage pain. However, everyone involved in wound management is in a position to recommend the use of analgesic medications and is responsible for understanding how the prescribed drugs interact with the patient, the wound, and the ability of the patient and the patient's caregivers to manage the wound.

General Anesthesia

Complex debridement may be performed in an operating room with the patient under general anesthesia. However, several issues need to be considered for general anesthesia. General anesthesia is not appropriate if the patient needs to be conscious to have verbal interaction with the surgeon during the procedure. Another form of anesthesia should be used if postrecovery residual effects, cardiopulmonary consequences, or maternal/fetal transfer of general anesthesia are problematic, or the patient clearly expresses a preference to be conscious.

Two methods of general anesthesia are used, inhaled and intravenous. In many cases, both are used. Inhaled general anesthesia is performed through an endotracheal tube (GETA) attached to the source of anesthetic gas. Either a gas or volatile liquid is placed into the device. An anesthesiologist or nurse anesthetist is responsible for monitoring the patient's response to anesthesia and making necessary adjustments. Inhaled anesthesia is often preferred because of the ease of adjustment. Volatile liquids such as halothane, enflurane, isoflurane, and methoxyflurane are aerosolized for GETA.

Intravenous (IV) anesthesia is useful due to its rapid induction of general anesthesia. Intravenous anesthesia alone may be sufficient for short procedures; for longer procedures general anesthesia is maintained with gas. Drugs used for IV general anesthesia include barbiturates such as thiopental. Adjuvants to general anesthesia include preoperative sedatives such as barbiturates, opioids, and benzodiazepines, especially diazepam. For certain procedures, neuromuscular blockers are indicated. Diazepam or other benzodiazepines may also be used as an adjuvant during local anesthesia to relax a patient. These adjuvants also improve the ease of administering general anesthesia through an endotracheal tube.

Inhalation anesthetics dissolve in membranes, altering the membrane fluidity and interfering with the opening of sodium and other ion channels. Because inhaled general

SHORT FORM MCGILL PAIN QUESTIONNAIRE

Date: _____

Name: _____

Check the column to indicate the level of your
pain for each word, or leave blank if it does not
apply to you.

	Mild	Moderate	Severe
1. Throbbing	_____	_____	_____
2. Shooting	_____	_____	_____
3. Stabbing	_____	_____	_____
4. Sharp	_____	_____	_____
5. Cramping	_____	_____	_____
6. Gnawing	_____	_____	_____
7. Hot-burning	_____	_____	_____
8. Aching	_____	_____	_____
9. Heavy	_____	_____	_____
10. Tender	_____	_____	_____
11. Splitting	_____	_____	_____
12. Tiring-exhausting	_____	_____	_____
13. Sickening	_____	_____	_____
14. Fearful	_____	_____	_____
15. Cruel-punishing	_____	_____	_____

Indicate on this line how bad your pain is—at the left end of line means no pain at all, at right end means worst
pain possible.

No Pain _____ Worst Possible Pain

S/33   A /12   VAS /10

Figure 10-2. Short form McGill Pain Questionnaire. (Reproduced with permission of author © Dr. Ron Melzack, for publication and distribution.)

anesthetics are highly fat soluble, they are stored throughout the body and wash out slowly in obese individuals. If the general anesthetic effects linger, leading to longer periods of immobility, an increase in the risk of pressure ulcers, accumulation of secretions in the lungs, and other problems associated with lack of mobility may occur. General anesthetics can cause confusion, sleepiness, and some patients develop temporary psychosis. Patients may also have temporary muscle weakness if a neuromuscular blocker is used; however, these are unlikely to be used for surgical debridement. Intravenous general anesthetics such as thiopental bind to receptors on chloride ion channels. Binding to these receptors decreases the probability of neurons depolarizing. At the proper dose, these drugs produce sedation or anesthesia. At greater doses, medullary paralysis and death may result.

Local Anesthetics

Local anesthetics work primarily as sodium channel blockers. Some of these drugs (notably lidocaine) can be used to treat arrhythmias also. To be useful, the local anesthetic must remain in the area of interest. These drugs can diffuse slowly from the tissue of interest, and diffuse more rapidly in areas of high blood flow. Application of heating modalities prior to injection of local anesthetics decreases their effectiveness. In some cases, the effectiveness of a local anesthetic is improved by co-injecting a vasoconstricting agent (epinephrine). In rare cases, accidental injection of lidocaine into a blood vessel during an attempt at infiltration may produce systemic effects. Central nervous system effects include somnolence, confusion, agitation, seizures, and respiratory depression. Cardiac effects consist of arrhythmias, decreased heart rate, and contractility. Local anesthetics can be administered by several routes including the typical infiltration of tissues with a hypodermic needle and syringe, topical (described more below), and transdermal (use of iontophoresis is described below). Local anesthetics are also used for peripheral nerve blocks. Brachial plexus block is especially useful for upper extremity surgery. Local anesthetics can also be administered via catheter to the epidural or subdural space for anesthesia of the lower extremities (epidural and spinal anesthesia).

Analgesia

Analgesics include opioids, nonsteroidal anti-inflammatory drugs (NSAIDs), and acetaminophen. Opioids bind to specific receptors in the spinal cord and brain to decrease the transmission of pain signals from the periphery to the cortex. NSAIDs are used for minor pain that may follow injury or surgery. With tissue injury or other causes of inflammation, the enzyme phospholipase A is activated, forming arachidonic acid. Arachidonic acid is then converted by 1 of 2 pathways. The enzyme cyclooxygenase produces the family of chemicals known as prostaglandins and thromboxane, and the enzyme lipoxygenase produces the various leukotrienes.

NSAIDs work by blocking the enzyme cyclooxygenase (COX), which decreases the production of prostaglandins and thromboxane from arachidonic acid. A major adverse effect of NSAIDs has been erosion of the gastric and duodenal mucosa. The lining of the stomach is protected by the local effect of prostaglandins in the stomach. Decreasing the production of prostaglandins by the stomach can lead to serious, even fatal damage. With the discovery of a second type of the COX enzyme, drugs that preferentially affect them have been developed. COX1 is present in the stomach, but COX2 is not and appears to mediate much of the prostaglandin production associated with pain and inflammation. New COX2 drugs have been approved for treating arthritis in individuals at risk for developing gastrointestinal ulceration by NSAIDs, but only celecoxib (Celebrex, Pfizer, New York, NY) is still available.

All true NSAIDs have 3 basic properties: analgesic, antipyretic, and antithrombotic. In some cases, NSAIDs will need to be avoided in patients with prolonged bleeding times. Acetaminophen does not meet all of the criteria for NSAIDs because it has analgesic and antipyretic properties only. Most NSAIDs and acetaminophen are generally effective against only mild pain, requiring the use of opi-

ate drugs for moderate to severe pain. However, ketorolac tromethamine (Toradol, Roche, Basel, Switzerland) is one NSAID that can be effective against moderate pain.

Although much of the inflammation caused by tissue injury may be attributed to leukotrienes, no lipoxygenase drugs have yet been approved as analgesics. Leukotrienes are involved intimately with airway inflammation and drugs either decreasing the production of or blocking binding sites for leukotrienes have only been approved for asthma at this time.

Opioid analgesics are naturally occurring substances derived from the opium poppy and are very effective against even severe pain. Semisynthetic opioids are produced by modifying naturally occurring compounds. However, natural and semisynthetic opioids have tremendous potential for dependency. Synthetic opioids relieve moderate to severe pain with fewer adverse effects or dependency.

Opioids are available in a number of formulations for different routes of administration. Opioids can be administered orally, intramuscularly, intravenously, and transdermally (fentanyl patch). Opioids bind to a number of specific types of opioid receptors, which tend to be localized to different locations in the brain and spinal cord. In addition, the various types of opioids bind better to different types of opioid receptors. Receptors are located within the substantia gelatinosa, the site of synapse between peripheral nociceptive neurons, on second order neurons in the tip of the posterior gray, and in multiple areas within the brain. Binding of opioids to the presynaptic membrane (release site of neurotransmitter from the nociceptive neuron) diminishes the release of neurotransmitter onto the second order neuron, and therefore, decreases the probability of perception of pain at the cortex. In addition, opioids hyperpolarize the postsynaptic membrane on the second order neuron, rendering the release of neurotransmitter by the peripheral nociceptor less effective in producing an action potential in the second order neuron, also decreasing the probability of relaying a pain message to the cortex. Binding of opioids by receptors in specific regions of the brain excites pain suppressing neurons. Opioids may also function peripherally by suppressing the release of substance P by peripheral nociceptors. Release of substance P is believed to perpetuate the pain caused by tissue injury and inflammation.

Issues Related to Use of Opioid Analgesics

Unfortunately, opioids have a number of adverse effects that vary tremendously in their severity among patients. Opioids are generally sedating and may even produce respiratory depression. Orthostatic hypotension produced by opioids requires the clinician to exercise care in assisting patients with transfers and ambulation. Nausea, vomiting, and constipation are common adverse effects. For this reason, opioids are commonly used in preparations designed to decrease gastrointestinal motility. Patients may be prescribed antiemetic drugs as needed when they are also taking opioid analgesics.

Some physicians, particularly those who prescribe opiates for patients with chronic pain, may require a pain contract. Failure to follow the contract results in the patient being denied any future opioid prescriptions. Patients must agree to take the prescribed medication at the dose and frequency prescribed and obtain them only from one pharmacy. The pharmacy is given a copy of the contract. Any medication that is lost or stolen will not be replaced. Patients are not to share pain medications with anyone else and they are subject to drug testing. Should any patients seem to require more medication to tolerate treatment, the clinician performing the wound care should contact the patient's physician directly and develop a strategy to improve the patient's ability to tolerate treatment. Outpatients using opioid pain medications should not be driving themselves to a clinic. Clinicians must determine whether someone is actually driving the patient to the clinic rather than simply trusting the patient. Asking to speak to a family member about home care is a nonthreatening way of determining that the patient has a driver.

Patient-Controlled Analgesia

The purpose of patient-controlled analgesia (PCA) is to maintain drug levels in a small range within the analgesic range. Compared with intramuscular (IM) injections typically given at 3 to 4 hour intervals, PCA will maintain a fairly steady analgesic effect, whereas repeated IM injections allow wide fluctuations in perception of pain just before and after injection. Moreover, peaks in plasma opioid concentration caused by IM injection have a greater potential for causing sedation, nausea, vomiting, orthostatic hypotension, and other adverse effects. A typical protocol for PCA includes a loading dose to achieve initial analgesia rapidly, a provision for demand dosing with lockout intervals over certain time frames such as 1 and 4 hours and a background infusion rate. The background infusion rate is provided to ensure that plasma opioid concentration does not fall below the therapeutic level, whereas the lockouts provide a safeguard against overdosing. The demand dose is available to the patient as needed, usually by pushing a wired remote button. The patient should be encouraged to use the available demand doses and should be instructed in the means by which the infusion pumps are controlled in terms of lockout intervals and background infusion. If patients are either too sedated or have too much pain, the PCA pump may require adjustment. For long-term use, access ports with central lines may be used for administering analgesia. Either opioids or local anesthetics may be used with a patient-controlled analgesia through either a central line or epidural catheter. Anesthetics cause loss of

both sensation and motor function, whereas opioids produce analgesia without loss of motor function. Care must be taken during transfers and ambulation in individuals receiving local anesthetics in an epidural or subdural line due to loss of lower extremity strength.

Anti-Anxiety and Sedative Medications

Benzodiazepines are the more commonly used anxiolytic/sedative medications. Benzodiazepines such as diazepam (Valium), alprazolam (Xanax), clonazepam (Klonopin), lorazepam (Ativan), and midazolam (Versed) are commonly prescribed as adjuvants to general or local anesthetics. Ativan and Versed also have the desirable effect of amnesia for the time of their effective use. Patients using these drugs can still be cooperative as well as being more tolerant of painful procedures. In particular, patients who become agitated during debridement may benefit from prescription of these drugs.

ELECTROTHERAPY

Whereas oral and injectable analgesic drugs require prescription by a physician and administration by a registered nurse, electrotherapeutic means of analgesia can be administered by a number of healthcare providers. The types of modalities available include transcutaneous electrical nerve stimulation (TENS), interferential current (IFC), and iontophoresis. TENS, as originally developed, was based on the gate control theory of pain described by Melzack and Wall in 1965. The basis of the gate control theory is that stimulation of larger afferent (sensory) nerves that enter at the same spinal cord level as the nociceptive neurons carrying pain signals diminishes perception of pain. Simple, well-known applications of the gate control theory of pain include rubbing a painful area and "running off" the pain.

Nociceptors as well as mechanoreceptors and thermoreceptors have 2 axons (pseudounipolar neurons) and a cell body that resides in a dorsal root ganglion (trigeminal ganglion for the face). The peripheral axonal process carries information from the periphery encoded as a frequency of action potentials propagated from the distal end to the cell body, which then continue from the cell body along the central axonal process to synaptic terminals in the dorsal gray matter, in particular the substantia gelatinosa. The outer white matter of the spinal cord consists of tracts of axons carrying information either from the brain to the spinal cord (descending tracts) or from the spinal cord to the brain (ascending tracts). The white matter of the spinal cord (as well as the brain) consists mainly of myelinated axons, where the fatty myelin substance creates the characteristic color of the outer part of the spinal cord and inner tracts through the brain. The gray matter of the spinal cord lacks the white color due to the relative lack of myelin in areas composed primarily of cell bodies of ascending interneurons that synapse with sensory neurons, cell bodies of motor neurons that synapse with descending interneurons, and cell bodies of local interneurons that allow the sharing of information within the spinal cord. Thus, the gray matter's color is the result of a sea of cell bodies with some myelinated axons running between them. The substantia gelatinosa has a clear appearance due to the very high proportion of unmyelinated neurons converging in this region.

Much of the sensory information reaching the cortex to provide conscious perception requires a chain of 3 neurons from the periphery to the cortex. Sensory neurons entering the spinal cord from the dorsal root ganglion are called first order neurons. Second order neurons synapse within the gray matter of the spinal cord and ascend in the white matter. Second order neurons typically terminate in the thalamus, synapsing with third order neurons that carry the information from the thalamus to the cerebral cortex. Some sensory systems deviate from this general framework and multiple other connections exist among areas of the cerebrum and cerebellum. Well-localized pain linked directly to a specific stimulus is carried in this 3-neuron type of arrangement. Pain that persists due to tissue injury or inflammation is carried through a different pathway in that second order neurons travel to the reticular activating system, leading to poorly localized pain with a greater persistence and emotional component.

A large number of synapses exist among neurons entering the substantia gelatinosa as well as binding sites for short-acting natural opioids (enkephalins). The gate theory of pain is based on the premise that stimulation of mechanoreceptive neurons with their cell bodies in the same dorsal root ganglion as the nociceptors of interest synapse with interneurons that can "close the gate" to pain information. These "gatekeeping" interneurons are proposed to release neurotransmitter on the synaptic terminals of nociceptors rendering release of neurotransmitter from the nociceptor more difficult. In addition, enkephalin appears to be released onto the postsynaptic membrane of the second order neuron that synapses with the nociceptor. Enkephalin release onto the second order neurons hyperpolarizes the postsynaptic membrane, diminishing the effect of neurotransmitter release by the nociceptor. Release of enkephalin, therefore, both decreases the probability of release of neurotransmitter by the nociceptor onto the second order neuron and decreases the effectiveness of the neurotransmitter released onto second order neurons. As a result, fewer action potentials are developed in the second order neurons and less pain is perceived at the cortical level.

Transcutaneous Electrical Nerve Stimulation

TENS devices are simple electrical stimulators that allow the amplitude, frequency, and duration of biphasic pulses to be adjusted. Lead wires are attached to self-adherent electrodes placed on the skin (Figure 10-3). In addition, several means of modulating the settings for amplitude, frequency and duration are typically found on commercially available units. For example, a given modulation setting may cause the pulse frequency to cyclically increase and decrease from a set value. Because of the nature of pain carried by the larger lightly myelinated Aδ nociceptive neurons and the unmyelinated C neurons, TENS application is typically directed at diminishing persistent pain associated with the more primitive C neuron and medial spinothalamic tract. Current generated by the TENS device depolarizes mechanoreceptors within the skin causing inhibition of second order neurons synapsing with nociceptors of the C type of neuron. As such, TENS may be useful for management of persistent pain associated with chronic wounds.

A simple means of passing current through the mechanoreceptors associated with the same dorsal root ganglion as the injury is to place electrodes around the site of injury. With a single channel device, electrodes may be placed either medially and laterally to the wound or proximally and distally. A 2-channel device allows electrodes to be placed completely around the site of injury. Other approaches include placing the electrodes over the peripheral nerve supplying the area if the nerve is sufficiently superficial, eg, peroneal, medial, ulnar, radial nerves. Electrodes can also be placed over the brachial plexus at Erb's point, between the clavicle and belly of the upper trapezius to manage pain throughout the upper extremity, analogous to the infusion of local anesthetic onto the brachial plexus. Some clinicians also attempt to manage pain by placing electrodes paraspinally at the level of the dorsal root ganglion of interest. Configurations used for TENS electrode placements are shown in Figure 10-3B.

Conventional TENS as originally developed uses biphasic pulses at a frequency of approximately 100 Hz, a pulse duration of about 80 milliseconds and an amplitude great enough that the patient perceives a vibratory stimulus (sensory level of stimulation), but not sufficiently strong to elicit contraction of muscle beneath the skin (motor level of stimulation). Low frequency TENS, as the name implies, is performed at a low frequency of 2 to 4 Hz. In addition, low frequency TENS is characterized by a greater pulse duration (approximately 250 milliseconds) and a greater intensity. The intensity is greater than motor, to the point that the patient can perceive stimulation of nociceptors (noxious level of stimulation). Most patients will perceive an uncomfortable, prickling sensation and many patients

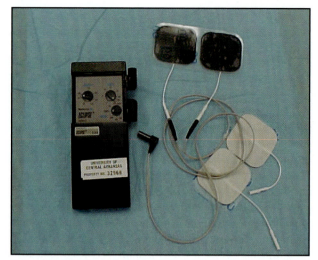

Figure 10-3A. Typical TENS unit.

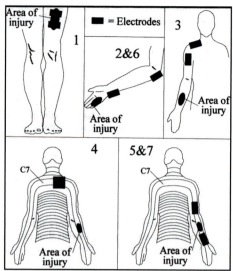

Figure 10-3B. Rationales for TENS electrode placement. The 7 rationales include: 1) Directly over the site of injury or pathology, providing the skin is intact; 2) Over the trunk of the peripheral nerve innervating the area of injury or pathology. The nerve must be superficial (eg, peroneal or ulnar nerve); 3) Over the nerve plexus from which the nerve innervating the area of pain originates. In particular, the brachial plexus can be very useful for pain anywhere in the upper extremity. An electrode is placed over Erb's point (the area between the clavicle and trapezius where the brachial plexus is the most superficial); 4) Over the sensory nerve roots innervating the site of pain (using a dermatome chart); 5) Within the same dermatome as the site of pain (assuming affected nociceptors are entering the same dorsal root as the stimulated mechanoreceptive neurons); 6) Over the motor point of an injured or painful muscle. The motor point is the location at which one obtains a muscle contraction with the lowest current. Presumably this location is directly over the nerve of the muscle, which also contains sensory neurons of the muscle (Aα fibers); 7) Arranged so that the current will run between 2 electrodes through the area of pain.

do not tolerate this type of stimulation well, preferring conventional TENS. Low frequency TENS is not explicable based on the gate control theory of pain. Some have suggested that this pattern of stimulation evokes release of natural opioids. The time frame of the onset of analgesia and persistence of pain relief is consistent with this idea.

During debridement, dressing changes, and any other procedures that create pain acutely, conventional TENS is less likely to be effective. Perception of pain occurring during a stimulus is conveyed by Aδ neurons to second order neurons running through the lateral spinothalamic tract to the thalamus and then relayed to the cortex by third order neurons. This pain is, therefore, localizable and graded to the intensity of the stimulus. This type of pain ceases when the stimulus is removed, but pain associated with tissue injury and inflammation and conveyed by C nociceptive neurons may follow at some later time.

Another mode of TENS called brief intense may be used for this acute aspect of pain. Brief intense TENS is produced by gradually increasing amplitude, duration, and frequency of pulses as tolerated by the patient. Done properly, brief intense TENS produces not just analgesia, but anesthesia. During brief intense TENS, wound debridement may be performed without pain. Following debridement, the TENS device can be reset to conventional settings to manage any pain that might result from tissue injury during debridement.

Interferential Current

Although IFC may be used for other purposes, it can be used for the same purpose as TENS. Whereas TENS transmits electric pulses produced within the stimulator and conducts them to body tissues through paired electrodes on the skin surface, IFC produces an interference pattern generated by crossing 2 alternating currents of slightly differing frequency through body tissues. The difference in the frequency of the 2 crossing currents produces a cycle of maximum constructive to maximum destructive interference and back to maximum constructive interference at a rate equal to the difference in frequency of the 2 alternating currents. Within each cycle, amplitude of the interference current ranges from an amplitude of nearly zero to an amplitude of nearly double the individual alternating currents. Although this cycle is

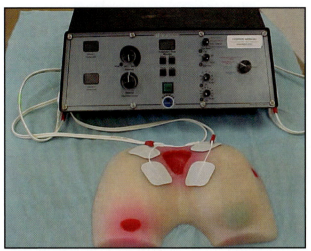

Figure 10-4. Set-up for interferential current treatment. Note the electrode placement pattern of two leads set perpendicular to each other.

constructed of 2 currents of 4,000 to 5,000 Hz, each cycle of interference from minimum to maximum and back behaves at the tissue level as an individual pulse. Each cycle is called a beat for the purpose of discussing the physiologic effects of IFC. The frequency of beats generated in the tissues is simply the difference in frequency of the 2 alternating currents. For example, if one current is 4,000 Hz and the other is 3,990, the beat frequency is 10 Hz and it will produce 10 muscle twitches per second if the intensity is great enough.

Producing IFC in the tissue requires 2 channels and 4 electrodes. Two electrodes from one lead are placed on the skin such that an imaginary line drawn between the two electrodes of the lead intersect a similar imaginary line between the electrodes of the other lead to form an imaginary perpendicular line. When done this way, the current generated in the tissue produces the beats as described above. The intensity of the IFC varies through the tissue in a cloverleaf pattern. Current intensity is greatest in the tissue between the imaginary lines and reaches a minimum directly along the imaginary lines. To improve the dispersion of current within tissue, a fluctuation of current amplitude causes a shift of the current distribution such that the "cloverleaf" pattern moves cyclically through the tissue.

Due to the way that IFC is generated, specific devices must be used to generate IFC. Several manufacturers produce portable IFC units that can be carried readily by patients. Set up for IFC is demonstrated in Figure 10-4. To generate analgesia with IFC, beat frequency and amplitude are set as they would be for conventional or low frequency TENS, except that with IFC no adjustment for pulse duration is available. Because of the way IFC is generated in the tissues, a much greater quantity of charge is

run through the tissue compared with the biphasic pulses of TENS devices, which makes IFC very useful for generating a brief intense type of effect. Another advantage of IFC compared with traditional biphasic TENS devices is the low skin impedance that results from the much higher frequency used in IFC. The lower skin impedance allows greater recruitment of mechanoreceptors before skin nociceptors are recruited. This allows the patient to tolerate enough current to achieve a greater anesthetic effect than can be generated by biphasic pulses of TENS devices. Moreover, IFC is designed to run current through a tissue of interest without the need to place electrodes directly on this specific area. Generating an anesthetic effect with IFC is fairly simple. Over the course of 1 to 2 minutes, current is increased gradually as tolerated by the patient until numbness is reported. Over this time, the patient will be able to tolerate increasing amounts of current either in the form of increased beat frequency or amplitude as the current is applied.

Iontophoresis

Iontophoresis is the use of direct current to drive ionized molecules transdermally. Although many types of compounds have been addressed in the literature for various ailments, modern iontophoresis is typically performed for driving dexamethasone, an anti-inflammatory drug into tissues to treat chronic musculoskeletal conditions such as tennis elbow. Iontophoresis units are now promoted for pediatric use as an alternative to infiltration with lidocaine prior to starting lines or suturing lacerations. Application of iontophoresis requires 2 electrodes. The solution of ionized medication is suffused onto a smaller active, absorbent electrode. Depending on the electrode size, 2 to 4 ml of solution is used. A larger dispersive electrode is placed on a nearby area. The correct polarity for the medication must be set on the device. Dexamethasone is driven across the skin with a negative electrode and lidocaine requires a positive electrode. Dosage of iontophoresis is quantified in units of mA x min, the product of current in mA and duration in minutes. Although not correct from a physics standpoint (Coulombs would be correct), using the mA x min unit allows the clinician to manipulate the 2 variables to maximize patient tolerance. For example, a dose of 40 mA x min can be generated with an intensity of 4 mA and a duration of 10 minutes, a current of 2 mA and duration of 20 minutes, or other suitable combination of current and duration.

TOPICAL APPLICATION OF LOCAL ANESTHETICS

Another alternative to systemic drugs is topically applied local anesthetic. Several preparations are now available. Both lidocaine and benzocaine are available in a spray. Lidocaine is also available in liquid and gel forms. For minor acute wounds, a combination of lidocaine, neomycin, polymyxin B, and bacitracin is available over the counter as Neosporin plus. Another preparation is EMLA (eutectic mixture of local anesthetic) cream. EMLA is a combination of 2.5% prilocaine and 2.5% lidocaine in an emulsion with a melting point below room temperature, which keeps both anesthetics in the liquid oil portion. This is commonly used for local anesthesia prior to using subcutaneous infusion ports attached to central lines for home or outpatient intravenous services. The cream stays in place on the skin and is absorbed sufficiently to avoid the need for infiltration of local anesthetics. EMLA is also packaged in a disk within an occlusive dressing with an adhesive tape ring. Lidocaine has a more rapid onset and prilocaine has a more prolonged effect. In practice, local anesthetic gel or spray is placed on the edges of wounds prior to painful procedures such as debridement, pulsatile lavage with concurrent suction, or may be done when dressing changes alone are painful.

OTHER INTERVENTIONS TO MANAGE PAIN

The Krasner pain model may be used to address pain within the plan of care. Wound pain in the Krasner model consists of chronic (persistent), noncyclic acute, and cyclic acute pain. Chronic or persistent wound pain that is not related to any specific event or known pain trigger is most likely due to the cause of the wound and, therefore, the underlying cause of the wound must be corrected to relieve the pain. Examples include compression therapy for venous ulcers, repositioning or teaching others to reposition patients with pressure ulcers, and protecting limbs with arterial disease. Noncyclic acute pain as described in the Krasner model is produced by obvious painful procedures that do not occur on a regular basis such as sharp debridement. The term *cyclical acute pain* describes what is experienced with routine occurrences associated with wound care such as dressing changes.

Using this framework, the treatment plan and how it is executed can be modified to reduce pain as much as possible within the plan of care. The type of debridement done may need to be changed to a less painful method. For example, necrotic tissue may still have viable nerves and blood vessels running through them. Both cutting and tugging on necrotic tissue to debride it with sharp instruments may be painful. Even the cutting of necrotic tissue that has no innervation may cause molecules from the tissue to be released on viable nociceptors, leading to pain. Likewise, dressings selected may influence the amount of pain experienced by the patient. Dressings that are allowed to desiccate and adhere to a wound can cause

much pain during removal. Soaking or gently irrigating the dressing may be necessary to avoid excessive pain. A different type of dressing that does not adhere to the wound may be required. Different types of dressings will need to be changed at intervals appropriate to their use. If the treatment plan allows, less frequent debridement and dressing changes should be performed should pain become a major issue. In some cases, simple changes in how debridement and dressing changes are performed can reduce pain. A patient may experience less pain if positioned appropriately and if touching the area of pain can be minimized.

A variety of nonpharmacologic methods for decreasing stress may be effective in managing pain. Application of cold (cryotherapy) or heat may reduce pain, but should be used judiciously due to the effects of temperature on blood vessels. Reducing blood flow may slow healing and increasing it with heat may lead to unwanted bleeding. Technology may be employed through biofeedback devices. Stress may also be reduced by carefully explaining procedures to patients and displaying empathy. Let the patient know that some patients seem to experience pain and you will do whatever you can to minimize it. Choosing a less stressful word such as discomfort might be more effective. If the patient does not ask whether a procedure will be painful, you should initiate the discussion rather than allowing the patient to be surprised. Some patients may not find a given procedure to be painful. Let the patient know what the typical range of responses to the procedure is. For example, before pulsatile lavage tell the patient that some people seem to find the procedure to be uncomfortable, but others actually find it to be soothing, like rubbing a painful area.

Along with this strategy, the clinician should offer the patient the opportunity to call "time out" during the procedure. The clinician must be willing to stop the procedure immediately and only resume when the patient indicates he or she is ready. A word or phrase such as "stop" or "time out" must be chosen before the procedure begins. Strategies for managing children are discussed in Chapter 16, special populations.

Some patients may benefit from soothing music or nature sounds; however, some patients may find this auditory stimulation to be annoying instead. Having a range of music or nature sounds increases the likelihood of finding the sound that most effectively reduces a patient's anxiety.

Biofeedback

Biofeedback presents 2 noninvasive and nonthreatening means of reducing pain. Because biofeedback empowers patients to voluntarily control some physiologic aspects that often contribute to the perception of pain, tolerance for painful stimuli may be increased. Both electromyographic (EMG) and thermal biofeedback may be used to train a patient to decrease stress, which in turn may be sufficient, or may be used in conjunction with other types of pain management. Other biofeedback techniques that could be employed are galvanic skin response and electro-encephalography.

Although EMG biofeedback is commonly used for muscle re-education by training a patient to increase the EMG signal detected, it may be used for relaxation by training the patient to decrease the signal of a muscle that becomes active during stress. A common target is the frontalis muscle. The patient attempts to decrease the signal during a stressful event such as wound debridement and thereby reduce the perception of pain. Focus on the signal of the biofeedback device may also act as a distraction from the painful event. EMG biofeedback uses a device that can be smaller than a TENS unit to which 3 leads are attached to electrodes. Some devices may use electrodes that are prepared with all 3 contacts on a single adhesive patch. Two leads are used to record the difference in potential created between them as electric current that signals muscle contraction passes by them. The third electrode is an indifferent electrode used to electronically eliminate electrical artifact due to radio signals, fluorescent lights, static electricity, and other extraneous electrical activity. The 2 active electrodes are generally oriented along the line of pull of the muscle of interest. The active leads must be placed relatively close to each other and should not be placed across the midline of the body or an electrocardiographic signal may be detected and obscure the skeletal muscle activity. The EMG signal may be displayed as a variety of visual or auditory means. Usually a number of different auditory signals are selectable, allowing the patient to choose one most suitable for the purpose of the device. Visual cues of muscle activity vary among devices, including bar graph types of displays, a series of lights, or a digital readout.

Patients may also be taught to regulate muscle activity through Jacobsen's exercises. Although a variety of ways are used to teach these exercises, the premise is that a person learns to self-detect muscle activity by progressively contracting muscles then relaxing them. During stress a person might be able to relax muscles voluntarily by learning to sense excessive muscle tension. Deep breathing, pursed lips breathing, and breathing techniques used in Lamaze natural childbirth education may also help.

Thermal biofeedback can be used similarly to reduce stress. A thermistor is attached to a finger, such as the third finger of the nondominant hand. The other end of the thermistor is plugged into a device that provides information about the finger's (or other body part's) temperature. The temperature signal, like EMG biofeedback, may be displayed in a number of ways in either or both auditory and visual means. The theoretical basis of thermal biofeed-

back is providing a means of sensing the activity of the sympathetic nervous system. A high level of stress activates sympathetic activity, which leads to a number of physiological changes. The sympathetic function addressed by thermal biofeedback is constriction of peripheral blood vessels. With low stress, little vasoconstriction of arteries serving the finger occurs, resulting in higher finger temperature than that of a person who is stressed. With stress, sympathetic nerves constrict arterial vessels supplying the fingers, resulting in decreased finger temperature. As with EMG biofeedback, the patient is to focus on the device in an attempt to decrease stress, which may decrease perception of pain. Some patients learn thermal biofeedback very quickly and can increase skin temperature within a few sessions, or possibly during the first session.

SUMMARY

Pain management is the responsibility of everyone involved in wound management. It may be provided by analgesic drugs prescribed by a physician, ranging from typical NSAIDs, ketorolac for moderate pain, or weak to strong opioids for moderate to severe pain. Analgesia can also be provided by electrotherapy, using TENS on the brief intense mode during debridement or conventional TENS for background relief. Interferential current has the advantage of being applied to the area surrounding the wound and the greater current passing through the wound. Local anesthetics can be applied to the edges of wounds undergoing debridement as a spray, gel, or cream.

QUESTIONS

1. Who is authorized to prescribe strong NSAIDs and opioids for pain relief? Why?

2. What are aspects of pain management that may be provided by anyone?

3. What electrotherapeutic devices are available to reduce pain? What is the basic mechanism by which these work?

4. Why is lidocaine used for short procedures and bupivacaine for longer procedures?

5. What is the significance of Erb's point for TENS application?

6. What types of nonpharmacologic methods are available for managing pain?

BIBLIOGRAPHY

Broadbent E, Petrie KJ, Alley PG, Booth RJ. Psychological stress impairs early wound repair following surgery. *Psychosom Med.* 2003;65(5):865-869.

Ciccone CD. *Pharmacology in Rehabilitation*. Philadelphia, PA: F.A. Davis; 1996.

Gatchel RJ, Mayer TG, Theodore BR. The pain disability questionnaire: relationship to one-year functional and psychosocial rehabilitation outcomes. *J Occup Rehabil*. 2006;16(1):75-94.

Gatchel RJ, Peng YB, Peters ML, Fuchs PN, Turk DC. The biopsychosocial approach to chronic pain: scientific advances and future directions. *Psychol Bull*. 2007l;133(4):581-624.

Gatchel RJ, Robinson RC, Pulliam C, Maddrey AM. Biofeedback with pain patients: Evidence for its effectiveness. *Seminars in Pain Medicine*. 2003;1:55–66.

Hockenberry MJ, Wilson D, Winkelstein ML: *Wong's Essentials of Pediatric Nursing*. 7th ed. St. Louis, MO: Elsevier Science; 2005.

Katzung BG. *Basic and Clinical Pharmacology*. East Norwalk, CT: Appleton & Lange; 1998.

Krasner D. The chronic wound pain experience: a conceptual model. *Ostomy Wound Manage*. 1995;41(3):20-25.

Melzack R. McGill Pain Questionnaire Short Form. http://www.health-sciences.ubc.ca/whiplash.bc/pdf/mcgill1.pdf. Accessed July 30, 2009.

Melzack R, Wall PD. Pain mechanisms: a new theory. *Science*. 1965;150(699):971-979.

Price P, Fogh K, Glynn C, Krasner DL, Osterbrink J, Sibbald RG. Managing painful chronic wounds: the Wound Pain Management Model. *Int Wound J*. 2007;4(suppl 1):4-15.

Reddy M, Kohr R, Queen D, Keast D, Sibbald RG. Practical treatment of wound pain and trauma: a patient-centered approach. An overview. *Ostomy Wound Manage*. 2003;49 (suppl 4):2-15.

Robinson AJ, Snyder-Mackler L. *Clinical Electrophysiology: Electrotherapy and Electrophysiological Testing*. Baltimore, MD: Williams & Wilkins; 1995.

Sibbald RG, Armstrong DG, Orsted HL. Pain in diabetic foot ulcers. *Ostomy Wound Manage*. 2003;49(suppl 4):24-29.

Wong on Web. http://www1.us.elsevierhealth.com/FACES/. Accessed August 25, 2009.

Wound Bed Preparation

Debridement is a time-honored and frequently performed aspect of wound management. However, for every individual patient, the clinician should ask why should I debride this particular wound and what is the optimal method?

REASONS FOR WOUND BED PREPARATION

Optimizing wound healing is an appropriate goal for almost any case. Because desiccated tissue acts as barrier to cell migration, its removal is a clear benefit to patients.

However, even moist necrotic tissue is problematic. Slough occupies space within a wound and thereby decreases the ability of cells to migrate. Devitalized tissue and damaged cells release chemical mediators of inflammation, delaying the onset of proliferation of new cells to fill a wound. Inflammation, in turn, leads to leakage of blood vessels in the wound bed, leading to loss of protein and fluid through open wounds. Leakage of proteins causes additional problems. Fibrinogen leaking onto the surface of the wound is converted into the hard, insoluble protein coat of fibrin on the surface of a wound. Chronic inflammation results in the production of molecules that further slow healing

Irion G.
Comprehensive Wound Management, 2nd ed. (pp 203-222)
© 2010 SLACK Incorporated

and aging of cells within the wound bed. Loss of protein from the vascular space leads to edema and malnutrition both locally in the dependent areas in which edema occurs and, in general, in the form of protein malnutrition. Most importantly, necrotic tissue provides an environment conducive to bacterial growth.

Debridement is also important to decrease the potential for infection. Dead tissue acts as a medium for infection and may hide infection, abscesses, tunnels, and sinus tracts. Rapid debridement can bring a wound into bacterial balance. In one series of patients, pressure ulcers that had a bacterial burden of greater than 100,000 per gram were sharply debrided. Of these, 96% remained at less than 100 per gram. According to Robson, the ideal environment is one in which the bacteria are in balance—not bacteria-free. Low levels of bacteria may accelerate certain aspects of wound healing, but a burden greater than 100,000 per gram severely retards healing. In particular, the production of proteases capable of breaking down growth factors and the attraction of neutrophils appear to be responsible. The presence of β-hemolytic streptococci is particularly problematic in even low numbers. Fibrinolysins, leukocidins, hemolysins, and hyaluronidase allow the bacteria to protect themselves from the immune system and spread through tissue. In addition to the benefits of debridement, we must also consider the risks associated with not debriding. These include slow healing, osteomyelitis, the need for amputation of an infected limb, advancing cellulitis, sepsis, and in extreme cases, death. On these bases, debridement generally meets the definition of medical necessity.

WOUND CLEANSING

Wound cleansing during the initial visit and at each dressing change has been recommended by the AHCPR. Prevention of injury during cleansing is emphasized. Some authorities recommend against using any direct scrubbing action on the wound. Others have even challenged the notion that wound cleansing must be done with every dressing change. However, the clinician who must assess the wound during a dressing change must cleanse the wound sufficiently to make appropriate decisions for further management. The AHCPR recommendation is for use of normal saline or certain types of specialized detergents with a mild irrigation pressure that allows wound cleansing without traumatizing the wound bed or driving bacteria into the wound. The recommended safe and effective ulcer irrigation pressure range is between 4 and 15 psi.

Irrigation

Simple cleansing can be performed with prepackaged, single dose, 8 psi sterile saline irrigation; irrigation bulbs

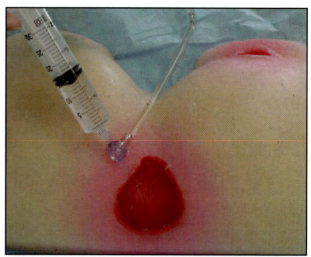

Figure 11-1. Irrigation syringe designed specifically for wound cleansing. A valve system allows the syringe to be filled from a source of sterile saline and the saline to irrigate at the appropriate pressure for safe wound cleansing.

produce too little pressure. A syringe and 19-gauge catheter or equivalent produces an appropriate pressure for irrigation (Figure 11-1). Devices designed specifically for cleansing teeth, such as Waterpik (Waterpik, Ft. Collins, CO), have been used for irrigation. These devices first gained popularity during the Vietnam conflict, but they are not designed to produce appropriate pressure. Irrigation devices should also have a splash shield to prevent spraying necrotic tissue and contaminated fluid over the treatment area. Several devices have recently been developed incorporating both the irrigation pressure desired and a splash shield. Pulsatile lavage devices deliver appropriate pressure and include splash shields and suction to aid in the removal of loosened necrotic tissue and to minimize the spray of contaminated fluid in the treatment area. When used specifically to remove necrotic tissue, pulsatile lavage is considered to be a form of debridement.

Wound cleansing may also be done with a minimal amount of mechanical force with gauze, cloth, sponges, and either normal saline or special detergents. The AHCPR recommends that clinicians not use antiseptic agents or disinfectants such as sodium hypochlorite, Dakin's solution, H_2O_2, iodine, acetic acid, or skin cleansers such as hexachlorophene and chlorhexidine, or povidone iodine scrub on pressure ulcers. Although these agents may be appropriate for initial cleansing of acute wounds, the principle for which the AHCPR panel recommended against use of antiseptic agents on pressure ulcers should be extended to other chronic wounds. The lack of understanding of the differences between gross contamination of acute wounds and colonization of chronic wounds is the most likely reason for referrals for cleansing wounds with these agents. AHCPR guidelines have suggested that irrigation pressure be between 4 and 15 psi. A pressure lower than 4 psi is believed to be ineffective at removing bacteria and debris from a wound bed. Pressures exceeding 20 psi are believed to drive bacteria into the wound.

More costly ways of cleansing a wound include whirlpool and pulsatile lavage with concurrent suction (pulsed lavage). Whirlpool treatment has only been recommended for cleansing pressure ulcers with thick exudate, slough, or necrotic tissue, but not for clean ulcers. Other methods that include a component of debridement, such as pulsatile lavage are more likely to be effective for this type of wound. Whirlpool can be useful to clean residues of materials such as silver sulfadiazine from full and partial thickness burns when simple irrigation is insufficient. Another benefit of using whirlpool for this type of injury is the ability of the patient to perform range of motion exercises in the moving water that would not be tolerated otherwise. Whirlpool and pulsatile lavage as used for debridement will be discussed further under debridement using hydrotherapy.

DEBRIDEMENT

Guidelines from organizations such as the ADA and the National Pressure Ulcer Advisory Panel encourage debridement in most cases. Payment for many adjunct therapies (see Chapter 14) will be denied if debridement is not performed. The AHCPR guidelines call for removal of any necrotic tissue from the wound if consistent with goals, to select the method most appropriate to patient condition and goals and the need to assess and control pain. Because of the availability of different methods for individuals with different treatment goals and in different settings, for example, inpatient versus home health care, the recommendation of AHCPR for debridement of pressure ulcers cannot be more specific. These guidelines also state that any one or a combination of sharp, mechanical, enzymatic, or autolytic debridement techniques may be used unless an urgent need for removal of devitalized tissue with sharp debridement arises. Indications for urgent sharp debridement include advancing cellulitis or sepsis. Sharp debridement is the most rapid means of debridement and is the most appropriate for debriding thick, adherent eschar and extensive quantities of necrotic tissue from ulcers. Smaller wounds may be sharply debrided at bedside. Extensive sharp debridement must be done in an operating room or special procedures room.

Sharp debridement must be done with sterile instruments. A clean, dry dressing should be applied for 8 to 24 hours if bleeding occurs. After bleeding ceases, moist dressings, if appropriate, should be used again. In addition, sharp debridement is reserved for individuals who meet licensing requirements and have demonstrated skill in this technique. Clean dressings may be used in conjunction with mechanical or enzymatic debridement techniques. A recommendation associated with debridement has remained controversial. Heel ulcers have received special consideration in terms of debridement. AHCPR guidelines state that heel ulcers with dry eschar should not be debrided if they do not have edema, erythema, fluctuance (boggy feel), and drainage. However, the guidelines also state clearly that such wounds should be assessed daily for complications that may require debridement. One source of the controversy is the singling out of heel ulcers. Wounds with dry eschar on other body parts are not addressed specifically. Another important recommendation (discussed further in Chapter 10) is pain management. Clinicians often resign themselves to pain during debridement. AHCPR guidelines very specifically recommend the prevention or management of pain associated with debridement as needed. Strategies for pain management are addressed specifically in Chapter 10. Arrange for patients to be medicated sufficiently ahead of time to allow maximal plasma concentration of any oral or injected analgesics. Oral medications will take much longer than those administered by intravenous or intramuscular routes.

Types of Debridement

Four basic types of debridement are typically described: mechanical (nonspecific), enzymatic (chemical), autolytic, and sharp. The type of debridement suitable for a given wound as with any intervention depends on the complete clinical picture including characteristics of the wound, characteristics of the patient, social and work responsibilities, resources available, and the setting in which the patient is being seen. Important factors to consider in deciding which type of debridement to use include the type of wound (etiology); the amount of necrotic tissue, which may not be observable initially; the condition of the patient, including terminal illness; the care setting, which includes time constraints on discharge; and clinician or caregiver experience. The clinician must examine the depth of the wound for necrotic tissue using good lighting and should be familiar with different tissue types. The clinician should consider patient preferences. Issues related to patient preference include the time frame for the plan of care, pain and psychological issues, and who will be performing the dressing changes.

Mechanical Debridement

To remove necrotic tissue from a wound quickly, mechanical shearing or scrubbing forces can be applied. Most of these techniques cannot selectively remove necrotic tissue and are often discussed as a means of nonspecific debridement. One simple technique is scrubbing the necrotic tissue with a saline-moistened gauze or other type of sponge. Rather than using direct scrubbing on the wound, some clinicians will utilize hydrotherapy and irrigation. Hydrotherapy and wound irrigation are useful for softening and mechanic removal of eschar and debris. A recommended method is irrigation through a 19-gauge angiocath, or equivalent, to produce an optimal irrigation pressure. Too little pressure is ineffective in removal of necrotic tissue, whereas excessive pressure may drive bacteria into the wound. However, when very rapid debridement is required, for example with advancing infection, sharp debridement is indicated, and nonselective, mechanical debridement should be stopped.

Dextranomers

Dextranomers are small beads, 100 to 300 nm in diameter, produced by the combination of dextran and epichlorohydrin, a polymerizing agent. Dextranomers are promoted for wound debridement. The beads are poured into wet wounds. The highly linked dextran molecules (long chain polysaccharide) allow dextranomers to absorb a large quantity of water. One gram of dextranomer can absorb 4 ml of water. Water is absorbed faster than it is released into the wound. As water is absorbed, microbes, protein degradation products, fibrin, and other molecules are taken up by dextranomers. These beads are rinsed out of the wound and changed daily. Dextranomers are nontoxic and reduce inflammation. Dextranomers may have an additional benefit of absorbing odors.

Wet-to-Dry Dressings

The wet-to-dry dressing remains a very popular technique, but is largely used inappropriately. A moistened gauze sponge (frequently 4 inches x 4 inches) is placed into the necrotic area and is allowed to dry completely. The adherent necrotic tissue is pulled out of the wound with the 4 x 4. This procedure can be very painful and is nonspecific in that healthy tissue may be removed along with the necrotic tissue. Wet-to-dry dressings should be changed every 4 to 6 hours using adequate analgesia. Although sharp debridement is likely to produce a better outcome, wet-to-dry dressing removal done properly can provide rapid debridement to prepare a wound for operative repair or to prepare a patient for discharge to home when the wound is clean and stable.

Clinicians should avoid placing a dry dressing on granulation tissue. Removal of dry dressings from granulation tissue causes bleeding and damages the new tissue. Wet-to-dry dressings are not cost-effective for small wounds or wounds with little necrotic tissue, nor do they have any place in a facility where sharp debridement could be performed. Ethical considerations contraindicate wet-to-dry dressings unless a clear benefit to the patient can be demonstrated. Pain and the loss of healthy tissue must be

counterbalanced with an improved outcome such as earlier discharge from the hospital to meet ethical standards. The use of wet-to-dry dressings under circumstances in which a gentler method yields a similar outcome must be considered unethical. The purpose of the wet-to dry dressing is also undermined when clinicians soak the dressing off the wound. If a referral is received requesting a wet-to-dry dressing and the clinician determines that this approach is inappropriate, the clinician should arrange a discussion with the referring physician explaining the appropriate options. Sharp debridement is more selective and less likely to cause pain and damage to granulation tissue.

Hydrotherapy

A typical hydrotherapy session is carried out in a whirlpool tank (Figure 11-2) for 20 minutes with water at a temperature generally in excess of body temperature. Agitation is directed toward the wound requiring debridement. A number of benefits, but also a number of detrimental effects, have been described for whirlpool treatments. In addition, several of the benefits commonly ascribed to whirlpool treatment have no sound physiological basis. Benefits of whirlpool therapy include moisture to soften and agitation to loosen adherent necrotic tissue, increased temperature to increase blood flow and presumably increase metabolic rate, and proliferation of granulation tissue and epithelial cells.

Clear detrimental effects include maceration of surrounding skin, dependent position of the lower extremities, potential occlusion of venous and arterial vessels in a limb hung over the edge of a whirlpool tank, increasing the demand for blood flow in a limb with arterial insufficiency and increased damage to burned tissue by the elevated temperature of a whirlpool. Systemic effects include a drop in blood pressure in patients with compromised cardiovascular systems or those taking antihypertensive medications. In addition, the benefits listed above must be analyzed more critically in light of a particular patient. First, other methods of softening and loosening adherent necrotic tissue are available and these methods may actually be faster or more cost effective. Wounds on certain areas of the body are not accessible to the agitated water. Elevated temperature increases circulation to a limb with normal, healthy blood vessels. Increased temperature raises metabolic rate, which, in turn, increases release of mediators of increased blood flow to the area. This effect, however, only occurs in a person with the ability to dilate blood vessels appropriately. In a person with arterial insufficiency, demand for blood flow is increased with increasing tissue temperature, thereby aggravating the arterial insufficiency. Long exposure to water creates maceration and the removal of oil from the skin may subsequently cause dry, cracked skin. Although tanks and turbines are disinfected between patients, contamination may occur

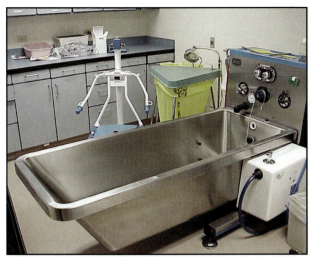

Figure 11-2A. Hydrotherapy tank typically used in wound care. The unit has a built-in water jet that allows the entire body to be submerged.

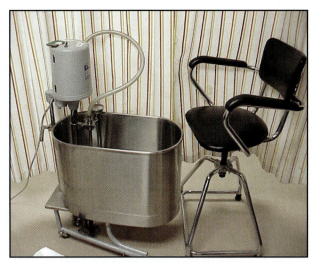

Figure 11-2B. Hand/foot tank may be used for wounds on the distal leg and foot and the distal forearm and hand.

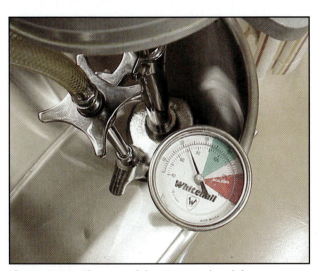

Figure 11-2C. Close-up of the air control and thermometer for the hand/foot unit.

between disinfection and patient treatment. *Pseudomonas aeruginosa* is particularly problematic with hydrotherapy. The presence of multiple wounds may result in cross-contamination. Moreover, as discussed in Chapter 2, growth of granulation tissue occurs most rapidly at normal body temperature. The elevated temperature of most whirlpools will not increase growth of tissue, but is more likely to retard growth. Temperature should be kept in a lower range between 92° and 96°F (33° and 35.5°C). Failing to pay attention to the temperature of water in the whirlpool may also lead to burns in individuals insensitive to temperature or cause deeper injury to an area that has been burned. Turbulence of the water in the whirlpool tank can aerosolize microbes and deposit them several feet away from the tank. Additives for infection control

discussed in Chapter 9 are frequently cytotoxic and may retard wound healing.

Contraindications and Precautions for Whirlpool Therapy

Patients with range of motion limitations or who exceed the weight limits of equipment such as lifts or chairs may not be able to get into a whirlpool tank. If any area of the body should not become wet such as a newly closed surgical incision, or the patient has a cast that cannot be protected from the water, an alternative treatment is needed. In addition, patients who are not allowed out of their rooms because of isolation or require a ventilator cannot be transported to a whirlpool tank. Patients may have allergies to additives to the whirlpool. Wounds that are actively bleeding or have proteinaceous exudate will cause large bubbles to form and possibly spill over the edge of the tank. A bottle of lotion or specific defoaming agent should be available during treatment. Because anything that is placed in a whirlpool tub may be deposited in the wound, patients with colostomies, gastrostomies, ileostomies, or incontinence should not be put in a full body tub. Care must be taken with central lines or other medical devices that pass through the skin. If possible, these areas are left out of the water and placed in a water-proof device such as a shoulder length glove. Otherwise, the patient should not be placed in the whirlpool tub. Even for patients without these issues, fecal material and bacteria and fungi from the rectum and genitalia may be deposited in the wound.

Pulsatile Lavage With Concurrent Suction

Pulsatile lavage devices offer a distinct advantage of portability. Patients in intensive care units, on isolation precaution, and those who are too difficult to move can be treated in their rooms. These devices operate under the same concept as carpet cleaners. They simultaneously irrigate with controllable pressure and remove excess fluid from the wound. This technique has become very popular and in many facilities, pulsatile lavage has totally or nearly replaced whirlpool treatments. Three major product manufacturers produce battery-operated devices. The AC pump device, Pulsavac (Zimmer, Ltd., Swindon, United Kingdom) was the first to gain widespread recognition. Zimmer also has a handheld, battery-operated portable version available. Versions of these devices are shown in Figures 11-3, 11-4, and 11-5. The original Pulsavac device was somewhat cumbersome to set up, requiring threading of tubing through the machine, but has been redesigned to improve its usability. Davol has a handheld battery-operated unit called the Simpulse (Davol Inc, Cranston, RI). The InterPulse (Stryker Instruments, Kalamazoo, MI) device is also a handheld, battery-operated unit.

Four basic components exist in all types of pulsatile lavage units—suction, adjustable pump, tip, and hand piece. Suction is provided by either wall suction or a portable pump (Figure 11-6). In the case of wall suction, a pressure regulator must be placed on the wall outlet. All hospital rooms have wall suction available and many have pressure regulators available in the rooms. In many outpatient locations, however, wall suction is not available. Portable pumps may be purchased for approximately $400. Often these are mounted onto a cart ($200), which can also be used to store supplies. A suction canister is placed between the pulsatile lavage unit and either the wall suction pressure regulator or the portable pump. The canisters are designed to collect fluid and prevent the movement of fluid into the suction pump. Setting up the suction aspect of the device does not require sterile technique and should be done before removing dressings from the patient. Hand pieces may have either fixed or variable settings. Placing the device into the variable mode allows the operator to vary the lavage pressure by altering the grip on the handle between high, medium, and low pressures or high and low settings. The fixed mode locks the lavage pressure into the high, medium, or low setting and requires the operator to depress a button to unlock the setting, similar to locking features on power tools such as drills.

As originally developed, all pieces of pulsatile lavage guns came directly in contact with either the patient or body fluids. These were designed for disposal with infectious waste. In the case of handheld, battery-operated units, everything used was to be thrown away after treatment. Although disposal of the complete unit was thought to be feasible for trauma surgery, reimbursement for non-surgical use made the devices cost-prohibitive if the hand piece could only be a single-use device. Battery-operated units have been redesigned with the suction tubing built into the disposable tip, rather than running through the

hand piece. With this arrangement, the hand piece can be reused on the same patient for multiple uses while the suction tubing, tip, and canister contents are discarded. Generally, a hand piece is reused until the batteries run down. It is then discarded and a new hand piece is used for the patient's next visit.

A variety of tips are available. Usually 2 sizes of tips with splash shields are available (Figures 11-3 and 11-4). A long flexible tip with a measuring guide is available for some models to allow lavage and suction of tunnels and tracts (Figure 11-5). The markings allow measurement of the depth of the tract or tunnel for evaluation purposes and to ensure that the tip is placed the correct distance into the defect for appropriate debridement. Splash shields are very flexible and their contours can be manipulated to approximate the shape of the wound. One hand is generally left on the tip to guide the tip across the surface of the wound with light pressure and to manipulate the shape of the splash shield to optimize cleansing. Manipulating the tip shape also minimizes the amount of fluid running out of the wound or being sprayed from the wound into the environment.

In addition to the obvious risk of splashing of fluid under pressure, fluid can become aerosolized and carry microbes a short distance. While using pulsatile lavage, PPE should be worn to minimize risks associated with splashing and aerosolization. A full mask or mask with built-in eye shield is preferred over separate mask and eye protection. The clinician's clothing needs to be protected to avoid transmitting anything that might be splashed or aerosolized during treatment (see Chapter 9). Several preparatory steps must be carried out before the actual process occurs. The bags of saline need to be warmed to skin temperature by approved methods. Some have proposed microwave ovens and others have used hot packs or blood warmers. The time required for microwave heating of saline bags varies with the size of the bag and power output of the microwave oven. Heating a 1-L saline bag with a typical small microwave oven is likely to require 1 to 1 1/2 minutes to reach body temperature. A biomedical engineer or technician can measure the temperature of saline bags to find the correct time. The patient needs to be draped appropriately, especially if the procedure is performed in the patient's bed. Sufficient clean towels are placed where fluid is likely to run off the patient and sterile towels are placed surrounding the wound. Also check the operation of the vacuum pump. You can put your hand over the end of the lavage tip to feel whether suction is adequate. You do not want to be surprised to find an inadequate vacuum source during the procedure. A plastic drape allowing visualization, but capable of containing splashes is supplied with the Davol Simpulse's tips. Some clinicians have developed their own drapes to contain fluid.

Figure 11-3. Inserting the tip on a pulsatile lavage hand piece.

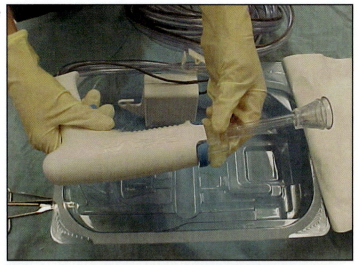

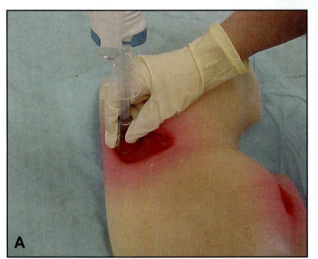

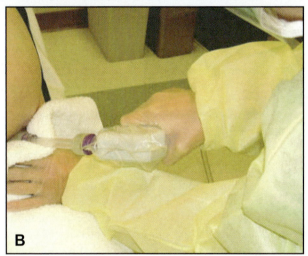

Figure 11-4. Use of a pulsatile lavage unit on a wound model. Note the one hand is used to both guide and contour the tip along the surface of the wound.

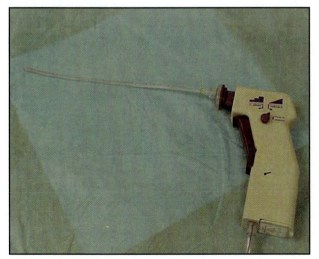

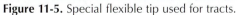

Figure 11-5. Special flexible tip used for tracts.

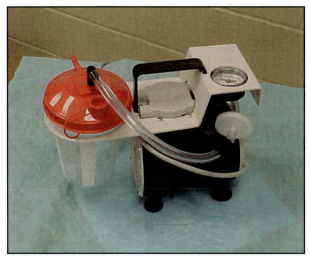

Figure 11-6. Example of a portable vacuum pump.

Table 11-1

Pulsatile Lavage Procedure

- Warm bags of sterile saline
- Drape patient
- Attach suction canister to regulator or portable pump
- Set the suction to desired vacuum and check for normal operation
- Hang bag(s) of saline
- Place hand piece and tip on sterile field
- Attach appropriate tip on hand piece
- Attach vacuum tubing to vacuum source
- Spike the bag(s)
- Remove lock pin if applicable
- Squeeze trigger to fill the incoming line with saline
- Begin lavage
- At end of procedure, release trigger
- Ensure wound is not full of fluid
- Turn off vacuum source and detach hand piece tubing from vacuum source
- Discard appropriate items in appropriate biohazard containers

The procedure should be explained thoroughly to the patient. Procedures for pulsatile lavage are listed in Table 11-1. The carpet cleaner analogy is generally sufficient. Any necessary medications should have been given to the patient in advance so that desired plasma concentrations exist at the time of the procedure. Topical application of local anesthetic may be used as needed by individual patients. The first step is attaching the suction canister to the vacuum source—either wall suction or a portable suction pump and set the regulator to the proper negative pressure. The bags of normal saline should be pre-warmed to skin temperature and hung on a pole to allow spiking. The hand piece is removed from the package and placed on a sterile field. The appropriate tip is then applied to the hand piece. The tip cannot be inserted incorrectly on the hand piece; it will only fit if the suction and spray are aligned properly. A different size or shape exists on the vacuum and spray openings. Identify the suction tubing coming from the hand piece and attach it to the vacuum canister on the port marked "patient" or "ortho." Another tube is attached between the suction pump and the port marked "suction." Next the tube running through the hand piece with a spike on its end is identified and inserted into a bag of sterile saline. Check for a lock pin on the hand piece before starting. The Davol Simpulse uses a black lock pin. Leaving the lock pin in place causes the tubing to fill as soon as the saline bag is spiked. The pin must be removed before saline runs out of the tip. The hand piece

trigger can be squeezed as the device is held over a water proof container until the tubing fills with sterile saline and begins to exit the tip. Care should be taken to prevent overfilling suction canisters. Be certain to select a large enough canister to hold a fixed volume of fluid used to irrigate the wound.

If a wound is smaller than the splash shield, no movement of the tip across the wound is necessary; however, making subtle changes in the direction of the pulsed fluid across the wound will enhance the shearing effect compared with holding the tip stationary. During the procedure, carefully follow the contours of the wound to avoid dragging the tip across the wound surface. Keep enough pressure to avoid leaking around the splash shield, but try to avoid hurting the patient by holding it down with too much pressure. The tip does not need to be moved briskly across the wound, but all areas that need lavage should be covered. Therefore, the tip may be held in various locations as opposed to scraping across the surface and inflicting pain. If the wound contour does not allow adequate suctioning, fluid will run out of the wound onto the patient as the towels become overwhelmed with fluid. If fluid leaks from under the splash shield, try to change the shape of the splash shield to prevent leakage. If that approach still causes fluid to leak around the splash shield, holding a towel around the splash shield will hold the fluid under it sufficiently to allow suction to carry the fluid out of the wound. This technique is demonstrated in Figure 11-4.

Also take care to avoid occluding the holes built into the splash shield. These holes allow air to be suctioned into the tip to prevent collapse of the tip and latching on to the wound, which may cause pain and bleeding. Latching on occurs on loose tissues that can be suctioned into the splash shield and block the holes in the splash shield. Two options for preventing latching are to maintain a finger tip under the splash shield so a continuous flow of air into the tip is ensured. The second method is stretching the loose tissue to pull it taut under the splash shield.

Flexible tips are used to irrigate and suction tunnels/tracts. To receive maximum effect, the flexible tip should also be moved within the tunnel/tract, rather than only irrigating the bottom. Careful probing of the wound ahead of time will allow the clinician to know how far to insert the tip. On occasion, the tip may not seem to go any farther. Clinicians will know to push the probe more if they already know how far it should go. Not knowing the depth of a tunnel, a clinician may have difficulty getting the tip into a tunnel and assume that the tunnel has closed. A flexible tip may need to be manipulated to maintain suction. A sound similar to that caused by a dentist's suction may be heard if suction is working well. The flexible tip can also latch onto the sides of a tunneling wound. If the irrigation solution runs out of the wound and no suctioning sound can be heard, give a gentle twist to permit suction to occur. With either type of tip, stop irrigation until the cause of fluid leakage can be determined.

Two potential issues to troubleshoot are the failure of fluid (effluent) to enter the suction canister and the failure of fluid to be pumped out of the hand piece. Effluent refers to the fluid coming off the wound to be captured in the suction canister. If the wound begins to fill with saline, stop the lavage and troubleshoot the lack of suction before excessive fluid spills out. Potential problems include not turning on the suction pump, incorrect placement of hoses, malfunction of the pump, and kinking or occlusion of a vacuum line. Suction canisters have a float valve that will seal off the suction source if too much volume enters the canister. The float valve prevents fluid entry into the pump itself. Suction will fail if the canister fills and the float valve inside the canister shuts off the suction source. This could happen if the canister is too small for the volume of saline used or by forgetting to replace a canister if a second bag of saline is used. Failure to hold the splash shield effectively over the wound can cause fluid to leak in spite of normal suction. Lack of fluid moving through the hand piece can be caused by twisting of the saline bag where the spike enters. If a bag is spiked by twisting only in one direction the supply line can recoil, causing the flexible area where the spike enters the bag to then twist and occlude. Lack of irrigation can also happen when one forgets to spike the second bag after the first is depleted and the suction canister is changed.

Following the procedure, lavage is terminated by releasing the trigger, moving the tip away from the patient in such a way as to minimize spilling fluid, and then the suction is discontinued. Do not turn off the suction pump with a glove that was used for the lavage procedure. Any tubing that has carried fluid from the wound must be discarded as well as the tip inserted into the hand piece. Suction canisters and saline bags are single use items. Regardless of how much saline is used or how much the canister is filled, these are to be discarded. Some suction canisters are permanent with disposable liners as opposed to a disposable canister. In that case, only the liner is discarded. Care should also be taken to avoid spilling the contents of the canister. The fluid within the suction canister is disposed of in a manner consistent with facility procedure. Facility procedure may allow the dumping of the contents in a sink or commode and the disposable canister in a biohazard bag. Another option is solidifying powder that forms a gel when added to the contents of the canister. A glass canister is placed in a container approved for return to central sterile supply after the fluid and liner are discarded.

Quantity of Saline and Number of Tips Used During Treatment

The amount of saline used depends on the size of the wound and the difficulty in removing necrotic tissue and debris. Although some clinicians might be tempted to use a single bag of saline for each patient, clinical judgment must be exercised and a reasonable quantity determined. In some cases, a full bag should not be used. Once the lavage stops removing necrotic tissue and debris, lavage should continue for a brief time to ensure that nothing else will be removed. For example, a small tract 4 cm deep might have copious purulent drainage and after 400 mL of lavage, the effluent is clear. Continuing to irrigate under pressure is unlikely to produce any further debridement, but it may instead damage healthy tissue within the wound and promote inflammation. On the other extreme, a person with confluent pressure ulcers of the sacrum and bilateral ischial tuberosities has a wound 20 cm across and ranging from 12 to 8 cm long. The wound bed is 60% covered in adherent yellow slough and drainage from the wound has been copious and yellow. Lavage with only 1 L of saline is unlikely to be as effective as 3 L. In addition, some patients will need lavage with both a splash shield and flexible tip. Patients with abscesses or pressure ulcers frequently have both large open areas and tracts. Sufficient saline should be used in both types of wounds and both tips should be used. Although the flexible tip does not suction well from a tract with a depth less than 3 cm, a splash shield tip is unlikely to be effective in debridement of a tract. In some cases such as dehiscent abdominal wounds, a tract runs between 2 openings of the wound. Lavage in one direction will demonstrate fluid running from the other opening. In such wounds, consider lavage from both directions to ensure that debris is not simply being forced to the other opening without being suctioned out of the wound. If one opening is higher than the other, consider lavage from the lower opening, then from the upper opening, to drive out any debris that might have lodged in the other end.

Frequency and Duration of Pulsatile Lavage Treatments

With the emphasis on earlier discharge from acute care hospitals, once a patient is referred for pulsatile lavage, the patient will likely be treated daily until discharge. In a small number of cases, the continued presence of foul odor and copious purulence dictates BID (twice daily) treatment. Pulsatile lavage may be discontinued during an inpatient stay under unusual circumstances. Possibilities include a wound that is already rather clean with very limited necrotic tissue, or a patient who has a protracted length of stay allowing treatment to reach its conclusion. Pulsatile lavage may be used to prepare a wound for grafting and treatment would be discontinued when the wound bed is deemed ready by the surgeon. Good communication between the clinician performing pulsatile lavage and those placing grafts is important to prevent premature grafting that fails because the wound is not ready. Pulsatile lavage may also be discontinued for surgical debridement and might be resumed after surgery. Again, good communication is important. A surgeon may assume that pulsatile lavage has been resumed when the clinician performing it has not been notified of the surgeon's desire to resume treatment.

For outpatients or those in longer-term care facilities, no hard rule for treatment frequency or duration exists. A patient with a large wound and a number of complications may need to be seen for several weeks, whereas a patient coming from a long inpatient stay might need very few treatments. The wound bed and the effluent from the pulsatile lavage should be described in documentation tying together the purpose of the treatment, the patient's condition, and need for continued treatment. Both persistent purulence and tissue necrosis should be considered. The discovery of a new tract or pocket of purulence should also be documented. Some insurance providers consider pulsatile lavage strictly as an instrument for debridement of necrotic tissue. The risk of not continuing treatment of a wound with persistent purulence must be emphasized. Without adequate documentation of the state of the wound, many treatment visits may be provided without reimbursement. Although a number of factors must be considered, a starting point for a plan of care is daily treatment for approximately 1 week, then every other day. Factors to be considered are the amount of necrotic

tissue, the amount of purulence, the quality of the effluent, and patient resources such as the patient's ability to care for the wound between treatments, transportation issues, and insurance coverage. A wound may have a bed that looks good to the unaided eye, but the canister contains tan, opaque effluent indicating a high bacterial burden that creates the risk of spread of infection. This wound should be treated at least daily. If a wound has mostly granulation tissue and only cloudy effluent, pulsatile lavage every other day is likely to be sufficient. When a wound is nearly or fully granulated and effluent is clear, wounds should show rapid reduction in size. When this occurs and the patient or care giver can manage cleansing and dressing changes, the patient should be discharged. Examples of effluent are shown in Figure 11-7.

Indications, Precautions, and Contraindications to Pulsatile Lavage

Pulsatile lavage with suction is a useful method of shearing bacteria and slough from the surface of wounds, including undermined areas and tracts. It is an excellent alternative to avoid the pitfalls of whirlpool treatments noted above. Pulsatile lavage can be directed to a specific site, therefore, fluid from one area of the body does not carry material into the wound. Because the devices are portable they can be taken to patients who cannot be transported. In some facilities, all pulsatile lavage treatments are done at bedside. Other facilities limit bedside treatment to those who cannot be transported due to use of a ventilator, isolation, or weight limits on transporting patients.

Pulsatile lavage does not replace sharp debridement, but is useful in conjunction with it. Pulsatile lavage is particularly good for neuropathic and venous ulcers, but is not useful over hard eschar. Irrigation and drainage wounds secondary to abscesses and dehiscent wounds are also good candidates, particularly where tunneling cannot be visualized between surface openings of dehiscent wounds. After surgical debridement of pressure ulcers and necrotizing fasciitis, pulsatile lavage can remove necrotic tissue that remains or that develops after surgical debridement.

No specific contraindications for pulsatile lavage have been described in the literature. As noted under indications for whirlpool, patients with burns or certain skin diseases over larger surface areas may be treated more effectively with whirlpool therapy instead of pulsatile lavage. Precautions for pulsatile lavage include use near internal organs and excessive bleeding. Care must also be taken with patients who have immune deficiencies. Such patients should wear face masks to avoid inhaling aerosolized microbes. Some facilities may require patients to wear face masks or require clinicians to use drapes that contain any aerosolization.

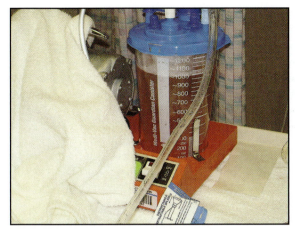

Figure 11-7A. Tan, opaque effluent demonstrating the need for at least daily treatment.

Enzymatic (Chemical) Debridement

Enzymatic debridement is indicated as an alternative for a patient who cannot tolerate sharp debridement or for the patient who has no time constraints or risk of infection and wishes an alternative to sharp debridement. This type of debridement may also be used in the acute care setting to complement other types of debridement. Enzymatic debridement works well in long-term facilities, home care, and outpatient settings, but only if the ulcer is not infected. The breakdown of tissue within the wound increases the risk of bacteria entering the circulation and causing sepsis. Because of the risk of sepsis with enzymatic debridement, the clinician needs to monitor for signs of sepsis. A more absorbent dressing must be used with enzymatic debridement such as a clean, moist dressing applied over the wound because of the increased drainage associated with enzymatic debridement as the chemical solubilizes the necrotic tissue. However, if moist dressings are left in place too long, they can desiccate and adhere to the wound. If the dressing becomes adherent, gentle irrigation to remove the adherent dressing is reasonable. Some clinicians use petrolatum-gauze products such as Adaptic (Johnson & Johnson, New Brunswick, NJ) or Xeroform (Kendall, Mansfield, MA) over the enzymatic debrider to minimize desiccation and adherence. Enzymatic debriders should be discontinued when the necrotic tissue is cleared from the wound, if signs of sensitivity are present, or the product fails to remove necrotic tissue within a 2-week trial period. These should also be discontinued in the presence of bacterial super-growth or tunneling to other body cavities. The use of enzymatic debriders is limited by the need for a physician's order and prescription.

At this time, collagenase and the combined preparation of the proteolytic enzyme papain with urea are the only chemicals available. Collagenase is effective because colla-

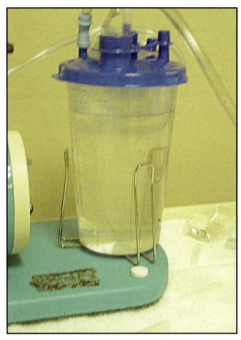

Figure 11-7B. Cloudy effluent demonstrating the need for every other day or 3 times per week treatment.

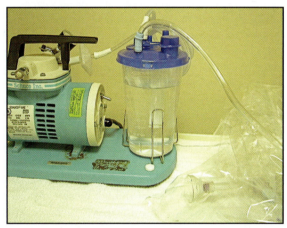

Figure 11-7C. Clear effluent suggesting re-evaluation of the need for continued pulsatile lavage.

gen makes up such a large proportion (75%) of dry weight of skin. Breakdown of collagen is generally believed to enhance migration of cells. Enzymatic debridement will be less effective if applied to wounds indiscriminately. Good results will only be obtained if the enzymatic debrider is used properly. Enzymes of any type are only effective within a certain range of pH and are inactivated by other chemicals and by a poor environment. Therefore, thorough cleansing of wounds should be done before application of enzymes. Because these proteins are effective only on the surface available to them, the clinician needs to crosshatch eschar to increase surface area. Crosshatching with a scalpel increases the number of edges of eschar over which the enzymatic debriders can function. When done properly, the enzyme converts one large mass of eschar into a large number of small areas of eschar that will lift off the wound or be solubilized. Enzymatic debriders require prescriptions from a physician; therefore, they are unlikely to be available at the first treatment session unless a physician writes a script before referring a patient.

Papain-Urea

Papain is a proteolytic enzyme obtained from the papaya. It degrades and liquifies nonviable proteins, including fibrin, collagen, and elastin. The urea component is stated to increase the effectiveness of papain by causing protein molecules of necrotic tissue to unfold, providing more area for papain to digest them. Papain-urea is applied twice daily following cleansing or debridement of the wound. For inpatients, nursing staff will need to provide at least one of the daily applications and for outpatients, the patient or a caregiver will need to administer the debrider application at least one each day, depending on the number of visits per week. Patients are instructed to wash their hands before and after applying papain-urea. When applied in a clinic, clinicians should not directly touch enzymatic debriders. They may be squeezed onto a tongue depressor or cotton-tipped applicator. Chemical debriders are to be applied directly to the wound and as much as possible, they should contact only necrotic tissue. Granulation tissue, any structures within the wound such as tendons or ligaments, and surrounding skin should be avoided. Usually saline-moistened gauze is applied over the enzymatic debrider, then a dry dressing to absorb drainage and protect the surrounding skin from maceration. A skin protectant may be needed on the surrounding skin, depending on the amount of drainage. Some patients may experience a painful or stinging sensation with application and some of them will not be able to tolerate papain-urea. In those cases, collagenase may be tried. Papain-urea is stored at room temperature away from moisture and heat. Papain-urea has the advantage of remaining active over a broader range of pH than collagenase. Papain-urea remains active within a pH range of 3 to 12, whereas collagenase is limited to a range of 6 to 8.

Papain-urea is available as Accuzyme, AllanEnzyme, Ethezyme 650, Ethezyme 830, Kovia, Pap-Urea, Ethezyme, Accuzyme SE, Kovia 6.5, and Paptase. One brand of papain-urea, Accuzyme contains a chlorophyllin-copper complex. The chlorophyll component is an effective deodorizer and, according to the manufacturer, this ingredient reduces fibrin formation and enhances the structural integrity of the deposited collagen matrix. This ingredient is also available in a spray as Accuzyme SE, which eliminates the need to make contact with the wound and may be less wasteful than application as an ointment. Papain-urea and papain-urea/chlorophyllin complex were removed from the 2008 Medicare Formulary Reference File (FRF), effective January 1, 2008. CMS removed all products without an approved FDA application. Collagenase ointment is the only enzymatic debrider listed on the 2008 Medicare Part D formulary file, which is likely to negatively impact the use of papain-urea in general.

Collagenase

This enzymatic debrider is available in a white petrolatum base as Santyl (Smith & Nephew, Largo, FL). The collagenase enzyme is produced by the bacterium *Clostridium histolyticum*. Collagenase may also produce erythema in some patients. Collagenase is indicated for enzymatic debridement in both chronic wounds and burn injuries. Collagenase is applied in the same manner as papain-urea onto necrotic tissue, but daily instead of twice per day. Collagenase may be applied a second time if the dressing becomes too wet. The manufacturer of Santyl states that topical antibiotic powder is to be applied to infected wounds prior to application of collagenase and collagenase is to be discontinued if infection does not respond to antibiotic powder. Hydrogen peroxide and heavy metals inactivate the enzyme. Topical medications and dressings containing silver must not be used with collagenase. Because the effectiveness of collagenase is limited to a pH of 6 to 8, acetic acid, Dakin's solution, or anything else with an extreme pH must not be present in the wound. Wounds need to be irrigated copiously to remove any acid or metal that might remain. Cleansing may be done with normal saline.

Autolytic Debridement

This type of debridement relies on the ability of the clinician to trap endogenous enzymes in an optimized environment by using occlusive dressings. The wound environment is also optimized by filling cavities loosely to prevent abscess formation, but not tightly to prevent granulation. If the wound is dry, the clinician should hydrate the wound to allow enzymes access throughout the wound bed. For a dry wound, a combination of hydrogel and film may be used as long as the surrounding skin does not become macerated. Foam or hydrocolloid dressings may be used to promote autolytic debridement in cases of greater drainage. However, occluding a wound for several days in an effort to promote autolytic debridement creates an exudate that others may mistake for pus. Others may need to show that the exudate simply rinses away and no odor remains with irrigation. Autolytic debridement is another alternative for the patient who cannot tolerate sharp debridement or other methods, but who also has no time constraints or risk of infection. Because the wound must be occluded with a synthetic dressing and occlusion promotes the growth of bacteria, autolytic debridement is contraindicated in infected ulcers.

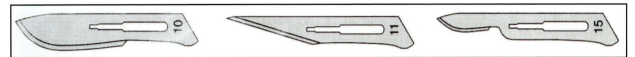

Figure 11-8. Scalpel blades commonly used for sharp debridement.

Sharp Debridement

The method of choice with risk of infection or progression of infection is sharp debridement. It may also be the method of choice for removing large quantities of necrotic tissue rapidly. This method may not be suitable for some individuals. In particular, this method needs to be used with caution in patients with bleeding disorders or anticoagulation. Sharp debridement is the most efficient means of removing necrotic tissues. However, it is also very demanding of resources including training of the clinician, tools, cost, and possibly the need for an operating or special procedures room. The person performing this procedure must have special credentials, training, and licensure. Those typically allowed to perform sharp debridement include physicians, physician's assistants, physical therapists, and advanced practice nurses. These individuals are required to have licenses issued by individual states. In addition, payers may require evidence of advanced training to receive reimbursement for sharp debridement. State practice acts may limit which healthcare providers are allowed to perform sharp debridement and may list additional requirements. Note that organizations such as the American Physical Therapy Association (APTA) have issued position statements regarding appropriate clinicians for performing sharp debridement. The APTA has taken a position that regardless of state practice acts that may allow physical therapist assistants to perform sharp debridement, it is only to be performed by physical therapists and not by physical therapist assistants because of differences in their education, particularly cadaver-based gross anatomy.

Sharp Debridement in the Operating Room

In certain cases, sharp debridement needs to be performed by a surgeon. These cases include those in which the procedure may cause severe pain, if extensive debridement is required, if the degree of undermining/sinus tract/tunneling is undetermined, if bone must be removed, if debridement must be done near vital organs, or the patient is septic. Surgical debridement should also be considered if the patient is immunosuppressed.

Bedside Debridement

In cases other than those described above, clinicians other than surgeons may perform the procedure. Tools typically used include curved scissors, forceps, curettes, scalpels with #11, #15, or #10 blades (Figure 11-8), silver nitrate sticks, and local anesthetic. The clinician may choose to use either lidocaine or benzocaine spray, lidocaine gel or eutectic mixture of local anesthetic (EMLA) cream, which consists of 2.5% lidocaine and 2.5% prilocaine. The clinician should create an optimal environment for the procedure including appropriate lighting, positioning, and infection control. Visibility of the wound is easily taken for granted. A procedure light and magnifiers greatly enhance the ability to discern colors and details in the wound bed. A comfortable position for both the patient and clinician should be assumed to prevent fatigue or other problems in both the patient and the clinician. Debridement is done with the principles of sterile technique. Sterile instruments must be used. Examination or sterile gloves may be used, depending on facility policy and the immune status of the patient.

Basic Techniques

In all cases, sharp debridement should be considered a highly selective form of debridement. As such, the clinician should endeavor to minimize damage to healthy tissue. Bleeding may obscure the clinician's vision. Because of the risk of bleeding during this procedure, the clinician should start debridement at the bottom of the wound and work toward the top. Other considerations include working from the center of the wound where the wound is less sensitive to pain to its periphery, which is more likely to be sensitive. A general rule to follow is to debride the areas likely to bleed or to be painful last. On occasion, these 2 rules may be in conflict. If so, consider how repositioning may allow both of these areas to be performed last. These problems can be minimized by using local anesthesia to reduce pain and silver nitrate sticks to stop bleeding.

Another consideration is to stay within a given plane to avoid spreading bacteria into lower layers. If a fascial plane is reached, one must stop and reassess the situation to determine whether deeper debridement is needed. Following sharp debridement with a high risk of bleeding, a dry dressing should be placed on the wound for 8 to 24 hours if significant bleeding occurs during the procedure. The wound may need to be packed (discussed in Chapter 12) more tightly to maintain hemostasis. The dressing may later be changed to an appropriate occlusive dressing (see Chapter 12). In many cases a wound may only require a single sharp debridement procedure. However, several procedures may be required for a number of reasons. Stopping may become necessary because of excessive pain or bleeding, fatigue of the clinician, or the patient

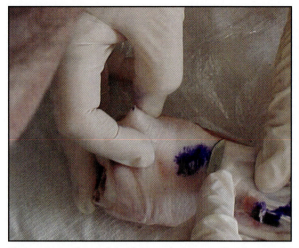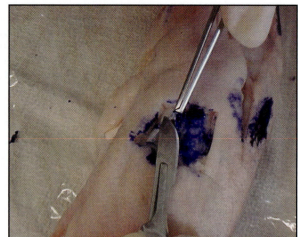

Figure 11-9. Sharp debridement being practiced on a pig's foot.

says to stop. Debridement may be continued later, particularly with a large wound, a wound with painful areas, and wounds that bleed. Moreover, areas that appeared to be viable one day may be necrotic the next day, requiring further debridement. Other forms of debridement may be necessary in addition to sharp debridement to prepare a wound for surgical closure or transfer of the patient's care. Wounds with excessive bioburden, but little necrotic tissue may require several days of pulsatile lavage with periods of sharp debridement. During debridement, care must be taken to avoid cutting into undermined or tunneled areas and in areas of purulent drainage where visibility is compromised. The clinician should never cut what cannot be seen. Reasons to stop debridement include exposure of tendons, bones, and blood vessels, excessive bleeding, the patient can no longer tolerate debridement, and the clinician's judgment. Because each compartment surrounded by fascia has its own blood supply and because fascia acts as a barrier for bacterial penetration, the clinician must pause and assess whether deeper debridement is warranted if a fascial plane is reached.

Instruments

Sharp debridement requires the use of PPE both to protect the clinician from body fluids and to protect the wound from contaminants on the clinician. The face should be protected with either a mask with built-in eye shield or a face shield. A cap, gown, and gloves are also needed. One may become complacent after debriding many wounds having never experienced any splash or spray from a wound. Unfortunately, the cost of one incident of blood splattering in a clinician's eye greatly exceeds any costs of being prepared. In a similar vein, a clinician who has been wearing PPE for pulsatile lavage might be tempted to take off this PPE before performing some minor sharp debridement. The risk of contamination

greatly outweighs any benefit of improving the clinician's comfort by removing PPE.

Instruments used for the procedure may include scissors, forceps, scalpel, curette, and hemostats. Scalpels should be used sparingly; they can cause too much inadvertent cutting and are difficult for the novice to control. However, they are useful for trimming callus and scoring eschar. An individual should have substantial experience in using a scalpel in a safe setting such as practice on a pig's foot (Figure 11-9) and scoring eschar and trimming callus before using a scalpel on the edges of necrotic tissue.

Forceps and scissors are available in a disposable suture removal kit or good quality surgical instruments may be obtained (see Figure 11-10). Although the initial cost of good surgical-quality instruments and cost of repeated sterilization following each procedure may influence administrators to choose disposable forceps and scissors, these instruments have such poor quality that they are not suitable for sharp debridement. If quality surgical instruments are used frequently the initial cost becomes offset to a large degree by their durability. Forceps that will hold tissue securely cost $40 or more and have the added cost of sterilization each time they are used. Forceps should minimally have serrated tips. Adson and other types of forceps with teeth on the tips will hold tissue better.

Scissors with good quality cutting edges are even more expensive and can cost $30 for small scissors up to $80 or more. Several types of scissors are used by clinicians. Scissors may have blunt tips, sharp tips, or one sharp and one blunt tip (blunt/blunt, sharp/sharp, or blunt/sharp, respectively). Curved scissors are preferred to flat scissors for two reasons. When cutting with the tips of curved scissors up, less risk of accidental injury by the tips occurs. When cutting with the tips down, cutting can be performed in a tighter area. Although the novice may wish to start with a pair of blunt/blunt curved scis-

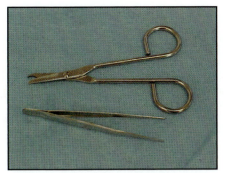

Figure 11-10A. Instruments used for sharp debridement: suture removal kit.

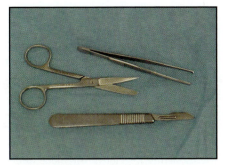

Figure 11-10B. High quality reusable surgical instruments suitable for sharp debridement.

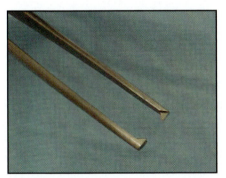

Figure 11-10C. Close-up of toothed tissue forceps. The teeth improve the handling of necrotic tissue.

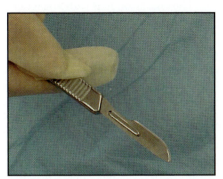

Figure 11-10D. Close-up of a #10 scalpel blade on a #3 handle, showing proper handling.

sors because of the safety issue, more experienced clinicians may prefer curved sharp/sharp iris scissors. Because iris scissors are smaller, the clinician is able to reach into tighter areas of the wound.

An alternative to using iris scissors in tight locations is a curette. A curette can scoop underneath adherent necrotic tissue, avoiding the awkward manipulation of scissors and forceps in a tight area, or trying to pick up adherent necrotic tissue with forceps and cut under it with scissors. Curettes come in a variety of sizes and composition. Sterilizable metal curettes have better cutting properties. Cheap dermal curettes with a metal loop do not cut as well as more expensive plastic versions. The curette works well with a technique similar to making melon balls. Holding the curette as a pencil, supination of the forearm cuts under adherent necrotic tissue.

Scalpel blades, like scissors, are available in several different types and operator preference plays a large role in the type used. The type of blade is identified by a number. Blades may have curved or straight cutting edges and are available in different sizes. Blade type may be selected based on particular tasks. In addition, different number blades fit onto different types of handles (also identified by number). Both the #3 and #7 handles fit a series of useful

blades for working in tight areas: the smaller #10, #11, and #15 blades. The #3 handle is familiar to most people. It is shaped to fit in the palm of the hand as well as being held with a pencil-like grip and has a serrated portion to aid grip with the thumb and index finger. The #7 handle also fits these blades, but it is a thinner handle and may not be as easy to grasp for the novice. The #4 handle fits the larger # 20, #21, #22, and #23 blades. The smaller #10 blade and larger #20 blade are versatile with a rounded cutting edge. The #11 blade has a triangular blade with a straight cutting edge and narrow tip. The #15 blade due to its small size is quite versatile. It has a curved cutting edge similar to a #10 blade, but is much smaller. It can fit into tighter areas, but will dull faster.

Any of the blades can be used for the basic sharp debridement techniques of scoring, shaving, and cutting, but some blades are better suited for certain tasks. The #11 blade with its straight cutting edge can be more difficult to handle for scoring or other cuts perpendicular to the surface, whereas the #10, #20, or #15 blades allow a more natural wrist and finger flexion motion for scoring. For shaving, a #11 blade can be used effectively for the sawing type of motion parallel to the surface. Curved blades do not supply as much cutting edge for this maneuver.

For fine work, a #15 blade works nicely, but because of its size it is not suitable for removal of a large amount of easily accessible necrotic tissue because it has a short cutting edge and dulls rapidly. Eventually, most clinicians will likely develop a personal preference for either a #10 or #11 blade. Just like scissors and forceps, scalpels may be either disposable or reusable. In either case, the blades are discarded after each use. Disposable scalpels come with blades already attached and both handle and blade are discarded without having to remove the blade, reducing the risk of injury by removing blades. In addition, disposable scalpels are very cost effective with a low purchase price and avoiding the cost and inconvenience of sterilizing the handles. The risk associated with changing blades is reduced by changing the blade with either hemostats or preferably, a scalpel blade remover available from surgical instrument suppliers. Because sterile technique is followed during sharp debridement, scalpel packages will need to be opened ahead of time or by another individual not involved in the sterile technique.

Bleeding

Bleeding is largely unavoidable if sharp debridement is to be accomplished effectively. Although necrotic tissue does not bleed, small viable blood vessels may still carry blood through necrotic tissue. Creating bleeding is not a requirement for good sharp debridement, but if some bleeding does not occur, some necrotic tissue will likely be left in the wound. With careful debridement, bleeding is usually stopped easily. Hemostasis is only problematic when clearly healthy tissue is cut or the patient is using anticoagulants or has a bleeding disorder. Sharp debridement may be done on patients at risk for excessive bleeding. Regardless of the reason, all bleeding during sharp debridement will stop eventually. With appropriate hemostatic measures, the amount of bleeding is usually insignificant from a hemodynamic standpoint. Several means are available to promote hemostasis. Silver nitrate sticks are similar to cotton-tipped applicators, with a small amount of silver nitrate on their tip, rather than cotton. They need to be touched briefly to small bleeds and may need to be moistened slightly with saline. Flushing the rest of the wound with saline minimizes the damage done to other areas of the wound. Pressure may be applied with a small piece of alginate dressing. For larger bleeds, pressure may need to be applied with 4 x 4 cotton gauze sponges. Copious bleeding may occur during the first visit of an inpatient after surgery. Blood-soaked dressings should cue the clinician that bleeding may still be occurring or may be easily initiated. In such cases, one should carefully remove any packing in the wound and be prepared to address any bleeding. Irrigate with normal saline if necessary to prevent tearing the wound bed with an adherent dressing and causing more bleeding.

Anatomic Considerations

Although debridement may be required on any body part, it tends to be needed more commonly in a few locations. These locations include common areas for pressure ulcers, such as the sacrum, ischial tuberosity, greater trochanter, and sites common for neuropathic ulcers such as the metatarsal heads. A particular concern is avoiding damage to flexor tendons of the foot. Knowledge gained from a cadaver-based anatomy course equips the clinician to navigate among important structures located in any region of the body. The clinician will be able to envision the location of arteries, veins, nerves, tendons, ligaments, and fascial boundaries. Knowledge of fascial compartments is particularly important in locating likely areas for tracts to form and where to direct pulsatile lavage to clear these tracts.

Low Frequency Ultrasonic Debridement

New devices have been developed that utilize ultrasound in the kHz range. This frequency of ultrasound allows energy to be focused on a small area. Nonviable tissue is destroyed with no appreciable injury to healthy tissue. Ultrasound may be transmitted by near contact with a probe (Sonoca, Söring, Quickborn, Germany) that constantly drips water that acts as the conductive medium for the ultrasound. These devices operate on the principle of cavitation created by the ultrasound. Cavitation destroys bacteria and fibrin deposits while penetrating into fissures within the wound bed. A variety of tips are available to suit the shape of the wound. The hand pieces are interchangeable and may be autoclaved after use. No consumable supplies are used other than normal saline; however, the device is very expensive (about $30,000). The Sonoca operates at 25 kHz. Intensity is adjustable, but frequency is not. The cost may be offset by the increased efficiency of debridement. The device has 3 modes. The contact mode as the name implies involves touching the wound with the tip to provide more energy. The noncontact mode is designed for more sensitive tissues. The dipped mode is used for wounds that can be filled with fluid such as deep wounds and subcutaneous defects that can be filled with fluid. The ultrasonic energy is transmitted through the fluid.

MIST (Celleration, Eden Prairie, MN) is a low-frequency, noncontact ultrasound device. The fluid is driven through the device onto the wound bed as a mist that vibrates at the frequency determined by the device. Celleration claims MIST to be a bioactive therapy that promotes wound healing at the same time that it removes bacteria, fibrin, and slough. The Sonoca device is considered to be high intensity, low frequency, whereas MIST is considered to be low intensity, low frequency ultrasound. Both manufacturers claim their devices to be painless, fast, and easy to use. Although the MIST device is somewhat less expensive, it uses consumable hand pieces that greatly increase the cost of treatment. To offset this cost, a new Category III CPT code 0183T is effective January 2008 for "low frequency, noncontact, nonthermal ultrasound, including topical application(s) when performed, wound assessment, and instruction(s) for ongoing care, per day."[1] Category III codes are temporary CPT codes designed specifically for emerging technologies. Celleration states that their device is the only low frequency ultrasonic device approved by the FDA for wound healing. Arobella Medical produces a low frequency device that combines sharp debridement. The Qoustic Curette (Arobella Medical, LLC, Minnetonka, MN) transmits low frequency ultrasound while the curette is used to debride sharply (Figure 11-11).

Jetox

Another approach to debridement is the technology of the Jetox-ND and Jetox-HDC instruments (TavTech, Ltd., Yehud, Israel). The Jetox-HDC was designed to more effectively treat difficult to debride wounds. This device sprays microdroplets of saline solution with a concentrated airstream. The microdroplets range in size from 5 to 100 µm and travel at supersonic speed (about 200 m/s). Jetox-ND is a lightweight, disposable, hand held device that uses compressed oxygen, saline bags, and a special nozzle to create its effect. The Jetox-HDC incorporates a suction component not present on the Jetox-ND. The microdroplets can be aimed precisely at necrotic tissue. The manufacturer states that the spray creates a peeling effect on necrotic tissue without injuring viable tissue beneath. Due to the nature of the spray, the treated area does not become covered with a layer of fluid as it does with other technologies—including pulsatile lavage and low frequency ultrasound—which allows for continuous loosening and removal of necrotic tissue. This device was developed in Israel and is distributed in the United States by DeRoyal.

The Jetox device (ND or HDC) is simply attached to an oxygen source by a luer connection. The Jetox-HDC is attached to a suction source, and a bag of saline is spiked. The valve to the oxygen source is opened and adjusted, depending on patient tolerance and condition of the wound. Contact is made between the Jetox tip and the area of the wound to be debrided. Treatment is continued until the wound is considered sufficiently clean. PPE must be worn during treatment as in any debridement procedure. When treatment is complete, the oxygen source and suction are turned off and the wand and tubing are discarded.

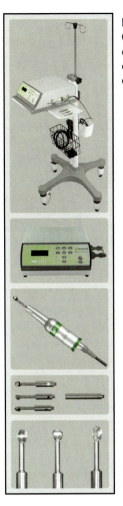

Figure 11-11. Arobella Medical's Qoustic Curette low frequency device that combines sharp debridement and ultrasonic debridement.

WHEN NOT TO DEBRIDE

Not all necrotic tissue needs to be debrided. Specific examples include stable heel wounds and severe arterial insufficiency. In addition, technical issues need to be considered. General guidelines for not debriding heel wounds include eschar that is firmly adherent, lack of inflammation of surrounding tissue, lack of drainage from below the eschar, and eschar that does not feel soft or boggy. Small wounds a few mm to cm with eschar may heal just as rapidly without debridement. Necrotic tissue caused by arterial insufficiency should not be debrided. In these wounds, a lack of blood flow not only retards healing, but prevents the immune system's handling of bacteria that may enter the wound. Moreover, exposure of necrotic tissue to surface bacteria presents the risk of potentially serious infection. As a general rule, the clinician should never debride what cannot be seen. As tempting as rapidly removing what is believed to be necrotic tissue may be, the clinician risks not only damage to healthy tissue, but also introducing bacteria into the blood. Reasons to stop debridement include exposure of tendons, bones, and blood vessels, penetration of a

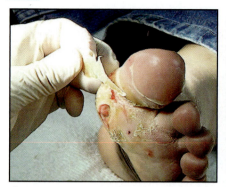

Figure 11-12A. Examples of wounds requiring debridement. Extensive callus on plantar surface of diabetic foot. A combination of peeling and shaving was used to remove callus.

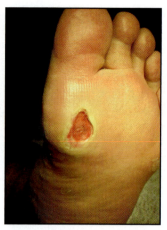

Figure 11-12B. Foot debrided of callus after multiple visits.

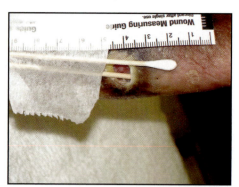

Figure 11-12C. Pocketing with nonviable tissue over pocketed area. All tissue overlying cotton-tipped applicator required debridement.

fascial plane, excessive bleeding, the patient can no longer tolerate debridement, and the clinician's decision to stop. On occasion, debridement beyond fascia may be required. Only physicians are licensed to cut healthy tissues; therefore, if a sinus tract or tunnel needs to be deroofed, the patient should be referred to a surgeon. Sharp debridement requires greater skill and, in some states, may require certain credentials and documented training.

LARVA THERAPY

The use of maggots (fly larvae) for tissue debridement has been traced to the Civil War. At that time, wound infection was a major cause of mortality. Wounds infested with maggots appeared to have a lower rate of infection and mortality than those that did not. The use of maggots declined with the introduction of antibiotics, but has survived and enjoyed a recent resurgence. Maggots used for wound debridement are sterile larvae of blowfly that can be obtained from specialized laboratories. The cost is approximately $75 per bottle of 200 maggots. Appropriate wounds include any chronic wound that does not require surgical intervention for debridement. Any wound for which autolytic or enzymatic debridement are suitable may be treated with maggots. Maggots perform highly selective debridement of necrotic tissue as well as maintaining a suitable level of bacteria in the wound. A number of protocols for using maggots have been developed. The maggots need to be contained over the wound and not allowed to migrate. They are typically left in place for 48 to 72 hours, so they need to be held in place securely. One approach is to use 2 hydrocolloid sheets. A hole approximating the size of the wound is cut in the first hydrocolloid sheet and applied around the wound. The bottle of maggots is applied to the wound and covered with a mesh material. A second hydrocolloid sheet, also with a hole in

it, is placed over the first to secure the mesh in place. The top hydrocolloid sheet is removed and discarded with the maggots and mesh between layers. The bottom hydrocolloid sheet is left. The procedure is repeated up to twice per week until the wound bed is completely debrided. Two to 6 applications may be necessary.

SUMMARY

The process of debridement is preceded by the development of a plan of care addressing why debridement is necessary and which method is most suited to reach the outcomes outlined. Examples of wounds requiring debridement are shown in Figure 11-12. Four types of debridement are described. Sharp, mechanical, enzymatic (chemical), and autolytic debridement are options determined based on the characteristics of the wound, characteristics of the patient and the facility and time constraints placed on wound debridement. In many cases, sharp debridement is preferred to manage risk of infection. Sharp debridement requires the use of sharp instruments to cut along the border between viable and necrotic tissue and a high skill level. Mechanical means of debridement include use of hydrotherapy, scrubbing, and irrigation. Autolytic debridement is a means of allowing the wound to clean itself with endogenous enzymes under an occlusive dressing. Enzymatic debridement involves the use of commercially produced enzymes requiring a physician's prescription to degrade necrotic tissue. Autolytic and enzymatic debridement are useful when time constraints and infection are not issues. Debridement is not performed on dry gangrene caused by arterial insufficiency and may not be necessary for stable heel ulcers. Sharp debridement is the preferred method for rapid removal of necrotic tissue, especially in cases of high risk of infection or neuropathic ulcers. Cutting is performed along the

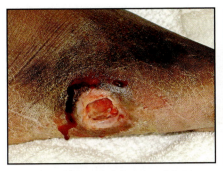

Figure 11-12D. Foot following debridement of waxy, necrotic tissue from foot in 11-12C. Debridement was performed by shaving waxy tissue with scalpel. Edges of viable tissue beveled.

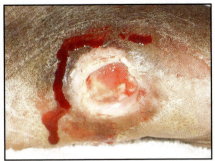

Figure 11-12E. Close-up of same foot as 11-12C and 11-12D. Note bleeding from edges of viable tissue.

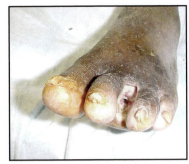

Figure 11-12F. Necrotic tissue appearing in third ray amputation. Although all apparent necrotic tissue is removed in surgery, tissue unable to survive following surgery appears as in photo and requires further debridement.

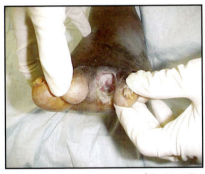

Figure 11-12G. Same wound in 11-12F following sharp debridement of necrotic tissue. Wound needs to be examined the following day for the appearance of further necrotic tissue requiring debridement.

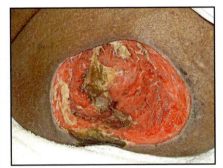

Figure 11-12H. Pressure ulcer over right greater trochanter. Yellow slough present at 12:00, 3:00, and scattered throughout; black eschar at 9:00; note necrosis of greater trochanter surface.

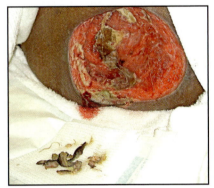

Figure 11-12I. Same wound as 11-12H following one episode of sharp debridement. Eschar and slough removed with scissors are shown in foreground.

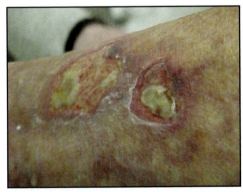

Figure 11-12J. Slough from leg wound removed by combination of pulsatile lavage and sharp debridement with forceps, scissors, and curette.

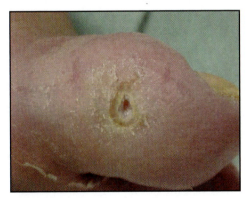

Figure 11-12K. Callus around wound on great toe, which was removed by peeling using forceps.

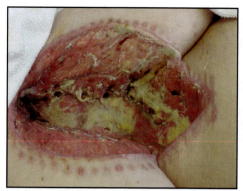

Figure 11-12L. Adherent yellow slough in dehiscent sternal wound. Slough removed by pulsed lavage, sharp debridement, and hydration of wound bed.

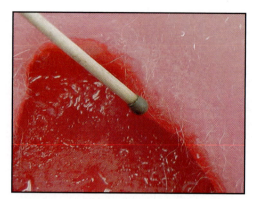

Figure 11-12M. Silver nitrate stick used in debridement and hemostasis. Tip is wet with normal saline and touched to area requiring debridement or hemostasis. Wound is then flushed with normal saline to remove residual silver nitrate.

margins between necrotic and viable tissue and bleeding is likely to occur. Bleeding may need to be controlled by silver nitrate sticks, alginate, or gauze. Dry dressings are placed on bleeding wounds for several hours to prevent hematoma formation.

QUESTIONS

1. What considerations are made before deciding to debride?

2. What are the major reasons for performing sharp debridement?

3. Why might autolytic debridement be preferred by some patients?

4. What is the rationale for not debriding dry gangrene?

5. Under what circumstances might hydrotherapy be a preferred method of debridement?

6. Discuss problems in using hydrotherapy for wounds caused by arterial insufficiency, venous insufficiency, and burns.

7. What are some of the major advantages of using pulsatile lavage? Disadvantages?

8. Name contraindications for bedside sharp debridement.

9. Under what circumstances is sharp debridement likely to require multiple sessions? Single sessions?

10. List advantages of #10, #11, and #15 scalpel blades.

11. List advantages and disadvantages of using iris scissors.

12. What are the advantages of curved scissors with blunt tips?

REFERENCE

1. 2009 Annual Update to the Therapy Code List. Available at http://www.cms.hhs.gov/transmittals/downloads/R1625CP.pdf Accessed September 9, 2009.

BIBLIOGRAPHY

AHCPR Supported Clinical Practice Guidelines. Available at: http://www.ncbi.nlm.nih.gov/books/bv.fcgi?rid=hstat2.section.4521. Accessed September 9, 2009.

APTA: Procedural interventions exclusively performed by physical therapists. HOD P06-00-30-36 (Program 32) [Position] http://www.apta.org/AM/Template.cfm?Section=Policies_and_Bylaws&TEMPLATE=/CM/ContentDisplay.cfm&CONTENTID=25681. Accessed September 25, 2009.

Arnall DA. Enzymatic debriders in wound care management. *Acute Care Perspectives.* 2000;8(2):12-21.

Callam MJ, Harper DR, Dale JJ, Ruckley CV, Prescott RJ. A controlled trial of weekly ultrasound therapy in chronic leg ulceration. *Lancet.* 1987;2(8552):204-206.

Eriksson SV, Lundeberg T, Malm M. A placebo controlled trial of ultrasound therapy in chronic leg ulceration. *Scand J Rehabil Med.* 1991;23(4):211-213.

Irion GL. Sharp debridement and consequences of coding and the APTA position statement. *Acute Care Perspectives.* 2000;8(2):1-6.

Johannsen F, Gam AN, Karlsmark T. Ultrasound therapy in chronic leg ulceration: a meta-analysis. *Wound Repair Regen.* 1998;6(2):121-126.

Peschen M, Weichenthal M, Schopf E, Vanscheidt W. Low-frequency ultrasound treatment of chronic venous leg ulcers in an outpatient therapy. *Acta Derm Venereol.* 1997;77(4):311-314.

Robson MC, Mannari, RJ, Smith PD, et al. Maintenance of wound bacterial balance. *Am J Surg.* 1999;178:399-402.

Schultz GS, Sibbald RG, Falanga V, et al. Wound bed preparation: a systematic approach to wound management. *Wound Repair Regen.* 2003;11(suppl 1):S1-28.

Dressings

12

OBJECTIVES

- List basic purposes of dressings.
- Distinguish desired characteristics for dressing acute and chronic wounds.
- Discuss appropriate conditions for occluding wounds.
- List types of nonocclusive dressings; discuss appropriate conditions for nonocclusive dressings.
- Discuss properties of different types of occlusive and semi-occlusive dressings including hydrogels, semipermeable film, hydrocolloids, alginate, hydrofibers, and composites.
- Discuss appropriate conditions for using each type of occlusive dressing.
- Describe alternatives for individuals who cannot tolerate adhesives.
- Discuss the types of secondary dressings and list purposes for using them.
- Discuss different types of tape relative to their appropriate use, including use on fragile skin.
- Describe the purposes of drains, retention sutures, and Montgomery straps.
- Remove sutures and staples.

Throughout history man has placed a wide variety of substances in, over, and on wounds in an effort to improve healing. Today, we enjoy a wide variety of materials that may be used as wound dressings. Clinicians are expected to make decisions concerning the optimal dressing for each patient. Each decision made in choosing a wound dressing must be based on a combination of many factors: pathophysiology of the wound, ease of use by patients, amount and quality of drainage, presence or absence of infection, depth, social and economic issues, and the properties of the dressing. Clinician preference, cost, and the opinion of a manufacturer's representative should not be determining factors. The purpose of this chapter is to develop a decision-making process by which a wound dressing may be chosen. More important, the process includes deciding when to use a different type of dressing as the wound and other factors may change. Four categories of products must be considered for their appropriateness on any given wound: dressings that cover wounds, dressings that fill wounds, products to protect the surrounding skin, and secondary dressings to hold dressings in place.

PURPOSES OF WOUND DRESSINGS

Armed with an understanding of the cause of the wound and possible complicating factors, we can begin

Irion G.
Comprehensive Wound Management, 2nd ed. (pp 223-246)
© 2010 SLACK Incorporated

Table 12-1

Purposes of Dressings

- Physical protection of wound, prevention of contamination
- Promote autolytic debridement
- Retain warmth, moisture, cells, enzymes, and growth factors in wound bed
- Fill dead space to prevent formation of hematomas, abscesses, tunnels, sinus tracts
- Management of drainage by absorption, evaporation, or occlusion

Table 12-2

Categories of Dressings Recognized by CMS

- Hydrogels: sheets
- Biologicals and synthetic membranes
- Impregnated
- Collagens
- Silicone gel sheets
- Contact layers
- Silver technology
- Elastic gauzes
- Transparent films
- Wound fillers

- Gauzes and nonwoven dressings
- Liquid skin protectants
- Hydrocolloids
- Moisture barriers
- Hydrogels: amorphous
- Therapeutic moisturizers
- Hydrogels: impregnated dressings
- Skin substitutes
- Oxygen reconstituted cellulose

the process of selecting a wound dressing. The next step is to understand the purposes, first of dressings in general, then the properties and purposes of specific classes of dressings. As we will see, even within a class of dressings, substantial differences in properties may make one brand of dressing more appropriate than another. Starting with the simplest purpose, dressings serve to physically protect the wound from the external environment and prevent contamination. Dressing selection usually differs between acute and chronic wounds. With acute wounds, the greatest concerns are infection and hematoma formation. In contrast, chronic wounds are usually colonized, although contamination with microbes new to the wound increases the risk of infection. The major concern with chronic wounds is optimizing the wound's microenvironment without compromising the integrity of the surrounding skin. A second purpose for dressings is promoting breakdown and removal of necrotic tissue. A third purpose is filling dead space in a wound to prevent the formation of hematomas, abscesses, tunnels, and sinus tracts. Managing drainage, whether purulent exudate or serous transudate, is

a fourth purpose. Dressings that hold fluid within wounds (occlusive and semi-occlusive dressings) promote healing by maintaining moisture, retaining growth factors and enzymes, and allowing autolytic debridement. Purposes for dressings are listed in Table 12-1

CLASSIFICATIONS OF DRESSINGS

Dressings may be classified by the way they are used to manage drainage. Categories of dressings recognized by CMS are listed in Table 12-2. A dry-to-dry dressing is placed on a wound dry and removed when it is dry. These are used to absorb very light drainage and promote hemostasis in acute wounds. These dressings may be used to cover acute wounds closed by primary intention or small acute wounds. This type of dressing is usually not employed for large or chronic wounds. A wet-to-wet dressing is moistened, usually with either normal saline or an antiseptic solution such as a triple antibiotic to soften eschar or treat an infected wound. A third type is the wet-to-dry dressing (Figure 12-1), which is used for nonselec-

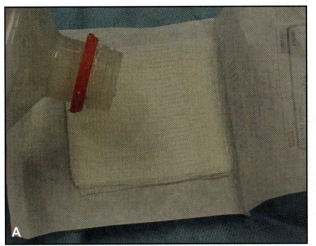 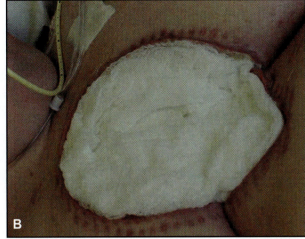

Figure 12-1. Saline-moistened gauze dressing. (A) Wetting a sterile 4 x 4 with sterile normal saline. (B) Bandage roll moistened with normal saline in dehiscent sternal wound.

Table 12-3

Types of Dressings

Non-occlusive	Occlusive & Semi-occlusive
Dry-to-dry gauze	Semipermeable foam
Contact layer	Semipermeable film
Wet-to-dry gauze	Alginate, hydrofiber
Wet-to-wet gauze	Hydrogel
Petrolatum gauze	Composite
Composite	Hydrocolloid

tive debridement of wounds with either large amounts of necrotic tissue or wounds that must be debrided rapidly. Microenvironmental (occlusive and semi-occlusive) dressings are designed to optimize the wound environment to promote healing. The term *occlusiveness* is quantified by the water vapor transmission rate (WVTR). Occlusive dressings do not allow anything to cross them in either direction. A truly occlusive dressing would have a WVTR of zero. Semi-occlusive dressings allow some movement of water vapor and other gases across them; therefore, they have a measurable WVTR. Occlusiveness exists on a continuum and is only one factor in choosing a dressing. In some cases, the occlusiveness of a dressing is obvious; in other cases, some dressings termed *microenvironmental dressings* may not be more occlusive than nonmicroenvironmental dressings. Differences in occlusiveness of different dressing types will be discussed with each type of dressing. Several subtypes of microenvironmental dressings also

are discussed (see Table 12-3). In addition to differences in the ability to retain moisture, other characteristics to consider are the ability to absorb drainage and to maintain the temperature of the wound bed.

NONOCCLUSIVE DRESSINGS

The mainstays of this category are products constructed of cotton gauze. Gauze sponges have a long history in wound care and many individuals who do not stay current with appropriate care may consider saline-moistened gauze to be a standard of care. Gauze products are readily permeable to bacteria, gas, and fluid and are, therefore, considered nonocclusive. They handle heavy drainage primarily by absorption. They are indicated for protecting acute wounds closed by primary intent, absorption of copious drainage and bleeding to prevent a hematoma. Nonocclusive dressings are also indicated for

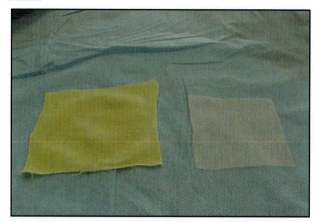

Figure 12-2. Examples of petrolatum impregnated gauze—Xeroform (yellow) and Adaptic (clear).

infected wounds and as a wet-to-dry dressing when rapid debridement is necessary. Gauze products include telfa pads, gauze sponges, and bandage rolls. Cotton gauze is reasonably absorbent and can be layered to provide sufficient absorption of copious exudate. Dry gauze performs acceptably well as a bacterial barrier when wounds are not draining. It loses its effectiveness as it soaks through with drainage. Wet gauze is not a good bacterial barrier because it can transmit bacteria through moisture into a wound. Gauze also permits uncontrolled evaporation of fluid from a wound as it wicks fluid, leading to desiccation of wound beds unless drainage is heavy. Desiccation leads to the additional problem of dressings adhering to desiccated, proteinaceous exudate. Removal of adherent dressings is associated with the release of bacteria into the air. Evaporation of fluid as it is wicked from the wound reduces its temperature, which will decrease the production of granulation tissue and the effectiveness of immune cells. Lowering the temperature of a wound has been shown to increase the risk of infection.

Because gauze dressings will adhere to desiccated fluid in wounds, telfa and related products have been designed to act as nonstick layers between the wound surface and the absorbent material. Unfortunately, these "nonstick" materials frequently fail to perform as advertised. Exudate is absorbed across the nonstick surface, dries across the pores, and then adheres to the wound bed. Other nonstick options include dressings coated with a petrolatum product. Vaseline gauze or Adaptic consists of white petrolatum coating a synthetic mesh. Xeroform has a yellow color due to the presence of bismuth tribromophenate, an antimicrobial in a petrolatum base applied to a fine mesh cloth. Although the petrolatum coating decreases the risk of adhesion, drainage can also dry across these perforations in the same manner described for telfa pads. Granulation tissue may grow through the perforations causing adherence and bleeding during dressing removal.

Another possible nonstick dressing is a contact layer, which is designed to allow water and electrolytes to cross the dressing, but not cells and proteins that are responsible for adherence of dressings to wound beds.

Cotton gauze material is woven, and based on the quality of its production, stray pieces of material can be shed from them into the wound bed. Contamination of the wound bed with small pieces of cotton shed from the dressing can promote chronic inflammation and stimulate copious drainage from the wound. The continual use of gauze in wounds promotes a vicious cycle of inflammation, copious drainage, and use of a dressing material that promotes inflammation. Cotton gauze can be useful as a dressing when ointments are used directly on the wound that require frequent dressing changes, for example, over silver sulfadiazine or over enzymatic debriding agents to minimize desiccation.

Petrolatum gauze (Figure 12-2) may be useful for protecting a wound from outside contamination, retaining moisture in a wound, and reducing the risk for adherence. Because cotton fibers are not directly in contact with the wound bed, irritation and drainage will be reduced compared with cotton gauze. However, petrolatum coated materials lack absorbency and require frequent dressing changes. These dressings are more occlusive than gauze sponges, so use with infected wounds must be done with caution.

Contact layer dressings and composites with contact layers are made of nonstick material similar to telfa, but with much smaller perforations that allow some evaporation of excessive moisture while minimizing risk of adherence. Some products such as Exu-Dry (Smith & Nephew, Andover, MA) combine a contact layer with a layer of highly absorbent material (Figure 12-3). This type of dressing has characteristics that are suitable for acute or infected wounds without the drawbacks associated with gauze, telfa, and petrolatum dressings.

MICROENVIRONMENTAL (OCCLUSIVE AND SEMI-OCCLUSIVE) DRESSINGS

Occlusive and semi-occlusive dressings offer some very important advantages for the wound, the patient and the clinician. These dressings are designed based on the principle that healing is the most effective if the wound microenvironment is optimized. Optimization of the wound microenvironment includes maintaining an appropriate moisture level and temperature, availability of macromolecules of healing (glycosaminoglycans, proteoglycans, and collagen), availability of growth factors (macrophage- and platelet-derived), acceptable levels of nonpathogenic microflora, and protection of environment from pathogens.

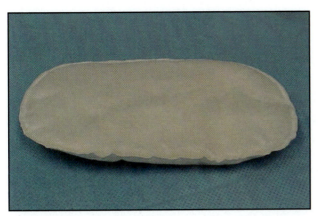

Figure 12-3A. Composite dressing: intact Exu-Dry dressing.

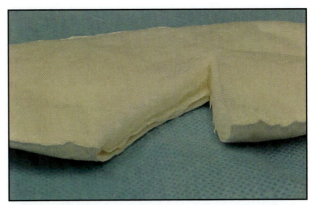

Figure 12-3B. Exu-Dry dressing cut in cross-section to reveal layers. Contact layer is on top.

Wound moisture is critical for migration of epithelial cells, movement of enzymes, growth factors, and structural molecules. An appropriate occlusive dressing maintains wound bed moisture while preventing accumulation of excessive moisture that can damage surrounding skin. An appropriate microenvironmental dressing also prevents desiccation that leads to scab formation. Desiccated fibrin and blood may act as a dressing to retain moisture below and to keep out pathogens, but slows epithelial cell migration as cells are forced below to resurface a wound.

Promoting autolytic debridement is an important indication for microenvironmental dressings. Autolytic debridement is able to proceed under these dressings due to the retention of fluid and enzymes under them. Although the properties of microenvironmental dressings are useful for chronic wounds, they may be harmful for infected wounds for the same reason that they promote autolytic debridement. Occlusive dressings should not be used over infected wounds as they will promote the growth of microbes with potential spread of infection. Some occlusive and semi-occlusive dressings are useful for acute wounds that have little necrotic tissue or drainage and they may be left in place for several days at a time. Many times, wounds will be closed when the occlusive dressing is removed. Another advantage of occlusive dressings is the decreased handling of the wound. Decreased handling minimizes inflammation, which, in turn, decreases drainage from the wound. Although some microenvironmental dressings are nonadherent, others are very adherent to the surrounding skin. Very adherent dressings should be reserved for wounds that may be left covered for several days with the goal of minimizing trauma. Certain microenvironmental dressings, especially hydrogels, are soothing to irritated wounds, especially burns, chemical burns, and radiation burns. Among the microenvironmental dressings, only alginates and their synthetic equivalents are not contraindicated for infected wounds.

Semipermeable Film Dressings

Many brands of semipermeable polyurethane films are now available. Film dressings have acrylic adhesive on them that allows them to adhere to skin, but not to wound beds. An example is shown in Figure 12-4. These dressings are semi-occlusive and allow some evaporation of fluid. However, they cannot absorb any drainage and will allow drainage to accumulate under them. Therefore, they are only indicated for minimal drainage as they cannot handle moderate or maximum levels of drainage. Should drainage become too great, the dressing will loosen and leak. Film dressings are particularly useful for superficial wounds or partial-thickness wounds with minimal drainage. They are useful as secondary dressings to hold a more absorbent material in the wound. Film dressings have a low coefficient of friction and can protect skin against friction injury. However, friction on the edges of a film dressing may dislodge it.

When applying film dressings, a margin of more than 1 inch (3 to 4 cm) of healthy surrounding skin should be covered. Because this type of dressing is quite adherent, frequent, repeated removal and will damage a patient's skin. A skin protectant should be applied to the surrounding skin (see skin protectants in Chapter 14). Skin protectants improve the adhesion of these dressings and decrease the probability of edges rolling up. Depending on the location of the dressing, films may need to be taped to prevent rolling up of edges. These dressings should not be used on infants and small children too young to understand the purpose of the dressing. Because these are made of polyurethane with an adhesive backing, they may be deliberately or accidentally removed and become a choking hazard.

To prevent skin injury, proper technique must be used when removing semipermeable films, especially to skin of elderly individuals. If pulled directly from the wound, the skin may adhere more strongly to the film dressing than

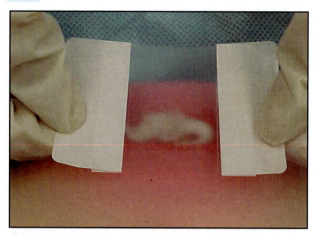

Figure 12-4A. Semipermeable film dressing applied as a secondary dressing over alginate wound filler.

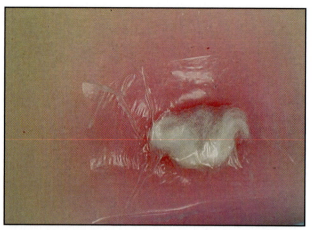

Figure 12-4B. Semipermeable film dressing in place. Placing a hand on the dressing to warm it for several seconds improves the adherence. The alginate filler is clearly visible beneath this dressing.

to itself, causing skin to tear, especially in the elderly or others with fragile skin. Skin should be stabilized when using an adhesive dressing to prevent excessive pulling on it. Proper technique to remove a film is to lift a corner and stretch the semipermeable film tangentially to the wound, causing the dressing to stretch and loosen. Pulling a film dressing back over itself can result in skin tears and denudation of the skin surrounding a wound. Semipermeable films in particular, and any dressing should be applied with care to avoid restricting adjacent parts of the body, particularly with sacral and coccygeal wounds. Care must be taken not to bridge the gluteal cleft with these dressings. If a semipermeable film is to be used in this area, a number of alternatives may be used. First, the dressing may be turned such that a corner of the dressing is placed in the cleft, between fingers, or toes or other areas. A second option is to cut a dressing into a valentine shape and apply the dressing with the point in the cleft. Placing 2 dressings with one on either side and overlapping in the middle to cover the entirety of the wound is another option. If placing a single piece of dressing material across an area such as the gluteal cleft cannot be avoided, start with the dressing folded and begin placing the dressing in the center and delicately smooth outwardly so that full mobility is unimpeded.

Semipermeable Foams

These semi-occlusive dressings manage drainage by absorption, evaporation and occlusion. An example is shown in Figure 12-5. They are the most absorbent of the microenvironmental dressings. A variety of foam thickness is available to manage a wide range of drainage. They will retain large quantities of fluid in the wound, absorb excessive drainage, and some brands allow substantial evaporation to occur as well. They are not as permeable to gas and water vapor as films, but are less occlusive than

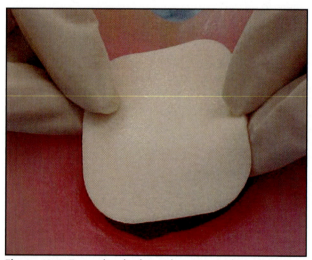

Figure 12-5. Example of a foam dressing used to cover a wound.

hydrogels or hydrocolloids (see below). Major advantages of foams, in addition to their absorbency, are the physical cushioning of wounds and thermal insulation to maintain the temperature of the wound closer to the optimal temperature for the growth of fibroblasts and epithelial cells. Manufacturers have constructed these dressings with a number of additives, including surfactants and detergents to help clean wounds, and charcoal to absorb odor. Charcoal can also be built into composite dressings.

Hydrogels

This material is available in 2 basic forms: sheets and amorphous. Examples of hydrogels are shown in Figure 12-6. Hydrogels are not generally used to manage drainage, but they provide some occlusion, absorption, and evaporation. The primary purpose of hydrogel is hydrat-

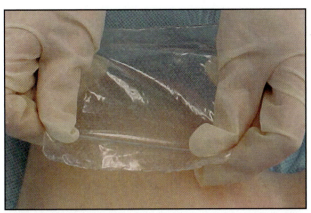

Figure 12-6A. Hydrogel sheet being applied over a wound model.

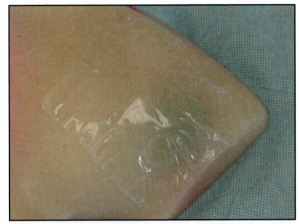

Figure 12-6B. Hydrogel sheet dressing in place.

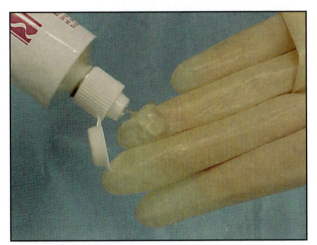

Figure 12-6C. Amorphous hydrogel used to moisten a dry wound bed.

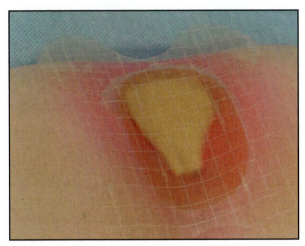

Figure 12-7. Thin hydrocolloid dressing used as a secondary dressing. The alginate filler can be visualized through a thin dressing.

ing dry wounds. In addition, hydrogel can be very soothing on wounds, especially abrasions, burns, and radiation burns. Hydrogel sheets may also be used on partial-thickness or full-thickness wounds. Sheets are also available over-the-counter in nonsterile form, which are very popular for cyclists and other athletes prone to abrasions. Due to their high water content, hydrogel sheets adhere to wounds without adhesives and are removed without trauma. However, they can slide off the wound, potentially requiring taping to keep them in place. The sheets come with polyethylene film on both sides. The inner film is always removed and the outer film may be removed to increase evaporative loss of fluid from the wound.

Amorphous gel is available in tubes and other squeezable containers for use in wounds with subcutaneous involvement. Amorphous gel is well suited for hydrating dry wounds. It is especially useful for protecting tendons, ligaments, nerves, and blood vessels from desiccation. A thin layer of amorphous gel may also be used to line cavities. Medicare specifically states that hydrogel should not

be used to fill a wound. In addition to hydrating a wound, hydrogel may soften and loosen slough. If the wound must be held open, another form of filler can be used on top of hydrogel. Hydrogel-impregnated gauze sponges are available and are used as electrodes for electrical stimulation as a means of increasing wound healing. Metronidazole gel is available for treating wounds infected with gram-negative bacteria. Amorphous hydrogel and hydrogel sheets can also be used as an interface for therapeutic ultrasound (see Chapter 14).

Hydrocolloids

Hydrocolloids are the most occlusive of the microenvironmental dressings and are easily distinguished by their appearance. Many brands and types are available (see Figure 12-7). They have a characteristic appearance with a distinctive tan color. This material comes in a variety of thicknesses. The thicker varieties are opaque and a deeper tan. Thin hydrocolloid sheets are a lighter tan color and allow limited visualization of the wound. This material is also capable of absorbing moderate drainage in addition to occluding the wound. As hydrocolloid absorbs water, it becomes lighter in color and softer, and should be changed when it becomes soft and white. These dressings are very adhesive and are designed to be worn for several days at a time, which leads to several precautions. First, these dressings should never be used on infected wounds. They are also not recommended for wounds with subcutaneous defects, including undermining, tracts, and tunnels. The outer surface is impermeable to water; therefore, hydrocolloid dressings can be worn in the shower if prolonged contact or soaking can be avoided.

Because of the adhesion of hydrocolloid sheets necessary to allow the dressing to stay in place for several days between dressing changes, hydrocolloids should only be used if the clinician is comfortable with allowing the wound to stay covered for 5 days or longer. Like semipermeable films, hydrocolloid dressing should have a margin of 2 to 3 cm of healthy skin beneath them coated with skin protectant. When hydrocolloid dressings are removed, the product of several days' worth of autolytic debridement trapped under them will have a mild odor and superficially resemble purulence. However, when the drainage is cleansed from the wound, the odor and soupy drainage will be gone, indicating that the wound is not infected. Hydrocolloids also have a low coefficient of friction, which minimizes friction injury to the area of the wound. The edges of hydrocolloid sheets will frequently roll up, especially when placed in locations where shearing forces are present with bed mobility. In these cases, clinicians frequently tape the edges of hydrocolloid sheets.

Application of skin protectant beneath hydrocolloid sheets prevents rolling the edges of hydrocolloid sheets and skin injury during hydrocolloid dressing removal. Hydrocolloids are also available for filling cavities and managing drainage. Hydrocolloids can be formulated in pastes, granules and spiral-cut sheets to fill a wound. These absorption products require a secondary dressing to hold them in the wound. The secondary dressing could be a hydrocolloid sheet, or something simpler such as film or gauze. These fillers will allow the absorption of greater drainage and will reduce the need for dressing changes. Decreasing the frequency of dressing changes increases patient comfort, patient adherence to the plan of care and decreases the opportunity for contamination and chronic inflammation caused by rough handling. Like semipermeable films, hydrocolloid sheets must also be removed carefully to prevent injury to the surrounding skin of the wound and a skin protectant is used to protect the skin from injury. Like film dressings, hydrocolloids can be cut in creative ways to make them fit over specific parts of the body such as the sacrum and toes. Cutting hydrocolloid dressings to allow dressings to conform well is shown in Figure 12-8.

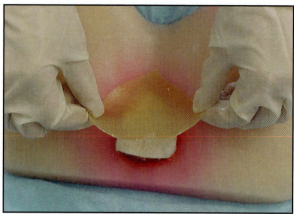

Figure 12-8A. Hydrocolloid sheet cut into a valentine shape to place over a sacral wound.

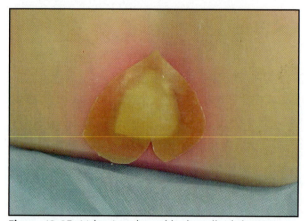

Figure 12-8B. Valentine-shaped hydrocolloid sheet in place.

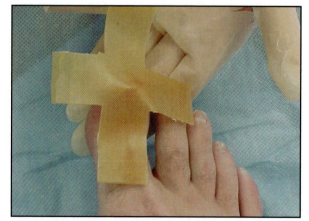

Figure 12-8C. Cross shape used for the end of a toe or finger.

Alginates and Hydrofibers

The most versatile of the microenvironmental dressings, alginates are derived from long-chain sugars obtained from sea weed and have the property of changing from a

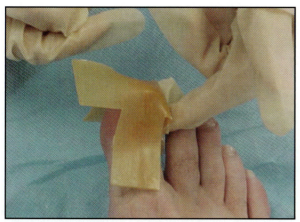

Figure 12-8D. Folding the tabs into place.

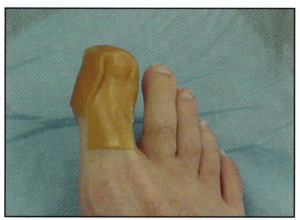

Figure 12-8E. Completed application of hydrocolloid dressing to the end of a great toe. Holding a hand over the hydrocolloid sheet to warm it increases the conformability and adherence of the dressing to provide a good fit over the irregular shape of the toe.

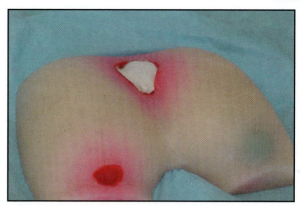

Figure 12-9A. Application of alginate or hydrofiber dressing. Alginate sheet was cut to fit a sacral wound.

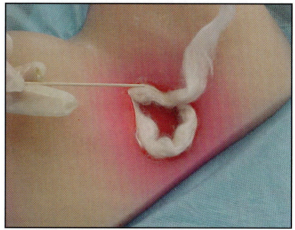

Figure 12-9B. Alginate rope placed loosely beneath undermined areas of a wound.

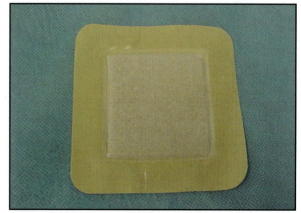

Figure 12-9C. Example of composite dressing combining alginate with foam.

fiber to a gel as it absorbs fluid. Alginate dressings can hold up to 20 times their weight in water and may desiccate wounds with little drainage. Hydrofibers are synthetic improvements on the older generation products. Examples are shown in Figures 12-4, 12-7, and 12-9. A composite dressing of alginate with polyurethane foam is shown in Figure 12-9C. With an appropriate secondary dressing, alginates and hydrofibers can be used with maximum drainage. This material has sufficient tensile strength that the gel formed by absorbing water is removed easily from the wound bed as a single piece. Following removal of the gelled alginate, flushing the wound with normal saline should remove any residue. Although some clinicians like to premoisten alginates to fill desiccated wounds, alginates were designed to absorb drainage, not hydrate wounds. A simpler and more cost-effective approach to wound hydration is coating the wound with amorphous hydrogel. Alginates and hydrofibers should not be used on dry wounds, hard eschar, or third-degree burns. If a

wound bed begins to dry, cease alginate/hydrofiber use and switch to a less absorbent dressing.

The secondary dressing used over alginate or hydrofiber can be selected based on the drainage. A semipermeable film can be used with minimum exudate (Figure 12-4), whereas foam, or absorbent secondary dressings may be used for copious drainage. If a hydrocolloid is used as the secondary dressing (Figure 12-7), the clinician must be willing to leave the dressing in place for several days. Alginates come in the form of sheets and ribbons, have remarkable tensile strength, and can be placed into undermined and irregularly shaped areas (Figure 12-9). Some clinicians have a habit of fluffing the alginate sheets before filling a cavity, but this practice is unnecessary. Alginate can be combined with collagen. As the alginate absorbs drainage, collagen is absorbed into the wound to promote healing.

ANTIBIOTIC CREAMS AND OINTMENTS

Antibiotic creams can be used as primary dressings. They generally require a secondary dressing, which, in addition to covering the antibiotic, is needed to absorb drainage from necrotic tissue and blisters and to protect the tissue below. Although antibiotic creams/ointments are generally associated with burn injuries, they can be used for other wounds. Silver containing creams are very expensive, therefore, other types of antibiotic creams or ointments are frequently used for other types of wounds.

Silver Sulfadiazine

This antibiotic in the form of a thick soothing cream may be considered to be a dressing. It is used primarily on burns with or without gauze to protect wounds, but may be applied to some types of acute wounds. Silver in the form of this cream, liquid silver nitrate, and silver salts are broad spectrum antimicrobials. However, silver impairs fibroblasts and epithelial cells. In spite of this, silver may lead to more rapid healing by avoiding chronic inflammation that might occur with high levels of bacteria or fungi on burn or other acute wounds. Silver sulfadiazine should be applied under clean conditions, with a thickness of one-sixteenth of an inch after hydrotherapy and debridement (Figure 12-10). It also needs to be reapplied to areas from which it has been removed by patient activity. The cream is to be left in place for 24 hours. Silver sulfadiazine is contraindicated for pregnant women, infants before the age of 2 months or premature infants because of the risk of kernicterus, brain damage caused by bilirubinemia. Although frequently used for many days, it should be discontinued when the risk of infection has passed, usually with complete debridement.

Mafenide Acetate

Mafenide acetate is provided as a 50 g packet of white, crystalline powder. It is best known as Sulfamylon. The

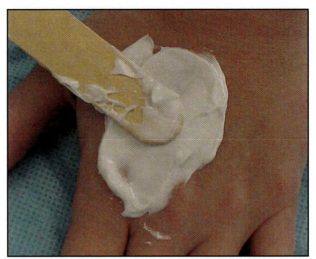

Figure 12-10. Application of silver sulfadiazine with a tongue depressor.

packet is mixed with 1 L of sterile water or normal saline to produce a 5% topical solution according to manufacturer instructions. The solution is stored at room temperature, and used within 48 hours after mixing. Mafenide acetate is also available as an 11% cream applied similarly as silver sulfadiazine. The primary use of Sulfamylon is on burn injuries as an alternative to silver sulfadiazine. A discussion of the uses of these 2 agents is found in Chapter 15 on burn injuries. Burn dressings are soaked with Sulfamylon to the point of saturation and then covered with another layer of dressings. The primary dressing is to be kept wet. The manufacturer suggests using a bulb syringe or irrigation tubing to moisten the primary dressing every 4 hours. Dressings are to be left over grafts up to 5 days at which time the graft should have taken. Patients may have allergic reactions or develop acidosis during Sulfamylon treatment. Sulfamylon is to be discontinued if an allergic response occurs. With acidosis, the treatment may be discontinued for 24 to 48 hours and possibly restarted.

Neosporin and Polysporin

Both of these are supplied in a petrolatum-based ointment. Although generic equivalents are available, the ingredients may vary among manufacturers. Neosporin consists of 3 antimicrobial agents, whereas Polysporin contains 2. Both contain polymyxin B and bacitracin. Neosporin contains neomycin in addition. These combinations provide broad spectrum coverage, but are too toxic, especially nephrotoxic and ototoxic, to be used in any manner other than topical. Bacitracin is a cell-wall-active agent effective against gram-positive organisms. Polymyxin B damages cell membranes of gram-negative organisms. Polysporin is claimed to be effective against *Staphylococcus aureus, Streptococcus* species, *E. coli, Hemophilus influenzae, Klebsiella* and *Enterobacter* species, *Neisseria* species, and *Pseudomonas aeruginosa*, but the manufacturer states that it is not effective against *Serratia marcesens*. As an ointment, it is used topically on minor wounds, particularly on the face and eye, where neosporin use is not recommended due to the possibility of allergic reactions to neomycin. Polysporin is also available as a powder, which is recommended for use with collagenase.

Neosporin, with the additional component of neomycin gives broader coverage. Neomycin is an aminoglycoside that impairs bacteria protein synthesis. It provides excellent coverage against gram-negative and weak coverage against gram-positive organisms. Other formulations of Neosporin are available. The pain relief variety has pramoxine, a local anesthetic, but does not include bacitracin due to chemical properties of the mixture. Neosporin has been promoted as a means of causing wounds to heal faster; however, the comparison has been done against wounds that did not use Neosporin and not against the petrolatum base without the antimicrobials. Both polysporin and neosporin are useful for patients to use at home. Patients need to be told to read the instructions and be specifically warned against any allergic reactions.

Cadexomer Iodine

Although iodine-containing antiseptics are not approved for use in wounds, cadexomer iodine has been designed specifically for wounds. Cadexomer iodine provides sustained release iodine rather than the large amount released from povidone iodine. It can be applied directly to wounds in the form of an ointment or a spray and is available on a sheet to be placed in wounds. As the material absorbs drainage, it forms a gel and releases iodine into the wound. Cadexomer iodine is indicated for wounds with heavy drainage, heavily contaminated wounds, and second-degree burns due to its ability to absorb drainage. Its absorptive nature is also useful in controlling odor and protecting surrounding skin from drainage. By maintaining a moist wound bed, cadexomer iodine promotes autolytic debridement. In addition, the gel is able to conform to the shape of the wound, which also assists in retaining fluid in the wound bed and off surrounding skin. The ointment form has a brown color and requires a secondary dressing. The gel needs to be replaced when it becomes a yellow or gray color.

Some potential issues with cadexomer iodine exist. The darkly pigmented gel obscures the wound bed and the color may alarm those who are not familiar with this product. Removing the gel from a wound may be uncomfortable for a patient. Cadexomer iodine must not be used on anyone with a known allergy to iodine. According to the manufacturer, the level of sustained release of iodine from cadexomer iodine does not lead to the cytotoxicity associated with povidone-iodine. Cadexomer iodine's uses include chronic wounds and infected wounds. The iodine component does not change the requirement of any systemic antibiotics.

SILVER DRESSINGS

Technology to vaporize silver salts and deposit nanocrystalline silver on materials has allowed silver options for alginates/hydrofibers, foam, and contact layers; their grayish hue makes them readily identifiable as containing silver. The nanocrystalline form of silver produces sustained release of silver on the wound bed. Contact layer types of silver dressings are wet with water, not with saline; dressings may need to be remoistened with water before they are changed. Silver dressings should not be used with enzymatic debriders; therefore, the clinician must decide which is more important because silver inactivates enzymatic debriders. Silverlon (Argentum Medical, LLC., Chicago, IL) is essentially a contact layer made with nylon mesh. Acticoat (Smith & Nephew, London, England) is indicated for burns, graft, and donor sites. It consists of a silver coating on a polyethylene mesh with an inner core of rayon and polyester for absorption. A newer version, Acticoat 7 is designed to be effective for up to 7 days; the original was approved for 3-day wear. Silver alginates and hydrofibers are changed as needed, but must be changed daily if the wound is infected. Other uses for silver dressings suggested by manufacturers include venous ulcers and use under negative pressure wound therapy (Chapter 14). Although the materials used in silver dressings appear to be effective bactericides *in vitro*, they have not been shown to produce more rapid healing than similar dressings without the silver component. In reimbursement situations that do not allow for the recovery of dressing material cost, the clinician must take into account the greater cost and use them judiciously.

OXYGEN RECONSTITUTED CELLULOSE AND MATRIX METALLOPROTEINASES

A common problem plaguing chronic wounds is the excessive level of matrix metalloproteinases (MMPs). MMPs are part of normal response to acute wounds and dissipate as the inflammatory phase of healing occurs. MMPs are a family of 26, possibly more, zinc-dependent proteolytic enzymes produced by multiple cells including neutrophils, macrophages, fibroblasts, and endothelial cells. These enzymes degrade proteins including collagen and growth factors. In chronic wounds, the level of MMPs exceeds that of acute wounds and they persist, creating a vicious cycle of tissue breakdown and chronic inflammation. Part of the regulation of MMPs is the production of tissue inhibitors of metalloproteinases, known as TIMPs.

At least 4 types of TIMPs have been identified, most importantly TIMP1 and 2. These are insufficient in many chronic wounds, leading to the development of dressings made of a material that controls MMP levels in wounds. Oxygen reconstituted cellulose (ORC) binds MMPs and forms a gel as it absorbs wound exudate. Promogran (Johnson & Johnson, New Brunswick, NJ) is a freeze-dried matrix of collagen and ORC that is placed in a wound as a thin hexagonal wafer.

DRESSING MATERIALS RELEASING GROWTH FACTORS AND COMPONENTS OF WOUND MATRIX

Living skin equivalents such as Apligraf (Organogenesis Inc, Canton, MA) and Integra (Integra LifeSciences Corporation, Plainsboro, NJ) could be considered as a dressing. These produce natural growth factors while protecting the wound and allowing native cells to reproduce and cover the wounded area. Living skin equivalents are discussed in greater detail in Chapter 2. Oasis (Cook Biotech Incorporated, West Lafayette, IN) performs many of the same functions as living skin equivalents. It is produced from porcine small intestine submucosa. This material can be implanted or applied topically. It provides a scaffolding for cell migration and release of growth factors that stimulate angiogenesis, granulation, and re-epithelialization. The porcine intestinal submucosa reduces MMPs, mediators of inflammation, and proteolytic enzymes of chronic wounds, creating an environment closer to that of an acute wound. Hyaluronic acid is also used as a wound dressing in Hyalofill (ConvaTec, Skillman, NJ). This material comes in sheets and ribbons similar in appearance to alginate. It is composed of a polymer that releases hyaluronic acid as it absorbs fluid and becomes a gel. Hyaluronic acid is believed to be released for 2 to 3 days into wounds. The manufacturer recommends it for neuropathic ulcers, pressure ulcers, traumatic, and surgical wounds.

HYPERTONIC SALINE

Dressings with hypertonic saline absorb exudate, bacteria, and solubilized necrotic tissue. Mesalt (Molnlycke Health Care, Göteborg, Sweden) is a dressing composed of sodium chloride bound to a synthetic gauze pad. It is simply placed into a wound, where it releases hypertonic saline into the wound. Drainage, bacteria, and other materials are then absorbed into the pad. This dressing is designed specifically for heavily draining wounds and should not be used on clean wounds with minimal drainage that could be injured by the hypertonicity produced by release of sodium chloride in a small volume of fluid.

USING DRESSINGS

A few general points about using dressings need to be addressed. The first important point is organization. Organizing the dressing change in advance is key to minimizing contamination of the wound. The clinician should gather all dressing materials and anything else that might be needed to evaluate the wound, especially if cleansing and debridement will precede the dressing change. Although a sterile field is not an absolute requirement (see Chapter 9), following the basic principles of maintaining a sterile field in a reasonable manner is good practice to prevent contamination of the wound. The time that packages are left open before being used should be minimized as much as possible. This can be achieved by having an assistant available, allowing the patient to be the assistant, or organizing the dressing change as carefully as possible. Sterile dressings must be used on acute surgical wounds, whereas clean dressings are allowable on chronic wounds. However, dressings are generally obtained in sterile packaging. Regardless of the requirement, as much care should be taken to meet sterile technique and maintain a clean environment for wound treatments.

Management of Cavities

Wounds with substantial subcutaneous involvement may require either packing or filling to optimize healing. The term *packing* is frequently used incorrectly to describe a process of placing dressing materials into a wound. Packing refers to a specific type of wound filling that is used to promote hemostasis and prevent hematoma formation, or to keep a wound open as it is prepared for delayed primary closure (tertiary closure). Removing postoperative packing can be painful for the patient. The wound is packed under general anesthesia, but is usually removed when the patient is conscious. Moreover, the wound is packed more tightly than could be achieved in a conscious patient. When removing packing, carefully determine the best direction to remove the packing material. On occasion, a surgeon may have changed directions while packing a wound, resulting in the formation of a knot. These are very difficult to remove, requiring patience and possibly cutting pieces from the packing material, whether packing strip or bandage rolls are used.

Packing prevents the wound from filling with granulation tissue and re-epithelializing so tertiary closure can be performed once the wound is clean and stable. Incision and drainage wounds created due to osteomyelitis are the usual type requiring packing. Filling, in contrast, is used strictly to allow dead spaces to heal from the wound bed, preventing premature closure of the wound surface over a dead space. Dead spaces such as this create an unacceptably high risk for forming a new abscess. Filling is done loosely to promote healing from the inside out, and to manage drainage in wounds with undermined or tunneled wounds or those with sinus tracts; packing such wounds will delay healing. However, inadequate filling of tracts may also allow the tract to close over a dead space. Therefore, filling tracts/tunnels requires a good feel for the bottom of a tract and pushing the material to the bottom first. Novices may be unwilling to push packing strip deeply enough due to the patient's reaction and must learn to focus on the important task of not allowing dead space beyond packing strip.

Selection of materials used for filling or packing wounds is largely determined by whether the wound is infected and the quantity of drainage from the wound. Packing strip is used for filling as well as packing tracts, tunnels, and other areas within a wound of substantial depth. In addition to physically filling cavities, packing strip wicks moisture and bacteria from the wound. Plain packing strip is dry woven cotton with great tensile strength with no possibility of breaking inside the wound or shedding stray fibers. A continuous 15 foot length is supplied in each bottle of packing strip. This material is available in various sizes such as 1/4 inch, 1/2 inch, 1 inch, and 2 inch. A popular option for infected wounds is iodoform, which is simply packing strip moistened with an iodine solution. Iodoform is available in the same sizes. Plain packing strip is commonly moistened before placing it into a wound. Normal saline or antibiotic solution might be used.

The procedure for placing packing strip into a tract is shown in Figure 12-11. Typical tracts are filled with 1/4 inch strip, but larger sizes may be used for larger defects. For a typical tract, packing strip can be lifted straight up from its bottle with cotton tipped applicators in a chopstick technique; forceps may be used instead. Having removed a previous piece of packing strip from a wound allows the clinician to estimate the length required for a dressing change. If precutting the length of packing strip, be sure to cut a greater length than necessary. Excess packing strip can be cut off, but being left with a piece that is too short requires removing the packing strip and starting anew with a longer piece. This length is cut with scissors that are either sterile or have been cleaned and subjected to high level disinfection. A cheaper option is the use of a scalpel blade.

The length of packing strip to be used is held in the nondominant hand and an end of the strip is held over the tract to be filled. A cotton-tipped applicator is used to push a folded over end of the strip to the bottom of the tract. The stick end is commonly used to push the strip unless the opening is large enough to accommodate the enlarged cotton-tip. For a much larger opening, a tongue depressor or gloved finger may be used instead. When using a cotton-tipped applicator, the applicator must be withdrawn carefully to avoid pulling the strip back out of

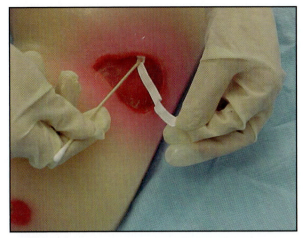

Figure 12-11. Technique for placing packing strip into a tunnel.

the wound. A twisting motion may be needed to push in the strip and withdraw the stick in a narrow tract. After withdrawing the stick end, the strip is folded over the end of the stick and strip is again pushed to the bottom. Repeat as many times as needed to fill the tract. By folding the strip over the end of the stick with each push, the strip becomes pleated within the tract, taking up the space of the width of the tract. When the tract is filled, cut the strip to leave 1/2 inch or 1 cm protruding to allow the strip to be removed at the next dressing change. Making certain that the strip is long enough to fill the wound allows the excess to be simply cut. If the strip is too short, it will need to be removed and the process repeated with a longer piece of strip. Never place a second piece on top of one already in the tract. It might not be found and removed during the next dressing change. An alternative technique is filling tracts directly from the packing strip bottle without cutting until the tract is filled. The problem with this technique is the potential for contaminating the strip as it is pulled from the bottle.

When wide tracts or other areas require filling, a larger width strip may be used, or a bandage roll may be substituted. A range of 1-inch, lightweight bandage roll through 4-inch, bulky bandage roll may be used, depending on the width to be filled. Although these may fill the area required, be aware that they are not designed specifically for this purpose. Packing strip is made specifically to prevent the loss of fibers in wounds, whereas bandage rolls may leave fibers. Undermined areas and open areas of wound may be filled with greater width packing strip, bandage roll, or gauze sponges (2 x 2 or 4 x 4), depending on the configuration of the wound. Be aware that the use of multiple gauze sponges in undermined areas creates the possibility of leaving one or more in the wound with the next dressing change. Using a single piece guarantees that no materials will be left in the wound. If a patient has multiple tracts, be particularly careful to leave the ends of packing strip where they cannot be missed and document the number carefully in case someone else will be removing them. Plain packing strip, gauze sponges, and bandage rolls are generally moistened with saline or an antibiotic solution, rather than placing dry materials into the wound. They should also be placed loosely into an infected undermined or open area, but are packed into a wound that is to be kept open for delayed primary closure. Always fill in one direction; choose one area to fill first and move consistently across the defect. Going back to an area that has already been filled may result in creating a knot that will be difficult to remove later. Also keep moist materials within the wound, avoiding surrounding skin. Prolonged moisture on surrounding skin is likely to cause maceration and delay re-epithelialization.

Gauze sponges and packing strip will need to be changed at least daily and possibly twice or more each day to remove infectious material. An alternative to gauze materials is alginate sheets or ropes (see Figure 12-9). Alginate and hydrofiber, have greater biocompatibility than gauze packing strip or sponges; therefore, they do not promote inflammation and prolonged heavy drainage. They are also removed easily from a wound, decreasing pain to the patient and trauma to the wound bed. An additional benefit is that alginates and hydrofibers will not wick fluid onto surrounding skin, which is a common problem with gauze leading to maceration. These materials may be used in infected wounds, but they must be changed at least daily. Also try to minimize the number of pieces of alginate/hydrofiber placed in the wound. If possible, use 1 piece to avoid leaving any behind with the next dressing change. Collagen sheets and ropes have the added advantage of the collagen being absorbed into the wound and possibly enhancing healing rate. Gauze should be avoided on granulation tissue. Clean wet wounds can be filled loosely with alginate or hydrofiber ribbon or sheet, hydrocolloid fillers or dextranomers. Dextranomers are described under mechanical debridement in the previous chapter. Wounds with dry wound beds can be lined with hydrogel to provide moisture to assist healing. Strategies for selecting wound dressings to meet goals for treatment are listed in Table 12-4.

SECONDARY DRESSINGS AND BANDAGING TECHNIQUE

Secondary bandages may have multiple purposes. They are used to hold the primary dressing in place, increase absorption, provide compression when needed, provide warmth and comfort to the area, and to physically protect or pad the area of the wound. Secondary dressings may consist of adhesive bandages, bandage rolls, gauze

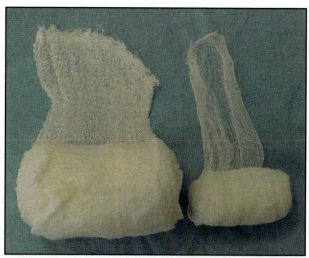

Figure 12-12. Two basic types of bandage rolls. Left: bulky bandage used for absorbency. Right: lightweight bandage roll to promote movement and give a neater appearance. These may also be used for packing wounds.

sponges (commonly 4 x 4) taped over the primary dressing, or one of a number of elasticized materials such as Flexnet, tubigrip, ACE bandages, or certain compression bandages. A tertiary dressing would be placed over a secondary dressing.

Bandage rolls are convenient to meet the most needs of secondary dressings. They come in various widths, although 4-inch bandages appear to be most commonly used. The width of the bandage used varies with the diameter of the body part being wrapped. In applications with smaller or large area diameter, sizes ranging from 1 to 6 inches may be used. A 1-inch bandage roll may be used on a finger or toe, a 2-inch bandage roll on a small hand, a 3-inch on a larger hand, a forearm, or distal leg. Four-inch bandages are generally used on feet, legs, or arms. Six-inch bandage rolls may be used on thighs, trunks, or unusually large distal extremities. The weave of the bandage roll determines many of its properties. A thinly layered interlocking weave provides elasticity to the bandage roll, whereas a loose, bulky bandage provides more absorption and insulation. Lightweight cotton bandages such as Kling (Johnson & Johnson, New Brunswick, NJ) or Conform Kendall, Mansfield, MA) allow mobility, but they are less absorbent than soft bulky bandage rolls such as kerlix, which are more absorbent and provide better padding, but provide less mobility. Soft bulky bandage rolls may be used for the specific purpose of limiting mobility on occasion. Bulky bandage rolls such as kerlix absorb, cushion, retain warmth, and can be used to immobilize a body part. Examples of bulky and lightweight bandage rolls are shown in Figure 12-12.

Three basic techniques for applying bandage rolls are commonly used. For all of these techniques, bandage rolls

Table 12-4

Dressing Decision Chart Based on Characteristics of Wound*

Type	Characteristics	Potential Problems	Goals	Dressing
Venous insufficiency	Shallow, granulating, moderate-heavy drainage	Maceration, lack epithelialization, edema of wound	Absorb drainage, reduce edema	Alginate/hydrofiber, foam or hydrocolloid, preferred: contact layer under multilayer compression bandaging
Neuropathic	Varied drainage depending on co-existing arterial disease and infection	Continued mechanical damage, possible concomitant arterial insufficiency, potential for infection	Prevent or manage infection, manage drainage, protect from trauma, debridement	Sharp debridement until necrotic tissue and infection cleared; determine dressing based characteristics
Dry shallow	Formation of scab	Lack of proliferation and autolytic debridement	Moisten	Hydrogel with transparent film
Moist shallow	Signs of chronic inflammation	Maceration of surrounding skin	Absorb drainage	Hydrocolloid or foam
Dry deep	Induration, erythema of surrounding skin	Lack of proliferation and autolytic debridement, dead space	Fill dead space, moisten	Hydrogel with transparent film
Moist deep	Copious exudate, maceration of surrounding skin	Maceration, lack of healing due to edema and damage to epidermis	Absorb drainage, fill dead space	Hydrofiber/alginate filler covered with hydrocolloid or foam
Deep infected	Odor, drainage, necrotic tissue	Spread of infection, lack of healing	Remove necrotic tissue, fill dead space	Sharp debridement moist gauze; brief trial of topical antibiotic
Deep, filled with necrotic tissue	Mild odor, yellow	Potential for infection, slow healing	Remove necrotic tissue, fill dead space	Debridement with dry dressing, enzymatic debrider with moistened gauze
Covered with eschar	Black or yellow covering, base of wound not seen	Potential for infection, slow healing	Remove eschar	Sharp debridement or crosshatch with enzymatic debrider; determined by depth and drainage

*This table is meant as a guideline only and serves as a starting point for a plan of care. Actual plans must take other factors into consideration such as the patient's resources and preferences. Plan of care should change as characteristics of the wound change.

should always be rolled on the patient's body from the bottom (see Figure 12-13A). Rolling from the top causes bandage rolls to catch on themselves causing uneven bandaging and possibly dropping of the bandage roll. A simple half-overlapping spiral is used for holding dressings in place and covering wounds (see Figure 12-13B). A figure 8 method has several purposes. It can be used to increase the amount of pressure under the bandage or may be used to allow more mobility at a joint. Wrapping around a knee or elbow in a figure 8 with a lightweight bandage roll allows flexion to occur more readily. A half-overlapping spiral with a bulky bandage roll can be used to inhibit movement at a joint. Another advantage of applying a bandage roll in a figure 8 is that it less likely to collapse with gravity on an extremity than a half-overlapping spiral. Rather than taping the top and bottom of bandages to a patient's skin, a figure 8 wrapping should be attempted first. Bandages can also be fan-folded (see Figure 12-13C) by folding it back over itself. Fan-folding is used to increase absorption and provide padding. Rather than use multiple gauze sponges and only part of a bandage roll, more efficient use of materials is accomplished by fan folding the bandage roll over the area requiring greater absorption or padding.

When using a bandage roll on the hand or foot, create a lock by making at least 1 turn (see Figure 12-13D) around the wrist or ankle. In general, we wish to keep the thumb separate from the other fingers to allow grasp (Figure 12-13E). Humidity can increase to a damaging level under bandage rolls. If toes or fingers are covered by a bandage roll, place 2 x 2s between toes or 4 x 4s between fingers to prevent maceration (Figure 12-13F). Bandage rolls and other secondary dressings may be dislodged easily between dressing changes. A plan for securing the secondary dressing should be considered before applying them. Strategies include placing a piece of tape above the heel or on the wrist just proximal to the hand to prevent loosening and migration of the bandage off the hand or foot (Figure 12-13G) and placing short pieces of tape perpendicular to the turns of the bandage to maintain the spatial relationship among these turns. On conical segments such as the thigh, leg, and forearm, the turns of the bandage may simply collapse with gravity loosening the bandage roll and causing it to fall off the body part. A combination of figure 8 and strategic taping can prevent the bandage roll from collapsing and unraveling. Figure 8 bandaging is shown in Figure 12-13H. Taping over either a primary dressing or a secondary dressing including bandage rolls should never be done circumferentially—one end of a piece of tape should never be arranged so it adheres to the other end. If swelling occurs, circumferential taping may lead to limb-threatening ischemia. A safe alternative is placing tape in a spiral such that the ends are still free to move relative to each other. Avoid finishing a bandage roll or leaving any folds under the foot where injury could occur. Ensure

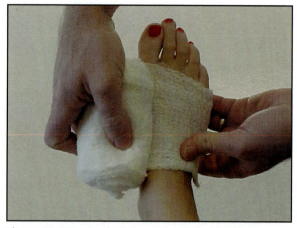

Figure 12-13A. Bandaging as a secondary or tertiary dressing. Proper technique involves rolling the bandage from the bottom.

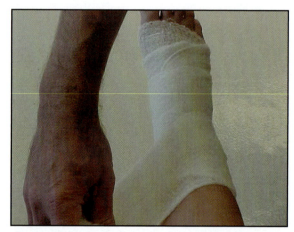

Figure 12-13B. Half-overlapping spiral technique.

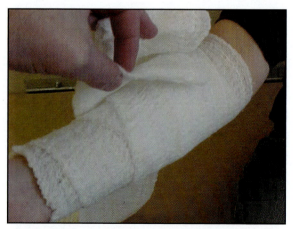

Figure 12-13C. Fan-folding to increase the layering, cushioning, and absorbency in the cubital fossa.

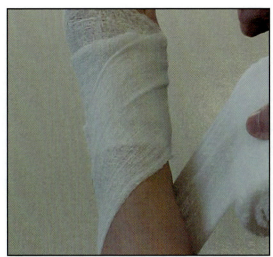

Figure 12-13D. Turning the bandage roll around the ankle to anchor it.

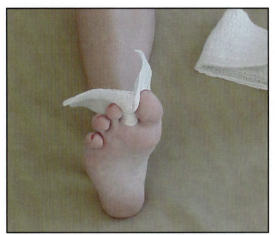

Figure 12-13F. Placing a 2 x 2 inch gauze sponge between toes to prevent maceration. Note technique that allows all 4 web spaces to be managed with only 2 gauze sponges.

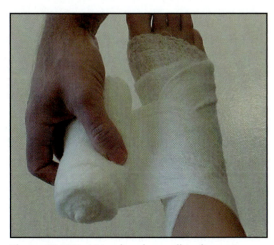

Figure 12-13H. Using bandage roll in figure 8 wrapping.

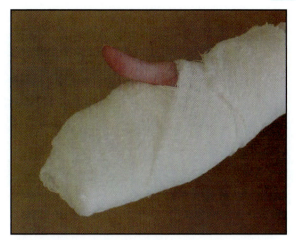

Figure 12-13E. Proper bandaging of the hand to allow free movement of an uninvolved thumb.

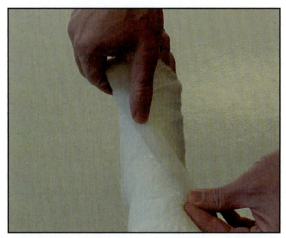

Figure 12-13G. Placing tape across turns of bandage roll to prevent bandage from loosening and falling onto foot.

that a person has footwear that will accommodate bandaging around the foot.

Taping

Four basic types of tape are used in wound care (Figure 12-14). They will be discussed in order of harshness to the skin. Silk tape such as the Durapore (3M, St. Paul, MN), is the most adhesive of the 4 types. Although it may cause minimal damage when used carefully and occasionally on young, healthy skin, it will tear weak, elderly skin and damage healthy skin with repeated use. It should be avoided for wound dressings because of cost and adhesiveness; unfortunately you may find that others may redress a wound on your patient using silk tape. Plastic tape such as the 3M brand, transpore, is still too adhesive and harsh for skin at risk for damage. It is convenient for use because it tears easily in both directions. Appropriate uses include

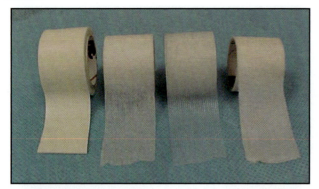

Figure 12-14. Types of adhesive tape. Left to right: foam, paper, plastic, and silk.

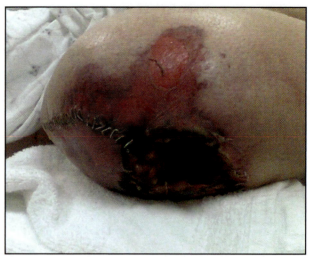

Figure 12-15A. Skin reaction caused by use of tape on a patient's skin.

taping secondary dressings to surfaces other than skin and anchoring a secondary dressing to itself, especially to make "racing stripes" (Figure 12-13G) on a bandage roll to prevent unraveling. Paper tape has low adhesion and is hypoallergenic. As such, it is usually gentle enough for repeated applications to healthy skin or occasional application to at-risk skin. It is a lower cost tape, but comes off skin easily. However, the use of skin protectant under paper tape greatly improves its adhesion. Appropriate uses include taping a primary or secondary dressing directly to the skin. The best type of tape to place directly on skin is an elastic foam tape such as the Microfoam (3M, St. Paul, MN). This type of tape has low, but adequate adhesion. It is gentle enough for daily or BID changes on at-risk skin and is comfortable and water resistant. Due to its elasticity, it conforms to irregular surfaces and stretches with swelling. However, it should not be stretched as it is placed on the skin. The recoil of the elastic tape causes shearing and damage to the skin. This type of tape is expensive and loses adhesion when repositioned. Its uses include taping a primary or secondary dressing directly to skin, especially at-risk skin or for those receiving frequent dressing changes.

TOLERANCE FOR ADHESIVES

Many individuals cannot tolerate the adhesives used on wound care products. One problem is the strength of the adhesive relative to the cohesiveness of the person's skin, especially elderly individuals. Younger clinicians with strong, supple skin may not foresee the damage that adhesive may have on older, drier, weaker skin. Many individuals also have immune reactions to adhesives (see Figure 12-15A). Wound dressings that are particularly problematic are semipermeable films and hydrocolloids, although other types of dressings may include adhesives. Semipermeable films are particularly problematic because they tend to be changed more frequently than other microenvironmental dressings. Even dressings that do not contain adhesives can

cause problems because of the need for taping to keep them in place or the use of secondary dressings with adhesives on them. A number of solutions are available. To protect skin from the mechanical aspects of aggressive adhesives, skin protectants can be used. Careful removal of semipermeable film by stretching as described above and leaving hydrocolloids in place as long as possible, then carefully removing them from the surrounding skin will minimize trauma (see Figure 12-15B to 12-15G). Alternatively, non-adherent dressings may need to be substituted for films and hydrocolloids. For dressings that require taping to hold them in place, a foam tape is the most appropriate, as long as the tape is not stretched as it is applied. Because foam tape is not as adherent as other types, a 2 inch width is usually necessary. Other options include the use of either bulky or elasticized bandage rolls, tubular bandages or net bandages (Figure 12-16). These may work well on areas of the body not subject to weight shifting and moving, but on highly mobile areas, the nonadherent dressing below is likely to shift.

ECONOMICS OF DRESSING CHANGES

One drawback of occlusive dressings is their cost. However, if we account for the faster healing under occlusive dressings and the greater frequency of nonocclusive dressing changes ($5 to $8.00 for a 4- to 7-day application) compared with the cost of gauze, the economic picture becomes quite different. The greatest cost of dressing changes does not come from the dressing itself, but the time for the dressing change to be performed. A wound being treated with nonocclusive dressings may cost $3.00 or more, depending on the number of gauze layers and the size of them. Moreover, the dressing change may be done twice each day at a cost of up to $6.00 in materials each

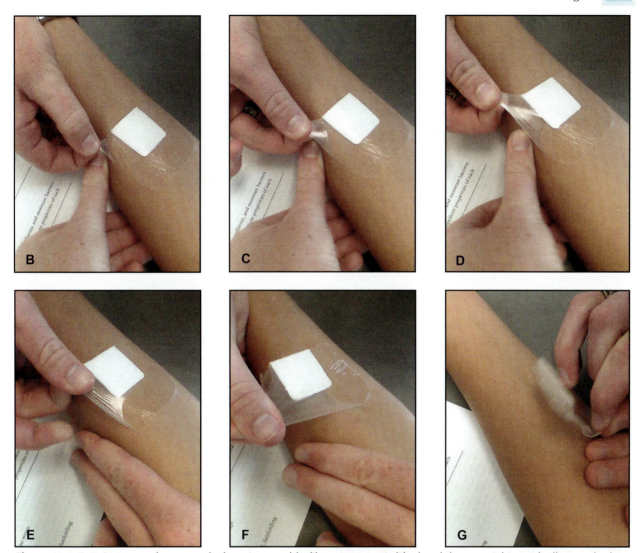

Figure 12-15B-F. Sequence for removal of semipermeable film. A corner is lifted and the material is gradually stretched to reduce the adherence of the dressing, while the skin beneath is stabilized to prevent injury.

day compared with $5 to $8 for the entire 5 days that a microenvironmental dressing is worn. Clearly, an occlusive dressing left in place for a number of days decreases costs related to clinician time and may actually decrease costs for materials.

For patients covered by Medicare Part B, additional reimbursement issues may need to be considered. Medicare Part B will reimburse only primary and secondary dressings for wounds that are caused by a surgical procedure, treated by a surgical procedure, or require debridement. Debridement must be performed by a licensed physician or healthcare professional as permitted by state law. Medicare will not reimburse for dressings used on skin conditions treated with topical medications, draining cutaneous fistulas, dressings used to protect a healed wound by reducing friction, shear, moisture, dress-

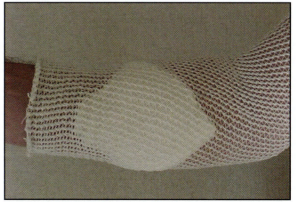

Figure 12-16A. Nonadhesive alternative for secondary/ tertiary dressings: stretch netting.

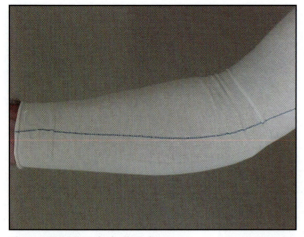

Figure 12-16B. Tubular bandage.

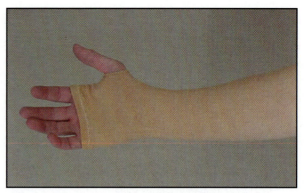

Figure 12-16C. Elasticized tubular bandage designed specifically for the hand and forearm.

ings over catheter insertion points, first-degree burns, skin tears, abrasion, venipuncture, or arterial puncture sites. For reimbursement, dressings must be ordered by a physician, nurse practitioner, clinical nurse specialist, certified nurse midwife, or physician's assistant, within state regulations. In addition, dressings will be covered only as long as medically necessary.

When procedures requiring the removal of a dressing are billed to Medicare, the cost of applying the dressing is considered incident to the charge and cannot be billed separately. Dressings ordered for home use by the patient for home dressing changes can be billed through the Durable Medical Equipment Regional Carrier (DMERC) based on a fee schedule established for each state by the use of a code from the Healthcare Common Procedure Coding System (HCPCS). No more than 1-month's supply may be ordered at a time. For these dressings, Medicare pays 80% of the fee schedule amount or the actual charge, if lower. For dressings with adhesive borders, no payment for other dressings or tape is allowed. Use of more than one type of wound filler or more than one type of wound cover is not allowed. A combination of hydrating dressing with an absorptive dressing on the same wound at the same time is not allowed. Dressing size should be based on the size of the wound. Medicare suggests that the size of wound cover be about 2 inches greater than the actual dimensions of the wound. In addition, Medicare does not cover skin sealants or barriers, wound cleansers or irrigating solutions, solutions used to moisten gauze, topical antiseptics, topical antibiotics, gauze and dressings used to cleanse or debride a wound but not left on a wound, elastic stockings, support hose, foot coverings, and leotards. Most of the unallowable items are either incident to other charges such as debridement or treatment of venous ulcers. For the most part, these regulations represent good clinical practice. However, note that at this time, dressings cannot be ordered by a physical therapist or occupational therapist. For optimal reimbursement, documentation of wound

characteristics must be congruent with the treatment plan. The DMERC will review documentation accompanying claims to determine medical necessity. Receiving reimbursement is likely to depend on the ability to document any specific or unique condition of the patient that requires an unusual product or combination of products. A letter of medical necessity from the ordering physician or other eligible clinician and the expected outcome of using the product are also necessary for reimbursement.

Characteristics, problems, and dressing decisions are expected to change through the course of healing. When wound characteristics change, the goals and dressing decisions should change. Note the DMERC guidelines for dressing changes outlined in Table 12-5. Your dressing choice and frequency of dressing changes should be guided by this table. Dressing decisions also need to be based on preferences of the patient, financial considerations, and the ability of the caregiver to apply the dressing appropriately.

DEVICES FOR SKIN APPROXIMATION

Clinicians may encounter additional means of approximating wound edges. In addition to sutures and staples, Montgomery straps, abdominal binders, and retention sutures may be used for dehiscent wounds or wounds at risk of dehiscence. Montgomery straps and retention sutures are described below, along with techniques for removing sutures and staples.

Montgomery Straps

Montgomery straps are commonly used for dehiscent abdominal wounds and may also be used for sternal dehiscence. Montgomery straps protect the healing wound from trauma caused by patient movement in bed, coughing, sneezing, and similar movement. They can be made with 2-inch silk tape laced with umbilical tape. Construction of Montgomery straps is demonstrated in

Table 12-5

DMERC Surgical Dressing Utilization Schedule

Type of Dressing	Drainage/Stage	Allowable Utilization
Alginate wound cover	Moderate-high, full-thickness, stage III or IV; not allowed for dry wounds or wounds covered with eschar	One per day
Alginate wound filler	Same as above	12 inches per day
Composite dressing	No specifics listed	Three per week
Contact layer	Used to line the entire wound	One per week
Foam	As primary on full-thickness wounds and stage III or IV pressure ulcers; as secondary for wounds with heavy drainage	Three per week
Gauze (nonimpregnated)	None listed	Six pads per day without border or one per day with border
Gauze (impregnated with other than water or saline)	None listed	One per day
Gauze (impregnated with normal saline or water)	None listed	Not covered; reimbursed at gauze rate
Hydrocolloid sheet	Light to moderate drainage	Three per week
Hydrogel sheet	Full-thickness wound with minimum or no drainage stage III or IV; not medically necessary for stage II	One per day without border; three per week for adhesive border
Hydrogel wound filler	Full-thickness wounds with minimum or no drainage stage III or IV; not medically necessary for stage II	Amount not to exceed amount needed to line the wound; additional amounts to fill a cavity are not medically necessary. Three ounces per wound per month
Specialty absorptive dressing	Moderate to high drainage stage III or IV	One per day without border; one every other day for adhesive border
Transparent film	Open partial-thickness; minimal drainage	Three per week

Adapted from LCD for Surgical Dressings (L11471): http://www.medicarenhic.com/dme/medical_review/mr_lcds/mr_lcd_current/L11471_2009-01-01_PA_2009-01_rev_2009-09.pdf

Figures 12-17A and 12-17B. A dehiscent sternal wound is shown in Figure 12-17C with completed Montgomery straps shown in Figure 12-17D. The skin can be protected by applying the tape onto hydrocolloid sheets placed on either side of the wound rather than directly on the skin. Montgomery straps are also available premade, but are rather expensive. Usually an ABD pad is the secondary dressing with either a saline-moistened gauze or alginate primary dressing, depending on the state of the dehiscent wound. Abdominal binders may be used in place of, or in conjunction with Montgomery straps as a means of preventing abdominal wound dehiscence.

Retention Sutures

A related intervention is the placement of retention sutures (see Figure 12-18). Retention sutures are also designed to reduce stress on edges of wounds. These are made of heavy material and are placed deeply within muscle or fascia, primarily in the abdominal wall. Indications for retention sutures are risk of dehiscence due to high

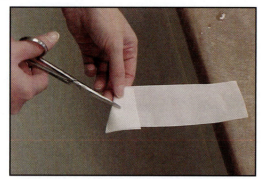

Figure 12-17A. Montgomery straps. Preparing an individual strap from 2-inch silk tape doubled over at one end to increase its strength and an opening cut for lacing the reinforced end.

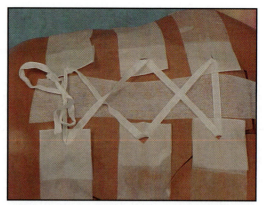

Figure 12-17B. Completed Montgomery strap made of 2-inch silk tape and 1/2-inch umbilical tape.

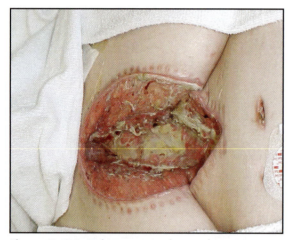

Figure 12-17C. Dehiscent sternal wound requiring Montgomery straps.

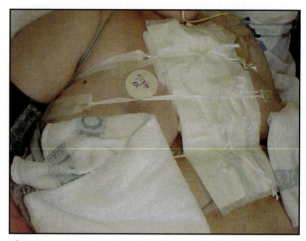

Figure 12-17D. Dressings in place over wound in 12-17C with Montgomery straps attached.

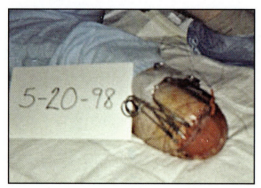

Figure 12-18. Retention sutures used on a dehiscent amputation wound. Sutures are drawn tight as edges become clean and granulated.

probability of poor wound healing (malnutrition, immune deficiency, use of corticosteroids), and increased intra-abdominal pressure from obesity or chronic coughing. They also may be used to assist healing by delayed primary intention. If used to prevent dehiscence, retention sutures are placed before regular sutures, then passed through a piece of tubing and tied after all appropriate layers are sutured, eg, peritoneum, muscle, fascia, subcutaneous tissue, and skin and left in place for up to 14 days. When retention sutures are placed around dehiscent wounds, they will be tightened by a surgeon to approximate clean edges as granulation proceeds. The process may advance from both ends of a wound toward the middle.

Staples and Sutures

In some practices, clinicians other than physicians may be requested to remove sutures or staples. These are typically removed after 7 to 10 days, depending on the stress placed on the skin and rate of healing at a particular site. Before removing them, one must determine whether sufficient healing has taken place. A tight healing ridge with minimal erythema should be evident. Obvious gaps and leaking of fluid contraindicate removal at that time. Signs of infection or nonhealing should be reported immediately to the referring physician. Slight erythema (1 to

2 mm) on the healing ridge and around each staple or suture is appropriate. A crust or scab on the surface may be cleansed with normal saline or tap water to determine whether sufficient healing has occurred.

Necessary materials are available in a disposable suture removal kit. The scissors in these kits have a hooked tip on one side designed to slip beneath sutures. The kit contains an alcohol skin wipe and a 2 x 2 for skin antisepsis before pulling sutures. Each suture is cut and pulled in the direction that maintains any knots above the surface. They should slide out readily with minimal pulling using the forceps in the kit. Sutures left in the skin too long may have substantial epithelialization that impairs suture removal. Some resistance also may be felt if crusts and scabs are not removed.

Staples are much easier to apply than skin sutures and will be used frequently by surgeons. The stapler bends the legs of the staple inward as it is pushed through the skin. These are easily detached with a surgical staple remover. Two prongs of the remover are inserted under the staple. When the handle is squeezed, the center of the staple is pushed down into a V-shape, which straightens the legs of the staple. As the tool is lifted from the skin, the staple's legs slide out of the skin. The staple is ejected from the tool and the process is repeated until all appropriate staples are removed. Removal with hemostats can be performed, but requires greater skill than using a tool specifically designed to remove staples.

SUMMARY

A number of decisions must be made regarding what dressing is appropriate for a given wound on a given person. A thorough history and physical examination, including issues that may dictate the need for more or less frequent dressing change and the ability to perform dressing changes must be done. With each dressing change the appropriateness needs to be reassessed. Nonocclusive dressings are appropriate for acute wounds, infected wounds, and wounds requiring rapid debridement or frequent inspection. Occlusive dressings are suitable for clean, stable wounds or wounds requiring autolytic debridement. Occlusive dressings range in properties from semipermeable films that retain fluid and allow some evaporation, foams that absorb large quantities of fluid, hydrogels that hydrate dry wounds, to hydrocolloids that absorb some drainage, but mainly hold drainage in place. Wound fillers are needed to occupy dead space in the wound. Alginates and hydrofibers are very absorbent, biocompatible, and suitable for wounds with heavy drainage. Hydrogels are useful for coating dry wounds. The use of moisture barriers and skin protectants helps protect surrounding skin from excessive moisture and the adhesion of

wound dressings. Most types of tape are too harsh for frequent use on skin, especially that of the elderly. Foam tape is preferred for direct skin contact. Silk tape is too harsh even for single use on healthy, young, skin. Harsh tape can cause skin tears of elderly skin. Secondary dressings are used in combination with primary dressings to meet the goals of the dressing. They range from simple bandage rolls to occlusive dressings. The proper combination of wound dressing materials cannot be dictated from a chart or company representative, but comes from consideration of all of the pertinent factors gleaned from a thorough history and physical examination.

QUESTIONS

1. Why are occlusive and semi-occlusive dressings inappropriate for infected wounds?

2. What risks to the surrounding skin are incurred in using an occlusive dressing that stays in place for several days? How can the risk be minimized?

3. Why do occlusive dressings lead to faster healing?

4. Why is hydrogel frequently used for neuropathic ulcers?

5. How do alginate/hydrofiber dressings protect surrounding skin?

6. What options do we have to minimize risk of injury to fragile skin when dressings must be applied?

7. Under what circumstances would a half-overlapping spiral be preferred over a figure 8 technique for a bandage roll? Under what circumstances would a figure 8 be preferred? A bulky bandage roll? A lightweight bandage roll?

CASE STUDIES

Based on the information given, choose an appropriate dressing, an interval for changing the dressing, and any progression in the dressing chosen.

1. An 80-year-old woman with a 40-year history of diabetes mellitus presents with shallow red wounds on the medial border of the left foot over the first metatarsal and below the medial malleolus. The wound has minimal drainage and the surrounding skin is dry. What long-term interventions need to be made to prevent such wounds from recurring?

2. A 90-year-old debilitated man is seen at bedside and observed to have a deep wound filled completely with gray necrotic tissue. He is also dependent in mobility. In addition to wound care, what other interventions are needed to promote healing and prevent other ulcers from forming?

3. A 35-year-old, 5 feet tall, 425-pound woman has a dehiscent abdominal wound with 25% granulation tissue, but 75% of dry necrotic tissue in the wound. What would you use initially? Once your initial goals are reached what would you do differently? What needs to be done with this person's nutrition at this time? At a later date?

4. A 25-year-old female cashier has had a wound superior to the medial malleolus for 2 years. The surrounding skin is indurated and stained a brownish-yellow color. The ulcer is irregularly shaped, shallow with nearly 100% granulation tissue within the wound. In addition to dressing changes, what other interventions are needed. What long-term intervention is necessary?

5. A 20-year-old man received a gunshot wound to the thigh. The wound is filled completely with a grayish yellow tissue and is foul smelling. The surrounding skin is hot, red, swollen, painful, and indurated with red streaks moving proximally. What type of dressing is needed? What other intervention is needed immediately given the signs evident on the surrounding skin?

6. A 25-year-old man decided to relieve the pressure in his overheated radiator by removing the radiator cap, and water sprayed over the entire anterior surface of the right upper extremity, chest, and axilla. The upper extremity displays redness from the elbow to the shoulder, and blistering from the elbow to the wrist. The radiator cap and rag protected his hand from burning. What dressing would you use initially? At what point would you discontinue this? What is likely to occur to the surrounding red areas on the arm, axilla, and chest over the next few days? Why would you extend the medication onto these areas?

7. A 55-year-old patient with a spinal cord injury has an ulcer on the ischial tuberosity with bone showing and surrounding areas of grayish yellow tissue. In addition to your dressing, what other interventions are necessary to prevent recurrence or occurrence on the other side?

8. An 85-year-old nursing home resident with poor mobility is left reclining in a chair almost all day long every day. He has a rounded triangular ulcer over the sacrum covered in hard black material. What needs to be done initially to remove the blackened material if signs of infection are present? What would you do if the wound appeared stable instead and you did not have any time constraints? What long-term interventions are needed to prevent recurrence?

BIBLIOGRAPHY

Ascherman JA, Jones VA, Knowles SL. The histologic effects of retention sutures on wound healing in the rat. *Eur J Surg.* 2000;166(12):932-937.

Demling RH, Niezgoda JA, Haraway GD, Mostow EN. Small intestinal submucosa wound matrix and full-thickness venous ulcers: preliminary results. *WOUNDS.* 2004;16(1):18–22.

Hodde, J. Naturally-occurring scaffolds for soft tissue repair and regeneration. *Tissue Eng.* 2002;8(2):295–308.

Hodde JP, Badylak SF, Brightman AO, Voytik-Harbin SL. Glycosaminoglycan content of small intestinal submucosa: a bioscaffold for tissue replacement. *Tissue Eng.* 1996;2(3):209–217.

Hodde JP, Ernst DM, Hiles MC. An investigation of the long-term bioactivity of endogenous growth factor in Oasis Wound Matrix. *J Wound Care.* 2005;14(1):23–25.

Hodde JP, Hiles MC. Bioactive FGF-2 in sterilized extracellular matrix. *WOUNDS.* 2001;13(5):195–201.

Kerstein MD. The scientific basis of healing. *Adv Wound Care.* 1997;10:30-34.

Kerstein MD. The scientific basis of healing: Erratum (missing table 2). *Adv Wound Care.* 1997;10:8.

McDevitt CA, Wildey GM, Cutrone RM. Transforming growth factor-b1 in a sterilized tissue derived from the pig small intestine submucosa. *J Biomed Mater Res.* 2003;67(2):637–640.

Mostow EN, Haraway GD, Dalsing M, Hodde JP, King D; OASIS Venous Ulcer Study Group. Effectiveness of an extracellular matrix graft (Oasis Wound Matrix) in the treatment of chronic leg ulcers: a randomized clinical trial. *J Vasc Surg.* 2005;41(5):837–843.

Niezgoda JA, Van Gils CC, Frykberg RG, Hodde JP. Randomized clinical trial comparing OASIS Wound Matrix to Regranex Gel for diabetic ulcers. *Adv Skin Wound Care.* 2005;18(5 Pt 1):258–266.

Parulkar BG, Sobti MK, Pardanani DS. Dextranomer dressing in the treatment of infected wounds and cutaneous ulcers. *J Postgrad Med.* 1985;31:28-33.

Rink AD, Goldschmidt D, Dietrich J, Nagelschmidt M, Vestweber KH. Negative side-effects of retention sutures for abdominal wound closure. A prospective randomised study. *Eur J Surg.* 2000;166(12):932-937

Solomon DE. An in vitro examination of an extracellular matrix scaffold for use in wound healing. *Int J Exp Pathol.* 2002;83(5):209–216.

Thomas Hess C. When to use transparent films. *Adv Skin Wound Care.* 2000;13:202.

Vazquez JR, Short B, Findlow AH, Nixon BP, Boulton AJ, Armstrong DG. Outcomes of hyaluronan therapy in diabetic foot wounds. *Diabetes Res Clin Pract.* 2003;59(2):123–127.

Veves A, Sheehan P, Pham HT. A randomized, controlled trial of Promogran (a collagen/oxidized regenerated cellulose dressing) vs standard treatment in the management of diabetic foot ulcers. *Arch Surg.* 2002;137(7):822–827.

Winter GD. Effect of air exposure and occlusion on experimental human skin wounds. *Nature.* 1963;200:378-379.

Scar Management

OBJECTIVES

- Instruct patients in methods to minimize scarring.
- Utilize methods to reduce the appearance of scars.
- Utilize methods to release adhesions due to cutaneous scars.
- Instruct patient/family/caregiver in scar management.

Scars have been discussed in Chapters 2 and 3 in the context of normal and abnormal healing. Full-thickness injuries heal with scarring, whether primary, secondary, or tertiary intention. Scar tissue lacks the strength and elasticity of normal skin and functions such as melanization, sweating, and oil secretion. Cosmetic issues include the lack of hair and altered pigmentation. The loss of elasticity and adherence of scar tissue to subcutaneous structures, especially to fascia may lead to decreased function upon closure of a wound. Immobilization during the formation and maturation of a scar frequently creates loss of range of motion following surgical procedures. Although healing by primary intention is less likely to create functional and cosmetic problems, prevention of complications and treatment to restore function may be necessary even with this

type of healing. This chapter describes the characteristics of scarring as they pertain to functional and cosmetic changes in the skin and methods of minimizing these changes and restoring motion of the skin.

NORMAL AND ABNORMAL SCAR FORMATION

Normal healing of superficial wounds occurs by re-epithelialization and, with time, remodeling of the dermis leads to normal skin appearance and function. With full thickness wounds, production of granulation tissue and wound contraction occur in conjunction with re-epithelialization. Myofibroblasts, fibrocytes, and colla-

Irion G.
Comprehensive Wound Management, 2nd ed. (pp 247-252)
© 2010 SLACK Incorporated

gen fibers produce a range of scar outcomes. Fibrocytes are a sub-population of white blood cells present in overabundance in abnormal scars. They have properties similar to fibroblasts including the synthesis of extracellular matrix macromolecules such as collagen. Fibrocytes are recruited to wounds and appear to be antigen-presenting cells like macrophages. These cells promote inflammation and may cause abnormal scarring due to their collagen production.

Optimal healing with a surgical incision produces a scar noticeable only with close inspection. Very large injuries, especially caused by burns, may produce massive scarring with tremendous loss of skin function and change in skin appearance. Burn scars, hypertrophic scars, and keloids were described in Chapter 3. These are the manifestations of overproduction of specific growth factors leading to suboptimal skin function. Hypertrophic scars become flatter and whiter over time, whereas keloids and burn scars maintain much of the initial function and appearance, with some decrease in the vascularity, but continued loss of normal skin contour and elasticity. Further, keloid scars may spread to adjacent uninjured skin and are likely to return if excised. Hypertrophic and burn scars may be excised and grafted if necessary.

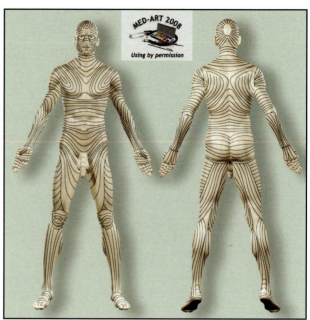

Figure 13-1. Langer's lines. (Used with permission of Davide Brunelli, MD. Available at www.med-ars.it/.)

HEALED VS CLOSED

Although considered by the general population to be synonymous, a closed wound may not be fully healed. The tensile strength of a scar is estimated to be 10% of uninjured skin when a wound is closed and becomes 80% under optimal circumstances. Remodeling of collagen fibers and restoration of skin elasticity and thickness allows skin to regain its tensile strength and perform its barrier function. These processes may require multiple weeks after closure, and in some cases, may not occur sufficiently on their own. Grafting or flaps may be necessary to produce sufficient coverage to restore sufficient skin function. Areas of particular concern are those with superficial bone such as over the olecranon and ulnar crest, the tibial crest and dorsum of the foot. The dorsum of the hand and other areas may also require surgical revision to achieve appropriate barrier function of the skin.

The orientation of a wound and its location also determine the quality of a scar. The skin's tension varies with location on the body along what are termed *Langer's lines*. On the trunk, neck, and extremities the lines run perpendicular to the long axis. The lines become oblique in rounded areas such as the pectoral, scapular, and gluteal (see Figure 13-1). For example, more tension is exerted horizontally on skin of the trunk and neck and less vertically in anatomical position. If possible, surgeons will create incisions along, rather than against Langer's lines. For example, a Cesarean section will be created with a slightly curved horizontal incision if medically feasible. Should a vertical incision be required, the scar will have more tension placed on it and will be more prone to being wide, thin, and weak. For the same reason, scars forming over bony prominences are subject to the same issues as discussed above and are less likely to heal completely when closed. Other issues with scar placement are discussed in by Wilhemi et al. In addition to Langer's lines, which were drawn based on studies of cadavers, guidelines described by Borges and Kraissl may be used in surgery to minimize scarring. Kraissl's lines are based on the direction of pull of muscles beneath the skin. Skin tension is considered to be at its minimum along lines perpendicular to the direction of muscle pull. For most areas, the lines are similar to Langer's lines. Another set of lines, particularly important for the face is Borges's lines. These lines run along furrows created naturally when skin is relaxed and skin is pinched. Multiple other guidelines are discussed in this reference.

POSITIONING/SPLINTING

Strategies for minimizing undesirable scar characteristics are based on minimizing unwanted stresses and increasing the stresses that produce a better quality scar. Body parts may be immobilized in splints, casts, or other orthoses. Although this strategy may be useful for optimizing scar quality, immobilization increases the risk of adhesions to subcutaneous structures, leading to pain and loss of range of motion and mobility. Abdominal scars decrease trunk extension leading to poor posture, secondary pain, and limitations of mobility throughout the upper and lower extremities. Scars affecting joints of the extremities lead to altered biomechanics with risk of injury to the joint directly affected and those involved in any compensatory motions. Methods for releasing adhesions are described below.

SURGICAL INTERVENTION FOR SCARS

A number of plastic surgery techniques are available to improve skin function impaired by scarring. Dysfunctional scars may be excised with or without grafting or flaps. More severe limitations caused by scarring are addressed with a technique known as Z-plasty. In this technique, a Z-shaped incision is made in scarred tissue. Tissue edges are rearranged in such a way that skin length is increased in functional directions (see Figure 13-2).

TOPICAL INTERVENTIONS

Pressure garments made of elastic material have been a mainstay of scar reduction for burn injuries. Pictures of common pressure garments are shown in Chapter 15. A custom-fit acrylic mask is used for the face rather than elastic material. Pressure garments are custom-made to exert approximately 18 to 30 mmHg pressure to involved areas. These are made of the same material used for compression hose for venous disease. The effectiveness of pressure garments on burn scarring, however, has been called into question. The uniformity of compression and the loss of compression over time within garments may decrease their effectiveness, and some studies have shown that those wearing pressure garments did not have better outcomes than those not wearing them.

Silicone sheets (Figure 13-3) can be used shortly after surgical incision to improve scar outcome. These sheets come in a variety of sizes and can be obtained at most pharmacies. They adhere to clean, dry skin and will continue to do so for several days. Depending on their location, they do not require any taping or secondary dressing to keep them in place unless they are placed on an area being sheared during sleep or a given activity. They are left on as much as feasible, but removed for bathing or any activity that might dislodge them, including sleep. Scars under silicone sheets are flatter and less discolored. Silicone sheets are expensive, but are reusable with proper care for several weeks. A given scar may require only a single sheet to obtain optimal results, but may need to be replaced if the adhesiveness of the sheet is lost. The mechanism by which silicone sheets work is unknown. A combination of chemical and physical properties is suspected. Silicone gel and sheets of other composition do not appear to be as effective as silicone sheets.

Another option for influencing scar composition is an ingredient of onions. However, onion extract in its com-

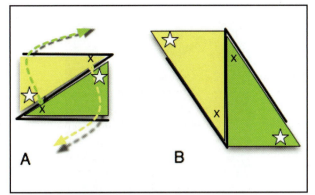

Figure 13-2. Z-plasty, a plastic surgery technique to improve the length and elasticity of tissue.

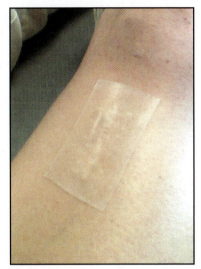

Figure 13-3. Silicone sheet used for scar modification.

mercial form has not been shown any more effective in the outcome of acute scars than simple petrolatum in a double blind, split scar study. Outcome in this study was defined as how pruritic, hypertrophic, erythematous, or painful a scar was. Other studies have shown onion extract gel to be better than placebo for scar coloration, but not for scar height, pain, or pruritus. These nonsurgical options are less expensive and invasive than the alternatives of surgical excision, intralesional corticosteroid injections, radiation, and laser treatment.

SCAR MOBILIZATION

Adherence of scars is quantified on a 3-point scale. A score of 3/3 indicates normal skin mobility. This is assessed at a comparable location deemed to be normal. Scores of 2/3 and 1/3 indicate mild and moderate hypomobility of the scar. Mobility should be assessed in every direction as adhesions may permit movement in some directions. For

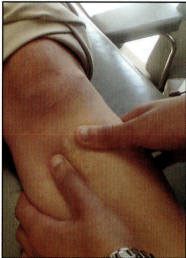

Figure 13-4A. Gentle massage to determine limits of scar excursion. Forces are increased to stretch scar as a form of massage.

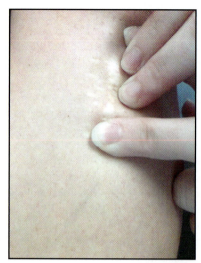

Figure 13-4B. Plucking an adherent scar. Two ends are fixed and the center (or other places as needed) are moved laterally to stretch adherent areas.

example, a scar may be fully mobile perpendicular to the wound, but immobile parallel to the incision, or mobile in only 1 of the 4 directions. The lack of any mobility is given a score of 0/3. Scar mobilization techniques are used for wounds that are sufficiently healed that aggressive mobilization will not tear through the scar. Generally this is the point at which any scabs have been shed. Areas of intact scab should not be mobilized directly, but other areas along the incision may be. Light massage-like mobilization 1 to 2 inches (2.5 to 5 cm) away from the incision may begin while scabs are intact. Prior to mobilization, desensitization may be required. This may be performed by simple massage of the area progressing to rubbing with a smooth surface cloth, progressing to a rougher object such as a washcloth.

As tolerated, the scar is pushed and pulled for several seconds in all directions that have limited mobility while feeling for the tension in the skin. Sufficient tension for blanching of the scar should be exerted and held. The feel of steadily increasing tension with stretch indicates that the scar tissue is within the elastic region of the length-tension relationship. A release in tension with further stretch is indicative of entry into the plastic region. If the plastic region is reached, improved scar mobility should be evident after treatment. Further stretch into the failure region may be difficult for patients to tolerate as it generally requires very aggressive mobilization through the elastic, plastic, and failure regions. A very abrupt release of tension may be palpated when the failure region is reached with full or near-full return of skin mobility in at least one direction.

The scar is then pushed or pulled in the opposite direction if necessary. Some degree of skin stretch should

occur to ensure entry into the plastic region. Intermittent stretching of the skin through functional movements that are restricted by the scar is performed throughout the mobilization session. Prolonged stretch of 15 to 30 seconds or longer may be combined with movement beyond blanching or the comfortable limit of stretch. Additional techniques such as contract-relax may be added by a physical therapist to counteract inhibition due to pain.

More aggressive scar mobilization is performed by plucking and rolling. Plucking refers to stabilizing 2 areas along a scar while pulling the scar perpendicular to the fixed spots as in plucking a string on a musical instrument. Rolling involves grasping a segment of scar and pulling the skin away from subcutaneous structures by rolling the skin between the thumb and index finger parallel to the incision. A more aggressive rolling technique along the length of the incision can be performed if tolerated by the patient. Patients are less likely to aggressively pluck and roll on their own. One should not expect progress with each session, but periodic improvements such as mobility being restored in one direction. Several sessions of aggressive scar mobilization may be necessary to restore skin mobility. In general, patients will require instruction and self-mobilization at home for good results. Relying strictly on the clinician to mobilize the scar will require either more prolonged or aggressive mobilization. Techniques are demonstrated in Figure 13-4.

PATIENT/CLIENT/FAMILY EDUCATION

In addition to techniques to prevent nonfunctional scars and to mobilize scars, education should include

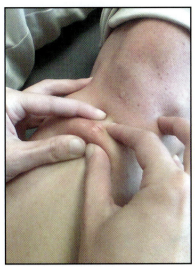

Figure 13-4C. Rolling an adherent scar. The scar is overlapped on itself while moving the fingers along the scar's length.

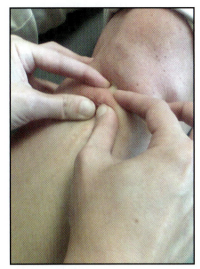

Figure 13-4D. A continuation of rolling the scar. In this case the scar is being mobilized from distal to proximal.

the effects of sun exposure on scar tissue. The lack of melanocytes and possibly other reasons, make this tissue more susceptible to sun injury. Covering skin or using a higher level of sun protection factor is necessary due to the greater risk of skin cancer in scar tissue than normal skin. Patients are also instructed in the need to lubricate scars to maintain moisture due to the loss of oil secretion, and to protect of the scar throughout the remodeling period as the tissue regains tensile strength. Itching (pruritus) is a common problem during the process of scar formation. Patients are advised to avoid scratching as this may lead to a vicious cycle of itching and scratching, injury to the skin or abnormal thickening of the skin. Alternatives to scratching include patting the area and, if ineffective, treatment with topical 5% doxepin cream (tricyclic that also blocks histamine receptors). Oral medications that may be used are gabapentin (anticonvulsant), ondansetron (serotonin blocker used to treat nausea), and diphenhydramine (histamine blocker).

SUMMARY

Scar tissue is the natural response to full-thickness skin injuries. Although most scars mature and remodel to return skin to near normal elasticity, some scars will present significant cosmetic and functional problems. Extensive scars and immobilization during scar formation are likely to create problem scars. Scar formation over bony prominences or other areas of natural skin stress and wounds perpendicular to Langer's lines (and other reference lines used

by surgeons) are also likely to cause problems. Options for preventing dysfunctional scars include splinting, pressure, and silicone sheets. Evidence for onion extract gel and pressure garments is not strong. Dysfunctional scarring may lead to loss of range of motion and secondary problems due to altered biomechanics in other areas. Scar mobilization techniques are described. These range from gentle massage-like movement to highly aggressive and painful rolling and plucking to free adhesions and restore skin mobility. Patient education about changes in the skin and protecting skin from sun and trauma as well as treatment of pruritus should be part of a treatment plan.

QUESTIONS

1. Why does scar management need to begin as early as possible?

2. What are the advantages and disadvantages of rolling and plucking scars?

3. What nonmanual options are available for modifying scars?

BIBLIOGRAPHY

Anzarut A, Olson J, Singh P, Rowe BH, Tredget EE. The effectiveness of pressure garment therapy for the prevention of abnormal scarring after burn injury: a meta-analysis. *J Plast Reconstr Aesthet Surg.* 2009;62(1):77-84.

Berman B, Perez OA, Konda S, et al. A review of the biologic effects, clinical efficacy, and safety of silicone elastomer sheeting for hypertrophic scar treatment and management. *Dermatol Surg.* 2007;33(11):1291-1302.

Brunelli, D. Langer's Lines. Available at http://www.med-ars.it/. Accessed September 9, 2009.

Chung VQ, Kelley L, Marra D, Jiang BS. Onion extract gel versus petrolatum emollient on new surgical scars: a prospective double-blinded study. *Dermatol Surg.* 2006,32:193-197.

Wilhelmi BJ, Blackwell SJ, Phillips LG. Langer's Lines: to use or not to use. Special topic. *Plast Reconstr Surg.* 1999;104(1):208-214.

Wynn TA. Cellular and molecular mechanisms of fibrosis. *J Pathol.* 2008;214(2):199-210.

Adjunct Interventions

14

OBJECTIVES

- Discuss indications for skin care products including therapeutic moisturizers, liquid skin protectants, and moisture barriers.
- Discuss the use of endogenous and exogenous growth factors to accelerate wound healing.
- Discuss indications, contraindications, and parameters for use of electrical stimulation with high voltage pulsed current and pulsed electromagnetic field.
- Describe the use of diathermy in wound healing.
- Discuss the use of ultraviolet C in wound management.
- Discuss the indications for negative pressure wound therapy.
- Discuss the theory of and uses of hyperbaric oxygen therapy.
- Discuss the theory of using therapeutic ultrasound and parameters for wound healing.

Debridement, dressing changes, patient education, and means to address the underlying cause of wounds are considered the primary components of wound care. Additional interventions may be appropriate on a case-by-case basis. These interventions constitute adjuncts to wound care. Adjuncts to be discussed below are topical agents including skin care products and growth factors and physical agents. Although many adjuncts are available, they are not substitutes for good wound management through debridement, appropriate dressing selection, offloading, compression therapy, and other means of addressing the underlying cause of a wound. A clinician should reassess the treatment plan before arbitrarily employing adjuncts.

SKIN CARE

A number of skin care products are designed to promote proper moisture levels in skin by adding moisture to skin, retaining moisture in the wound, or by protecting the skin from exposure to excessive moisture or aggressive adhesives used on some dressings. Three categories of skin products are classified by CMS. These skin products are not used directly on wounds, but to protect skin at risk for injury or to protect surrounding skin from damage from excessive wound drainage or from adhesives used for dressings. The categories are therapeutic moisturizers, moisture barriers, and liquid skin protectants. Other ingredients that

Irion G.
Comprehensive Wound Management, 2nd ed. (pp 253-268)
© 2010 SLACK Incorporated

Table 14-1

Categories and Ingredients of Skin Care Products

Category	Typical Ingredients
Emollient	Aloe vera, glyceryl stearate, lanolin, mineral oil
Humectant	Propylene glycol, glycerin
Preservative	Methylparaben, quaternium-15, propylparaben
Skin protectant	Allantoin, calamine, cocoa butter, dimethicone, glycerin, kaolin, white petrolatum, zinc oxide

may be present in skin care products include antimicrobials, detergents, humectants, preservatives, and surfactants.

Several lay terms may be used for skin care products. An emollient, by definition, is used to soften skin. Emollient typically refers to lotions used to moisturize dry skin, but in some cases, a product called an emollient could also be used as a moisture barrier. Humectants, such as glycerin, are designed to protect skin integrity by maintaining normal skin moisture. These agents could also be considered a type of skin protectant.

Skin care products are also classified by the terms *lotion*, *cream*, and *ointment*. This classification is determined chiefly by the concentration of solids and the fraction of water within the product. A lotion has a high water content and low concentration of solids. A product classified as a lotion is designed primarily for moisturizing skin that has lost moisture due to dry air or frequent hand washing. Lotion is important for both healthcare workers and for at-risk patients to prevent cracking of skin. Typical ingredients in lotions are water, mineral oil, stearic acid, glycerin, petrolatum, triethanolamine, magnesium aluminum silicate, glyceryl stearate, dimethicone, carbomer, methylparaben, DMDM hydantoin, aloe vera, and tetrasodium EDTA. In particular, aloe vera has been suggested to promote wound healing. Aloe vera gel is available commercially, but is not currently recommended by any wound guidelines. Aloe vera gel has also been shown to reverse the retardation of healing caused by the antiseptic, mafenide acetate.

Creams are thicker in consistency with less water than lotions and are frequently combined with solids such as zinc oxide. Ointments consist of substances that repel water and adhere to the skin. Common ingredients of ointments include petrolatum, mineral oil, lanolin, dimethicone, zinc oxide, and glycerin. Ointments and creams are used as moisture barriers for either protecting the skin around a draining wound or for protecting the perineum of individuals with urinary or fecal incontinence. Common skin care products and their typical ingredients are listed in Table 14-1.

The characteristics of various lotions, creams, and ointments can be tested easily by rubbing a small quantity on your own hand and dropping water on them. An ointment that will function well as a moisture barrier causes water to bead and run off the skin, whereas lotions designed as therapeutic moisturizers will allow water to remain on surfaces. Depending on the purpose of the substance, characteristics of the patient, and cost, different brands of ointments, creams, or lotions may be better suited for a particular patient. Various products may have ingredients better suited for therapeutic moisturizers or for a moisture barrier and some have a combination of both properties, and these substances have a wide price range.

Optimizing healing of wounds includes maintenance of an optimal level of wound moisture. Wound moisture is necessary for migration of epithelial cells, movement of enzymes, growth factors, and structural molecules. However, excessive moisture damages surrounding skin. Maceration may be prevented by less frequent and gentler dressing changes and treatment of the wound to decrease inflammation. However, less frequent dressing changes allow more drainage to accumulate beneath the dressing. A dressing and wound filler must be selected to allow an optimal combination of dressing wear, gentle handling of the wound, and protection of the surrounding skin from excessive moisture. In many cases, the clinician is faced with the choice of more frequent dressing change and promoting inflammation, or leaving a dressing in place and causing maceration. An option to lengthen dressing wear time without increasing risk of maceration is to apply a moisture barrier or skin protectant to the surrounding skin and a dressing capable of retaining drainage within the wound. A number of products are available for this purpose. An ointment with a substantial petrolatum, dimethicone, or zinc oxide component is useful as a barrier to water, causing beading and run-off necessary to keep fluid off the skin. Examples of skin care products are shown in Figure 14-1.

Liquid skin protectants, also known as skin sealants and skin protectors, have multiple purposes. Specifically, they are designed to protect skin from adhesives used for wound dressings. Secondly, they do not allow fluid from the wound to accumulate on the skin. They consist of molecules (butyl ester of PVM/MA copolymer) in a liquid vehicle that polymerize when exposed to air. Application of skin protectant is shown in Figure 14-2. Isopropyl alcohol is commonly used in skin protectants, which can cause pain if it gets into the wound or cracks in the surrounding skin. Nonsting formulations that do not use alcohol are also available. With a skin protectant in place, the adhesive of dressings does not contact the skin directly. When the adherent dressing is removed, the skin is less likely to be damaged. In addition, the polymer retains moisture in the skin and keeps moisture off the skin. Skin protectants should always be used under any self-adherent dressings or tape to prevent damage during removal, especially transparent films and hydrocolloid dressings because of the stronger adhesive used on them. Using skin protectants, the problem of protecting the skin from moisture leaking from the wound onto the surrounding skin and protecting the skin from aggressive adhesives can be accomplished simply with a single product.

Common skin protectants include Skin-Prep (Smith & Nephew, London, England), Allkare (Convatec, Skillman, NJ), Sween Prep and 3M No Sting Barrier Film (3M, St. Paul, MN). Skin protectants come in swabs, wipes, and squeeze containers. Regardless of the type of applicator, the material must be allowed to dry before a dressing is applied. Although adhesive removers are available, removal of skin protectants is not necessary with each dressing change. They should simply be re-applied as necessary. Adhesive removers are made of SD alcohol, propylene glycol monomethyl ether, decahydronaphthalene, ethyl acetate, and stearic acid. Frequent use of these can dry and damage skin. The use of a skin protectant can actually reduce the need for adhesive removers. Adhesive removers are typically used for removing dressings with aggressive adhesives. Use of a skin protectant under the adhesive allows the dressing to be removed without adhesive remover by gently lifting a corner and stretching the dressing material parallel to the skin surface.

Because therapeutic moisturizers and moisture barriers prevent dressings from adhering to skin, special measures need to be used if these substances are placed on skin surrounding a wound when a self-adherent dressing is to be used. Several means are available for securing dressings in these cases. A simple approach is to extend the dressing beyond the skin protected by these moisture barriers. This approach requires the moisture barrier be extended no farther than the beginning of the adhesive border of the dressing or to skin that can tolerate the increased moisture that may reach beyond the moisture barrier. A second

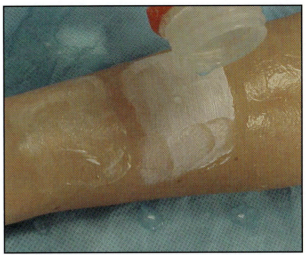

Figure 14-1. Examples of skin care products from left to right: moisturizing cream, protective cream, and protective ointment.

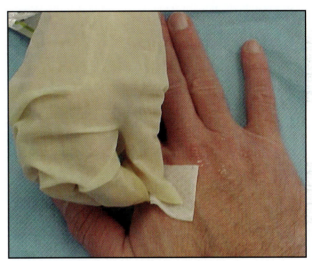

Figure 14-2. Application of skin protectant.

approach is to use a sufficiently absorbent dressing, or a dressing supplemented with another absorbent material, eg, alginate beneath a hydrocolloid dressing to prevent moisture from reaching the unprotected surrounding skin. A third approach is to secure a nonadherent dressing with elasticized netting or tubing. The clinician needs to exercise judgment as to the appropriate body part and person. For example, using this approach on the heel or elbow of a person who shifts position in bed frequently is likely to allow the dressing to shift off the wound, whereas this approach would work well on a nonweightbearing surface, away from joints, or in a person with limited mobility. A fourth approach is to use an elasticized bandage, a lightweight bandage roll, or a bulky bandage roll to secure a nonadherent dressing. Elasticized bandages or bandage rolls have the advantage of also managing edema, but may

Table 14-2

Strategies for Preventing Maceration

- Apply moisture barrier extending only to adhesive border of dressings or tape
- Fill wound with more absorbent material that does not wick onto skin
- Apply moisture barrier and use nonadhesive dressing with stretch tubing or netting
- Apply moisture barrier and use nonadhesive dressing with bandage roll
- Apply skin protectant on skin where drainage may accumulate

cause excessive pressure and limit the ability to monitor the wound. Bulky bandage rolls have the advantage of absorbing drainage that may leak from under the dressing to protect surrounding skin. Elasticized netting, tubing, and bandages come in a variety of sizes to allow wounds on any body part to be managed this way. A fifth approach is to use a liquid skin protectant as described above to protect the skin from both moisture and aggressive adhesives. The strategy used will depend on a number of factors, such as body part, characteristics and availability of different types of dressing, patient preference, and mobility, and numerous other issues. Strategies to prevent maceration of surrounding skin are listed in Table 14-2.

Wound Cleansers

AHCPR guidelines include cleansing of wounds with each dressing change. Two competing goals must be reconciled in deciding whether to cleanse the wound. For the clinician to perform a limited evaluation with each dressing change, the wound bed must be clearly visible. On the other hand, cleansing with each dressing change may cause tissue trauma and promote chronic inflammation. Because each patient presents with a different set of priorities, and priorities are likely to change through the healing process, the clinician should make a careful assessment of the need for cleansing. A reasonable philosophy to follow is that a dressing should be chosen to minimize the frequency of dressing change, but with each dressing change the wound bed should be clearly visualized to determine whether any changes in the plan of care are necessary. Cleansing may become necessary if the clinician cannot make a judgment due to lack of wound bed visibility. If possible, the dressing should be chosen to fit the number of days before the next evaluation or the patient or caregiver will be required to change a dressing and monitor the progress of the wound.

A number of products are available for cleansing wounds. Many forms of debridement also cleanse wounds, eg, whirlpool, irrigation, pulsatile lavage. The use of these is discussed in Chapter 11. Cleansers are designed to remove materials other than adherent necrotic tissue, which includes drainage, desiccated tissue, blood, adher-

ent macromolecules, and foreign materials. Cleansers range from normal saline to complex mixtures of detergents, chelators, surfactants, and preservatives including poloxymer, hydroxypropyl methylcellulose, potassium sorbate, DMDM hydantoin, methylparaben, D-panthenol, zinc gluconate, magnesium gluconate, and malic acid. Normal saline is least likely to cause tissue trauma and inflammation. Application of saline as a cleanser may be done by simply pouring normal saline over the wound or by using a low-pressure means such as an irrigation bulb. Higher-pressure irrigation can be performed with a saline-filled syringe with a small catheter attached. Another option is squeezing a bag of normal saline after removing one of the plugs from the bottom of the bag. Some studies have indicated that simple tap water is just as safe and effective as sterile normal saline on chronic wounds. Although some individuals use hydrogen peroxide as a cleansing agent because the effervescence may lift materials from the surface of the wound, this approach is not recommended because of the cytotoxicity of hydrogen peroxide. Ingredients found commonly in wound and skin cleansers are listed in Table 14-3.

Commercially available cleansers have a range of tissue toxicity; a number of these agents are listed in the AHCPR guidelines for treatment of pressure ulcers. Soaps and detergents dissolve in both water and lipid-containing substances such as cell membranes. Therefore, no soap or detergent is completely safe on wounds. In Chapter 9, infection control, soaps, and detergents are discussed as antimicrobial methods. By interrupting the surface tension created by hydrogen bonds of water molecules, surfactants allow soaps and detergents to bind to molecules in the wound. Chelators such as EDTA bind metal ions to remove them from the fluid, which softens hard water and improves the effectiveness of soaps and detergents. The combination of detergents, chelators, and surfactants makes specialized wound cleansers more effective than normal saline, but these chemicals may injure cells in the wound. Some dressings have these ingredients built into them in an attempt to accelerate the healing process by removing foreign and degraded materials from the wound fluid.

Table 14-3

Ingredients in Wound and Skin Cleansers

Category	Ingredient
Antimicrobial	Benzalkonium chloride, benzethonium chloride, benzoic acid, hexyl-resorcinol, malic acid, methylbenzethonium chloride
Chelators	Disodium EDTA
Detergents	Ammonium lauryl sulfate, sodium lauryl sulfate
Surfactant	Poloxymer, polysorbate 20

SKIN CLEANSERS

Skin cleansers are designed for use on at-risk skin and are often promoted as complementary products with skin protectants or therapeutic moisturizers. They are designed to be more gentle and effective than typical skin soaps and detergents. In particular, they are used for individuals with fecal and urinary incontinence. Both urine and feces are acidic, and fecal material is often very adherent. Frequent episodes of fecal incontinence throughout the day can lead to rapid breakdown of the perineal skin. Unfortunately, frequent cleansing with bath soap and scrubbing with rough wash cloths or towels to loosen fecal material can worsen skin damage. Skin cleansers, as described for wound cleansers, contain detergents, surfactants, and chelators. In addition, they are designed to neutralize the acid pH of urine and feces to reduce damage to the perineum.

GROWTH FACTORS

As of this writing, one form of growth factor has both FDA approval and coverage by CMS. According to the manufacturer, 99% of insurance plans cover it. Regranex (Ortho-McNeil, Raritan, NJ) is a 1% becaplermin gel, the trade name for platelet-derived growth factor (PDGF). The PDGF is generated by recombinant DNA technology, in which the B chain of PDGF has been inserted in a yeast, *Saccharomyces cerevisiae*.

Regranex has been approved for neuropathic ulcers with good circulation. This indication is based on research performed years ago showing that PDGF is deficient in poorly controlled diabetes mellitus. Replacement of endogenous PDGF promotes wound healing in individuals with diabetes mellitus, but becomes less effective if the person also has peripheral arterial disease. Regranex is provided in a gel that is to be applied in a thin film once daily and covered with a moist dressing. Because a thicker

coating provides no increased benefit and it is very expensive, it should be applied carefully. It must be refrigerated between uses. The effectiveness of PDGF is dependent on thorough debridement. It is ineffective if placed on necrotic tissue.

The FDA has recently required a boxed warning on the label of Regranex related to the increased risk of cancer mortality in patients who have used 3 or more tubes of Regranex. Use of Regranex was not associated with an increase in cancer incidence, but those who used three tubes or more had a 5-fold increase in cancer mortality. According to the manufacturer, it is not to be used in any area with a malignancy. The FDA does not recommend Regranex for patients with known malignancies. In clinical studies, 2% developed an erythematous rash near the wound to the gel base of Regranex.

An alternative to Regranex is the on-site production of platelet-rich concentrate from a patient's blood. A number of companies make devices to create it. Research is continuing on other growth factors and cytokines to facilitate healing.

PHYSICAL AGENTS

Therapeutic modalities using temperature, light, and other electromagnetic fields have been in use for more than 100 years, and some for centuries. Physical therapists are trained and licensed to apply these physical agents for a variety of indications. Nearly every possible modality available has been used in an attempt to facilitate wound healing. Cryotherapy is used for acute injuries to reduce pain and edema. Infrared light has been used in the past to dry wounds in an effort to prevent infection. This may have been useful in military situations in which triaging required some means of caring for wounds that were not considered as serious as those that required immediate attention; however, this is no longer a meaningful therapy. The forms discussed below include ultraviolet C, diathermy, ultrasound, electrical stimulation, and pulsed electromagnetic field. Other adjuncts to wound care to be discussed are hyperbaric oxygen therapy, negative pressure wound therapy, and application of leeches.

Ultraviolet C

Ultraviolet C (UVC) has a long history of topical use from cold quartz lamps for its fungicidal effect. Current recommendations for generating a bactericidal effect for cold quartz lamps is exposure for 72 to 180 seconds with the lamp 1 inch from the wound surface. Instructions provided by manufacturers for specific devices should be followed. Newer forms have been approved by the FDA for bactericidal use on open wounds. UVC has a wavelength between 200 and 290 nm. In contrast to UVA, which is used to activate chemicals in the skin such as psoralens for treating conditions such as psoriasis, and UVB used to activate melanocytes, UVC is directly toxic to susceptible bacteria. Wavelengths between 250 and 270 nm have the greatest bactericidal effect with a peak effect at the wavelength of 266 nm. The new UVC devices have guide bars so the wand can be rested over the wound, rather than requiring the operator to hold the lamp a given distance from the wound. UVC is particularly effective against methicillin-resistant *Staphylococcus aureus* (MRSA) and vancomycin-resistant *Enterococcus faecalis* (VRE) with a 99.9% kill rate using an 8-second exposure of UVC at a wavelength of 254 nm, an output of 15.54 mW/cm and distance of 1 inch. VRE were reduced to 99.9% with only 5 seconds of exposure. Exposures for 90 seconds and 45 seconds were required for 100% kill of MRSA and VRE, respectively.

Diathermy

By the definition employed by the FDA, diathermy devices cause "heat to go through" tissue. The FDA lists 3 types of diathermy: short wave, microwave, and therapeutic ultrasound. Microwave diathermy is no longer widely practiced and ultrasound is addressed specifically below. The benefit of diathermy as a heating agent is the ability to generate heat deep within the tissue, whereas the depth of heating of other modalities such as hot packs and whirlpool therapy is limited to superficial tissues. The Federal Communications Commission is responsible for ensuring that radio frequency emitting devices do not interfere with each other and has assigned an operating frequency of 27.12 MHz to short wave diathermy; however, some older short wave units may use the previously approved operating frequency of 13.56 MHz. Microwave diathermy has been assigned operating frequencies of 915 MHz and 2,450 MHz, the same as microwave ovens used for cooking. The FDA suggests that any diathermy device should be capable of producing heat in tissue within a range of 104°F to 114°F at a depth of 2 inches within 20 minutes and power output maintained below the pain threshold of the patient.

Short wave devices use coils and electronic controls to create an electromagnetic field that induces a current in the target tissue. Most short wave devices have 2 heads that can be positioned and operated independently. This configuration allows 2 areas of a body to be treated simultaneously or one area to be treated from 2 different directions. Application of very high frequency current creates heat in tissue. Heat may be used to raise tissue temperature to core temperature, which is the temperature at which cells replicate the most rapidly. Although diathermy is designed specifically for heating tissue, protocols suggested for applying diathermy to wounds call for a lower intensity—below that required to heat tissues. To further reduce the heating effect and optimize nonthermal effects, short wave diathermy is pulsed at a frequency between 700 and 7000 Hz. However, the mechanism by which "nonthermal" diathermy is suggested to facilitate wound healing has not been elucidated. The literature at this time does not contain sufficient randomized clinical trials to support the use of diathermy to augment wound healing.

A major advantage of diathermy is the ability to deliver the energy to the tissues surrounding the wound without actually touching the wound. Lack of patient contact with the device both protects the wound and the equipment from contamination. The diathermy drums (Figure 14-3) are placed near, but not touching the wound. A number of precautions must be observed when using diathermy. Diathermy must not be used over anything that is fluid-filled or metal. Check the patient for jewelry, ask specifically about any metal implants: orthopedic hardware such as prostheses, pins, screws, plates, and rods; pacemakers, defibrillators, intrauterine devices (IUD), cochlear implants, bone growth stimulators, deep brain stimulators, spinal cord stimulators, other types of nerve stimulators, dental fillings, metal sutures, or anything else that might contain metal. Even if the patient states that an implanted device has been removed, diathermy should not be administered unless you can be certain that all leads that had been attached were also removed. Leads may be left implanted after the device has been removed, or leads may have been partially removed. A safer policy is to never use diathermy for a patient who has ever had a metal implant. Have the patient remove any clothing with zippers or other metal fasteners. Be very specific about questions; some patients may forget about screws or rods left in bones unless asked specifically about them. Also check for zippers on pillows or any metal on the surface of the treatment table. Metal can become very hot and burn the patient, or may cause metal components of prostheses or orthoses to fail. The importance of determining the presence of implants cannot be overemphasized. Two cases of patients with deep

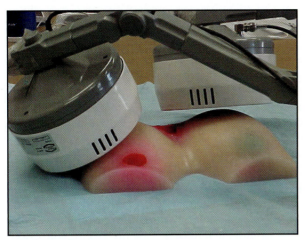

Figure 14-3A. Application of diathermy to a wound without towel.

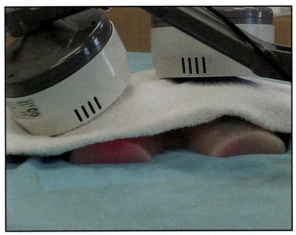

Figure 14-3B. Application of diathermy to a wound using towel.

brain stimulators receiving shortwave diathermy have been reported. Both received severe injury to the area of the brain where leads were implanted, resulting in a comatose state. Moisture in wounds, especially under dressings may be heated sufficiently to burn the patient. Dressings need to be removed and drainage absorbed as much as possible before treatment begins. Fluid filled areas include the eyes, heart, pregnant uterus, effusions, hematomas, and abscesses.

As with electrical stimulation, diathermy is provided for approximately 1 hour either daily or 3 times per week, depending on the patient. The Magnatherm (International Medical Electronics, Ltd., Kansas City, MO) device is designed specifically for enhancing wound healing. The protocol described by the manufacturer requires the patient be kept relatively still for more than 30 minutes and must, therefore, be positioned comfortably. Usually, positioning should not be a problem, because the arms on most diathermy devices are easily adjusted to accommodate most positions. Wounds need to be cleansed thoroughly before treatment begins to remove any substances that might absorb heat. If a wound needs to be covered, dry gauze may be used. In addition, the diathermy drum will need to be separated by either a folded towel or multiple towels to a thickness of about 1 to 1.5 cm. Some individuals have recommended that surgical caps be used to cover the drums. If this alternative is used, ensure that the drum does not make contact with the open wound, especially if the wound is wet. The drum typically needs to be kept an additional centimeter above the surgical cap.

The patient is to receive 5 minutes of treatment at a frequency of 5000 Hz at power level 12. This high frequency will produce heating of deep tissue. The protocol finishes with 25 minutes of exposure at the nonthermal frequency of 700 Hz and power level 12. Treatment is scheduled for

twice daily for 15 to 30 minutes for 1 to 4 weeks, depending on the size of the wound and complicating factors. Following treatment, the wound needs to be dressed as quickly as possible to retain the thermal effect of the treatment. The clinician should choose a dressing that is suitable for frequent dressing changes, yet optimizes the wound environment.

The risks and benefits of diathermy as an adjunct to wound care must be weighed carefully. The lack of scientific evidence of benefit and the risks associated with its use should be considered. To emphasize this point, one should realize that higher intensity diathermy is used surgically to coagulate tissue.

Therapeutic Ultrasound

Ultrasound (US) refers to sound waves with a frequency greater than what can be perceived by the human ear (20 to 20,000 Hz). Ultrasound used to create an image, such as echocardiography to examine the heart or to view fetal development is called diagnostic US. Therapeutic US is used to treat patients. The FDA considers therapeutic US to be a form of diathermy.

Ultrasound is generated by the application of a high frequency current to a crystal. The crystal vibrates due to what is called the reverse piezoelectric effect. The piezoelectric effect is produced when pressure is placed on a crystal to produce an electrical current. This effect is the basis of the phonograph. As described with diathermy, US can be used to heat tissue or can be used at a lower intensity or duty cycle (fraction of time that the US is activated) in an effort to assist healing of soft tissue injuries such as strains, sprains, and tendinitis. Ultrasound has also been proposed as a means of assisting healing open wounds. However, this modality has not been recommended by AHCPR due to lack of randomized controlled trials to demonstrate its effectiveness. Although a number of case studies supporting the use of US have been published, several randomized controlled trials have been done and have failed to show increased healing. Several studies investigating the effects of US at the cellular level have been published as well. Some of these demonstrate severe cellular damage created by US.

Application of Ultrasound to a Wound

For US to be transmitted to the wound bed, a coupling medium is required. Ultrasound does not conduct well through air, but does conduct well through water or water-based gel. Two approaches may be used to transmit US. One approach is placing the patient and the US head underwater. A second option is filling a deep wound with sterile US gel as a coupling agent. A shallow wound can be covered with a hydrogel sheet. Sterile saline may be used in the place of hydrogel, but saline is more difficult to keep in place.

Ultrasound can be provided at different frequencies, notably either 1 or 3 MHz. Higher frequency US does not penetrate tissues as deeply as lower frequency US. Clinicians have suggested using 3 MHz US on superficial wounds and 1 MHz on deeper wounds. The method of determining duration of treatment is based on the size of the US applicator. The recommendation is to move the US head over a site 1.5 times the size of the applicator for 1 to 2 minutes, then proceed to another site. For a small wound, the treatment can be done in a reasonable time. However, for a large wound, the duration of treatment required by this scheme may become excessive. For example, using a typical 10 cm^2 applicator on a 300 cm^2 wound, 20 areas would be created, requiring 20 to 40 minutes. The suggestion has also been to gradually increase time to 3 minutes per treatment area. For intensity, both pulsed and continuous modes have been described. Continuous US is more likely to create a heating effect, which may be desired or undesired. Acute injuries are typically treated with a low intensity (~0.5 W/cm^2), whereas chronic wounds may be treated with a somewhat higher intensity, approaching 1 W/cm^2. Intensity will depend on whether pulsed or continuous US is used and the duty cycle. One suggestion is to use pulsed US at an intensity of 1 W/cm^2 with a duty cycle of 25%. Suggestions given in the literature for the onset and frequency of treatment sessions is for BID treatments until the inflammatory phase is over, then reducing treatments to 3 per week. For chronic wounds the same sources suggest 3 treatments per week. A Cochrane Database report found 8 eligible trials of ultrasound as an adjunct to healing of venous ulcers. All 8 were found to have a medium to high risk of bias and no single study could demonstrate any statistically significant result. Pooling data from all eligible studies showed a possible weak effect of ultrasound on healing this type of ulcer.

Electric Stimulation

High voltage pulsed current (HVPC), formerly known as high-voltage pulsed galvanic, is the only type of stimulation presently available that has been consistently shown to improve wound healing. A number of early studies are supportive of low-intensity direct current, however, devices of this type are not generally available. On the other hand, microcurrent types of devices, which generate intensities in the microamperage range and various waveforms have been shown to be ineffective in promoting wound healing.

Several parameters must be used to describe a treatment protocol. Intensity may be quantified either in units of current (milliamps) or the electromotive force causing charge to flow (volts). For most devices intensity refers to current in milliamps, but HVPC devices are set in volts. Some devices will only have a knob or other adjustment marked current or intensity with a relative scale. If these devices are used, the intensity is adjusted to give a response that is determined by what the clinician observes, such as a minimally observable contraction, or to the patient's subjective response.

Intensity determines the type of neuron recruited by current. Although transcutaneous current recruits neurons based on diameter, the distance of the neuron from the source of current is also important. Based on size alone, the first neurons recruited by transcutaneous current would be the motor neurons signaling muscles to contract. The next group of neurons recruited would be sensory neurons indicating mechanical stimulation of the skin. Small sensory neurons carrying information about pain, temperature, and crude touch would be recruited last. However, because motor neurons are located subfascially, and many sensory neurons are located suprafascially, information carried by large sensory neurons is perceived at a lower intensity than that required to produce a motor response. The intensity required to recruit small sensory neurons in the skin may overlap with motor neurons, so a strong motor response may recruit an intolerable number of nociceptors, whereas a milder motor response is generally tolerable. As a general rule, the typical recruitment pattern produced by transcutaneous current is (1) the larger mechanoreceptive neurons located within the skin, (2) the large motor neurons beneath the skin, and (3) pain-receptive neurons in the skin. These 3 levels of intensity are termed *sensory*, *motor*, and *noxious*, respectively. Although the patient's perception tends to be dominated by the type of neuron newly recruited at each level of intensity, these levels are cumulative and overlap.

The second parameter is the frequency of pulsed current. Frequency of pulsed current is usually given in Hz (cycles per second). The frequency of pulsed current determines the quality of muscle contraction. Low frequencies create single twitches. Intermediate frequencies create undulating contractions called unfused tetanic contractions in which a slight relaxation occurs between stimuli. High frequencies produce tetanic contractions. The need to use the relative terms *low, intermediate,* and *high frequency* is due to the properties of different muscles. For example, hand and forearm muscles may tetanize at 15 Hz, whereas quadriceps may require 50 Hz for a tetanic contraction. For the purposes of wound healing, the frequency is generally much in excess of that needed for a tetanic contraction. A continual tetanic contraction would be very uncomfortable for the patient; therefore, electrodes are placed, if possible, away from muscles, and intensity is adjusted to a value that does not exceed a minimally visible muscle contraction.

The third parameter is the pulse duration or width. In general, increasing pulse width produces the same effect as increasing pulse intensity. Compared with devices used for neuromuscular electrical stimulation and transcutaneous electrical nerve stimulation, the pulses used for wound repair are very short, but the intensity is very high.

Waveform describes the combined effects of intensity, duration, and rise and fall times of pulses. The waveform of HVPC is generally described as triangular, although this term imprecisely describes the waveform. The pulses have a rapid rise and a slower decay and are paired. This waveform is often termed *twin peaks.* The rapid presentation of the second peak causes the 2 spikes to behave as a single electrical event. Therefore, in HVPC terminology, each set of 2 spikes is considered as a pulse with 2 phases. The timing between the 2 phases is adjustable on some devices as either the interphase or intrapulse interval. A shorter intrapulse interval increases the effectiveness of the pulses, but can be more uncomfortable for the patient.

Polarity describes the direction that ions or electrons travel relative to electrodes. A cathode attracts positive ions, or repels electrons. Anodes attract electrons and negative ions and repel positive ions. For historical reasons, the anode is termed the *positive electrode* because of its effect of driving positively charged particles away from it, and the cathode is termed the *negative electrode.* A number of studies have been performed with either positive or negative polarities for the electrodes attached to the wound. Other clinicians have started with a positive electrode over the wound and, based on a number of criteria, switch to a negative polarity. Other parameters include the duration of individual treatment sessions, the frequency of treatments and the number of treatments given.

General Technique

A typical HVPC device is depicted in Figure 14-4A. Twin-peak pulses are used at an amplitude and frequency of approximately 100V and 100 Hz, with pulse duration of approximately 50 μs. However, pulse duration and the interphase (or intrapulse) interval are fixed on many devic-

es. A variety of means for setting up the patient have been described. A typical set up is shown in Figure 14-4B. The positive electrode is placed over the wound with the negative electrode attached to the patient distally. Usually, the electrode that is not over the wound has a larger surface area to minimize current density and therefore, any electrical effects in the area used to complete the electrical circuit. A typical protocol for using electrical stimulation to augment wound healing is given in Table 14-4.

Electrodes

Several types of electrodes have been described. One approach to a wound with subcutaneous tissue loss is to place saline- or hydrogel-moistened gauze into the wound and attach the lead wire with an alligator clip. A number of manufacturers distribute hydrogel impregnated gauze for this purpose (See Figure 14-4C). The other lead wire is attached to a larger electrode. If this second electrode is large enough, one may consider the second electrode to be the indifferent electrode. Note the large indifferent electrode in use in Figures 14-4B and 14-4C. A typical protocol is to use a positive electrode in the wound for 1 hour either daily or 3 times per week, depending on the circumstances of the patient. When the wound does not continue to close at the accelerated rate, the polarity of the electrodes is switched to negative. The reversal of electrode polarity is to continue until the wound is either healed or progressing and stable enough to allow care to be completed by the patient at home. The size and distance between electrodes is adjusted based on the depth of the current desired. Superficial wounds should be treated with smaller electrodes placed close to each other. In the case of a deep wound, larger electrodes placed farther apart are used to drive current more deeply through the tissue of interest.

Electrode arrangements can be monopolar, bipolar, or multipolar. Due to the nature of electricity, any current will be bipolar, ie, electricity will flow from one area to another. The simple bipolar arrangement consists of 2 equally sized electrodes that will produce an equal flow of charge per surface area (current density) at both electrodes. Monopolar electrode arrangement is not truly monopolar, but behaves as if only one electrode is active. The monopolar effect is generated by creating a much greater current density at of the electrode of interest. Current density of the indifferent electrode is reduced by using a much larger electrode as shown in Figure 14-4B and 14-4C. The current is dispersed over a greater surface area, and therefore, the indifferent electrode is also commonly called a dispersive electrode. A multipolar arrangement is produced by arranging multiple electrodes for each polarity; this may be done using a bifurcated lead or a multichannel device.

The impedance of tissue beneath each electrode may vary tremendously from one place on the body to another.

Table 14-4

Typical Protocol for Electrical Stimulation for Wound Healing

- Polarity: initially positive; switch to negative when necrosis gone
  - » Switch to negative if healing reaches plateau
- Pulse rate: 100 Hz (some protocols are as low as 30 Hz)
- Amplitude: several volts below contraction
  - » Expected to be in range of 100-200 volts
  - » Depends on nature of tissue beneath electrode
  - » May be less than 100 V depending on patient tolerance
- Waveform: twin-peak
- Location
  - » Bipolar: one electrode on either side of wound
  - » Monopolar: active (negative) in wound, large dispersive distant on intact skin

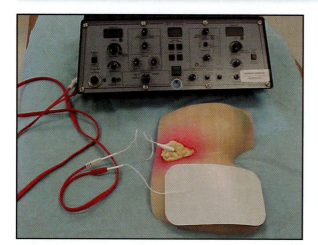

Figure 14-4A. Set-up of HVPC on a wound model.

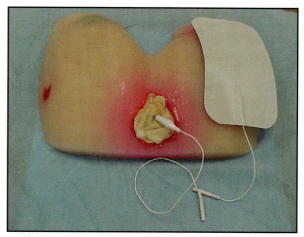

Figure 14-4B. Set-up of HVPC on wound model. Close-up of electrode placement.

Certain areas will cause discomfort or will diminish current. In general, the clinician should avoid dry skin, callused areas, bony prominences, and motor points. Placement of electrodes over these areas or over breaks in the skin will either cause patient discomfort and cause the clinician to reduce current to suboptimal levels, or will force the clinician to increase current to the point of patient discomfort. No conclusive data exist on optimal locations of electrodes. Several researchers have suggested that the dispersive electrode should be placed proximal to the wound.

Pulsed Electromagnetic Field

An alternative to HVPC is pulsed electromagnetic field (PEMF). PEMF is generated in the same manner as diathermy, but at a much lower frequency that does not produce heat. The optimal frequency for wound healing appears to be 15 to 20 Hz. Rather than placing electrodes in or around a wound, PEMF generates a current within tissue by alter-

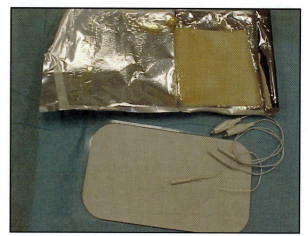

Figure 14-4C. Set-up of HVPC. Close-up of electrodes.

nating an electromagnetic field around the wound. A great advantage of PEMF over typical neuromuscular electrical stimulators is that PEMF does not require electrodes and can be used over clothing, bandages, casts, and so forth. PEMF has been used as a replacement for bone stimulators with implanted wires and has now been approved for the same purpose as HVPC for open wounds.

Several studies have shown increased rate of angiogenesis and wound healing, increased tensile strength of closed wounds, and increased release of FGF-2 with PEMF. Use of FGF-2 neutralizing antibody negates the effect of PEMF, suggesting the major effect is mediated through FGF-2. Changes in other angiogenic growth factors also occur with PEMF. Effects other than these growth factors and angiogenesis may be responsible for some aspects of faster and stronger wound healing.

PEMF is applied through 1 of 3 basic mechanisms. A ring that encircles a body part would only be used in a clinic and not for home use. Hand-held devices can be either held for the prescribed time or strapped on a part of the body. Suggested use for hand-held devices is holding the device over the area for 30 to 45 minutes, 1 to 3 times per day. Specific home use devices are made with an enclosed coil and battery that can be attached over the body area of interest with a strap or bandage roll. These devices may be left running until the battery fails. PEMF and other radiofrequency devices are not to be used on patients with pacemakers, implanted defibrillators, or similar implanted electronic devices.

Hyperbaric Oxygen

Oxygen is a required nutrient for survival of most tissues over an extended time. Specific to wound healing, oxygen is necessary for collagen production, neutrophil function to reduce risk of infection, and macrophage function in autolytic debridement. Moreover, high oxygen levels destroy anaerobic bacteria. On the other hand, high oxygen levels slow formation of new capillaries, cause arteriolar constriction, and may cause oxygen toxicity. The basic concept of hyperbaric oxygen (HBO) is to increase the oxygen available for wound healing. Claims made for HBO include increased antibiotic efficacy, fibroblast proliferation, collagen production and strength, production of growth factors, growth factor receptor sites, and elevated tissue partial pressure of oxygen. HBO been demonstrated as an effective treatment for a large number of conditions including decompression sickness, gas embolism, gas gangrene (clostridial myonecrosis), and carbon monoxide and cyanide poisoning.

Two types of HBO have been described. Systemic administration requires placing the patient in a chamber to accommodate the entire body. The gas composition inside the chamber is changed to 100% oxygen and is pressured to further increase the amount of oxygen within the chamber. A second type of HBO called topical HBO is administered by use of a plastic bag or other device attached to the skin over a wound. Whole body HBO is still recommended by those in this field, as opposed to topical HBO performed with extremity chambers or spot-chambers for areas such as the sacrum. A large number of case studies has been published, but randomized clinical trials showing efficacy of topical HBO are lacking.

Increases in PO_2 of inspired air at normal atmospheric pressure have a negligible effect on the amount of oxygen carried by the blood due to saturation of hemoglobin. Under normal circumstances, nearly 100% of oxygen carried by the blood is bound to hemoglobin. Once hemoglobin is saturated with oxygen, very little additional oxygen can be added to the blood. However, administration of 100% oxygen under 2 to 3 atmospheres of pressure can produce such a tremendous increase in arterial PO_2 that the amount carried by the blood improves. As arterial PO_2 increases, so does the distance that oxygen can diffuse from capillaries, which should be beneficial in any disease process in which diffusion of oxygen from capillaries is compromised.

Different types of systemic HBO chambers are available in different facilities. The type generally used for wound management consists of a clear tube accommodating one individual. Large chambers that accommodate multiple individuals are used for underwater physiology or treatment of decompression sickness (the bends or caisson disease) from too rapid ascent during deep sea diving or excessive exposure to hyperbaric environments. Typical systemic HBO treatments consist of 100% oxygen pressured to 2.0 to 2.5 atmospheres (2 to 2.5 times atmospheric pressure) for 2 hours daily or twice a day. Normal partial pressure of oxygen in the environment is approximately 760 x 0.21, or 160 mmHg. Partial pressure of oxygen in a whole body chamber may be as high as 1500 to 2000 mmHg. However, exposure to such high partial pressure of oxygen can cause oxygen toxicity, which needs to be monitored. Protocols may vary among facilities and type of wound.

Specific types of wounds appear to respond well to HBO. Crush injuries incurred within a few hours may benefit from the combination of pressure to reduce edema in the enriched oxygen environment and decreased leukocyte adherence. Similarly, skin flaps and grafts that are compromised by neutrophil accumulation during ischemia may benefit from this treatment. HBO has also been suggested for treatment of radiation necrosis and refractory ischemic ulcers. Wounds covered by CMS include necrotizing fasciitis, osteomyelitis, and crush injuries. See Table 14-5 for complete list of covered diagnoses. CMS has agreed to cover HBO for diabetic wounds of the lower extremities. Coverage requires that the patient have a Wagner grade III

Table 14-5

Diagnoses Covered by CMS for HBO Treatment

- Acute carbon monoxide intoxication
- Decompression illness
- Gas embolism
- Gas gangrene
- Acute traumatic peripheral ischemia as an adjunctive treatment when loss of function, limb, or life is threatened
- Crush injuries and suturing of severed limbs as an adjunctive treatment when loss of function, limb, or life is threatened
- Necrotizing fasciitis
- Acute peripheral arterial insufficiency
- Preparation and preservation of compromised skin grafts
- Chronic refractory osteomyelitis, unresponsive to conventional medical and surgical management
- Osteoradionecrosis as an adjunct to conventional treatment
- Soft tissue radionecrosis as an adjunct to conventional treatment
- Cyanide poisoning
- Actinomycosis, only as an adjunct to conventional therapy when the disease process is refractory to antibiotics and surgical treatment
- Diabetic ulcers of the lower extremity Wagner grade III or higher unresponsive to standard treatment

or higher, and failure to progress during 30 days of standard wound care. CMS coverage also requires the use of an FDA-approved HBO chamber for treatment. Coverage is ceased if wounds fail to improve within 30 days of HBO treatment. Although CMS recognizes that HBO treatment may require several months, average treatment time is expected to be 2 to 4 weeks. Unfortunately, the failure of wounds to heal is generally more complex than insufficient delivery of oxygen to tissues, which makes indiscriminate application of HBO to ischemic ulcers suspect. Moreover, the amount of time that can be spent in a hyperbaric chamber is limited. The effectiveness of HBO depends on proper patient selection. Poor delivery of oxygen to tissues is generally caused by arterial disease, which may be improved by surgery, rather than intermittent exposure to a source of enriched oxygen.

Negative Pressure Wound Therapy

In many deep wounds, edema and accumulation of drainage within the wound slows the delivery of nutrients necessary for healing. A constant, negative pressure device applied to the wound with a drainage system can be used to enhance the wound environment by removing excessive fluid. Devices consist of a pump, tubing, reservoir, and special foam type of dressing (Figure 14-5A). The dressing is cut to fit the wound and is placed into a wound with a film cover to seal the vacuum created by the pump

(see Figure 14-5B and 14-5C). Constant suction is applied to the wound until the wound's dimensions decrease sufficiently that the foam dressing can no longer fit in the wound. A smaller piece of foam may then be used to continue therapy. The appearance of a wound following negative pressure wound therapy (NPWT) is shown in Figure 14-5D.

CMS covers NPWT in either the home or an inpatient facility. For home care, chronic stage III or IV pressure ulcers, neuropathic ulcers, venous or arterial insufficiency ulcers, or chronic (defined as CMS as being present for at least 30 days) ulcer of mixed etiology may be covered. Coverage requires evaluation, care, and wound measurements by a licensed medical professional, application of dressings to maintain a moist wound environment, and debridement of necrotic tissue if present, and evaluation of and provision for adequate nutritional status. Requirements also include attempts to use standard treatment or they must be ruled out for medical reasons. Specifically for pressure ulcers, the patient must have been appropriately turned and positioned, the patient must have used a group 2 or 3 support surface (low air loss or air fluidized) for pressure ulcers on the posterior trunk or pelvis (not required if the ulcer is not on the trunk or pelvis), and the patient's moisture and incontinence have been appropriately managed. Requirements for coverage for neuropathic ulcers are evidence that the patient participated in a comprehensive

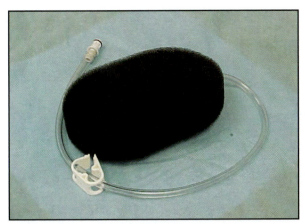

Figure 14-5A. Close-up of negative pressure wound therapy open cell foam dressing.

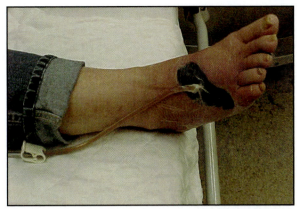

Figure 14-5B. Negative pressure wound therapy attached to the dorsum of a neuropathic foot.

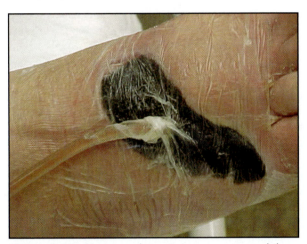

Figure 14-5C. Close-up of negative pressure wound therapy showing the evacuation of fluid from the wound.

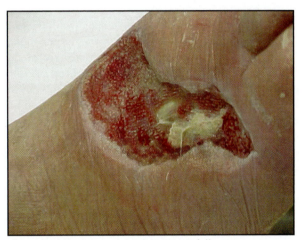

Figure 14-5D. Same wound as 14-5C following treatment with negative pressure wound therapy.

diabetic management program, and offloading the foot has been done. For venous insufficiency ulcers, compression bandages and/or garments must have been consistently applied, and leg elevation and ambulation have been encouraged. Inadequate documentation that wounds have failed to respond to standard care for the etiology will result in denial of payment.

Coverage for inpatient NPWT requires that treatments listed in the previous paragraph were either tried or ruled out for medical reasons and NPWT, in the judgment of the treating physician, is the best available treatment option. Coverage for inpatients includes complications of a surgical wound (primarily dehiscence), or complications of a traumatic wound such as the need for preoperative flap or graft, and medical necessity for accelerated formation of granulation tissue that cannot be achieved by other available treatments. For these approved inpatient conditions, coverage may be continued in the home.

Documentation, evaluation, and care must be performed by a licensed healthcare professional which may be a physician, physician's assistant, registered nurse, licensed practical nurse, or physical therapist. Denial may occur if debridement of necrotic tissue is not attempted, untreated osteomyelitis is present in the vicinity of the wound, cancer is present in the wound, or if a fistula to an organ or body cavity is present in the vicinity of the wound. For continued coverage, changes in the ulcer's dimensions and characteristics must be documented on at least a monthly basis. Medical necessity no longer exists if no measurable wound healing has occurred in either surface area or depth of the wound after 4 months, including any time NPWT has been used as an inpatient. Coverage is limited to a maximum of 15 dressing kits and 10 canister sets per month, unless documentation that a large volume of drainage, defined as greater than 90 ml per day is provided.

Application of NPWT

The system consists of a pump, which is durable equipment, and the foam dressing and canister, which are considered consumable supplies. Application should be done following standard infection control procedures. The wound should be cleansed or debrided as needed prior to application; NPWT is contraindicated for necrotic wounds with eschar. The surrounding skin is also cleaned thoroughly so the semipermeable dressing used in the NPWT application will adhere to the skin surrounding the wound. The procedure should be explained thoroughly to the patient and the patient positioned so the dressing can be placed in the wound without risk of it falling out during application. The patient should also be made as comfortable as possible and lighting should be adequate. Once the patient is in position, a new canister is placed in the NPWT pump and the open-cell foam dressing is cut with aseptic technique to a size slightly smaller than the wound. The foam dressing is then placed in the wound and the evacuation tube is connected to the dressing. At this point, the semipermeable film dressing that comes with the foam dressing material is placed over the foam and the tubing. The film dressing is then smoothed to ensure a seal around the wound and dressing. When a good seal appears to be in place, the evacuation tube is connected to the canister in the NPWT pump. The power is then turned on and diagnostics are run automatically by the device. A typical set up generates a negative pressure of 125 mmHg. NPWT is delivered for 48 hours continuously, then the dressing is removed and the wound is cleansed and reevaluated. As needed, NPWT is continued. The canister may be used for up to one week or until full. NPWT is discontinued when goals set for NPWT are reached. Goals may include wound closure, sufficient cleanliness of the wound or reduction in wound size to allow delayed closure. NPWT is generally stopped if no positive results are demonstrated in 1 to 2 weeks despite optimal care.

Types of Foam Used for NPWT

Two basic types are available for use. In addition, foam used for NPWT may be obtained preshaped for specific areas such as the abdomen, hand, and heel. The original black polyurethane foam has large pores, allowing negative pressure to be distributed throughout a covered wound site, even allowing multiple pieces to be linked within or between wounds. The polyurethane foam is flexible and easily trimmed to fit, but small particles of this foam can detach during trimming. This foam should never be cut over a wound, and any cut edges should be rubbed to remove any loose pieces that might come off while in the wound. The large pores reduce the tensile strength, so placing it into tunnel creates the risk of it breaking in the tunnel and leaving material behind. Polyvinyl alcohol (PVA) foam is white, has a greater density than the polyurethane foam, and has smaller pores. The greater tensile strength of white PVA foam allows filling of tunnels and undermined areas without fear of the foam tearing or breaking and being left in the wound. Polyurethane foam

is also available with silver, eliminating the need for a separate silver dressing to be used.

LEECHES

Application of leeches for medicinal purposes originated more than 500 years ago. Although the original goal was to restore health by bringing the body's 4 humors back into balance, current use is directed at overcoming venous congestion following reattachment surgery. Repair of injuries that involve reattachment of blood vessels such as gunshot wounds of the foot and crush injuries may also be indications for leech therapy. The leech used in current practice is *Hirudo medicinalis*. These leeches can be ordered from a small number of suppliers for overnight delivery and kept for several weeks in a ventilated refrigerator until needed. The saliva of leeches also has anticoagulant properties, which may diminish the risk of thrombosis of reattached digits, ears and skin flaps. Although some patients may not relish the idea of leeches being attached to them, the leech bites are usually painless, but may leave a characteristic "Y" shaped scar. Because leeches may attempt to migrate to other areas, a protective barrier must be applied around the area of interest. A small risk of infection or allergy also exists.

As needed, leeches are removed from the refrigerator and the skin is cleaned thoroughly with normal saline. A barrier is made from a 4 x 4 gauze sponge with a hole cut in the center and reinforcement with a towel. The leech should be transferred to the area of interest with forceps and guided as needed to the correct area. If the leech does not show interest, the skin may need to be pricked to draw a drop of blood to the area. The leech will feed for about 20 minutes and perhaps longer. The leech should be allowed to release the skin and should not be forcefully removed. When full, the leech will detach, but if pulled, mouth parts of the leech may be left in the wound and cause infection. The detached leech is then placed in a cup, covered in alcohol and discarded in an appropriate biohazard container.

Application of leeches may be difficult for the clinician. Because patients may be reluctant to agree to leech therapy, an unsteady or squeamish clinician may cause the patient to refuse an important therapy. Hematocrit and appearance of the site should be monitored regularly to ensure that excessive blood is not lost and the reattached body part is maintaining good circulation.

SUMMARY

Topical agents other than debridement and antiseptics are discussed in this chapter. Currently, one form of growth factor is available. Regranex is indicated for slow healing neuropathic ulcers in the presence of adequate blood flow and debridement. It contains platelet-derived growth factor, which is deficient in diabetes mellitus. Skin products include therapeutic moisturizers to prevent damage to skin by drying, moisture barriers that protect the surrounding skin from wound moisture, skin protectants that prevent damage by adhesives and fluid, and skin and wound cleansers. Skin and wound cleansers contain special ingredients to facilitate cleaning of wounds.

Several adjunctive therapies have been promoted to aid wound healing. Good evidence for the use of electrical stimulation and pulsed electromagnetic field exist and these are reimbursable through CMS. The evidence for diathermy and ultrasound is not as good and these carry risk of injury to the patient. Ultraviolet radiation may be a useful alternative to the use of antiseptics for controlling the growth of bacteria on the surface of wounds. Hyperbaric oxygen may be useful for wounds such as neuropathic ulcer, but evidence is lacking to support HBO for indiscriminate treatment of chronic wounds. Negative pressure wound therapy can be useful, especially for large dehiscent wounds and can be used for other types to stimulate production of granulation tissue.

QUESTIONS

1. What is the purpose of using platelet-derived growth factor for neuropathic wounds? Why is it not indicated for other types of wounds?

2. What is the purpose of a therapeutic moisturizer? What might occur if they are not used when indicated?

3. How can one maintain optimal fluid level in a wound without damaging the surrounding skin? What are common ingredients to find in this type of product?

4. What purposes are played by surfactants and chelators in wound and skin cleansers?

5. Which adjunctive therapies have received support from CMS?

6. Contrast diathermy and pulsed electromagnetic field therapy.

7. For what types of wounds would leeches be appropriate?

8. Contrast the purposes of systemic and topic hyperbaric oxygen therapy.

9. What potential benefits may be derived from HBO?

10. What are some of the possible drawbacks?

BIBLIOGRAPHY

AHCPR Supported Clinical Practice Guidelines. Available at: http://www.ncbi.nlm.nih.gov/books/bv.fcgi?rid=hstat2.section.4521. Accessed September 9, 2009.

Al-Kurdi D, Bell-Syer SE, Flemming K. Therapeutic ultrasound for venous leg ulcers. *Cochrane Database Syst Rev.* 2008;(1): CD001180.

Callaghan MJ, Chang EI, Seiser N, et al. Pulsed electromagnetic fields accelerate normal and diabetic wound healing by increasing endogenous FGF-2 release. *Plast Reconstr Surg.* 2008;121(1):130-141.

Crow L. New wound therapy offers treatment advantages for PTs. *Acute Care Perspectives.* 1999;7(2):10-11.

FDA Public Health Notification. Diathermy interactions with implanted leads and implanted systems with leads. http://www.fda.gov/cdrh/safety/121902.html. Accessed May 12, 2009.

Heggers JP, Kucukcelebi A, Listengarten D, et al. Beneficial effect of aloe on wound healing in an excisional wound model. *J Altern Complement Med.* 1996;2(2):271-277.

Hudson M. What's old is new again. Leech and maggot therapy: wound care in the 90's. *Acute Care Perspectives.* 1999;7(2):15-17.

Kalliainen LK, Gordillo GM, Schlanger R, Sen CK. Topical oxygen as an adjunct to wound healing: a clinical case series. *Pathophysiology.* 2003;9(2):81-87.

Medical Coverage Policies. Blue Cross/ Blue Shield of Rhode Island. https://www.bcbsri.com/BCBSRIWeb/plansandservices/services/medical_policies/VacuumAssistedWoundClosure.jsp Accessed July 4, 2008.

Medicare Coverage Issues. Transmittal 129. https://www.cms.hhs.gov/transmittals/downloads/R129CIM.pdf. Accessed May 12, 2009.

Rossi F, Elsinger E. Topical hyperbaric oxygen therapy for lower extremity wound care: an overview. *Podiatry Management.* 1997; November: 110-111.

Sheffield PJ. Tissue oxygen measurements with respect to soft tissue wound healing with normobaric and hyperbaric oxygen. *HBO Review.* 1985;6:18-43.

Smith PD, Kuhn MA, Franz MG, Wachtel TL, Wright TE, Robson MC. Initiating the inflammatory phase of incisional healing prior to tissue injury. *J Surg Res.* 2000;92(1):11-17.

Strauch B, Patel MK, Navarro JA, Berdichevsky M, Yu HL, Pilla AA. Pulsed magnetic fields accelerate cutaneous wound healing in rats. *Plast Reconstr Surg.* 2007;120(2):425-430.

Tepper OM, Callaghan MJ, Change EI, et al. Electromagnetic fields increase in vitro and in vivo angiogenesis through endothelial release of FGF-2. *FASEB J.* 2004;18(11):1231-1233.

Wieman TJ, Smiell JM, Su Y. Efficacy and safety of a topical gel formulation of recombinant human platelet-derived growth factor-BB (becaplermin) in patients with chronic neuropathic diabetic ulcers. A phase III randomized placebo-controlled double-blind study. *Diabetes Care.* 1998;21(5):822-827.

Young SR, Dyson M. Effective therapeutic ultrasound on the healing of full-thickness excised skin lesions. *Ultrasonics.* 1999; 28:175-180.

Thermal Injuries

15

OBJECTIVES

- Discuss first aid for burn injury.
- Describe typical medical management of severe thermal injury.
- Describe types of skin grafting/replacement available.
- Discuss how skin grafting affects exercise programs.
- Discuss appropriate exercise for individuals with thermal injuries.
- Discuss scar management following thermal injury.

FIRST AID FOR BURNS

First aid for burns should be taught at an early age to everyone. The first thing that should be done is to stop the burning process as quickly as possible to minimize burn injury and to remove the person from the source of heat. Should clothing become ignited the person must follow the basic rules of "stop, drop, and roll" to extinguish any flames. Other than high voltage electric shock, ignition of clothing produces the most severe burn injuries. After any flames are extinguished, all burned clothing must be removed. Smoldering clothing continues to transfer heat to the body. In some cases clothing may adhere to the skin, especially those made of synthetic fibers. If so, what is not adherent should be cut, if possible. Cool water, not cold water or ice, should be poured over burned area for 3 to 5 minutes. Cold water is capable of increasing the injury produced by heat.

In the case of a chemical injury, the area should be flushed continuously with cool water for 30 to 40 minutes. However, one must be careful not to flush chemicals onto areas of the body not already contaminated. Contact lenses should be removed before flushing. In the case of chemical injury, the label should be read and instructions should be followed if they are available. Otherwise, a poison control center must be contacted and instructions followed if the substance can be described to them.

Jewelry, belts, or anything else that could constrict should be removed as soon as possible; swelling occurs rapidly and can be severe. Ointments, butter, or anything else that is not sterile should not be applied to the burn to prevent infection of the damaged tissue. Burns should then

Irion G.
Comprehensive Wound Management, 2nd ed. (pp 269-276)
© 2010 SLACK Incorporated

be covered with a soft, clean, dry dressing, bandage, or sheet and the person kept warm while emergency personnel are en route. Medical attention should be summoned as soon as possible.

For minor burns, an antiseptic spray or cream with local anesthetic may be applied to the wound, along with a sterile dressing to protect the wound. If the wound does not appear to heal or if it appears to weep or have a foul odor, the injured individual should seek medical attention.

In the case of an electrical injury, the person in contact with electricity should not be touched until the source of current is disconnected. At that time the primary concern is circulation and breathing. With high voltage injuries, cardiopulmonary resuscitation may be required.

BURN INTERVENTIONS

Treatment of the burned person may include some or all of the following depending on the extent and severity of burns. Medical management includes emergency care, pain management, surgical debridement, and grafting. Physical therapists and other healthcare providers may be involved in further debridement, dressing changes, exercise, positioning, splinting, and scar management. Persons with small, partial-thickness wounds may require no emergency medical procedures, only pain medications and either brief inpatient or outpatient care for debridement, dressing changes, exercises, positioning, splinting, and scar management.

Medical Management

Major burns due to a combination of severity and body surface area are life-threatening and may have complications requiring emergency care. Life-threatening complications of burn injuries include hypovolemic shock due to fluid loss through wounds, the osmotic effect of dead tissue, loss of plasma proteins from damaged blood vessels, injury to airways and lungs due to heat and inhaled toxins, which may lead to the development of acute respiratory distress syndrome (ARDS), and burn infection. Burn infection may be caused by loss of the first barrier to infection, the presence of necrotic tissue, decreased blood flow to the burned area, and immune suppression. Following burn infection, bacteremia, especially if gram negative organisms are involved, may produce septic shock and death. In particular, fungal infections are problematic. Those with large, full-thickness wounds will receive emergency care, including an intravenous line, copious quantities of intravenous fluid, immediate cleaning, weighing, and debridement as tolerated, with surgical debridement as soon as the patient is medically stable. These patients will also receive nutritional support and will have an elevated room temperature to compensate for the patient's hypermetabolic

state. Hospitalization is expected to be approximately 1 day for each percentage of body surface area burned, plus 5 days for each grafting procedure, barring serious complications. Many individuals are hospitalized for months and may be intubated several times during the course of hospitalization. Wound infections will also add to the length of stay.

Debridement and Cleansing

Debridement and cleansing may be the responsibility of physical therapists, occupational therapists, or burn technicians and may involve whirlpool therapy. The type and extent of debridement or cleansing depend on the severity of the wound in terms of the depth of injury and the percentage of body surface area burned. Small, partial-thickness wounds may be cleaned and debrided on a once or twice daily basis. Large full-thickness wounds may be surgically debrided to the extent possible immediately upon arrival in a burn center. During hydrotherapy or other cleansing, water temperature should not exceed body temperature; excess heat can exacerbate damage to reversibly damaged cells. Breaking of blisters of superficial partial-thickness wounds continues to be controversial. The fluid in these blisters is considered sterile, so rupturing the blisters exposes necrotic tissue to environmental flora and increases the risk of infection. On the other hand, rupturing blisters and removing necrotic tissue decreases the risk of infection; moreover, several mediators of inflammation present within the blister fluid slow wound healing. Eventually with debridement all blisters will rupture as surrounding skin peels off into the blister. Whirlpool or cleansing with a basin and sterile saline to continue debridement, and remove topical medications and remaining contaminants may precede dressing changes. Silver sulfadiazine may be covered with a dressing or left uncovered. A simple bandage roll may suffice to protect the silver sulfadiazine from being removed by normal contact of the extremity during activity. Other options include sulfamylon and silver dressings described in Chapter 12. In the case of superficial partial-thickness burns with blisters, fan-folding the bandage roll or placing multiple gauze sponges over the blisters may be necessary to absorb drainage that might occur should the blisters rupture. Once necrotic tissue is debrided, the risk of infection is decreased substantially as is the need for silver sulfadiazine. Wounds should be evaluated at least briefly every time dressings are changed as wounds may evolve over a period of 3 to 4 days after the injury.

Grafting

Large, full-thickness burns can only regenerate from the edges; therefore, re-epithelialization is usually too slow to be feasible. Moreover, repair by secondary intention is more likely to lead to unacceptable wound contraction and loss of function. Persons with large, full-thickness burns will need skin grafts to cover their wounds. The types of grafts available include an autograft taken from unburned areas of the patient's own skin (donor site). The thighs, buttocks and trunk are the most common, but the site chosen depends on the size of the wound and what areas are not burned. An allograft is skin derived from another person, usually a cadaver. A patient receiving such a graft may need immunosuppressive drugs to prevent rejection. A xenograft is taken from another species, usually pigs. Artificial skin and cultured skin may be used when not enough viable skin is available for grafting. Over several weeks a small area of skin can be grown into a large sheet under culture conditions. Living skin equivalents (Apligraf, Integra, and others) may be used for several days until grafting can be performed. Removal of skin is done under anesthesia with a device called a dermatome. Either a full-thickness or split thickness may be cut. A full-thickness graft removes the entire thickness of the reticular dermis and is required for areas such as the face, neck, and flexor surfaces such as the elbow and axilla due to the superior functional and cosmetic results. Split thickness grafts are cut approximately 0.017 inch in thickness and may be either placed as a sheet or meshed before attaching them. One or more partial-thickness sheets are taped or stapled to the recipient site.

The recipient site must be clear of necrotic tissue and care taken to avoid accumulation of blood or serum under the graft. A sheet graft initially adheres to a site by a fibrin clot. Later, blood vessels invade the sheet and either anastomose with existing vessels in the sheet, or form new vessels in the sheet. The advantage of a sheet is a cosmetically better result, but accumulation of fluid under the graft or infection will cause failure of the graft to take. A meshed split thickness graft can be stretched to cover as much as 3 times the size of the donor site, which increases the efficiency of wound coverage. Applying a split thickness, meshed graft converts a single large wound into multiple small wounds with a short distance for cells to migrate to fill the wound. In addition to the greater coverage of a meshed graft, fluid will not accumulate beneath and cause graft failure. Healed split thickness grafts usually produce a characteristic diamond pattern on the healed skin (see Figure 15-1). Full-thickness donor sites are covered with a split thickness graft to heal the donor site. Split-thickness grafts can be harvested repeatedly after 10 to 14 days to cover more areas (Figure 15-2). This process allows autografting to cover large areas. Several reasons exist for failure of skin grafts to take. As discussed above, grafts first adhere to the recipient site by fibrin clot and within several days blood vessels invade the graft and collagen fibers form between the graft and underlying tissue. Inadequate excision or debridement of necrotic tissue from the

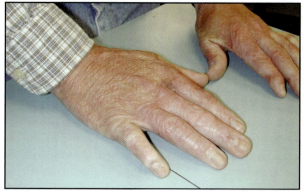

Figure 15-1. Healed split-thickness graft of the hand. Courtesy of Arkansas Children's Hospital, Little Rock, AR.

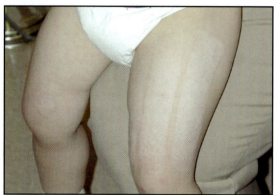

Figure 15-2. Donor site for partial-thickness grafting. Note healing, which will allow this area to be repeatedly harvested for partial-thickness grafting. Courtesy of Arkansas Children's Hospital, Little Rock, AR.

underlying tissue, inadequate contact of the graft due to accumulation of blood or serum, infection, and excessive mobility of the graft on the site are the primary reasons for grafts to fail. In many facilities stretching and active exercise of the grafted areas are discontinued for 3 to 5 days for upper extremity and trunk grafts and 7 to 10 days for lower extremity grafts. Other facilities allow active movement within the range of motion within the limit of staple pain on the day following grafting.

Range of Motion, Positioning, and Splinting

Exercise, positioning, and splinting are performed to avoid contractures and edema. Patients will generally hold limbs in the position of greatest comfort rather than move through a range of motion. Unwillingness to move a limb or an area of the trunk and neck is a risk for contracture; therefore, when only one side of a limb is burned, the simple solution is to splint or position so that the burned surface is put on a stretch. A second consideration for preventing contractures is knowing the propensity of given body segments to develop contractures. The most likely areas are the hand, axilla, neck, elbow, and foot. Contractures on the face may occur at the epicanthus, the commissures of the mouth, and lower lip. Burns to the anterior or lateral neck will cause flexion or lateral deviations of the head. Patients need to be positioned with the neck extended and rotated to the opposite side of any scar formation. This position may be accomplished by the use of two mattresses on the bed with the body supported by the upper mattress and the head by the lower. Contracture of the anterior axillary fold will primarily limit shoulder abduction, whereas scarring of the posterior axillary fold will limit shoulder flexion. Patients will need to have the shoulders placed in abduction and/or flexion with burns to these areas to reduce the risk of contractures.

The affected upper extremity may be placed in a tubular stocking and suspended from an overhead frame or from IV poles to achieve the desired position. Burns involving both the neck and axilla on the same side are particularly troublesome. Stretching the axilla places the skin of the neck on slack and stretching the neck requires the axilla to be placed on slack. Obviously, the patient should not be placed permanently in either position, but a schedule must be developed to accommodate the positioning needs for both body segments. The hand is at risk for a number of deformities. Formerly, the functional position of the hand was promoted for cases in which the hand was very likely to become contracted. The functional position is considered to be thumb opposition, slight wrist extension, and slight finger flexion to promote grasp and allow the patient to reach the mouth for feeding and grooming. The palm is very adherent and taut and left untreated, burn injury can produce finger flexion and opposition contractures. A burn of the palm will require a full-thickness graft to decrease the risk of contracture. The skin of the dorsum of the hand can accommodate substantial swelling, which, in turn, can produce a variety of deformities of the fingers. Untreated swelling of the dorsum of the hand produces a claw hand deformity with metacarpal-phalangeal extension and proximal and distal interphalangeal joint flexion. Injury to the relatively superficial extensor tendons of the hand can also produce boutonniere, swan neck, or mallet finger deformities.

Burns of the lower extremities may produce contractures into hip abduction and flexion and knee flexion, but the foot is at greatest risk of loss of function. The foot can develop either a contracture into dorsiflexion or plantar flexion, depending on the surface injured. Plantar flexion contractures are common problems when both sides are involved and the patient is bed bound. The weight of the foot compounded by sheets and blankets over the foot place the foot in a plantar flexed position. Simple low-temperature thermoplastic splints placed on the foot are

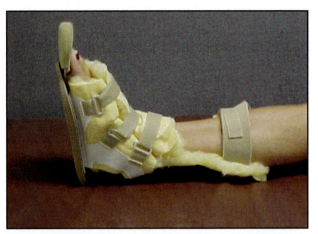

Figure 15-3. Multipodus foot orthoses phase II (Restorative Care of America, St Petersburg, FL) for preventing contracture of the ankle.

generally inadequate to overcome the forces of plantar flexion and more sophisticated and expensive devices are needed to prevent loss of dorsiflexion (see Figure 15-3).

As a general rule, if a patient is burned on both a flexor and extensor surface, one may choose to splint or position the joint in extension because of the greater ease of stretching tissue back into flexion than stretching back into extension. Frequent range of motion into both directions becomes even more imperative in this situation to minimize shortening in either direction. If possible, one should position the patient's body segments to avoid dependence of burned area and promotion of edema. In addition, skin creases above and below the burned area should be evaluated. As scarring and wound contraction proceed, the reservoir of skin elasticity is taken up in all directions from the site of injury. A potential complication that needs to be addressed in treatment planning is that skin elasticity is not equal in all directions of the body. Langer's lines (refer to Figure 13-1) represent a graphical means of discussing this phenomenon. Along the extremities, the skin is generally more extensible in a proximal-distal direction than in a medial-lateral direction. On the trunk, head and neck, the skin is more extensible in the cephalic-caudal direction than medially and laterally. Scars oriented vertically on the trunk or extremities have greater tension that those running along Langer's lines (horizontally). Some of Langer's lines are curved or oblique, especially at the transitions between body segments. Lines in these areas correspond to large muscles below. Over the gluteal, pectoral, and scapular regions, lines run perpendicular to the line of pull of these muscles. A scar forming along the line of pull of these muscles has greater stress on it than one forming perpendicular to the line of pull. Because the skin has more tension along these lines than between them, a round wound preferentially contracts perpendicularly to these lines, resulting in an oval scar that is elongated along a Langer's line instead of a round scar. Another manifestation of tapping into the skin's reservoir of elasticity is the loss of extensibility at adjacent skin creases. If a burn occurs over 3 adjacent skin creases such as the wrist, elbow, and shoulder, the middle joint is most affected by loss of extensibility and, in the case in which 2 adjacent surfaces are injured, the more proximal joint is more likely to lose extensibility.

Exercise

Although prevention of contracture needs to be the primary goal of therapy, strength and cardiovascular condition need to be maintained as much as possible. For smaller wounds treated in the whirlpool tank for debridement, active range of motion exercises can be done at the same time. Many patients who otherwise could not tolerate active movement of a hand or other body part can do so in the turbulent water. The patient needs to start moving the affected segment early. As the wound evolves and nerves regenerate, the patient may become increasingly unwilling to move affected parts of the body. Because of the potential for loss of extensibility throughout a limb due to scarring, active range of motion of other joints in the same extremity must also be encouraged in spite of pain. The type of exercise used to promote range of motion may range from passive range of motion, in which the movement is performed without any effort by the patient, to active-assisted range of motion in which the patient's movement is guided and assisted as necessary by another person. If the clinician is familiar with them, PNF (proprioceptive neuromuscular facilitation) patterns can be used to more efficiently stretch several joints at once with movement in 3 planes simultaneously. Active range of motion is performed by the patient, but the patient may receive verbal or tactile cues to guide the motion. A person who is unresponsive can only receive passive range of motion. However, the force placed on the healing skin cannot be gauged well by the person performing the passive range of motion and the movement can be excessive.

Range of Motion

During range of motion exercise, the clinician needs to monitor the patient for skin blanching, complaints of pain, excessive force needed to move a body segment, and signs of apprehension from the patient. Generally, the blanching, pain, excessive force, and signs of apprehension will occur at the same point in the stress-strain relationship of the skin when the slack has been taken out of the affected skin and it is stretched into the linear portion of the stress-strain relationship. The type and location of the pain reported by the patient also guides the force applied. Pain in the area of limited skin movement accompanied by tightness and blanching indicates the need to reduce

force. A pain caused by movement, especially compression of the tender skin overlying a moving body segment, is not an indication to stop exercise. Finally, if a patient demonstrates optimally expected range of motion, but the skin over the area blanches, the patient will continue to need therapy until the body segment can be moved independently through the range of motion without blanching.

Active range of motion exercises are least likely to harm healing tissue and grafts, but may be too difficult for a given individual to accomplish, especially one with an altered nutritional status, diminished strength, severe pain, and already limited range of motion. Active assisted range of motion is often an intermediate step in the progression to active range of motion exercises. When the patient is near the end of safe range of motion, the patient will cease moving the limb, letting the clinician or caregiver know that appropriate range of motion has been achieved. Active range of motion exercises are generally indicated if edema needs to be reduced in a particular body segment, if tendons are exposed, and during the first week after a skin graft. The muscle pumping effect assists in the removal of excessive fluid from the body part. An additional benefit of active rather than passive range of motion, particularly in PNF patterns is return to normal neuromusculoskeletal function.

Active-assisted range of motion exercise is typically indicated for a person with sufficient strength and coordination to follow verbal and tactile cues, but who already has elevated metabolic demands such that active exercise may increase cardiovascular demands excessively. Passive range of motion becomes necessary in certain cases that are rather obvious, such as peripheral nerve injury or other loss of motor input to the limb, including the use of general anesthesia. Passive range of motion may also be indicated for areas that need more extensive tissue elongation or an area of escharotomy. In addition, if the patient cannot tolerate active assisted range of motion due to excess metabolic demands, passive range of motion may be necessary for a number of days.

Passive range of motion exercises should not be performed in the cases of finger burns with an indeterminate depth due to risk of tendon injury, in areas of heterotopic ossification, exposed tendons, or in extremely resistive or combative patients. Range of motion exercises may be done while the patient is in full dressings, but performing range of motion exercises during dressing changes has the advantages that the clinician can see the skin's response to the motion and the patient will have received analgesia for the dressing change. If the burn wounds are covered, active range of motion exercises are preferred to avoid excessive force that cannot be adequately monitored.

More forceful, passive range of motion can be performed more readily while the patient is under anesthesia. Other advantages to range of motion during anesthesia include the ability to more accurately determine the available range of motion and identify soft tissue restrictions, rather than limitations due to weakness or pain during active motion. Moreover, because the patient cannot feel the tissue mobilization, more thorough stretching can be performed. Disadvantages of performing passive range of motion during anesthesia include the potential for excessive movement that may result in joint dislocation, fractures, tearing of compromised ligaments and tendons, and tissue separation.

To recover lost range of motion, prolonged low load stretch is preferred. This prolonged low load stretch can be accomplished with the use of a dynamic splint, which uses springs or similar devices to move an extremity toward the desired position or a CPM (continuous passive movement) machine. A CPM moves the affected extremity through a range of motion that can be specified in terms of its starting and stopping angle and the speed through which the extremity is moved. Gravity assisted range of motion can be accomplished by positioning a patient such that gravity pulls the desired body segment in the desired direction. For example, a person with decreased knee extension may lie in prone with a weight attached to the foot. If this type of therapy is used, the clinician needs to monitor for blanching and skin dryness to prevent cracking of the relatively weak and brittle scar tissue of a healed burn injury. Cracking and bleeding of burned skin are common complications of attempts to restore range of motion. Care to prevent these complications should be taken, but these may not be avoidable.

Strengthening

Strength training is needed to avoid loss of lean body mass and creation of negative nitrogen balance. With increased demands for protein and calories to repair a wound, the resultant hypermetabolic state can lead to wasting of muscles. The patient can be instructed in simple exercises that combine ROM and strength. Avoid exercises that place frictional or shearing forces on grafted skin and donor sites.

Cardiovascular

Cardiovascular exercise is needed to maintain or improve cardiopulmonary function. Upright positioning progressing to ambulation and other cardiopulmonary training is needed to improve hematocrit and plasma volume. While working to achieve improved orthostatic tolerance, the clinician should monitor vital signs, especially if the patient experienced extensive burns or has been medically unstable. The patient may not initially be able to tolerate an upright position for ambulation. The clinician may need to wrap the lower extremities in elasticized bandages to maintain central venous pressure in upright positions. The patient may need to start with sitting up, dangling legs, or a tilt table protocol to develop sufficient

orthostatic tolerance for cardiopulmonary training. If the patient lacks the mobility to reposition, a tilt table may be necessary to provide upright positioning. Burns may have destroyed large numbers of sweat glands, diminishing a patient's ability to dissipate heat. During exercise, avoid overheating the patient. Have a fan available and provide rest and water breaks during the activity. Upper extremity ergometry is particularly useful for burn rehabilitation for several reasons. Movement of the upper extremity ergometer encourages upper extremity range of motion. Because the patient is in a seated position the patient can take frequent rest breaks as needed, and with the lower extremities wrapped, the patient is better able to tolerate upright positioning in addition to the cardiovascular training that can be provided.

Scar Management

Burn wounds, more so than other types, are likely to result in proliferative scarring. Pressure garments are typically used to minimize over-repair. Examples of pressure garments are shown in Figure 15-4. Garments are specially measured and custom-made to exert equally 35 mm Hg pressure on recovering skin. Garments are available for any body part with delivery of a custom garment in 24 to 48 hours. Rather than elasticized garments, clear acrylic masks are used to exert pressure on the face in an effort to minimize scarring. Patients are encouraged to begin use of compression garments within 6 months of injury and to continue use up to 2 years if the scar is still actively in the remodeling stage and highly vascularized to receive better results. Pressure garments are worn 23 hours per day and only taken off for bathing. However, little research is available to demonstrate the efficacy of them. The mechanism by which pressure affects scar formation is not fully understood. Some literature is suggestive of a hypoxic effect on fibroblasts, diminishing collagen formation. Another theory suggests a mechanical effect that prevents the formation of whorls of collagen and promotion of flatter ribbons of collagen fibers. Some recent research reports have questioned whether sustained pressure is actually effective in reducing scarring associated with burn injuries. Other treatments proposed to reduce scarring of burn injuries include friction massage and ultrasound to the scars, neither of which is feasible with large areas of burns. Other options for scar management are discussed in Chapter 13.

SUMMARY

Burns are common injuries, although the vast majority of them are minor and self-treated. Major burns are severe injuries requiring intensive care and rehabilitation. Therapy for burn injuries includes wound debridement,

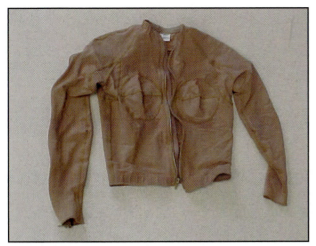

Figure 15-4A. Compression garment: jacket.

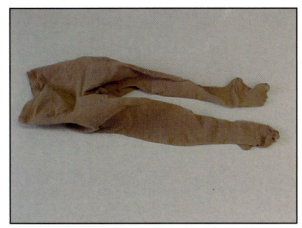

Figure 15-4B. Compression garment: leggings.

dressing changes, exercise, positioning, and splinting. Debridement and dressing changes for large full-thickness injuries are usually performed by technicians in burn centers, but less severe injuries may be managed in a physical therapy inpatient or outpatient clinic. Grafting, exercise, positioning, and splinting are performed to minimize loss of elasticity of the skin. If possible, the injured area is kept on stretch, but both surfaces may be injured and clinical decisions to minimize loss of function must be made. Critical areas include the neck, axilla, elbow, and foot. The appropriate use of active, active-assisted and passive range of motion are described. In addition to range of motion, exercises must be directed at maintaining muscle mass and cardiovascular function.

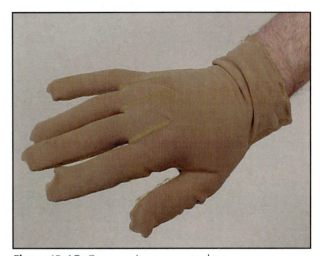

Figure 15-4C. Compression garment: glove.

QUESTIONS

1. List complications of burn injuries that frequently cause mortality.
2. Under what circumstances are full-thickness grafts required?
3. Why do full-thickness wounds need to be grafted?
4. Why must patients not be allowed to stay in their preferred position following burn injuries?
5. How can patients with burns be mobilized if their blood pressure falls with standing?
6. What option is available for providing gravitational stress to an immobile patient with burns?
7. What concerns do we have concerning thermoregulation after a burn injury?

BIBLIOGRAPHY

Anzarut A, Olson J, Singh, Rowe BH, Tredget EE. The effectiveness of pressure garment therapy for the prevention of abnormal scarring after burn injury: a meta-analysis. *J Plast Reconstr Aesthet Surg.* 2009;62(1):77-84.

Committee on Trauma. American College of Surgeons: Guidelines for Operation of Burn Units Chicago, American College of Surgeons, 1999.

Oliveira GV, Chinkes D, Mitchell C, Oliveras G, Hawkins HK, Herndon DN. Objective assessment of burn scar vascularity, erythema, pliability, thickness, and planimetry. *Dermatol Surg.* 2005;31(1):48-58.

Richard RL, Staley MJ. *Burn Care and Rehabilitation: Principles and Practice.* Philadelphia, PA: FA Davis; 1994.

Staley MJ, Richard RL. Burns. In: Sullivan SB, Schmitz TJ, eds. *Physical Rehabilitation: Assessment and Treatment.* 5th ed. Philadelphia, PA: FA Davis; 2006.

Van den Kerckhove E, Stappaerts K, Fieuws S, et al. The assessment of erythema and thickness on burn related scars during pressure garment therapy as a preventive measure for hypertrophic scarring. *Burns.* 2005;31(6):696-702.

Special Cases

OBJECTIVES

- List factors that should raise the suspicion of a wound with an unusual cause.
- Describe the characteristics of epidermolysis bullosa and its treatment.
- Describe unusual characteristics suggestive of malignancy, pyoderma gangrenosum, calciphylaxis, and vasculitis.
- Describe risks of skin injury secondary to obesity and to the need for intensive care.
- Discuss means of optimizing wound management at the end of life.
- Discuss modifications of interventions necessary for the elderly patient.
- Describe prevention of skin injury in elderly persons.
- Discuss means of optimizing wound management in children.

This chapter deals with situations that represent special care, or situations that may not be commonly addressed. Topics include wounds with unusual causes (epidermolysis bullosa, malignancy, pyoderma gangrenosum, calciphylaxis, and vasculitis), considerations relevant to patients receiving intensive care, skin of obese individuals, wound care of children, elderly, and those at the end of life.

WOUNDS WITH UNUSUAL CAUSES

Many of the wounds presented to clinicians have a routine etiology. These wound etiologies were discussed in Chapter 7. Sometimes, however, the etiology of the wound is not readily discerned, or the diagnosis given is not consistent with the clinical signs or the wound's heal-

ing trajectory. Wounds with etiologies other than those covered in Chapter 7 are commonly discussed as "unusual wounds." Although these wound etiologies may be rare, given such a large number of unusual etiologies, approximately 10% of leg ulcers are due to an unusual cause.

Suspecting Unusual Causes

In general, if a wound etiology is identified correctly, a certain rate of healing (healing trajectory) is expected with provision of optimal care. Several factors are suggestive of unusual wound etiologies. These include an increase in size despite appropriate therapy, the presence of excess granulation tissue (fungating), a change in bleeding, drainage, odor, pain, an unusual location, and failure to heal. Pruritus (itching) is a common phenomenon as wounds heal.

Irion G.
Comprehensive Wound Management, 2nd ed. (pp 277-294)
© 2010 SLACK Incorporated

Itching that occurs in conjunction with abnormally slow healing should also raise suspicion of an unusual wound. Biopsy of such wounds is generally in order, unless the etiology is diagnosed by the appearance of other clinical signs discussed below.

Infection

Bacterial infections are common. Typical culprits are MRSA and ß-hemolytic strep. An infection caused by a protozoan carried by the sandfly (Leishmaniasis) produces a characteristic wound. This wound has an appearance similar to impetigo with crusting, but the presence of shallow ulcers should raise suspicion of an etiology other than impetigo. Impetigo is more common among children and is characterized by superficial honey-colored crusting as described in Chapter 7.

Fungal Infections

Fungal infections of the skin are common, producing conditions such as athlete's foot, in which superficial fungal species inhabit the nails or epidermis. In more severe cases, a fungating mass called a mycetoma may produce a disfiguring ulcerated mass. The seemingly uncontrolled granulation characteristic of such wounds gives rise to the term *fungating*. However, a fungating wound may be caused by malignancy (see malignancy below).

A particular type of fungal infection of the foot is known as a eumycetoma. A similar infection caused by bacteria is termed *mycetoma*. The bacterial form is about 3 times as common as the fungal form. The contour of the foot or hand may eventually become distorted with one or multiple elevated and ulcerated areas. Initially patients may relate a history of a painless swelling of the affected area and may report a penetrating injury in the same area. The disease may progress for several years with the development of painless nodules, and may progress to extreme edema, induration, ulceration, and sinus tract development. A history of multiple closure and development of new ulcerations may be reported with localized spread of the infection. Symptoms of pain and systemic infection are unusual, but pruritus is common. Eumycetomas are generally more localized and less progressive than mycetomas. In cases of greater spread of the infection, lymphadenitis, lymphangitis, and lymphedema may occur, particularly if a secondary bacterial infection develops. Greater spread is associated with immunosuppression and may include development of pulmonary infection in those with HIV infection.

Species of fungus typically involved include *Madurella grisea, Madurella mycetomatis, Leptosphaeria senegalensis*, and, mostly, *Scedosporium apiospermum*. This type of infection occurs mainly in arid and semi-arid regions. Infection is usually the result of spores entering breaks in the skin during agricultural work. Infections typically occur in the foot and may occur in the hand due to the nature of its pathogenesis. Infection may spread proximally along the leg or forearm. Mycetoma (bacterial) has the same pathogenesis as the fungal form (eumycetoma). Bacteria may include *Actinomadura madurae, Actinomadura pelletieri*, and *Streptomyces somaliensis*. Treatment may include antifungals such as ketoconazole, itraconazole, localized surgical excision, or may require amputation. An infection called actinomycosis is caused by species of *Actinomyces*, particularly *Actinomyces israelii*, and produces a suppurative infection involving sites other than the hands and feet.

Mycetoma is relatively rare in the United States, but is endemic in Mexico. Other countries include India, Sudan, Somalia, Mauritania, and Senegal. A diagnosis of mycetoma should be considered for patients with foot or hand wounds as described here who have emigrated from latitudes between 15 degrees south and 30 degrees north. Mycetoma is twice as common in men, and usually occurs in those between the ages of 20 and 50 with occupational exposure to spores from contaminated soil.

GENETIC DISORDERS

Two major genetic diseases are associated with unusual wounds. The blistering disorder, epidermolysis is a collection of diseases of both recessive and dominant inheritance. Sickle cell disease frequently produces leg ulcers that may not be diagnosed properly.

Epidermolysis Bullosa

Epidermolysis bullosa (EB) is not a singular disease, but is a collection of genetic diseases leading to bulla formation secondary to defects in the basement membrane zone. The disorders are usually diagnosed at or shortly after birth. They are mostly autosomal dominant and have a range of severity. Autosomal recessive types of EB tend to be more serious than dominant.

The vast majority of cases (92%) are the mildest form, termed *epidermolysis bullosa simplex* (EBS). EBS is an autosomal dominant disorder with several subtypes of varying severity, depending on the mutation of specific keratin subtypes. The mildest forms affect the skin only with intraepidermal blistering and healing without scarring. Mild EBS may not be diagnosed until adulthood and, in some cases, it is not diagnosed in a parent until a child is diagnosed with EBS. Other forms of epidermolysis bullosa produce skin separation in different structures. Forms other than EBS are more severe and may include organ involvement. Separation occurs in the lamina lucida of the basement membrane in junctional EB, in the lamina densa in dystrophic EB, and through hemidesmosomes in hemidesmosomal EB. Specific molecular defects have been isolated in these disorders with research ongoing to replace defective genes.

Any form of EB places infants at risk for infection, and possible sepsis and death. Metastatic squamous cell carcinoma may be lethal in those with the autosomal recessive dystrophic EB during late teens through early adulthood. EBS, the autosomal dominant form of dystrophic EB, and milder forms of junctional EB may not shorten lifespan if sepsis is avoided.

Wound healing is impaired to varying extents in different types of EB. Loss of barrier function and the presence of serum on the skin places the skin at risk of infection. Some subtypes of EB have immunologic and gastrointestinal defects that increase susceptibility to infection and impair nutritional status. Cleansing of denuded areas with application of topical antimicrobials and occlusive dressings are typically required. The application of adhesives should be strictly avoided.

Squamous cell carcinoma may develop in areas of chronic denudation of those with dystrophic EB. Although squamous cell carcinoma generally occurs in sun-exposed areas of fair-skinned individuals, those with dystrophic EB may develop tumors on any area, not necessarily those with sun exposure. This malignancy has a peak incidence in the 20s through 30s, which is earlier than squamous cell carcinoma usually appears in the general population.

Sickle Cell Disease

Sickle cell disease (formerly known as sickle cell anemia) results from homozygous inheritance of HbS, a defective form of hemoglobin. The defect is the result of a single amino acid substitution that reduces the solubility of hemoglobin. The presence of a large number of malformed (sickle-shaped) red cells leads to obstruction of small vessels, with the potential for thrombosis and ischemic injury downstream of occlusions. The shortened life-span of abnormal cells produces hemolytic anemia. The sickling process that frequently occurs with sickle cell anemia may be precipitated by multiple factors, particularly events that produce dehydration and acidosis, such as viral illness, vomiting, and insufficient hydration when working outdoors. Other stressors such as fatigue, exposure to cold, and psychological stress may precipitate a crisis.

Approximately 0.15% of African Americans are homozygous for HbS, resulting in sickle cell disease; approximately 8% are heterozygous carriers. Heterozygous individuals have about 30% to 40% of HbS and are usually not affected with the significant morbidity associated with homozygosity. A heterozygous individual is said to have the sickle cell trait. Morbidity can occur under severe conditions such as high altitude flight without adequate pressurization of the cabin. Sickle cell disease has variable morbidity and mortality. Although sickle cell disease is a chronic disorder, morbidity is associated with injuries accumulated by multiple exacerbations or sickle cell crises.

Life expectancy is approximately 60 years with mortality due to several causes. About 30% die during an acute crisis, despite the lack of known organ damage. Infection causes most of the mortality in young children, whereas stroke, trauma, acute chest syndrome (see below), splenic sequestration crisis, and aplastic crisis cause mortality in teens and young adults.

Differing types of sickle cell crises tend to occur at different ages. The most common type is vaso-occlusive, which is very painful and may require strong analgesics. Vaso-occlusive injury is particularly severe in bone marrow. Infants are most prone to occlusions in the small bones of the hands and feet, producing pain and edema. Older children may have more joint pain. Older patients may develop acute chest syndrome, characterized by fever, chest pain, dyspnea, and coughing. Acute chest syndrome appears to be caused by a combination of pneumonia and vaso-occlusive disease affecting the lungs. Acute chest syndrome leads to hypoxia and is a life-threatening situation. Abdominal pain similar to acute abdomen with pain, distention, and abdominal rigidity is caused by occlusion and infarction of abdominal organs and the mesentery. Splenic sequestration crisis is a consequence of vaso-occlusive disorder affecting the spleen. Occlusion of splenic sinusoids results in trapping of blood within the spleen. This syndrome may progress slowly with complaints of fatigue and left-sided abdominal pain. Progression of the crisis can result in infarction of the spleen and hypovolemic shock. Similarly, priapism can result from occlusion of venous sinuses. Left untreated, thrombosis and necrosis may occur. Occlusion of cerebral vessels leads to neurologic symptoms related to the vessels affected, ranging from temporary focal defects to life-threatening stroke. Aplastic anemia crisis is more common among infants and children. Anemia can become severe with reticulocytopenia and very little production of red cells. Patients become severely ill, develop tachycardia and pallor. Crises are frequently due to parvovirus B19, the cause of "fifth disease" in children.

Sickle Cell Disease Related Leg Ulcers

Ulcers of the lower extremities are common in adolescents and young adults. The most common location is proximal to the lateral malleolus. Individuals may have a number of ulcers at various stages of healing located on both lower extremities. These ulcers appear to be the result of vaso-occlusive disease, but the reason for their location is not readily explained. Sickle cell ulcers are shallow with dimensions of 10 to 20 cm across. Their typical appearance consists of adherent yellow slough with small areas of granulation tissue visible within the slough. A black halo immediately around the wound is usually present due to accumulation of hemosiderin in the skin. Many patients have been self-managing these ulcers for

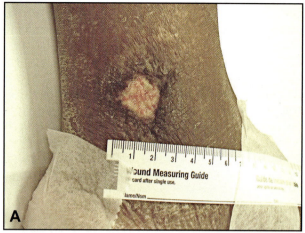

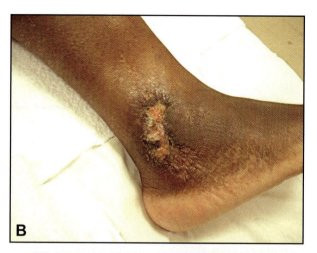

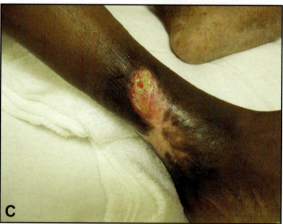

Figure 16-1. Sickle cell ulcers. (A) Note characteristic appearance and location. These ulcers may appear on other parts of the body. (B) Larger ulcer in same location. (C) Healed sickle cell ulcer over lateral malleolus with new ulceration proximal to it. Patient had multiple other healed ulcers.

months or years before closure of these wounds. Examples of leg ulcers associated with sickle cell disease are shown in Figure 16-1.

Aggressive debridement of these ulcers is difficult due to the intensity of pain experienced by many patients, especially if treatment is occurring during hospitalization for a crisis. Pulsatile lavage may also be poorly tolerated. Collagenase is more likely to be accepted as a treatment. A dressing that does not adhere to the wound bed is important with this type of ulcer. While the wound is covered with slough and receiving collagenase debridement, normal saline-moistened 2 x 2s may be used. As slough is debrided, granulation tissue must be protected. Even hydrogel and xeroform may adhere to granulation tissue between dressing changes. Vaseline gauze or a contact layer with a bandage roll may be more successful. In some cases, patients may benefit from compression bandaging or an Unna's boot if significant edema is present. Follow-up visits to ensure effective home care of the clean, stable wound should be scheduled if possible. Patients may experience regression of the wound with suboptimal care. Many individuals may be seen repeatedly as inpatients due to recurrent sickle cell crises and may demonstrate regression of a wound.

NEOPLASTIC DISEASE

Skin lesions produced by neoplastic disease include basal cell carcinoma, squamous cell carcinoma, melanoma, Kaposi's sarcoma, and cutaneous T cell lymphoma. Cancer resulting from chronic wounds is termed *Marjolin's ulcer*.

Basal Cell Carcinoma

Basal cell carcinoma (BCC) is the most common form of skin cancer with approximately 1 million new cases per year in the United States. It is frequently described as having a pearly appearance. Raised, translucent lesions with fine, visible blood vessels are common, but BCC may present as a nonspecific lesion on sun-exposed skin. Other presentations include an open wound that bleeds and crusts but does not heal, a reddish patch that itches or crusts, a pearly appearance with darker pigmentation, a pinkish neoplasm with an elevated, rolled border and crusted central indentation, and possible surface blood vessels, and a hypopigmented patch that has the appearance of a healed scar.

Common areas include the face, particularly ears, nose, and lips, the dorsum of the hand, and posterior cervical area. These areas tend to be exposed to sunlight because of geometry and occupational sun exposure. Although BCC is rarely metastatic, it can be highly invasive and erode a large area of continuous skin if untreated. The term *rodent ulcer* has been used in the literature to describe the appearance of untreated BCC. If the etiology is uncertain and the lesion is observed on typical areas of excessive exposure to sunlight, a biopsy can be used to diagnose BCC. Treatment by excision is generally curative.

Squamous Cell Carcinoma

Squamous cell carcinoma (SCC) is the second most common form of skin cancer. Its etiology is similar to that of BCC. SCC also generally occurs on sun-damaged skin. A precancerous lesion called actinic keratosis may precede development of SCC. Additionally, SCC may occur years later in skin damaged by exposure to sunlight, ionizing radiation, and skin that has recovered from a burn injury. Like BCC, SCC on sun-damaged skin is rarely metastatic, but the rate of metastasis is much greater on skin injured by ionizing radiation or burns. Risk of SCC is also increased by immunosuppression. Metastasis is also more likely to occur on modified skin and mucosa (20% to 30% as opposed to 0.5%). The treatment of SCC is also simple excision. More invasive treatment including chemotherapy may be necessary if metastasis occurs.

The usual appearance of SCC is a crusted/scaled patch with an inflamed base. However the appearance might also appear to be a simple bite reaction, scaling, or other trauma (Figure 16-2). The lesion in Figure 16-2 was initially diagnosed as an insect bite, but confirmed as SCC following biopsy. Presence on sun-damaged, radiation-damaged, or healed areas of burned skin should increase the suspicion of SCC. In both BCC and SCC, wounds will not heal and may increase in size.

Actinic Keratosis

This lesion is the result of sun damage, particularly on fair-skinned individuals. Scaling appears on typical sites of sun injury due to dysplastic cell proliferation in the dermis. These lesions are excised either sharply or by cryosurgical removal before SCC develops. Fair skinned individuals with a long history of sun exposure may require annual inspection of sun exposed skin and excision of multiple actinic keratoses.

Melanoma

Although not as common as BCC and SCC, melanoma is more likely to metastasize; mortality increases as vertical growth toward the dermis occurs. As a tumor of melanocytes, melanoma begins in the epidermis and proliferates into the dermis. It spreads to other parts of the body, especially liver, brain, and lung by entering the lymphatic system. Intracutaneous metastasis producing satellite tumors indicates a very poor prognosis. Melanoma is excised and regional lymph nodes may be removed as well, leaving wounds in both areas.

Melanoma has a variety of presentations. In contrast to common moles (nevi), melanoma has unusual characteris-

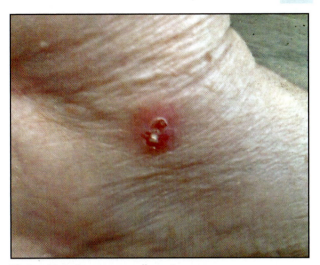

Figure 16-2. Squamous cell carcinoma.

tics. It may be much larger, more irregular, have variegated coloration, be more elevated above the skin, ulcerate, and bleed. The color can range from a tan to almost black with surrounding halo of hypopigmented skin. The appearance of a new mole on an adult that has some of the characteristics listed above should raise suspicion of melanoma. Early excision before the tumor invades the dermis and cells gain access to the lymphatic system is critical.

Kaposi's Sarcoma

Prior to the rapid proliferation of HIV in the 1980s, Kaposi's sarcoma was rare. It was originally described by Kaposi as occurring only in older Italian and Jewish men with decreased immunity. Kaposi's sarcoma is a form of cancer caused by Human Herpes Virus 8 in persons with compromised immunity. In addition to AIDS, the use of some transplant rejection drugs such as cyclosporin has also increased the incidence.

It can produce large and multiple patches or nodules of such colors as red, purple, brown, and black. Lesions may remain intact, or become ulcerative, fungating lesions. An example is shown in Figure 16-3. The rate of growth is also variable. In its original description, it was found to be slow growing (indolent) and unrelated to mortality. In AIDS and transplants, it may grow explosively leading to significant morbidity and mortality. Lesions are most commonly found on the lower extremities, face, mouth, and genitalia. Involvement of the mouth, gastrointestinal tract, and respiratory tract leads to significant morbidity including difficulty eating and speaking, malnutrition, weight loss, nausea and vomiting, intestinal obstruction, dyspnea, and hemoptysis.

The cancer cells are derived from lymphatic endothelium, producing vessel-like structures that fill with blood and produce the characteristic coloration of the lesions.

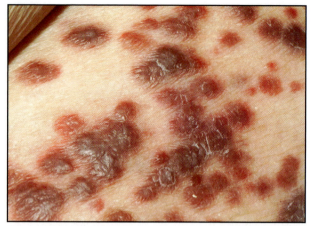

Figure 16-3. Kaposi's sarcoma.

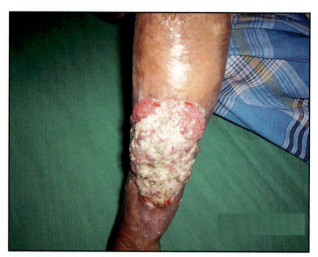

Figure 16-4. Marjolin's ulcer.

Kaposi's sarcoma is not directly treatable. If the cause of immunosuppression can be addressed, eg, antiviral treatment for AIDS, the lesions can be controlled and may regress to a large extent in a large number of patients.

Cutaneous T Cell Lymphoma

Mycosis fungoides is the most common form of cutaneous T cell lymphoma (CTCL), a form of non-Hodgkin's lymphoma. Its name was given in the original description of skin lesions with a mushroom-like appearance in the literature. Mycosis fungoides is primarily a disease of men over the age of 50. In the milder form of CTCL, erythematous patches/plaques are present and the onset is usually between 45 and 55 years of age. Disease manifestations are due to infiltration of the skin with CD4+ lymphocytes. A more severe form of cutaneous T cell lymphoma called Sezary syndrome has a later onset and is characterized by tumors and erythema caused by the presence of microabscesses in the skin, as well as a large number of the abnormal lymphocytes in the blood.

Stages of CTCL

The premycotic stage consists of small erythematous patches, most commonly on the chest and buttocks, that are easily confused with eczema or psoriasis. The plaque (infiltrative stage) is characterized by irregularly shaped erythematous plaques. The buttocks, skin folds, and face are the most common sites. In the tumor stage, raised ulcerating plaques are seen and the disease may have entered lymph nodes. In Sezary syndrome, the entire skin may become erythematous and thickened, with pruritus and exfoliation.

Pruritus occurs in many, but not all cases. Diagnosis must be made with skin biopsy. A number of treatments may be used including ultraviolet light, cancer chemotherapy, radiation therapy, interferons, and retinoids. With treatment, the disease may be stabilized or go into remission; however, mortality for mycosis fungoides is

about 50%. If these treatments are not effective, the drug vorinostat may be used.

Marjolin's Ulcer

Chronic wounds are not necessarily stable. Although some individuals may have open wounds for years and not become septic, a small number of these cases develop malignant cells. The usual cause is chronic osteomyelitis. Inadequate treatment of soft tissue wounds or other causes such as hematogenous spread from another site allow bacterial infection to linger within bones. Bacteria then develop biofilms within the osseous site, rendering systemic antibiotics useless against them. The chronicity of the infection does not allow healing of the overlying soft tissue. Patients may simply bandage open wounds and allow them to drain for years. Due to the constant presence of growth factors and compromised immunity, or perhaps other factors, cells within the wound lose control of normal growth and become malignant. This wound containing malignant cells is termed *Marjolin's ulcer*.

The typical Marjolin's ulcer is found on a lower extremity of a man between the ages of 40 and 70 and the wound has been present from 20 to 50 years. The wound is characterized by excessive granulation, frequently described as "exuberant." In spite of the amount of granulation occurring, the wounds do not close or re-epithelialize (Figure 16-4). The granulation tissue continues to build in the area in large, uneven heaps. These are usually squamous cell carcinoma. The metastatic rate for Marjolin's ulcer (30%) is much greater than that of squamous cell cancer in general. These wounds should be readily recognized as suspicious for Marjolin's ulcer by appearance and duration of the wound. A biopsy is done to confirm the suspicion. Wide excision may be curative, but amputation may be required in some cases. The underlying cause of the ulcer must also be addressed, generally by debridement or amputation of the infected bone.

AUTOIMMUNE DISEASES

Diseases affecting the skin may be due to autoimmune disorders that affect specific components of the skin. A large number of vasculitides may produce ulcerations of the skin. Other diseases, including pyoderma gangrenosum and erythema nodosum, appear to have immune components, but their mechanisms remain elusive.

Vasculitis

As autoimmune disorders, vasculitides tend to cause systemic signs of inflammation such as joint and muscle pains, lymphadenitis, fever, and malaise. Many vasculitides have been described in the literature. A number of them have skin involvement and may present as skin lesions/rashes that do not respond to normal treatment. In general, treatments for vasculitides involve immune suppression through corticosteroids or drugs used for organ transplants. Diagnosis generally requires biopsy. Those vasculitides that are more likely to affect the skin include hypersensitivity vasculitis, microscopic polyangiitis, polyarteritis nodosa, rheumatoid vasculitis (associated with rheumatoid arthritis), Churg Strauss vasculitis, Wegener's granulomatosis, cryoglobinemia, and Henoch-Schönlein purpura. Buerger's disease (thromboangiitis obliterans) is discussed below under vaso-occlusive disorders. Behçet's syndrome is discussed below.

Behçet's Syndrome

Behçet's syndrome is a rare disease primarily affecting young adults (20s to 30s). Signs include mouth sores, skin rashes and lesions, and genital sores. The distribution and severity of these lesions vary from person to person, and signs may remit and recur. Oral ulcers begin as raised lesions and ulcerate. They may occur on the lips, gums, and tongue. Skin lesions vary from acne-like to red, raised, tender nodules. Similar ulcers may occur on the vulva and penis. These ulcers heal in 7 to 10 days, but recurrence is common. An additional sign of Behçet's syndrome is uveitis. Although uveitis occurs with many other diseases, the combination with skin and oral ulcers should raise the suspicion of Behçet's syndrome. Uveitis in Behçet's syndrome causes erythema, pain, and blurred vision along with characteristic fundoscopic changes. Joint pain, particularly the knee, is another indication of Behçet's. Arthralgia is remitting and recurring. This disease can also cause aneurysm or thrombosis of blood vessels, digestive, and nervous system complications. In addition to the typical signs of Behçet's syndrome, a positive pathergy test assists in the diagnosis. To conduct this test, an injury to the skin is created with

a sterile needle. A skin lesion such as a reddened nodule 2 days later constitutes a positive pathergy test. Like other vasculitides, Behçet's syndrome is treated with corticosteroids or immunosuppressant drugs. An additional drug that may be used is interferon-α, which suppresses excessive immune response.

Pyoderma Gangrenosum

Pyoderma gangrenosum (PG) is a disorder of unknown etiology characterized by the development of skin ulcerations unrelated to other known causes of wounds. Patients may describe a small wound attributed to a spider bite or trauma that has progressed to a large, deep ulcer. Ulcers produced by PG have a characteristic appearance with violaceous, undermined borders (Figure 16-5). Any wound with this appearance should raise a high level of suspicion of PG. In addition, the skin surrounding wounds associated with pyoderma gangrenosum often demonstrate pustules, scabs, and scars from old wounds. PG is a rare disorder with an incidence of about 1/100,000 per year. The mortality of PG is very low; however, death might occur due to complications of treatment or due an underlying disease associated with PG.

A history of systemic diseases, notably autoimmune disorders, is associated with pyoderma gangrenosum in about 50% of cases. In addition to complaints of pain from the ulcer, the patient may experience arthralgia and malaise. Associated systemic diseases include inflammatory bowel diseases, rheumatoid arthritis, and hematologic diseases such as leukemia. Another important characteristic of PG is pathergy. Pathergy in PG specifically refers to the characteristic worsening or development of new wounds with skin trauma. Efforts to debride, forcefully clean, or graft the area are likely to cause the wound to worsen. Grafting is likely to cause the wound to increase in size and may cause PG at the donor site. No laboratory testing is available to diagnose PG, and no characteristic histology can be seen through examination of biopsies. Biopsy is useful only for ruling out other possible disorders. Diagnosis of PG requires a high level of suspicion due to the appearance of the wound and the exclusion of any other causes, particularly malignancies of the skin.

Treatment of PG includes protection of the wound while treating the underlying autoimmune disorder. Medical therapy involves systemic immunosuppression, which might include cyclosporine, oral corticosteroids, and infliximab. Infliximab and related drugs inhibit TNF. This drug is currently indicated for use in rheumatoid arthritis and Crohn's disease. Topical and injected corticosteroids might also be used in the treatment of PG. During wound healing, aggressive debridement is contraindicated.

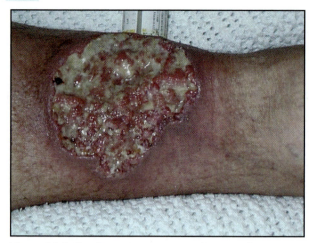

Figure 16-5. Pyoderma gangrenosum showing characteristic undermined violaceous borders.

Erythema Nodosum

This condition is a relatively rare reaction, usually occurring on the anterior surface of the legs of young women. The condition appears to be a delayed hypersensitivity reaction (type IV immune injury) associated with a recent systemic infection, exposure to drugs, and other disorders associated with the immune system. In some cases it may be idiopathic. An inflammatory reaction originating in the subcutaneous tissue produces raised red areas 2 to 6 cm in diameter and a few millimeters high. Joint pain commonly accompanies the appearance of nodules. Immune complexes unique to erythema nodosum have not been found, but may be found when this disorder is associated with specific autoimmune disorders such as inflammatory bowel diseases.

In a typical case, nodules begin to appear along with nonspecific signs of systemic inflammation, particularly fever and generalized aching. Arthralgia may occur before nodules appear, concomitant with nodules, or may not occur at all. Individual lesions develop initially into tense, indurated, and tender nodules over approximately 1 week. Over the next week, the lesions become boggy, but are not suppurative and do not ulcerate. They recede over several more days. New lesions may occur over a period of several weeks. Erythema nodosum lesions preceded by an infection clear in less time than those occurring idiopathically. Idiopathic erythema nodosum lesions may continue to erupt for 6 months. The initial red color fades to blue after the first week, then becomes progressively yellow producing the same color changes seen with an ecchymosis. The skin over the lesions regains normal color and the epidermis peels as in a superficial-thickness skin injury such as sunburn.

Arthralgia is experienced by about half of those with erythema nodosum. It may appear more than 2 weeks before lesions are discovered. A nondestructive edema with erythema and joint effusion typically occur in knees or ankles, but other joints may be involved. This arthralgia resolves in several weeks with residual joint discomfort possibly continuing for several months. Triggers for erythema nodosum include Strep infections, sarcoidosis, *Mycoplasma pneumoniae* infection (walking pneumonia), and *Campylobacter jejuni*, a common cause of food poisoning and a trigger for Guillain-Barre syndrome. Pathogenic fungi such as Coccidioidomycosis (San Joaquin Valley fever), Histoplasmosis, and Blastomycosis may also trigger an episode of erythema nodosum. Drugs triggering the disorder are sulfonamides, gold compounds, sulfonylureas, and oral contraceptives. Autoimmune disorders associated with erythema nodosum include ulcerative colitis and Crohn's disease, sarcoidosis, and Behçet disease. Lymphoid cancers including Hodgkin's disease, non-Hodgkin's lymphoma, and acute myelogenous leukemia may be preceded by an episode of erythema nodosum.

Diagnosis of erythema nodosum is generally made on the basis of history and physical examination. Biopsies are generally not useful as the lesion is subcutaneous. This disorder has no specific treatment. NSAIDs may be used to alleviate pain associated with tense, indurated lesions. Otherwise, the process is allowed to run its course.

CALCINOSIS CUTIS

Calcinosis cutis is a term representing a number of disorders characterized by deposits of calcium in the skin. Four classes of calcinosis cutis have been described: dystrophic, metastatic, iatrogenic, and idiopathic. The dystrophic form is due to injury leading to calcium deposits. Tissue trauma may result from any of a large number of causes, including neoplastic disease, acne, insect bites, varicose veins, autoimmune disorders, burn, or mechanical trauma. Injured tissue promotes binding of phosphate to denatured proteins, followed by binding of calcium to phosphate, and precipitation of crystals. Metastatic calcinosis cutis is caused by metabolic disorders resulting in hypercalcemia, hyperphosphatemia, or both. The high concentration allows calcium-phosphate crystals to precipitate in body fluids as hydroxyapatite or amorphous calcium phosphate.

Although calcinosis cutis is a benign process, patients may develop painful lesions and, depending on the location of lesions, joint mobility, or compression of neurons may produce additional pain. Lesions may ulcerate and become infected. In metastatic calcinosis, the underlying disorder such as chronic renal failure or parathyroid disease may cause substantial morbidity. Usually calcinosis lesions have a gradual onset and are asymptomatic. A preexisting injury may be associated with a dystrophic lesion. Idiopathic calcinosis cutis is not associated with tissue injury or metabolic disease producing elevated calcium or phosphate concentration. Iatrogenic calcinosis cutis is produced by treatment for another condition.

Diagnosis of calcinosis cutis is generally straightforward with the clinical presentation and a biopsy of a lesion displaying calcium deposits. Lesions may be located dermally or subcutaneously, but are readily accessible for biopsy. Lesions of calcinosis cutis vary with the etiology. Patients generally present with multiple firm papules or nodules distributed in areas typical for the etiology. Some types produce palpable crystalline material on the lesion's surface. Lesions may ulcerate and chalky crystal accumulation can be observed within the ulcerated lesion. Lesions of this appearance are also characteristic of gout. Severe calcinosis can affect blood vessels leading to ischemia and gangrene. Dystrophic lesions are limited to specific, localized area of tissue injury. Metastatic lesions tend to be large and symmetrically distributed. They are commonly located in the areas of larger joints, especially knees, elbow, and shoulders. If dystrophic cutaneous calcinosis is present, visceral and blood vessel deposits are very likely present and will lead to significant morbidity and mortality if the underlying cause is not adequately treated. Idiopathic calcinosis cutis may occur anywhere, but is usually limited to one area. Iatrogenic calcinosis cutis is essentially the same process as dystrophic, but the trauma is caused by treatment for another disorder that has traumatized the skin.

Treatment for calcinosis cutis is frequently of little value. Treatment is directed toward the underlying cause if it can be identified. Injection of corticosteroids into lesions may produce some benefit. Surgical excision of lesions may be indicated if they lead to excessive pain, recurrent ulceration and infection, or some functional impairment. However, recurrence frequently occurs following excision and excision may stimulate further calcinosis exacerbating the problem. Localized wound care of open lesions to prevent or clear infection may become necessary.

Calciphylaxis

Calciphylaxis is a specific type of calcinosis associated with end-stage renal failure. Calcification of blood vessels and subcutaneous tissue produces significant lesions that erode the skin revealing large chalky subcutaneous deposits several centimeters across (Figure 16-6). The lesions of calciphylaxis are frequently bilateral and fairly symmetric. Lesions seem to develop suddenly and skin necrosis may proceed rapidly over the course of several days. The wound bed changes over the course of several days from yellow to brown and black with desiccation of necrotic tissue. Disease characterized by lesions located on the lower extremities has a much lower mortality than disease

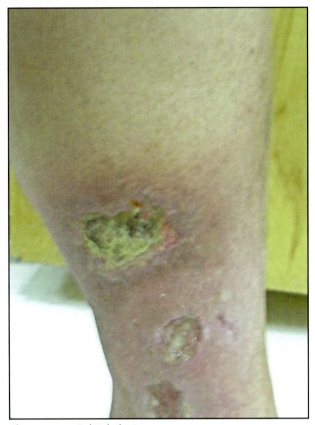

Figure 16-6. Calciphylaxis.

producing lesions on the trunk. Mortality is high with distal involvement (45%) and approaches 100% with trunk involvement. Because of the intense pain of the lesions and the high mortality, aggressive debridement and dressing changes in an effort to produce a clean, stable wound bed appropriate for healing is generally not a reasonable goal, particularly for lesions on the trunk.

The mechanism of calciphylaxis remains a mystery. Components of the disorder include chronic renal failure, hypercalcemia, hyperphosphatemia, excessive calcium-phosphate product, and secondary hyperparathyroidism. These problems of calcium and phosphate metabolism are common in end-stage renal failure, but only a small fraction (1% to 4%) of those with end-stage disease develop calciphylaxis. Additional factors that might trigger calciphylaxis in end-stage renal failure such as inherited immune components or comorbidity have not yet been identified. Mortality is associated with both sepsis due to infected skin lesions and from organ failure. Calciphylaxis is more common in women (3:1) than in men, and mostly in middle age. Longer-term dialysis appears to increase risk. Calciphylaxis may appear in spite of a patient receiving a renal transplant.

Medical care for calciphylaxis is primarily supportive. Treatment may include efforts to improve control of calcium and phosphate homeostasis and elimination of any of the trigger factors listed above. Administration of intravenous sodium thiosulfate may help by increasing the solubility of calcium deposits in tissues to allow excretion of excessive calcium. Another potential strategy is infusion of low-dose tissue plasminogen activator.

If aggressive debridement becomes necessary to avoid sepsis, debridement under general anesthesia is recommended due to the extensive and painful nature of the lesions. Negative pressure wound therapy (Chapter 14) following thorough debridement may be followed by grafting in select cases.

VASO-OCCLUSIVE DISORDERS

A large number of diseases may produce ischemia of the limbs. Atherosclerosis is the most common and is discussed in Chapter 7. Occlusive disease caused by autoimmune vasculitis was discussed above; distal peripheral microembolism, and thromboangiitis obliterans are discussed below.

Distal Peripheral Microembolism

Distal peripheral microembolism ("blue toe syndrome/ trash foot") is not a disease, but a phenomenon caused by embolization of atherosclerotic debris into small arteries and arterioles. By definition, microemboli are pieces of atheromas less than 1 mm in diameter. The release of atherosclerotic particles into the blood may occur spontaneously, but most cases of this syndrome are believed to be iatrogenic, caused by endovascular approaches to revascularization of the lower extremities. This syndrome has a wide range of morbidity with ischemia and infarction of a limited number of small areas or widespread embolism resulting in multisystem organ failure. The degree of injury produced by microembolism depends on both the quantity and composition of the emboli. Small emboli consisting of platelets and fibrin could be lysed with only reversible cell injury to distal tissues, whereas a large cholesterol embolus is more likely to cause irreversible injury with tissue necrosis.

Although other types of atherogenic microembolism have been described, the type that might be seen as an usual cause of foot wounds is a subtype of peripheral atheroembolism. In particular, microembolism originating from the aortoiliac arteries produces what is known as blue toe syndrome or trash foot. Other described types are renal syndrome and visceral syndrome. The term *blue toe syndrome* is due to cyanosis that may develop in the most distal vessels, which can be occluded by multiple emboli. Showers of atherosclerotic debris may produce tender, mottled areas of cyanotic and cool areas of various sizes, and sluggish capillary refill in the foot as well as toes. With accumulation of ischemic injury, tissue

necrosis may occur, producing ulcerations. The term *trash foot* is frequently applied to feet displaying this necrosis.

The treatment of distal peripheral microembolization has been compared with frostbite, with delayed debridement and amputation only after clear demarcation between viable and necrotic tissue. In both frostbite and distal peripheral microembolization, arterial inflow to the tissue and perfusion to surrounding tissue is adequate, but areas fed by localized branches of the microcirculation are occluded, leading to direct necrosis and later reperfusion injury if the embolus is broken down restoring blood flow. If possible, the source of microemboli is removed and heparin administered to stabilize plaque. Patients may be treated with aspirin and dipyridamole, but warfarin appears to cause increased risk of microembolism in a large percentage of patients at risk.

Buerger's Disease

Thromboangiitis obliterans is a vaso-occlusive, nonatherosclerotic disease primarily of middle-age male tobacco smokers. The disease had been described earlier in Germany in 1879, but Buerger's paper gathered sufficient attention that this disease is most commonly associated with his name. Buerger's disease is uncommon, but given a population of patients presenting with signs of peripheral arterial disease, a greater number will seem to be afflicted. The prevalence of Buerger's disease is estimated to be about 15 cases per 100,000 people. Although mortality due to Buerger's disease is unusual, gangrene of extremities requiring amputation occurs in almost half of those diagnosed. Mortality and severe morbidity may result from sepsis caused by infection of gangrenous extremities. The disease is believed to be caused by a combination of genetic predisposition from inheritance of specific types of antigens and exposure to cigarette smoke.

In Buerger's disease, patients will begin to display signs of peripheral arterial disease such as paresthesia, cold extremities, and weak pulses. Ulcerations of the digits are another sign of vaso-occlusive disorder, but they are not exclusive to Buerger's disease. These also occur in Raynaud's disease, scleroderma, and lupus. Migratory, superficial venous thrombosis occurs in approximately 50% of those with this disorder. Involvement of arterial vessels of organs may occur in a small number of those affected. Buerger's disease is more likely to be suspected if an onset of arterial disease is seen in men younger than 45, the patient smokes, and displays Raynaud's phenomenon. This disease is more common in men, but the difference in prevalence may simply reflect a lower prevalence of smoking in women.

No specific laboratory tests are currently available for Buerger's disease, but tests are likely to be performed to rule out other vaso-occlusive disorders such as one of the vasculitic disorders. To rule out lower extremity atherosclerosis in patients with physical signs of lower extremity ischemia, the Allen test can be performed. The diagnosis of Buerger's disease is more likely with a positive Allen test in addition to a history of smoking and the presence of lower extremity arterial ulcers. In the Allen test, the patient flexes the fingers into a fist to evacuate blood from the hand. A clinician occludes the radial and ulnar arteries simultaneously with his/her thumbs. When the arteries to the hand are occluded, the patient relaxes the hand and the clinician releases the ulnar artery while continuing to compress the radial artery. Failure of rapid refill of the hand indicates occlusive disease of the ulnar artery. The procedure is then repeated, but with release of the radial artery while maintaining compression of the ulnar artery as a test for the radial artery's patency.

Acute Buerger's disease is characterized by inflammation and thrombosis of small and medium diameter arteries. Often the inflammation and injury spreads to adjacent veins and nerves. As the disease progresses to the subacute phase, organization of thrombi occurs. Blood vessels may be totally occluded, but some will regain partial arterial flow due to canalization of thrombi. In end-stage disease, blood vessels are fibrosed with no possibility of ever conducting blood again. As more vessels undergo this process, the patient develops signs of arterial disease such as claudication during exercise. With progression of the disease, pain at rest, skin changes, and skin and soft tissue ulceration requiring amputation of the affected limb will occur in a large fraction of patients.

At this time, no pharmacologic treatments have been found effective, despite research into seemingly every possible mechanism of maintaining blood flow. Surgical revascularization is unlikely to be successful given the diffuse effects of the disease, and is only practical in cases in which bypassing discrete focal lesions can restore blood flow. The only treatment known to be effective is smoking cessation. Smoking cessation is imperative, but can be difficult. Of those who can successfully cease smoking, 94% avoid amputation, and all of those who cease before any gangrene develops appear to avert amputation. In comparison, 43% of those who continue to smoke will require an amputation within 8 years of symptoms. Risk of amputation exists even in those who switch to chewing tobacco or nicotine replacement therapies. Many of those who eventually require an amputation will progress to multiple amputations including bilateral upper and lower extremity amputations. Part of patient education is that amputation may be avoided if tobacco use is ceased. In addition, patients must avoid second-hand smoke. Smoking cessation by social contacts and family members may be necessary for multiple reasons: avoidance of second-hand smoke, avoiding temptation to resume, and having a social support system. Although amputation may be avoided with complete smoking cessation, Raynaud's phenomenon and intermittent claudication may persist.

Digital Ischemia Secondary to Vasopressor Administration

In cases of cardiovascular shock (hypovolemic, cardiogenic, neurogenic, or septic), adequate blood pressure for survival may require administration of drugs such as dopamine that result in severe vasoconstriction of small arteries of the distal areas of the extremities. If the patient survives, varying degrees of ischemic injury may occur, which may require amputation of gangrenous fingers, toes, or more proximal areas. An example of digital gangrene secondary to pressor-administration for septic shock is shown in Figure 16-7.

Warfarin-Induced Skin Necrosis

This condition is rare, occurring in 0.01% to 0.1% of those receiving warfarin anticoagulation treatment, usually obese women. Shortly after the initiation of anticoagulation with warfarin (Coumadin, Bristol-Myers Squibb Company, Princeton, NJ), hemorrhagic blisters evolve into large open wounds involving the full thickness of the skin and subcutaneous fat. In some cases, patients may have received multiple courses of warfarin before the condition develops. The wounds appear primarily in fatty areas such as the breast, buttocks, and thighs, often in a bilaterally symmetrical pattern. Wounds are attributed to a hypercoagulable state due to genetic deficiencies in proteins C or S, or other hypercoagulable states due to antithrombin deficiency and lupus anticoagulants combined with a large loading dose of warfarin. A rapid decline in factor VIII and protein C upsets the balance of coagulation and anti-coagulation leading to transient hypercoagulability and thrombosis of fatty tissues. Wounds may appear similar to necrotizing fasciitis or pressure ulcers, but a history of recent initiation of oral anticoagulation and biopsy should lead to diagnosis of warfarin-induced skin necrosis. Reversal of warfarin with administration of vitamin K combined with anticoagulation with heparin may limit the amount of skin necrosis. Wounds may be several centimeters in diameter and depth. Similar to other wounds associated with vascular occlusion, they are very painful rendering bedside debridement extremely difficult without adequate pain management. Patients usually recover, requiring debridement and skin grafts, but some cases of mortality have been reported.

Extravasation Necrosis

This form of skin necrosis results from the extravasation of intravenous fluid. Extravasation is the escape of fluids into surrounding tissue by leakage or accidental injection of fluid into tissue surrounding a vein. Extravasation is estimated to occur in 0.1% to 6% of patients receiving intravenous lines. Fluids that cause pain in patients with

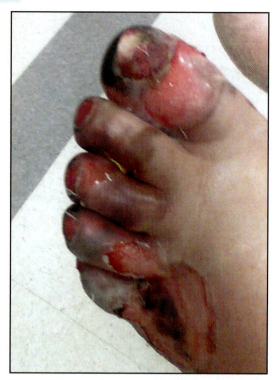

Figure 16-7. Digital gangrene secondary to pressor-administration for septic shock.

normal cognitive function are unlikely to create serious damage because patients will complain of pain and the problem will be corrected quickly. Both the volume of intravenous fluid allowed to run into the interstitial space and the physicochemical composition of the fluid determine the degree of injury. Skin necrosis may occur within hours or be delayed several days, depending on the nature of what is extravasated.

Normal saline and other isotonic fluids produce little or no injury, unless a massive quantity of fluid is extravasated. Hypertonic glucose solutions, calcium chloride/gluconate solutions, sodium bicarbonate solutions, and chemotherapeutic drugs are the most likely substances to cause severe skin necrosis. Hypertonic fluids move more fluid into the interstitial space than isotonic fluids due to a direct osmotic effect, then indirectly due to the osmotic effect of cell death. Movement of hypertonic fluid into the interstitial space may create a positive feedback in terms of osmotic effect, fluid movement into the interstitial space, pressure, and cell death within the compartment. Some cancer chemotherapeutic drugs act as irritants, but many cause cell death directly. Tissue necrosis accelerates if thrombosis of vessels occurs within the compartment. Skin necrosis may be severe even with salvage of the remainder of the limb. The range of injury may be limited to edema, erythema, pain, and burning sensation. Dry desquamation and blistering may occur with greater injury, especially

with chemotherapeutic agents. Full-thickness wounds with eschar formation and absence of granulation tissue will occur with greater injury. More severe injury may be accompanied by additional complications of compartment syndrome such as paralysis, sensory loss, and amputation.

BARIATRICS

The topic of bariatrics in wound management becomes more important as obesity has become more prevalent. Two-thirds of the population is estimated to be over-weight and one-half of the population is considered obese by Center for Disease Control (CDC) standards. According to the CDC, overweight for an adult is defined as body mass index (BMI) between 25 and 29.9, and obese is defined as BMI greater than or equal to 30. BMI is computed as weight in kilograms divided by the square of height in meters (kg/m^2). For example, a person who is 100 kg and 2 meters tall has a BMI of 25 (220 pounds and 6 feet 7 inches). Increasing body weight carries the risk of comorbidity associated with wounds. These include cardiovascular disease in general, lipid disorders, coronary artery disease, and hypertension. Additionally, being overweight requires a greater cardiac output to supply increased body mass, may obstruct venous and lymphatic vessels of the extremities, and compromises the ability to determine blood pressure by sphygmomanometry. The inability to produce sufficient diaphragmatic excursion due to obesity leads to chronic hypoventilation, which is termed *obesity hypoventilation* syndrome or Pickwickian syndrome. Obesity is also associated with obstructive sleep apnea, which can produce severe hypoxemia during sleep and arrhythmias. Orthopnea may also develop for the same reasons as Pickwickian syndrome and obstructive sleep apnea. Following surgery, the obese individual may experience prolonged recovery from general anesthesia. Chemicals used for general anesthesia are highly lipid soluble. Greater fat mass yields a large reservoir of general anesthetic that can impair the patient's ability to achieve full arousal and an obese individual can remain groggy for an extended period after surgery. This condition is known as resedation phenomenon and may lead to extended periods of immobility and increased risk of perioperative pressure ulcers.

Perineal skin is placed at risk due to the greater effects of incontinence. Cleaning the perineal area is more difficult due to obesity, and decreased mobility secondary to the combination of illness or injury with increased weight may lead to *functional incontinence*, a term describing insufficient mobility to reach appropriate toileting facilities.

Other issues associated with obesity are the greater prevalence of type 2 diabetes mellitus, gall bladder disease, and gastroesophageal reflux disease. Nutritional deficits are common due to the effects of unbalanced diet or episodes of severe caloric restriction. Although weight loss is a good long-term goal, an obese individual is susceptible to protein malnutrition when illness or injury is experienced. Negative nitrogen balance can occur even with an abundant supply of adipose tissue under these conditions. Consultation with a clinical dietician is necessary to ensure proper dietary therapy. During recovery from an illness or injury, recovery of mobility and exercise tolerance may be very slow because of the greater body mass in the face of a period of inactivity and loss of muscular strength. Obesity is often associated with emotional and financial stressors that may impair efforts to provide optimal wound care.

Skin Changes With Obesity

Tension placed on skin due to obesity increases the risk of skin tears. Other skin changes that may be related to tension placed on the skin include benign neoplasms called acrochordons (skin tags), acanthosis nigricans, hyperkeratosis, xerosis (excessive skin dryness), skin infections with *Staphylococcus*, *Streptococcus*, and *Candida* species, and intertrigo. Acanthosis nigricans is a hyperpigmented, velvety-textured area of skin commonly located on skin flexures, especially the nape of the neck and axillae. Acanthosis nigricans is also associated with diabetes mellitus and certain forms of cancer. It is believed to be caused by excessive serum insulin that stimulates abnormal skin growth secondary to insulin resistance. Acanthosis nigricans may be hereditary, idiopathic, or be associated with gastric cancer or polycystic ovary syndrome.

Skin tags have many similarities to acanthosis nigricans. They are distributed on the neck, axillae, and groin. They are also commonly found on eyelids. They may also be called pedunculated papillomas or fibroepithelial polyps. Because they are innervated, anesthesia is required for their excision. In addition to their association with obesity, skin tags are associated with pregnancy and polycystic ovary syndrome.

Xerosis associated with obesity leads to easy fissuring and portals of entry for bacteria and fungus. Bunching of unstretched skin results in skin folds that accumulate warmth and moisture, creating an environment suitable for bacterial and fungal growth. Intertrigo is the rashlike injury to such skin. The skin deep within folds can be extremely erythematous and malodorous. Skin under breasts and pannus is particularly prone to intertrigo. Pannus is the skin fold of the abdomen that may cover the pubic, inguinal, and anterior thigh skin. Zinc oxide or other skin protectants used for incontinence may be used in these areas. Topical antibacterial or antifungal medications may also be used. Silver-containing alginate dressings have also been proposed as a means of controlling intertrigo.

Although the presence of subcutaneous adipose tissue between skin and bony prominences provides cushioning and theoretically reduces the risk of pressure ulcers, severe obesity can create so much skin tension that the benefit of subcutaneous cushioning is lost. Instead, the skin is pulled so taut that pressure below the skin is actually increased. Massive pressure ulcers on areas such as the low back/upper gluteal, sacral, and ischial tuberosities may occur when a tremendously obese individual loses mobility for an extended period. Wounds greater than 10 to 15 cm (4 to 6 inches) deep may occur at the low back in very large, immobile individuals. Other at-risk sites include where medical devices, tubes, and lines are left under the skin. Skin over the greater trochanters may also be injured by seating in wheelchairs that are too narrow. Placing the person in a reclined position is an even greater risk for the obese person as shearing on the skin becomes greater due to the increased body mass. Skin is also at risk due to difficulty in repositioning a heavy person. Skin is subjected to greater friction and the effectiveness of repositioning may be compromised. Although areas of contact with the support surface might appear to be moved, the same bony prominences and skin may remain in contact with the support surface. The inability to see where the patient is in contact with the mattress and the movement of large amounts of tissue above the surface can be deceptive. To be certain that the person has actually been repositioned, a person may need to be pulled across the bed with a draw sheet and a wedge placed beneath him or her.

Surgical intervention such as gastric bypass, gastric banding, or similar procedures may be used to induce malabsorption as a means of reducing body weight. Although many patients who undergo these procedures have no postoperative morbidity, many will have difficulty with healing of surgical incisions, infection, and dehiscence of surgical wounds. Successful weight loss may exacerbate or induce intertrigo as subcutaneous fat is lost and skin folds overlap more than they did preoperatively. Removal of pannus (panniculectomy) may be considered cosmetic and not covered by insurance, although presence of pannus remains a risk to skin integrity.

Problems with healing occur due to diabetes, cardiovascular disease, and poor skin quality (xerosis, intertrigo, and other skin infections). In addition, the ability to obtain appropriate skin and subcutaneous tissue approximation postoperatively may lead to development of seromas and hematomas with risk of infection and dehiscence.

INTENSIVE CARE UNITS

Another area of concern is intensive care units (ICUs). Patients in ICUs have approximately double the risk of pressure ulcers of other patients in a given facility. Skin is at greater risk due to decreased health in general, with frequent malnutrition, decreased mobility, and the presence of multiple medical devices attached to the patient. The patient's diminished health and nutrition reduces the skin's tolerance for unrelieved pressure and shear. Medical device positioning is a particular area of concern as 50% of hospital-acquired pressure ulcers are caused by medical devices such as Foley catheters and intravenous lines. Friction from passive repositioning and shearing from the patient being placed in a reclining position for cardiovascular conditioning also increase the risk of pressure ulcers. As patients become very ill and develop organ failure, skin injury becomes more likely. Low blood pressure and cardiac output reduce perfusion of skin. Higher extraction of oxygen secondary to low cardiac output leads to hypoxia of the blood perfusing the skin. Venous return from the lower extremities is compromised from compression of blood vessels due to poor positioning in bed. Decreased venous return further reduces any problems with oxygen delivery caused by low cardiac output. Edema of the extremities caused by decreased venous return produces further venous compression and difficulty transporting nutrients to the skin.

Interventions for patients in the ICU include providing more frequent and meticulous skin examination. Appropriate cleaning after episodes of incontinence and use of skin protectants can reduce the risk of injury. Foley catheters and rectal tubes or pouches may be necessary to prevent injury to the perineal skin. Positioning a person in bed requires greater care to avoid injuries to the skin. Following repositioning, the linens under the patient should be checked to avoid wrinkles and bunching of the sheets, blankets and underpads. Underpads should also be changed frequently to prevent retention of fluid against the skin along with inspection of the bed itself for any foreign objects. Caps from medical devices, pieces of food, and cellular telephones have been found under patients turned to receive wound care.

LIFESPAN

Lifespan considerations include limiting injury to skin of the elderly and optimizing wound healing in children. The properties of aging skin were discussed in Unit I. Important points to the discussion of proper care for skin of the elderly are discussed below. Fetal wound healing is discussed in Chapter 2.

Aging Skin

A number of aspects of the gross morphology of aging skin are clearly evident. These include decreased moisture content manifested as greater roughness and scaliness of the skin, decreased elasticity manifested as wrinkling and laxity, the accumulation of benign neoplasms and increased risk of malignant neoplasms. Some of these effects, however, do not simply appear to be the effect of aging, but are due to the accumulation of sun damage. At the microscopic level, flattening of the dermal-epidermal junction can be observed with effacement of dermal papillae. The height of dermal papillae decreases 55% from the third to ninth decade. As this change occurs, the surface between the vascularized dermis and the epidermis decreases. Several changes observed in the skin of the elderly result from the decreased contact between these layers. The area available for nutrient transfer, the number of actively reproducing keratinocytes within the stratum basale, and decreased resistance to shearing result from this loss of contact surface between the dermis and epidermis.

Aging Epidermis

The thickness of the stratum corneum remains unchanged with aging, but an increased size and variability of cells is observed. In addition, the number of melanocytes decreases at a rate of about 10% to 20% per decade. Consistent with the decline in the number of melanocytes is a decreased number of nevi. As a result of the decline in the number of melanocytes, the skin has a progressively decreased protection from UV light. In addition, the resident macrophages of the epidermis, the Langerhans cells experience a 20% to 50% decrease.

Aging Dermis

As opposed to the epidermis, the dermis experiences a significant decrease in its thickness, averaging about 20%. This decrease in thickness produces the transparent appearance of elderly skin. Due to a 30% decrease in mast cells, less inflammation results from UV exposure. In addition, regression of the dermal vascular bed and decreased blood flow to appendages leads to gradual atrophy and fibrosis of appendages. A remodeling of elastic fibers into thicker, disorganized elastic fibers results in diminished elasticity and increased risk of tearing.

Functional Changes in the Skin

A 30% to 50% decrease in epidermal turnover has been described from the third to the eighth decade. In addition, a decreased repair rate has been quantified as both decreased wound tensile strength and collagen deposition. Dry, inelastic skin, with larger, more irregular epidermal cells leads to decreased barrier function. Moreover, decreased sensory perception increases the risk of injury to skin by mechanical forces such as pressure. Decreased sebum, estimated to decline by 23% per decade, allows the skin to become dry. Due to decreased numbers of Langerhans cells, immunity within the skin declines, putting the skin at higher risk of infection. Due to the more rigid, less elastic, drier nature of elderly skin with decreased contact area between the dermis and epidermis, the skin of elderly individuals tears and bleeds easily. Skin tears and multiple ecchymoses are commonplace in the skin of the elderly, especially those with multiple intravenous lines, and with the use of tape used to hold IV lines in place.

Modifications for the Care of Aging Skin

Foremost, the choice of wound products to be used on the skin of the elderly must take into account the fragile nature of the skin. Moreover, because of decreased inflammation, greater risk of malnutrition and dehydration, the clinician must assume a longer period for healing. Therefore, dressings that need to be changed frequently or have strong adhesive need to be used with care or avoided. Tape of any kind must be used judiciously. In particular, silk and plastic tape should not be used. Alternatives such as stretch netting should be considered. When occlusive dressings are chosen, hydrocolloids and semipermeable films should be used only if nonadherent hydrogel sheets are not practical. If films or hydrocolloid sheets are to be used, skin protectant needs to be placed on the surrounding skin. In addition, the absorbency of the dressing needs to be optimized. Although thin hydrocolloid sheets permit better visualization of the wound, thicker hydrocolloid sheet may be necessary to prolong time between changes. Filling the wound with an absorbent material such as alginate or hydrofiber can also prolong wearing time of hydrocolloid and semipermeable film dressings. When these dressings are removed, care must be taken to avoid injury to the skin. The skin should not be pulled with the dressing as it is removed. Gentle peeling of hydrocolloid sheets or stretching of a semipermeable film tangentially to the skin surface as the skin is held in place may reduce the risk of injury.

Cleansing of wounds needs to be done as gently as possible. Pulsatile lavage with suction may be done at a lower impact pressure or replaced by gentle irrigation as necessary. Mechanical damage and maceration can result from vigorous whirlpool therapy for cleansing or nonselective debridement. In the case of many elderly patients, the clinician must consider the risks and benefits of different types of debridement. Frequently, orders are received for whirlpool and wet-to-dry dressings on the wounds of the elderly. Additives to the whirlpools or topical agents placed on the wound may cause severe injury to the wound or surrounding skin. Elderly patients with wounds who are in the terminal stage of an illness may not benefit from the full range of options available from the clinician. The clinician must ask him- or herself what benefits will the patient receive from any given intervention. In many cases, wound healing is not achievable due to the nutritional or cardiopulmonary sta-

tus of the patient, and goals are limited to reducing the risk of infection and managing drainage and odor of the wound. In these cases, treatment consisting of optimizing autolytic debridement is appropriate, unless the wound is infected or infection is imminent.

Prevention of Skin Injury in the Elderly

In addition to selecting wound care products carefully, a number of other forms of skin protection should be considered. The skin of the elderly tends to become dry, brittle, and may fissure and tear with minor trauma. Therapeutic moisturizers may be necessary, especially during the winter or in low-humidity environments. Bed frames and rails should be inspected for sharp edges and padded as needed.

Optimizing Wound Healing in Children

In general, wound healing is more rapid in children than in adults. However, younger children present challenges to wound management. Permission to evaluate and treat children must be obtained from an appropriate adult, usually a parent. Children may not fully understand the interventions and may be fearful and reluctant to receive interventions, particularly pulsatile lavage, sharp debridement, and packing/unpacking wounds. The presence of parents to calm children needs to be assessed on a case-by-case basis. Although some parents may be able to calm a child sufficiently for interventions to be provided, some parents may create a negative environment by being too permissive and allowing tantrums, or by being too harsh and increasing the child's anxiety. Children may be more cooperative if they have the opportunity to inspect or play act any interventions ahead of time with appropriate considerations for infection control. Children should never be left alone in a treatment room as they may become curious and either hurt themselves or contaminate equipment and supplies.

Any parent/guardian in the treatment area will require face masks for protection from airborne microbes along with the patient. Other PPE will depend on the possibility of secondary contamination. In general, clothing worn by the patient's parent can be treated as the clothing from the patient. If another person with compromised immunity may be exposed to the clothing of the parent, the parent should either wear PPE or change clothing before encountering anyone with compromised immunity.

Very young children, such as infants, may be difficult to manage as nothing can be explained to them. Infants may also be more susceptible to infection than older children. Clinicians with any signs of respiratory disease should avoid treating infants, children with decreased immunity, or children with sickle cell disease. Rooms used with children should be thoroughly disinfected before and after treatments, especially when hydrotherapy from either whirlpools or pulsatile lavage is used.

Dressings chosen for a child, as those chosen for the elderly, should minimize frequency of changes and trauma. However, another consideration may be the durability of dressings for highly active children. Children may be encouraged to avoid physical activity that may disturb wound dressings, but the frequent reality is that this advice will be ignored. Dressings that can stand up to potential physical activity should be chosen. In addition, parents should be instructed early in reinforcing or changing dressings, including principles of sterile technique, disinfection of any scissors or other instruments, and contingencies for changes in the wound's status.

END OF LIFE

When discussing skin and wound care at the end of life, the focus changes from restorative to palliative care. In the common situation of restorative care, focus is placed on the return to former level of function including closure and healing of wounds. However, in palliative care the focus is the support of patients and caregivers and providing comfort rather than cure.

Pressure Ulcer Risk Factors at End of Life

With terminal disease, as well as any condition resulting in diminished mobility, several risk factors for pressure ulcers increase. Patients may develop hip and knee contractures, becoming contracted in the fetal position. When this occurs, the only turning surfaces available expose the sacral and greater trochanter areas to even greater risk because no good turning surfaces become available, leading to the inevitable development of pressure ulcers in these 3 sites. Pressure ulcers may develop in other susceptible locations in the sidelying or Fowler's position (recumbent with hips and knees flexed). With multisystem failure imminent, supply of nutrients and removal of wastes are compromised in the forms of heart failure, end-stage renal disease, hypoventilation, acidosis, malnutrition, and a generalized compromise of homeostatic mechanisms. Risk of skin injury is increased with urinary and fecal incontinence expected to occur in association with immobility and loss of homeostasis.

Definition of Skin Failure

Skin failure may be considered to be part of multisystem organ failure. As the largest organ of body, the skin becomes susceptible to failure for several reasons. Acute failure may result from a medical crisis leading to lack of perfusion in conditions such as hypotension or compart-

ment syndrome. Acute illness resulting in anemia, malnutrition, or immobilization also may place skin at risk. Skin injury due to chronic disease may result from prolonged immobilization, decreased skin perfusion due to chronic heart failure, and malnutrition due to disease involving the alimentary tract. Chronic illnesses may be accumulated, eg, congestive heart failure, renal failure, anemia, immobility, incontinence, and other diseases that predispose one to skin injury. Most commonly, acute illness superimposed on chronic disease is likely to lead to skin injury. A person with poorly controlled diabetes mellitus, for example, may fracture a hip, develop an infection, experience a deep vein thrombosis, pulmonary embolus, and multiple other problems resulting in a downward spiral of health that might not have occurred but for the underlying chronic disease of diabetes mellitus.

Kennedy Terminal Ulcer

The classic sign of skin failure occurs in the sacrococcygeal area and has been dubbed the *Kennedy terminal ulcer*. Like many stage IV pressure ulcers, the resulting skin failure seems to occur suddenly, likely also due to necrosis occurring deeply at first. In most cases, the skin in the sacrococcygeal area becomes red, purple, then black within hours and results in a pear shaped ulcer. This ulcer, indicative of the skin failure component of multisystem failure, is often observed within 24 hours of death.

Palliative Care

Palliative care is provided to individuals known to have a terminal condition. Under Medicare hospice rules, time of death is expected to be within 6 months as certified by a physician. Many individuals may exceed the expected lifespan or may decline more rapidly. Hospice care paid by Medicare may be provided through either home or inpatient care. Under hospice, patients may not receive treatments specific to cure of a condition, but may receive services that provide improved quality of life by increasing patient comfort and pain relief.

Healing of ulcers already present may not be a reasonable expectation, depending on the underlying disease. If a patient has a condition decreasing perfusion to the area of a skin injury due to peripheral arterial disease, low cardiac output, or hematocrit, healing is not expected. If the patient does not have skin injury already, measures to decrease risk of pressure ulcers are in order. The patient's sensation, mobility, skin condition, including moisture, friction, and shear need to be assessed. The level of activity in bed (or out of bed if possible) and nutrition, hydration, and body weight should be part of the examination as well. Issues related to risk of pressure ulcers in bedbound or chairbound individuals are discussed thoroughly in Chapter 7.

After physical examination and discussion of patient and caregiver needs and abilities, appropriate goals for palliative wound care may be determined. The most common goals include preventing deterioration and infection of the wound and minimizing risk of skin injury elsewhere. Because healing may not be a reasonable goal, clinical decisions should be weighted toward patient comfort and minimizing pain. For example, aggressive sharp debridement and frequent dressing changes may not be in the patient's best interest. If a wound is deteriorating and infection is likely to spread, however, aggressive debridement may be necessary. Managing odor and drainage take greater precedence for reasons of the patient's psychosocial well being. Preventing the loss of a social support system due to odor or unpleasant appearance of wound drainage should be addressed in the plan of care.

Dressings used in palliative care should be chosen to minimize the number of changes and pain during them. Dressings that reduce odor and more effectively manage drainage may also be chosen. However, dressings must be chosen also to minimize risk of infection. Decreased immunity may be associated with terminal conditions. Several strategies for odor control are available. Because decreasing risk of infection takes precedence over healing in this state, using cytotoxic agents such as acetic acid or Dakin's solution can be appropriate. Other choices include silver and other antimicrobial dressings. Even in the case of a noninfected wound, the accumulation of drainage under an occlusive dressing may produce an unpleasant odor. Several dressings are available with charcoal to absorb odor and allow dressing changes to be done less frequently. Some compromise between pain management and pain may become necessary when debridement or cleansing the wound are the only means available to control odor and infection. Another solution to odor control is the placement of charcoal or cat litter designed to absorb odors under the patient's bed.

SUMMARY

Multi-organ system failure may include skin failure. In palliative care one must determine the needs and priorities of both patients and caregivers. The need for aggressive debridement must be weighed against patient discomfort. Dressings should be chosen that minimize trauma, but do not promote pain, leakage, or odor. Cues for unusual wounds include an appearance or location that is out of the ordinary, failure to heal or worsens over time, and abnormal appearing granulation tissue. In these cases a biopsy should be performed by an appropriate clinician to rule out neoplastic, infectious, or inflammatory disease.

QUESTIONS

1. Why do obesity and intensive care increase the risk of pressure ulcers?
2. What characteristics should cue you to look for an unusual cause of a wound?
3. How does the patient's imminent death affect a treatment plan for a wound?
4. Why should aggressive debridement be avoided in sickle cell disease?

BIBLIOGRAPHY

Ad-El DD, Meirovitz A, Weinberg A, et al. Warfarin skin necrosis: local and systemic factors. *Br J Plast Surg.* 2000;53(7):624-626.

Baldwin KM, Ziegler SM. Pressure ulcer risk following critical traumatic injury. *Adv Wound Care.* 1998;11(4):168-173.

Bostanjian D, Anthone GJ, Hamoui N, Crookes PF. Rhabdomyolysis of gluteal muscles leading to renal failure: a potentially fatal complication of surgery in the morbidly obese. *Obes Surg.* 2003;13(2):302-305.

Centers for Disease Control and Prevention. Defining Obesity and Overweight. http://www.cdc.gov/nccdphp/dnpa/obesity/defining.htm. Accessed May 14, 2009.

Chan YC, Valenti D, Mansfield AO, Stansby G. Warfarin induced skin necrosis. *Br J Surg.* 2000; 87:266-272.

Compher C, Kinosian BP, Ratcliffe SJ, Baumgarten M. Obesity reduces the risk of pressure ulcers in elderly hospitalized patients. *J Gerontol A Biol Sci Med Sci.* 2007;62(11):1310-1312.

DeFranzo AJ, Marasco P, Argenta LC. Warfarin-induced necrosis of the skin. *Ann Plast Surg.* 1995;34(2):203-208.

Falabella A, Falanga V. Uncommon causes of ulcers. *Clin Plast Surg.* 1998;25(3):467-479.

Fife C, Otto G, Capsuto EG, et al. Incidence of pressure ulcers in a neurologic intensive care unit. *Crit Care Med.* 2001;29(2):283-290.

Hafner J, Schneider E, Burg G, Cassina PC. Management of leg ulcers in patients with rheumatoid arthritis or systemic sclerosis: the importance of concomitant arterial and venous disease. *J Vasc Surg.* 2000 Aug;32(2):322-329.

Hahler B. An overview of dermatological conditions commonly associated with the obese patient. *Ostomy Wound Manage.* 2006;52(6):34-40.

Halabi-Tawil M, Lionnet F, Girot R, Bachmeyer C, Levy PP, Aractingi S. Sickle cell leg ulcers: a frequently disabling complication and a marker of severity. *Br J Dermatol.* 2008;158(2):339-344.

Jacob SE, Weisman RS, Kerdel FA. Pyoderma gangrenosum—rebel without a cure? *Int J Dermatol.* 2008;47(2):192-194.

Kennedy Terminal Ulcer. http://www.kennedyterminalulcer.com/ Accessed May 14, 2009.

Labropoulos N, Manalo D, Patel NP, et al. Uncommon leg ulcers in the lower extremity. *J Vasc Surg.* 2007;45(3):568-573.

Langemo DK, Brown G. Skin fails too: acute, chronic, and end-stage skin failure. *Adv Skin Wound Care.* 2006;19(4):206-211.

Lichon V, Khachemoune A. Mycetoma: a review. *Am J Clin Dermatol.* 2006;7(5):315-321.

Mert A, Kumbasar H, Ozaras R, et al. Erythema nodosum: an evaluation of 100 cases. *Clin Exp Rheumatol.* 2007;25(4):563-570.

Mumcu G, Inanc N, Yavuz S, Direskeneli H. The role of infectious agents in the pathogenesis, clinical manifestations and treatment strategies in Behçet's disease. *Clin Exp Rheumatol.* 2007;25(4 Suppl 45):S27-33.

Murakami Y, Shibata S, Koso S et al. Delayed tissue necrosis associated with mitomycin-C administration. *J Dermatol.* 2000;27:413-415.

Naylor WA. A guide to wound management in palliative care. *Int J Palliat Nurs.* 2005;11(11):572, 574-579.

Panasiti V, Devirgiliis V, Borroni RG, et al. Management of skin ulcers in a patient with mycosis fungoides. *Dermatol Online J.* 2006;12(2):16.

Rashtak S, Pittelkow MR. Skin involvement in systemic autoimmune diseases. *Curr Dir Autoimmun.* 2008;10:344-358.

Rogge FJ, Pacifico M, Kang N. Treatment of pyoderma gangrenosum with the anti-TNFalpha drug - Etanercept. *J Plast Reconstr Aesthet Surg.* 2008;61(4):431-433.

Schrijvers DL. Extravasation: a dreaded complication of chemotherapy. *Ann Oncol.* 2003;14(Supplement 3): iii26–iii30.

Schue RM, Langemo DK. Pressure ulcer prevalence and incidence and a modification of the Braden Scale for a rehabilitation unit. *J Wound Ostomy Continence Nurs.* 1998;25(1):36-43.

Seaman S. Management of malignant fungating wounds in advanced cancer. *Semin Oncol Nurs.* 2006;22(3):185-193.

Trent JT, Kirsner RS. Wounds and malignancy. *Adv Skin Wound Care.* 2003;16(1):31-34.

Wilson JA, Clark JJ. Obesity: impediment to postsurgical wound healing. *Adv Skin Wound Care.* 2004;17(8):426-435.

Nonpatient Interventions

Having a grasp of the science behind wound management, the etiology, and interventions, we now must consider dealing with additional issues. Because each patient is unique, we learn to adapt our set of interventions to optimally meet the patient's needs. Although our thought may be very clear to ourselves, we also need to communicate effectively with many parties. The chapter on documentation discusses issues related to putting our thoughts to paper so others may understand our thoughts. These parties include members of our own profession, other healthcare providers, those who make reimbursement decisions, and even juries. Additionally, we want to develop a clear plan of care that will address as many factors as possible that we then have to elaborate in our documentation. Chapter 17 deals in general with documentation issues, including legal issues, and chapter 18 deals more specifically with developing a plan of care that is optimally effective in terms of patient outcomes and costs of providing care. At times, meeting regulations and maximizing reimbursement for service rendered can seem at odds. However, with experience and careful planning, especially if we can better account for psychosocial issues impacting our patients, we will frequently be able to maintain fiscal responsibility while providing the best possible care for our patients. Chapter 19 addresses a number of important regulatory, reimbursement, and psychosocial issues that will allow clinicians to become more proficient and efficient.

Documentation

Documentation 17

Objectives

- Describe elements of the medical, family medical, social, work, and home history to document in an initial evaluation.
- Discuss use of photography for documenting wound management.
- Discuss potential problems that substandard documentation may cause.
- List the 4 necessary components for proving a civil court action.
- Discuss how proper documentation can minimize the risks of denial of payments and lawsuits.

THE NEED FOR DOCUMENTATION

The old axiom has been "If it hasn't been documented, it wasn't done." We have now evolved to optimizing documentation of patient care to maximize reimbursement. Increasingly, we also need to document carefully to avoid legal pitfalls. Regardless of the motivation for documentation, the underlying reason for documentation is to provide a clear road map of where we expect patient care to go, any detours, and the final destination. This is true whether one clinician is in a position to provide care through discharge, or multiple clinicians must be involved. The plan of care (Chapter 18) is developed from a simple flow of thought from what has already been documented.

Many facilities use forms for documenting wound management. Some are universal forms; others use forms specific for wound etiology, eg, a form for thermal injuries, another for pressure ulcers, another for venous ulcers. The advantage of etiology-specific forms is that they can be more efficient and readable because they contain only information pertinent to the type of wound. The information requested on the form is more likely to be relevant to the patient, and the clinician will not forget to ask certain questions or perform certain tests relevant to the etiology of the wound. For example, a pressure ulcer form may contain one of the risk assessment tools such as the Braden or Norton scale, and a form for neuropathic ulcers would contain the elements of foot screening. Another advantage

Irion G.
Comprehensive Wound Management, 2nd ed. (pp 297-320)
© 2010 SLACK Incorporated

of an etiology-specific form is that it can usually be printed on a single sheet. A single sheet is more likely to be read by other members of the wound management team and other parties who have an interest in the care provided. However, information should not be crammed into a single page such that the readability of the form is compromised. Etiology-specific forms become a problem when the clinician does not know the true cause of a wound. A clinician may not reach an accurate diagnosis even after the form has been completed, especially if a wound presents a difficult differential diagnosis. A compromise is the use of a generic wound-care form supplemented with an etiology-specific form. An example of a generic integumentary documentation form is given in Figure 17-1. Supplemental forms specific to venous disease, pressure ulcers, thermal injuries, and neuropathic injuries are given in Figures 17-2, 17-3, 17-4 and 17-5, respectively.

Proper documentation can be difficult if a logical sequence is not followed. In this chapter the concepts of the *Guide to Physical Therapist Practice* are used as a basis for documentation. This system is based on continuous development and testing of hypotheses of causal and contributing factors that have led to the patient's current state of health. The clinician must then select tests to confirm, refute, or modify hypotheses regarding these causal and contributing factors. As the clinician takes a verbal history or reads a history from another source, the process of developing hypotheses is already occurring.

Frequently, a referring clinician has provided a diagnosis for the patient's condition. This referring diagnosis may be a good starting point, but must not be the sole focus of the patient history or physical examination. On occasion, the referring diagnosis may be incomplete or inaccurate. In particular, the clinician must be wary of less common etiologies that may masquerade as common types of wounds. To a great extent, the clinician must perform a complete physical examination and take a history as if none had been done by another clinician already. Failure to confirm data collected by another clinician produces the potential for casually accepting a referring diagnosis and missing a critical piece of information that either generates the diagnosis or contributes to the patient's condition.

For example, a patient may be referred with a diagnosis of cellulitis superior to the medial malleolus with wounds that have remained open for 2 years. Despite the referring diagnosis, the prudent clinician becomes suspicious of venous disease, so the questions and testing start down the road of confirming contributing factors for venous disease rather than accepting the diagnosis of an infection. If the patient reports a history of diabetes, the clinician will immediately begin asking questions related to both neuropathy and peripheral arterial disease. In both of these cases, the clinician will perform an examination

of the peripheral circulation to rule out arterial disease, a contraindication for compression.

ELEMENTS OF THE HISTORY

For facilities other than acute care hospitals, a standardized history form becomes increasingly important. Hospital-based facilities will have a history and physical examination section on the patient's chart that should contain all relevant information. Information critical to the treatment plan for the wound, however, should be kept in a centralized area of the chart so an individual taking over care of the patient will not be required to read an entire chart. In addition, the hospital chart provides lab values and lists medications. This information can supplement what is on the history. For example, a history of congestive heart failure or rheumatoid arthritis may not be explicitly documented in the history and physical, but medications listed in the chart may cue the clinician to inquire about these conditions.

In an outpatient facility, the standardized history form can be useful if done carefully. An example of an outpatient history form is given in Figure 17-6. Often, simply asking a patient to fill out the form is not sufficient. With an exhaustive listing of possible ailments, patients are likely to run down the list of irrelevant items quickly and miss an important problem that should have been identified. Key items should be confirmed verbally with the patient and, if possible, with a family member or caregiver, and the patient should be asked directly whether he or she has any medical conditions that might be related to the wound.

Important questions are generated by both the etiology of the wound and any additional diagnoses listed in the history. In particular, questions related to diabetes are critical. Anyone who reports a history of diabetes mellitus should be asked about glycemic control, including current blood glucose and HbA1c to determine short- and long-term glycemic control.

Questions about standing and walking are particularly important for lower extremity ulcers. A person with wounds consistent with venous disease needs to be asked about standing. A person with apparent neuropathic ulcers needs to be asked about walking, shoes, offloading techniques used, and other items discussed in Chapter 7. Also the patient should be asked about any symptoms that accompany walking that may be suggestive of intermittent claudication.

Questions about lifestyle, general health, vision, balance, and available care at home are important in developing a treatment plan that can be followed by the patient and any caregivers. Information to be documented was discussed thoroughly in Chapters 5 (history) and 6 (physical examination). Examples of completed documentation forms are given in Figures 17-7 to 17-11.

GENERIC INTEGUMENTARY DOCUMENTATION FORM

Patient_____ Age_____ M F   Clinician_____ Date_____

History
Chief complaint_____
Home arrangements_____
Support system_____
Occupation/education/hobbies/home activities_____
_____
Ambulation required for lifestyle_____
Standing required for lifestyle_____
Current lifestyle limitations_____
Medications_____
Past medical history _____
Previous treatment for condition_____
Review of Systems
Neuromuscular_____
Musculoskeletal_____
Cardiopulmonary_____
Integumentary_____
Physical Examination
Wound photo or drawing here:

Color_____ Odor_____ Drainage _____ Extent_____
Shape_____ Tissue in wound   Black_____ %   Yellow_____ %   Red_____ %
Surrounding Skin
Texture_____ Temperature_____ Swelling: - +   ++   +++   ++++
Color_____ Hair/nails_____ Ecchymosis_____ Hemosiderin_____
Demarcation_____ Maceration_____ Epiboly_____
Diagnosis Impaired integumentary integrity with:
_____Risk of injury   _____Superficial injury
_____Partial-thickness injury   _____Full-thickness injury
_____Full-thickness injury and subcutaneous involvement
Prognosis: Within_____days weeks months, and within_____visits, the patient is expected to:
_____
Plan of Care
Patient and family/caregiver education_____
Procedural interventions_____ frequency_____ duration_____
_____ frequency_____ duration_____
Signature_____ Date_____

Figure 17-1. Generic integumentary documentation form contains a short section for history and physical examination items most directly related to the cause of the wound and several blanks to be filled with words, checks, or "+" signs. The use of this form does not presume any diagnosis or etiology. Instead, the form is a means of keeping the clinician "on track" using the *Guide to Physical Therapist Practice*. The therapist collects data and performs special tests as needed to rule in or rule out the wound's cause. In the diagnosis section, the clinician chooses with a check mark one or more of the 5 listed diagnoses based on impairments and the guide. The prognosis derives from the diagnosis and the special circumstances of the patient. The plan of care includes patient/family/caregiver education and procedural interventions. To an extent, "goals" are part of the prognosis section; specific documentation requirements may require goals related to functions necessary to the patient (eg, the patient will be able to stand for an 8-hour shift without complaining of pain; the patient will have sufficient range of motion for self-feeding). The final section is only present to allow individuals with a need to know what direct or "procedural" interventions are being performed for the patient, how frequently, and an expected time at which the intervention will no longer be needed. If documentation of functional outcomes is needed, a general initial evaluation form may also need to be used.

SUPPLEMENTAL DATA FOR DIAGNOSIS OF VENOUS ULCERS

Patient_____ Clinician_____ Date_____

Alternatives to standing _____

Location(s)_____

Status of surrounding skin_____

Size of wound(s)	Length_____cm	Width_____cm	Depth Partial-thickness	Full-thickness
Ankle brachial index	Right_____	Left_____		
Temperature of right foot	normal	increased	decreased	
Temperature of left foot	normal	increased	decreased	
Capillary refill (right)	normal	sluggish	absent	
Capillary refill (left)	normal	sluggish	absent	
Foot volume	Right_____	Left_____		
Wound bed	% Red_____	% Yellow_____	% Black_____	
Color of granulation tissue	red	pink		
Drainage	minimal	moderate	copious	

Color of drainage _____

Compression therapy (specify)_____

Signature_____ Date_____

Figure 17-2. Supplemental data for diagnosis of venous ulcers is used for the patient who is determined by the clinician to have venous ulcers. This form is meant to supplement the generic integumentary documentation form. These items are more directly related to venous ulcer risk factors, prevention of recurrence, and appropriate treatment. Note in particular the items to rule out arterial insufficiency. These items include ankle brachial index, foot temperature, capillary refill, and color of granulation tissue. Items used to confirm the suspicion of venous ulcers are also listed and will be illustrated in Figure 17-8.

A list of prescription drugs, over-the-counter medicine, and herbal remedies should be obtained. Often, patients will not remember all of the medications by name. Asking patients to bring in and show all of their medications will improve the accuracy of the drug review. Many patients are proactive and carry a list of their medications with them. Other patients are extremely careless with medications. An extreme example is a patient who kept all of his medication in a single bag and took pills of different shapes and colors as he saw fit.

ELEMENTS OF THE PHYSICAL EXAMINATION

The physical examination performed during the initial visit will be much more comprehensive than that of subsequent visits. In particular, general health and mobility, and possible complicating factors that may influence the patient's ability to follow a treatment plan need to be explored. Subsequent visits must have some element of examination, but they are focused more on whether the prognosis developed from the initial visit is still appro-

priate and gives the clinician the opportunity to explore complications not foreseen during the initial evaluation. General mobility should be evaluated and documented, even if the patient has no mobility. The lack of mobility weighs heavily in the prognosis of certain types of wounds, especially pressure ulcers. The quality of gait is also important, particularly for the person with neuropathic feet. The loss of proprioception leads to unsteady gait, loss of heel-toe progression and, in extreme cases, a wide-based gait with slapping of the foot onto the floor. Inability to control the foot and ankle during gait are high-risk factors for the person with neuropathy due to increased shearing forces on the plantar surface.

Strength, range of motion, sensation, and reflexes need to be addressed. The extent of this aspect of the evaluation needs to be ascertained at the time of the evaluation. Limited range of motion of the foot is also a major prognosticator of neuropathic ulcers. Sensory tests can be done quickly and can distinguish between small and large sensory neuron loss. Reflexes are particularly diagnostic of large neuron deficits in neuropathy, but may also be informative for patients with other pathologies. Strength testing of the

SUPPLEMENTAL DATA FORM FOR PRESSURE ULCERS

Patient_____ Clinician_____ Date_____

Stage of ulcer (identify location on figure at right with wound number)

Identify location(s) of pressure ulcers

1.	I	II	III	IV	Partially filled	Filled	Covered
2.	I	II	III	IV	Partially filled	Filled	Covered
3.	I	II	III	IV	Partially filled	Filled	Covered
4.	I	II	III	IV	Partially filled	Filled	Covered
5.	I	II	III	IV	Partially filled	Filled	Covered

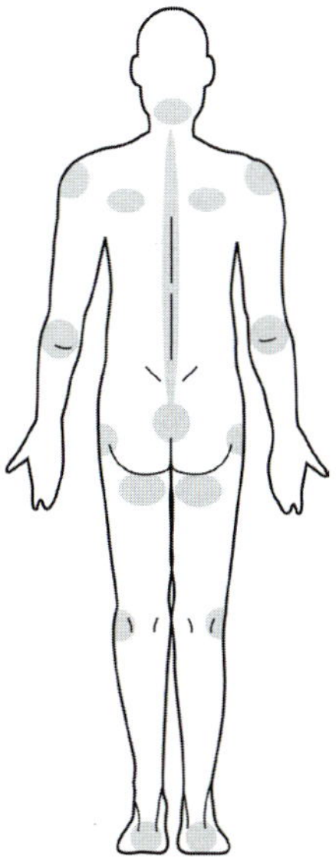

Size of ulcer (using identification key on right)

1.	Length_____cm	Width_____cm	Depth_____cm
2.	Length_____cm	Width_____cm	Depth_____cm
3.	Length_____cm	Width_____cm	Depth_____cm
4.	Length_____cm	Width_____cm	Depth_____cm
5.	Length_____cm	Width_____cm	Depth_____cm

Tunneling, sinus tracts, undermining

1.	Distance_____cm	Direction_____:00	Drainage_____
2.	Distance_____cm	Direction_____:00	Drainage_____
3.	Distance_____cm	Direction_____:00	Drainage_____
4.	Distance_____cm	Direction_____:00	Drainage_____
5.	Distance_____cm	Direction_____:00	Drainage_____

	1	2	3	4	5
Odor	_____	_____	_____	_____	_____
Drainage	_____	_____	_____	_____	_____
% R, Y, B	_____	_____	_____	_____	_____
Surrounding skin condition	_____	_____	_____	_____	_____

Signature_____ Date_____

Figure 17-3. Supplemental data form for pressure ulcers is used for the patient with pressure ulcers. The first area includes information on the depth and degree of healing of up to 5 ulcers. Sadly, many patients will have more than 5 ulcers and a second or third supplemental data form for pressure ulcers may be used. Depth of the ulcer is indicated by using Roman numerals I through IV. As discussed in Chapter 7 and elsewhere in the text, many clinicians have difficulty handling documentation of a healing pressure ulcer. The last 3 columns of "Stage of ulcer" allow the clinician to document the progress of the wound in addition to the original depth of the injury by which the wound is meant to be staged. To the right, a figure used in Chapter 7 is placed on the form. Note that only a posterior view is used. In this view, wounds on the posterior side of the body and right and left sides can be circled, enumerated, and a line drawn to the circle or ellipse. This view covers a large fraction of pressure ulcers, including the problem areas of the occiput, epicondyles of the elbow, sacrum, ischial tuberosities, and heels. If a wound is located on the anterior surface, a note can be written to indicate that the wound is not on the visible side and give a brief description (eg, chin and a line drawn to the figure to indicate the location on the anterior side). Due to the prevalence of tunneling, sinus tracts, and undermining with pressure ulcers, a section has been devoted to describe them.

foot is similarly important, particularly for the individual with peripheral neuropathy. Loss of intrinsic foot muscle strength precedes critical foot deformities. Ankle-brachial index is considered to be a minimum standard for any patient with lower extremity ulcers. Suspected peripheral arterial disease should be quantified this way for possible referral to a vascular surgeon. A person with diabetes mellitus presenting with neuropathy of the lower extremities is at high risk for peripheral arterial disease and should be tested. Moreover, the person with venous ulcers needs to be tested to rule out arterial insufficiency before initiating compression therapy.

text continues on p. 311

SUPPLEMENTAL FORM FOR THERMAL INJURY

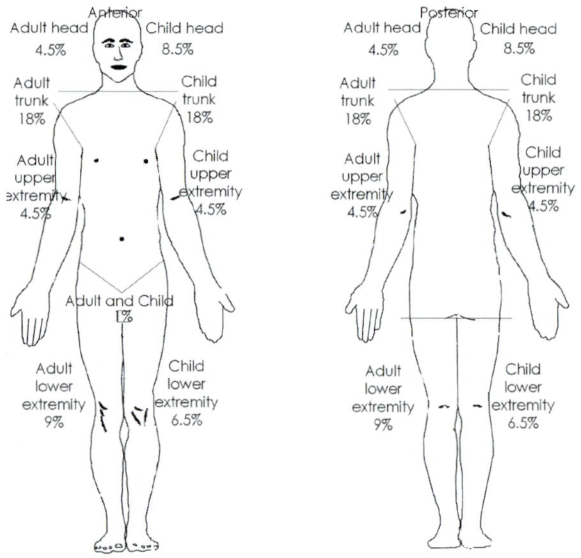

Indicate locations and depths of thermal injuries on the figure to the left.

- - Superficial thickness (1st degree)

//// Superficial partial thickness (2nd degree)

\\\ Deep partial thickness (deep dermal)

xxx Full thickness

Anterior

Adult head 4.5%   Child head 8.5%

Adult trunk 18%   Child trunk 18%

Adult upper extremity 4.5%   Child upper extremity 4.5%

Adult and Child 1%

Adult lower extremity 9%   Child lower extremity 6.5%

Posterior

Adult head 4.5%   Child head 8.5%

Adult trunk 18%   Child trunk 18%

Adult upper extremity 4.5%   Child upper extremity 4.5%

Adult lower extremity 9%   Child lower extremity 6.5%

	RUE	LUE	RLE	LLE	Anterior trunk	Posterior trunk
Deficits in range of motion	____	____	____	____	_____	_____
Deficits in strength	____	____	____	____	_____	_____
Active exercise	____	____	____	____	_____	_____
Active assisted exercise	____	____	____	____	_____	_____
Passive stretch	____	____	____	____	_____	_____
No movement allowed	____	____	____	____	_____	_____

Deficits in tolerance for bed mobility, bed exercise, position changes, ambulation (specify)_____
_____

Indicate special positioning needs _____

Signature_____   Date_____

Figure 17-4. Supplemental form for thermal injury consists of figures to indicate the extent and depth of thermal injuries, including burns, scalds, and frostbite. This form may also be applicable to chemical and radiation injuries. Different patterns of shading are used to indicate the depth of injury. In some cases, the actual depth may not be certain, especially in the case of distinguishing a deep partial-thickness from a full-thickness wound. A key for the shading is given on the right. The next section is a table with a synopsis of neuromusculoskeletal impairments and appropriate types of movement for the 6 areas of the body, used as headings for the table. In many cases, thermal injuries are limited to 1 or 2 of the segments. For the deficits in range of motion and deficits in strength rows, the clinician may enter a ✓ to indicate a deficit, a Ø to indicate no deficits in that body region, or may explicitly state a movement or muscle group affected. The next 4 rows of the table use the same 6 body regions and a ✓ is entered in 1 of the 4 rows under each column heading. At a glance, a clinician will know whether active range of motion, active assisted, passive, or no movement is appropriate for the 6 regions. The clinician may make a note to indicate situations in which different types of movements are appropriate for different areas in 1 of the 6 categories given. For example, an injury may create a situation in which active range of motion is required for the hand, passive stretching is appropriate for the elbow, and active range of motion is appropriate for the shoulder. Moreover, certain directions of movement (eg, abduction or flexion) may need to be done in different ways. The next section addresses bed mobility, bed exercise, and ambulation.

SUPPLEMENTAL FORM FOR NEUROPATHIC ULCERS

Patient_____ Clinician_____ Date_____

Location(s): Indicate location of wounds on the diagram below and create a numeric key if there are multiple wounds.

Wound #	1	2	3	4	5
Wagner grade	_____	_____	_____	_____	_____
Size	_____	_____	_____	_____	_____
% Red	_____	_____	_____	_____	_____
% Yellow	_____	_____	_____	_____	_____
% Black	_____	_____	_____	_____	_____

Indicate location of callus on the diagram below with the symbol /////

Reflexes: AJ right   present   diminished   absent   AJ left   present   diminished   absent

Foot deformities (specify)_____

Gait deviations (specify)_____

Pulse (right)   4   3   2   1   0   (specify artery palpated)_____

Pulse (left)   4   3   2   1   0   (specify artery palpated)_____

Capillary refill (right)   normal   sluggish   absent

Capillary refill (left)   normal   sluggish   absent

Ankle brachial index   Right_____   Left_____

Right foot temperature   normal   decreased   increased (specify temperature)

Left foot temperature   normal   decreased   increased (specify temperature)

Sensory testing (indicate on the diagram below + for intact, +/- for diminished, - for absent

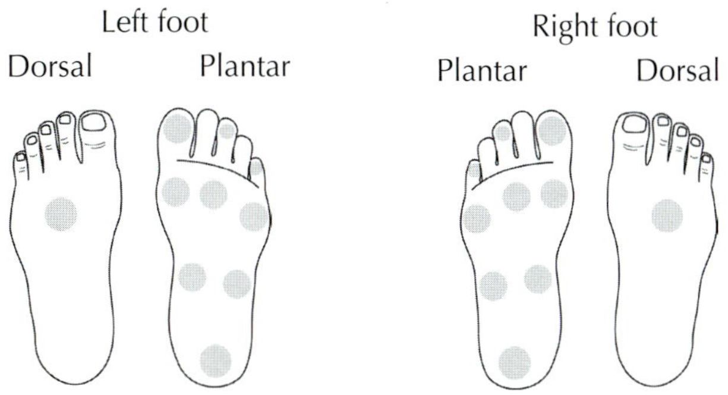

Left foot
Dorsal   Plantar

Right foot
Plantar   Dorsal

Signature_____   Date_____

Figure 17-5. Supplemental form for neuropathic ulcers. The term *diabetic foot ulcer* does not recognize that diabetes mellitus can cause both neuropathy and arterial insufficiency. The first item is the Wagner grade, in which 0 is an injury with intact skin; 1 is a shallow ulcer; 2 is a deep ulcer; 3 indicates infection of the wound or surrounding/underlying structures, especially osteomyelitis; 4 pertains to gangrene of the forefoot; and 5 indicates gangrene to most of the foot. The next section is used to document standard tests and measures for neuropathic ulcers and requires the filling of blanks or circling of items. The last item is a map of the feet. Four maps are given. On the left side are views of the plantar and dorsal left foot, and the right foot is on the right. The circles on the foot indicate the standard locations for sensory testing using a monofilament. The plantar foot has 9 locations and the dorsal foot only one. In addition to the labels placed on the form, contours on the plantar figure and toenails on the dorsal figure are given to help identify the surface of the foot.

SAMPLE HISTORY FORM

List present conditions being managed by a licensed health care provider (physician, physical therapist, occupational therapist, speech therapist, audiologist, podiatrist, nurse, osteopath, psychologist, or other).

_____
_____

List current medications including prescriptions, over-the-counter medications, herbal or other self-administered remedies, and any dietary modifications. Obtain and review use of all of your medication bottles prior to filling out this part of the form.

_____
_____

List any surgical procedures and the condition for which they were performed.

_____
_____

List previous medical conditions, treatments received for them, and the outcomes of treatment.

_____
_____

Family History (circle all that apply):

Heart disease   Diseases of arteries or veins   Stroke   Diabetes   Respiratory disease

Have you been told that you have heart, lung, blood vessel, endocrine, digestive, kidney, skin, or any other disease?   yes   no

If so specify _____

Do you presently have any of the following symptoms (circle all that apply):

Chest pain	yes	no
Shortness of breath	yes	no
Dizziness or feeling faint	yes	no
Difficulty sleeping while lying flat in bed (need to raise head to breathe)	yes	no
Swelling of the legs, ankles, or feet	yes	no
Palpitations or abnormal heart rhythm	yes	no
Pain or cramping of legs with activity that is relieved by rest	yes	no

Loss of sensation of any part of the body	yes	no	specify_____
Coldness of any part of the body	yes	no	specify_____
Frequent urination	yes	no	
Getting up at night to urinate	yes	no	
Elevated blood sugar	yes	no	don't know
Night sweats	yes	no	
Change in appetite	yes	no	specify_____
Change in sleep pattern	yes	no	specify_____
Fever	yes	no	
Changes in pattern of bowel movement or urination	yes	no	

Specify the change _____

Unusual bleeding or discharges	yes	no	specify location _____
Pain resistant to over-the-counter medications	yes	no	
Pain that wakes you at night	yes	no	
Pain that does not change with activity or position	yes	no	

If yes to any of the last three questions above, specify the location of your pain _____

Red streaks	yes	no	specify location _____
Swollen lymph nodes/glands	yes	no	specify location _____
Changes in skin texture	yes	no	specify location_____
Loss of body hair	yes	no	specify location _____
Thickening of nails	yes	no	specify location _____

Figure 17-6. Sample history form. This form is made available to the patient before the first clinical visit to ensure accuracy, especially for list of medications. On clinic visit, review the form with the patient and assess the patient's understanding of the items on the history form.

Case #1, Generic Integumentary Documentation Form and Supplemental Data Form for Diagnosis of Venous Ulcers (Figures 17-7 and 17-8)

A 42-year-old man (Figure 17-7) was referred with a diagnosis of cellulitis of the distal tibia. Although the true etiology was immediately obvious, the data collection began with a history. During the history, the initial suspicion of venous insufficiency was repeatedly reinforced. The chief complaints of discomfort to mild-moderate pain, the location described by the patient, and discoloration were all consistent with venous ulcers. The 6 items in Figure 17-7 are designed to help the clinician understand the individual's situation as it may affect prognosis. The patient's domicile and the presence of a small number of steps were not consequential, although numerous combinations of a particular type of domicile and lifestyle could create difficult situations. The patient had several family members at home and all were agreeable to keeping the patient on-track with the treatment plan. Cost issues were not a major concern, which allowed the patient sufficient access to the clinician to ensure that the treatment plan would be carried out to its completion. Although the patient's condition did not prevent the patient from working, he was uncomfortable and sometimes in pain at work, and he rarely engaged in his normal recreational activity. He mostly stayed at home and watched television, which put his cardiopulmonary status at risk. Knowing that the patient was basically on his feet most of the day during his normal routine and how his condition had been limited dictated an aggressive treatment plan and modifications at his place of work.

The review of systems included basic tests as described in the *Guide to Physical Therapist Practice*. This patient was in good health except for the history of hypertension and venous insufficiency. The neuromuscular and musculoskeletal systems were noted to be within normal limits (WNL). Because blood pressure was not completely under control with medications, and venous engorgement was noted in both legs, current BP as well as the venous problem were noted in the cardiopulmonary line. The ulceration and presence of skin changes were noted under integumentary. No integumentary problems were noted elsewhere on the patient.

The observation of the wound was then recorded using the CODES system described earlier in this book. This information, in conjunction with the history and condition of the surrounding skin, easily led to the etiology of this ulcer. The impairment-driven diagnoses based on the *Guide to Physical Therapist Practice* could then be chosen. This patient was still at risk of further ulcerations, so this diagnosis was checked in addition to the full-thickness injury. The patient's prognosis was based on his generally good health and apparent willingness to adhere to the treatment plan. This was tempered by the patient's working condition, which is discussed further in the supplemental venous ulcer form. The procedural interventions are listed along with the frequency and duration. The compression bandaging needed to be changed more frequently initially until the venous insufficiency was better controlled and the drainage diminished.

GENERIC INTEGUMENTARY DOCUMENTATION FORM

Patient __Stan Jones__   Age _42_ (M)   F   Clinician _Linda Smith_   Date _7/4/01_

History

Chief complaint _Discomfort, weeping wound on leg, and discoloration around wound_

Home arrangements _Mobile home, 4 steps with single rail, step mother, 2 teenage brothers, 10-year-old sister live with pt_

Support system _Relatives living with pt, employer provides health insurance_

Occupation/education/hobbies/home activities _Cashier in convenience store, hunting, fishing, rebuilding autos_

Ambulation required for lifestyle _Primarily stands at cash register for 8-hour shift, sometimes with recreational activities_

Standing required for lifestyle _Stands almost entirety of waking hours_

Current lifestyle limitations _Discomfort to minor pain at work, has curtailed recreational activities_

Medications _Zoloft, Xanax, Prazosin_

Past Medical History _Recurrent leg ulcers, anxiety, HTN_

Previous treatment for condition _W/P, wet-to-dry dressings_

Review of Systems

Neuromuscular	_WNL_
Musculoskeletal	_WNL_
Cardiopulmonary	_BP: 130/90, dilated, tortuous superficial leg veins in both legs_
Integumentary	_Wound on medial, distal right leg, skin changes documented below_

Physical Examination

Wound photo or drawing here:

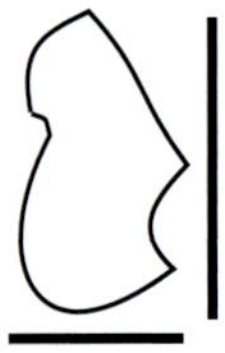

10.2 cm

6.4 cm

Color _red_   Odor _Ø_   Drainage _copious serous_   Extent _see diagram, full-thickness_

Shape _irregular_   Tissue in wound: Black _0%_   Yellow _10%_   Red _90%_

Surrounding skin:

Texture _flaky_   Temperature _33.5°C_   Swelling: -   +   ++   (+++)   ++++

Color _brown/yellow_ Hair/nails _WNL_   Ecchymosis _wound edges_   Hemosiderin _✓_

Demarcation _poor_   Maceration _✓_   Epiboly _Ø_

Diagnosis   Impaired integumentary integrity with:

✓ Risk of injury   __ Superficial injury

__ Partial-thickness injury ✓ Full-thickness injury

__ Full-thickness injury and subcutaneous involvement

Prognosis   Within _3_ days weeks (months) and within _20_ visits, the patient is expected to: Demonstrate preventive care, have full wound closure

Plan of Care

Patient and family/caregiver education _Causes and care for venous ulcers including self-performance of compression therapy_

Procedural interventions _debridement_	frequency _3-5 days_ duration _3 weeks_
compression bandaging	frequency _3-5 days_ duration _3 months_
Pt will be fit for custom stockings when leg volume normalizes	frequency _once_ duration _1 visit_

Signature ____ *Linda Smith, PT* ____   Date _7/4/01_

Figure 17-7. Example of a generic integumentary documentation form. The forms have been designed to reduce redundancy as much as possible without sacrificing the "at a view" features of the forms.

SUPPLEMENTAL DATA FORM FOR DIAGNOSIS OF VENOUS ULCERS

Patient __Stan Jones__ Clinician __Linda Smith__ Date __7/4/01__

Alternatives to standing __Store manager has agreed to allow pt to rotate between cashier work and stocking__

Location(s) __R medial leg, just proximal to medial malleolus__

Status of surrounding skin __Hemosiderin staining, flaking, and weeping__

Size of wound(s): Length __10.2__ cm Width __6.4__ cm Depth partial-thickness (full-thickness)

Ankle brachial index Right __1.1__ Left __1.0__

Temperature of right foot (normal) increased decreased

Temperature of left foot (normal) increased decreased

Capillary refill (right) (normal) sluggish absent

Capillary refill (left) (normal) sluggish absent

Foot volume right __1480__ left __1320__

Wound bed % red __90__ % yellow __10__ % black __0__

Color of granulation tissue (red) pink

Drainage minimal moderate (copious)

Color of drainage __clear__

Compression therapy (specify) __4-layer compression bandaging prn, estimate 3 to 5 days between changes initially; fit for custom stocking when volume normalizes__

Signature_____ *Linda Smith, PT*_____ Date __7/4/01__

Figure 17-8. Example of the venous ulcer form. This form is used if the patient is determined to have venous ulcerations. It is designed to eliminate lengthy descriptions and features components pertinent only to venous ulcers, including preventive measures and treatment specific to venous ulcers. In this example, the location of the wound proximal to the medial malleolus and condition of the surrounding skin are both consistent with venous ulcers. The next items are used to rule out arterial insufficiency. In this patient's case, we can see a normal ankle-brachial index, normal foot temperature, and normal capillary refill so we can assume that compression therapy is appropriate for this patient. Using a foot volumeter to quantify swelling of the lower extremities, clearly the right lower extremity is swollen. As detailed in the generic form, no edema had been observed in the left lower extremity but venous engorgement has. This is a clear sign that the left lower extremity is at risk and the patient should be fitted with a custom stocking if feasible or use one of several alternatives discussed in Chapter 7 to reduce the risk of venous ulcers of the left leg. Note the blank for color of granulation tissue. This is another check for arterial insufficiency. Beefy, red granulation tissue, as in this example, indicates normal arterial inflow to the wound. Pink granulation tissue, on the other hand, is indicative of diminished arterial supply to the wound. Copious drainage is also consistent with uncontrolled venous pressure, although a recent dressing change could deceive the clinician. The clinician must ascertain when the current dressing was applied to estimate the degree of drainage. The last line is complementary to the treatment plan on the generic form. Because of the establishment of venous hypertension as the underlying cause of the wound, the specific form of compression therapy, rather than other forms of intervention described on the generic form, is specified on the supplemental venous ulcer form.

SUPPLEMENTAL DATA FORM FOR PRESSURE ULCERS

Patient Tom Gray   Clinician Jack Wilson   Date 9/30/01

Stage of ulcer (identify location on figure at right with wound number)

1.	I	II	III	(IV)	partially filled	filled	covered
2.	I	II	III	(IV)	partially filled	filled	covered
3.	I	(II)	III	IV	partially filled	filled	covered
4.	I	II	III	IV	partially filled	filled	covered
5.	I	II	III	IV	partially filled	filled	covered

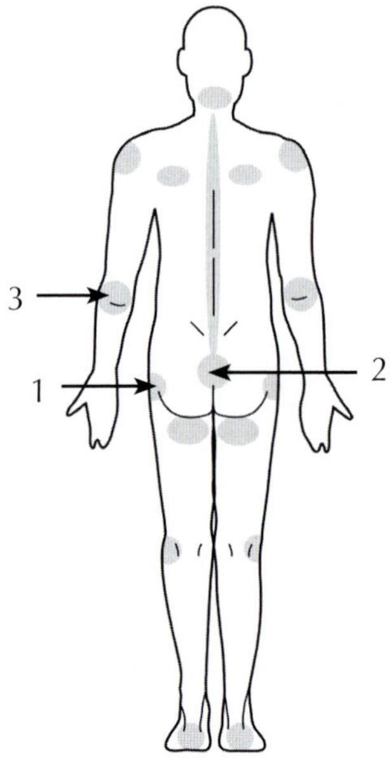

Size of ulcer (using identification key on right)

1.	Length 5.0 cm	Width 3.5 cm	Depth 6.2 cm
2.	Length 4.6 cm	Width 3.0 cm	Depth 1.0 cm
3.	Length 2.1 cm	Width 1.7 cm	Depth N/A cm
4.	Length ____ cm	Width ____ cm	Depth ____ cm
5.	Length ____ cm	Width ____ cm	Depth ____ cm

Tunneling, sinus tracts, undermining

1.	Distance 2.0 cm	Direction 12 :00	Drainage purulent
2.	Distance 2.8 cm	Direction 1 :00	Drainage gray
3.	Distance ____ cm	Direction ____ :00	Drainage _____
4.	Distance ____ cm	Direction ____ :00	Drainage _____
5.	Distance ____ cm	Direction ____ :00	Drainage _____

	1	2	3	4	5
Odor	foul	slight	N/A		
Drainage	purulent	min, serosang	N/A		
% R, Y, B	10, 50, 40	10, 80, 10	N/A		
Surrounding skin condition	inflamed	inflamed	WNL		

Signature   *Jack Wilson, RN, WOCN*   Date 9/30/01

Figure 17-9. Example of the pressure ulcer form. This is a relatively simple form that takes into account the frequent multiplicity of pressure ulcers. Space for information for 5 ulcers is available. In the first section, the stage of the ulcer as defined by NPUAP (discussed in Chapter 7) and how much healing has occurred are documented.

Case #2, Supplemental Data Form for Pressure Ulcers

The patient described in Figure 17-9 had 3 ulcers in very common locations and common stages for these locations. The wounds at the left greater trochanter and sacrum had been monitored but not aggressively treated before referral due to the patient's general poor health. Because bone was visible in both, the staging was very straightforward. The epidermis covering the medial epicondyle of the left elbow had been denuded with some injury into the dermis. The elbow ulcer was, therefore, a stage II. This patient was fairly emaciated and fortunate to have only these 3 ulcerations. This woman had severe contractures of both hips and knees and severely altered mental status. Due to the patient's history and armed with the knowledge of the mechanism of pressure ulcers, the trochanteric and sacral wounds were probed for undermining and tunneling. The undermining would have been drawn on the generic form, and the supplemental form would indicate the size, direction, and drainage with the undermined areas. Both the undermined area and the visible area of the trochanteric ulcer were purulent. Thus, the patient was brought into the hospital for sharp debridement, although the decision had to be made for the patient due to her altered mental status. The sacral wound, on the other hand, was less problematic and the decision was made to treat this wound as well. The sacral wound needed cleaning, as it was filled with old, grayish, necrotic tissue. This residual necrotic tissue was likely the cause of the continued inflammation. The elbow wound was simply cleaned and protected.

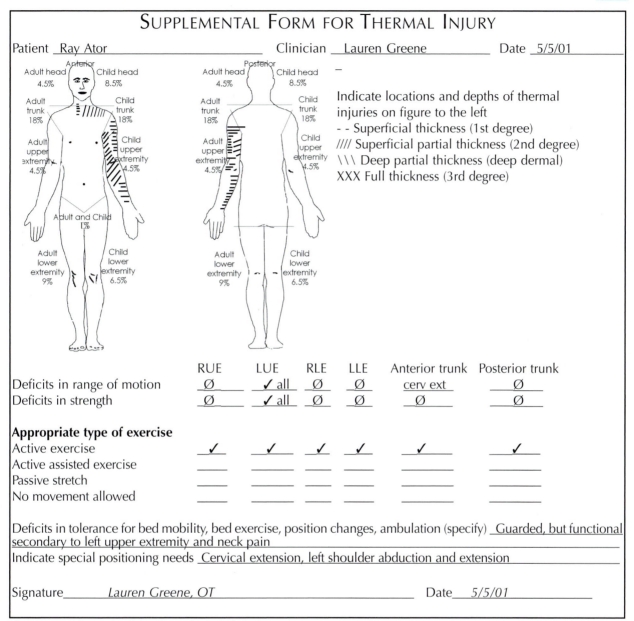

SUPPLEMENTAL FORM FOR THERMAL INJURY

Patient __Ray Ator__   Clinician __Lauren Greene__   Date __5/5/01__

Anterior
Adult head 4.5%   Child head 8.5%
Adult trunk 18%   Child trunk 18%
Adult upper extremity 4.5%   Child upper extremity 4.5%
Adult and Child 1%
Adult lower extremity 9%   Child lower extremity 6.5%

Posterior
Adult head 4.5%   Child head 8.5%
Adult trunk 18%   Child trunk 18%
Adult upper extremity 4.5%   Child upper extremity 4.5%
Adult lower extremity 9%   Child lower extremity 6.5%

Indicate locations and depths of thermal injuries on figure to the left
- - Superficial thickness (1st degree)
//// Superficial partial thickness (2nd degree)
\\\ Deep partial thickness (deep dermal)
XXX Full thickness (3rd degree)

	RUE	LUE	RLE	LLE	Anterior trunk	Posterior trunk
Deficits in range of motion	Ø	✓ all	Ø	Ø	cerv ext	Ø
Deficits in strength	Ø	✓ all	Ø	Ø	Ø	Ø

Appropriate type of exercise

	RUE	LUE	RLE	LLE	Anterior trunk	Posterior trunk
Active exercise	✓	✓	✓	✓	✓	✓
Active assisted exercise						
Passive stretch						
No movement allowed						

Deficits in tolerance for bed mobility, bed exercise, position changes, ambulation (specify) __Guarded, but functional secondary to left upper extremity and neck pain__

Indicate special positioning needs __Cervical extension, left shoulder abduction and extension__

Signature__Lauren Greene, OT__   Date__5/5/01__

Figure 17-10. Example of the thermal injury form.

Case #3, Supplemental Form for Thermal Injury

The patient described in Figure 17-10 received a scald injury from opening the radiator cap after his car overheated. He used a rag to open the radiator cap, thereby avoiding injury to his left hand. The sleeveless undershirt he was wearing protected most of his chest from injury, but exposed his axilla and neck. Although these are critical injuries for functional activity, the depth of injury was superficial and he healed nicely in 2 weeks, regained full function, and returned to work in 3 weeks. Generally speaking, full-thickness injuries are much more likely to result in contractures than partial-thickness injuries. However, superficial partial-thickness injuries are very painful, and the patient could only tolerate small areas of debridement at a time, even with opioid analgesia. The deficits observed in range of motion were due to pain with movement rather than injury to the skin. The patient was encouraged to perform left upper extremity and cervical range of motion exercises. He was only admitted overnight but was seen daily as an outpatient after his discharge. The patient was instructed to maintain his head in extension and alternate between full and 90 degrees of shoulder abduction to prevent taking the neck off stretch.

SUPPLEMENTAL FORM FOR NEUROPATHIC ULCERS

Patient___Brad Smith___   Clinician___Jim Brown___   Date__12/7/01__

Location(s): Indicate location of wounds on figure below and create numeric key if multiple wounds

Wound #	1	2	3	4	5
Wagner grade	3	___	___	___	___
Size	5 cm x 3 cm	___	___	___	___
% Red	90	___	___	___	___
% Yellow	10	___	___	___	___
% Black	0	___	___	___	___

Indicate location of callus on the diagram below with the symbol /////

Reflexes: AJ right   present   diminished   (absent)   AJ left   present   diminished   (absent)

Foot deformities (specify)___Hammer toes bilaterally_____

Gait deviations (specify) ___Nonambulatory_____

Pulse (right)   4   3   2   (1)   0   (specify artery palpated)__DP_____

Pulse (left)   4   3   2   (1)   0   (specify artery palpated)__DP_____

Capillary refill (right)   normal   (sluggish)   absent

Capillary refill (left)   normal   (sluggish)   absent

Ankle brachial index   right__0.5_____   left__0.6_____

Right foot temperature   normal   (decreased)   increased __30.4°C__

Left foot temperature   normal   (decreased)   increased __30.2°C__

Sensory testing (indicate on the diagram below + for intact, +/- for diminished, - for absent

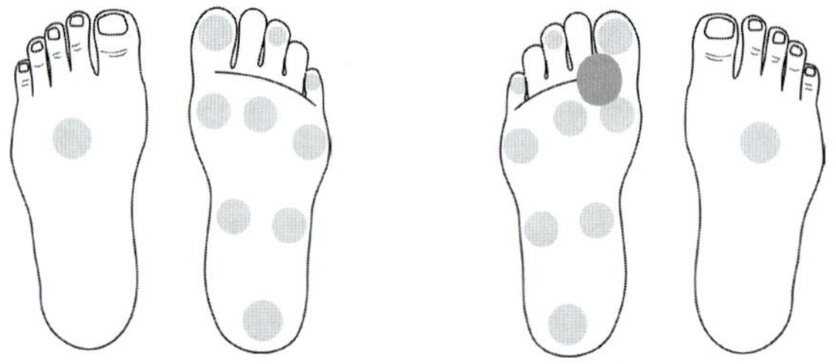

Left foot   Right foot
Dorsal   Plantar   Plantar   Dorsal

Signature___*Jim Brown, DPT, CWS*_____   Date___12/7/01___

Figure 17-11. Example of the neuropathic ulcer form.

Case #4, Supplemental Form for Neuropathic Ulcers

The patient described in Figure 17-11 had no sensation on either lower extremity below the knee and eventually required bilateral amputations. The patient had not been ambulatory and was in general poor health, including kidney failure, for which he was receiving hemodialysis. On the generic form, multiple ulcerations including a previous ray amputation on the other foot would have been noted. On this admission, he had osteomyelitis of the second metatarsal, which eventually was amputated. The color of the tissue within the wound was pink instead of red due to his arterial insufficiency, which coexisted with his neuropathy. He had no reflexes, no intrinsic muscle strength (which produced hammer toes), and a weak pulse bilaterally. Moreover, the suspicion of arterial insufficiency was confirmed with the low ankle brachial index, decreased foot temperature, and as would be noted on the generic form, thickened toenails bilaterally. Wound management in this case was limited to preparation of the wound for delayed primary closure following the amputation. This included twice a day W/P and packing with saline-moistened gauze until the surgeon deemed the site ready for closure.

continued from p. 301

The wound itself and the surrounding skin need to be described thoroughly during the initial evaluation and during each dressing change. For this reason, a section on a hospital chart needs to be devoted to this aspect. Even if the dressing is not changed, the expectation is that at least the dressing be examined during each nursing shift for an inpatient. In settings outside a hospital, documentation of the wound and surrounding skin needs to be done for each visit. If the patient or a caregiver is tending to the wound between visits, the clinician needs to take a report from the patient or caregiver and document this report in the permanent record. The ability of the patient or caregiver to provide necessary care at home needs to be documented so the plan of care can be adjusted as needed.

Because a substantial amount of information is present on the initial evaluation, clinicians may be tempted to write excessively concise notes. An example of such a note is given in Figure 17-12. At a minimum the location, color, odor, drainage, extent, and surrounding skin are documented. Anything that alters the diagnosis or prognosis must be stated explicitly as diagrammed in Figure 17-12. Any changes in the patient's other abilities from the initial evaluation should be examined on a regular basis by physical examination or interview as set by facility procedures or as deemed necessary by the clinician. In addition to the physical examination of the wound, the patient should be interviewed, at least briefly during each visit, to determine whether changes have occurred since the initial evaluation and previous visits, and whether any change is due to the etiology of the wound or related to work, home, recreation, or resources. When this information is documented appropriately, the need for modification of the plan of care can be justified to all parties, including payers. If the patient or a caregiver is responsible for some aspects of wound management between visits, the adherence to the treatment plan should also be documented. The clinician needs to check for signs of nonadherence that might include the patient's knowledge of the details of the treatment plan, the condition of the wound, the condition of dressings, wear on shoes, changes in blood glucose, or other details relevant to the treatment plan. If the treatment plan outside the clinic is not being followed, modifications are likely to be needed. Careful documentation of nonadherence may be necessary to institute required changes in the treatment plan. If nonadherence is due to physical limitations, the patient may need to be seen more frequently in the outpatient or home health setting. A change from autolytic debridement to sharp debridement may be necessary if the patient is not willing or able to perform the necessary dressing changes, or is unable to maintain the integrity of the dressings. The patient may also need to be referred to a social worker or case manager to address deficits in social or financial support necessary to follow the treatment plan.

The treatment plan should be a logical extension of the history, physical examination, diagnosis, and prognosis. If these are documented carefully, the medical necessity and details of the treatment plan should be clear to any third party payers. In addition, other clinicians who may need to take over care of the patient will be better able to execute the plan. Bear in mind that due to personal preferences of the patient, clinician, or caregiver, some details of how the plan is executed may vary from the initial plan. Documentation may be in either the well-established SOAP (subjective, objective, assessment, and plan) format or some other form, such as a narrative, following the language developed in the *Guide to Physical Therapist Practice*. The subjective portion corresponds roughly with the history taken from the patient. The objective section contains components of the history taken from medical records and the physical examination. The assessment section of a soap note will contain elements of diagnosis and sometimes elements of the prognosis. The plan section of a SOAP note contains the treatment plan, although some individuals will place functional objectives and goals with the "A" section. Comparing these 2 approaches, some aspects are common to them, but a number of items fall into different categories. For example, the information taken from the patient and that taken from medical records go into different parts of the SOAP note, whereas history is a complete section using the *Guide* approach. A comparison of documenting with these 2 approaches is given in Table 17-1.

PROGNOSIS

Prognosis is done fairly readily based on the *Guide to Physical Therapist Practice* integumentary practice patterns B through E. Practice pattern A is related to prevention of loss of integumentary integrity. Some of this pattern's elements may be important for a given patient who already has a wound to prevent recurrence of the wound or development of a wound in another location. A thorough history and physical examination will help determine whether any of the potential complications listed in the prognosis section of the preferred practice patterns might extend the time frame or lead to a new episode of care. The clinician needs to assess adherence constantly and, if necessary, modify the treatment plan to make adherence achievable so the prognosis can become achievable. The modifications may either increase or decrease the time frame and may limit some of the outcomes originally expected. An example of a shortened time frame is one in which autolytic debridement was initially proposed, but due to complications, sharp debridement was substituted in the treatment plan.

When developing the prognosis, one must be clear what the clinician's role in the episode of care is. In many

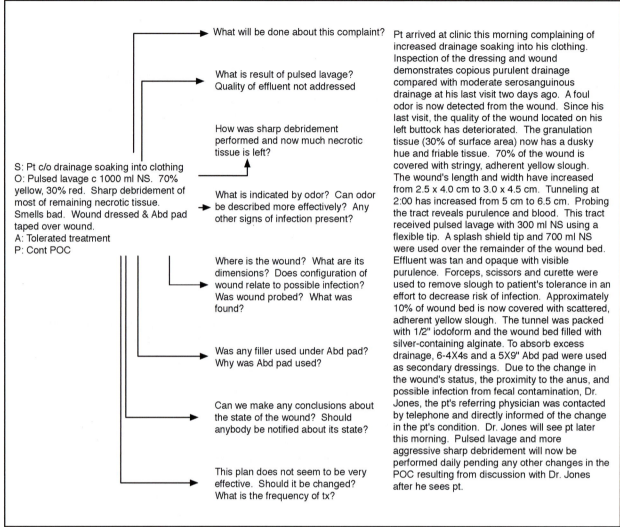

What will be done about this complaint?

What is result of pulsed lavage? Quality of effluent not addressed

How was sharp debridement performed and now much necrotic tissue is left?

S: Pt c/o drainage soaking into clothing
O: Pulsed lavage c̄ 1000 ml NS. 70% yellow, 30% red. Sharp debridement of most of remaining necrotic tissue. Smells bad. Wound dressed & Abd pad taped over wound.
A: Tolerated treatment
P: Cont POC

What is indicated by odor? Can odor be described more effectively? Any other signs of infection present?

Where is the wound? What are its dimensions? Does configuration of wound relate to possible infection? Was wound probed? What was found?

Was any filler used under Abd pad? Why was Abd pad used?

Can we make any conclusions about the state of the wound? Should anybody be notified about its state?

This plan does not seem to be very effective. Should it be changed? What is the frequency of tx?

Pt arrived at clinic this morning complaining of increased drainage soaking into his clothing. Inspection of the dressing and wound demonstrates copious purulent drainage compared with moderate serosanguinous drainage at his last visit two days ago. A foul odor is now detected from the wound. Since his last visit, the quality of the wound located on his left buttock has deteriorated. The granulation tissue (30% of surface area) now has a dusky hue and friable tissue. 70% of the wound is covered with stringy, adherent yellow slough. The wound's length and width have increased from 2.5 x 4.0 cm to 3.0 x 4.5 cm. Tunneling at 2:00 has increased from 5 cm to 6.5 cm. Probing the tract reveals purulence and blood. This tract received pulsed lavage with 300 ml NS using a flexible tip. A splash shield tip and 700 ml NS were used over the remainder of the wound bed. Effluent was tan and opaque with visible purulence. Forceps, scissors and curette were used to remove slough to patient's tolerance in an effort to decrease risk of infection. Approximately 10% of wound bed is now covered with scattered, adherent yellow slough. The tunnel was packed with 1/2" iodoform and the wound bed filled with silver-containing alginate. To absorb excess drainage, 6-4X4s and a 5X9" Abd pad were used as secondary dressings. Due to the change in the wound's status, the proximity to the anus, and possible infection from fecal contamination, Dr. Jones, the pt's referring physician was contacted by telephone and directly informed of the change in the pt's condition. Dr. Jones will see pt later this morning. Pulsed lavage and more aggressive sharp debridement will now be performed daily pending any other changes in the POC resulting from discussion with Dr. Jones after he sees pt.

Figure 17-12. Example of poor documentation with demonstration of reworking into an effective progress note.

cases, the clinician in the acute care hospital is not expected to achieve complete healing of a wound, but to achieve a clean and stable wound, ready for some type of surgical repair such as grafting; or the goal is preparing the patient for discharge or transfer to the appropriate destination such home with self-care or caregiver, or to a different type of facility. In other cases, typical of hospital- or resident-based facilities, one clinician may work with the patient temporarily and another, who may be from a different discipline, takes over care once characteristics of the wound meet the established criteria. In an outpatient setting, the clinician will need to vary frequency of visits and discharge the patient from the clinician's care as the characteristics of the wound change. Regardless of the setting, a time frame for complete healing or a prognosis for optimum condition of the wound should be developed. Variance from the final predicted outcome after discharge may be grounds for a new episode of care.

MEDICAL NECESSITY

A document giving the plan of care and showing medical necessity must be generated for Medicare and other reimbursement. To meet Medicare's criteria for medical necessity, documentation should support that 1) the treatment is necessary, 2) improvement of the condition is expected, 3) the treatment is being provided by the proper clinician, and 4) the condition will not improve or will become worse if treatment is not provided. Within the initial evaluation document, a succinct argument framed by the principles of medical necessity should be provided. A well-written plan of care describes the optimum combination of appropriate wound care and the reality of how the plan interacts with the patient. With sufficient experience, the plan of care will flow readily from the history and physical examination.

Given 2 patients with identical characteristics, 2 different plans of care are likely to be needed. Variance in the

Table 17-1

Comparison of SOAP Note Documentation to Use of Guide Language

SOAP Format	Common Elements	Guide Language
Subjective	Chief complaint, history of the complaint, lifestyle, work, school, play	History
Objective	Review of systems, routine screening tests, tests specific to rule in/out suspected diagnosis	Physical examination
Assessment: diagnosis or a description of the cluster of signs and symptoms; outcomes, functional goals and time frames		Evaluation: mental process, not written, in which information is analyzed critically
		Diagnosis: identifying a cluster of signs and symptoms, often identified as a practice pattern
		Prognosis: expected outcomes and time frame for achievement; discussion of complications
Plan	Specific interventions including patient education, behavior modification, direct interventions, eg, debridement and frequency and duration	Plan of care

plan of care should be viewed as accommodations to the unique combinations of patient characteristics, including physical condition, resources, and lifestyle. Differences in plan of care among patients with the same etiology should be supported explicitly by documentation. Although the accommodations may seem straightforward to the treating clinician, another person reading the documentation needs to read the explicit reasons to make appropriate decisions on reimbursement, the need for additional diagnostic testing, or the need for additional interventions such as surgery. These accommodations for individual differences need to be written with the concept of medical necessity in mind. Explicitly describe why each accommodation is necessary for the patient to benefit from the proposed plan of care. A well-documented initial evaluation that outlines the reasons for the choices made will generally meet all the goals of documentation, including reimbursement, the ability of other clinicians to understand the treatment plan, and improved clinical decision making.

PHOTODOCUMENTATION

The phrase, "a picture's worth a thousand words," is commonly used. This is frequently true in the case of open wounds. Words alone may fail to describe the appearance and the progression of healing adequately. In many cases, a hand-drawn diagram may be adequate, but in others, the quality of the wound needs to be captured more thoroughly. Photography is especially important for the wound containing vast amounts of necrotic tissue. In these cases, wounds frequently become much larger before they can heal. A good quality photograph can show changes in the quality of the wound, and demonstrate complications that may not have been foreseen by others. This extra information can help the clinician explain the need for extended periods of care or the need to reevaluate the prognosis or plan of care.

The first question that most clinicians have regarding photodocumentation of wounds is the most appropriate type of camera. One may choose among digital, 35-mm film, and instant film (Polaroid) cameras. Both advantages and disadvantages exist for each type.

Polaroid pictures have the distinct advantage of providing an instant, permanent record of the wound. Within 1 minute the clinician knows whether a suitable image has been obtained. Polaroid cameras are also simple to operate. All the clinician needs to do is to aim and push one button; the cameras focus automatically. However, a

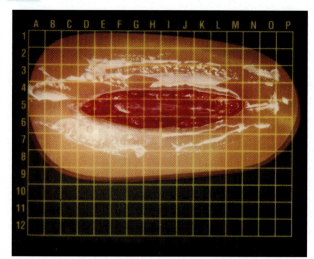

Figure 17-13. Example of Polaroid photo developed on grid film.

standard Polaroid camera cannot be focused at a suitable distance for most wounds. To allow close-up photography, a special lens system must be attached. Another advantage is special grid film available for Polaroid cameras. As the film develops, a grid is formed on the film (Figure 17-13). In addition, a mechanism for ensuring that the camera is held at the same distance from the wound with each photograph is available. With Polaroid's light-lock system, nothing touches the patient and the camera can be held with both hands. The light-lock system consists of 2 beams of red light within the lens adapter that are activated by the press of a button. The camera is then moved to a distance from the subject that causes the 2 beams to converge. If the camera is held too close or too far from the subject, 2 separate beams can be seen. However, instant photographs have several disadvantages. The resolution and color of an instant photograph are usually inferior to those of a 35-mm camera. The cost of an individual photograph is expensive (about $1.00 each). No negative is available to make copies or slides and the film itself is bulky. Over time, the photographs are likely to degrade. Although this may not seem important over the course of perhaps several weeks, photographs may be needed for reimbursement or legal reasons many months or even years afterward.

The standard for quality photography has been the single lens reflex camera using 35-mm film. These cameras are very expensive. Lower cost 35-mm cameras designed for casual consumer use as opposed to medical photography are unlikely to give the quality photograph desired. A single lens reflex camera itself may cost $400 or more, and the lenses needed add to the expense. Ideally, the camera would be equipped with several lenses. For most wounds, a 105-mm lens is appropriate. This size lens allows the photographer to remain at a suitable distance from the subject

to avoid distortion of the image's shape and colors that can be produced by photography with smaller lenses. A 35-mm lens allows the entire subject to be photographed and a 60-mm lens is suitable for large areas of the body. In addition to the expense of the camera, suitable lights and a light meter are needed for optimal quality photographs. Although the film itself is not expensive, processing can be. One may choose to develop film or send it to a film processor. Processing becomes more expensive per picture if the entire roll of film is not used. A major decision point for use of 35-mm film is the volume of photography done. In a clinic where photographic documentation is infrequent, 35-mm photography becomes impractical. The clinic will be faced with the choice of either paying for partial rolls to be processed, or with a delay in obtaining the photographs. The major risk in use of photographic film is the potential loss of information, which increases with the delay between taking the photograph and processing the film. Imagine having 2 weeks of photographs on a roll of film that is taken for processing and none of the photographs develop! Learning to use a single lens reflex camera also requires time, patience, and many rolls of film. The novice needs to take practice pictures under a systematic variety of film, lenses, lighting conditions, aperture settings, and film speeds before actual photographs of patients should be taken. Once optimal settings are determined, the photographer can be reasonably sure of good quality photographs in the future. Training multiple clinicians in a given facility becomes very expensive.

The newest way of photographing wounds is the digital camera. Digital cameras combine advantages of instant and 35-mm photographs. The clinician will know immediately whether the image is adequate. A wide range of price and resolution is available. Generally, higher resolution digital cameras are more expensive. A balance needs to be struck between the required resolution and price. A camera with a zoom feature is desirable, especially for smaller wounds. In addition, one must decide on a medium for transferring the picture from the camera. Digital cameras now have the capacity to store hundreds of photographs at a time. Secure data (SD) cards and other memory devices holding 2 gigabytes are very affordable. Transferring the photographs may be done in a number of ways including card readers, USB, firewire, and wireless connections. One must then consider how to store the digital pictures. At a minimum, photographs should be stored on a secure computer within the department. In addition, one may choose to print the picture or upload it to a computerized documentation system. Because the photographs do not require the purchase of film or the cost of film processing, digital photography is the most cost-effective means of photodocumentation. Another major advantage of digital photography is the ability to make as many copies of the picture as needed. One may track the progress of a wound by arranging a series of digital photographs in either a video display or hard copy.

Although the same rules of photography using 35-mm film apply, another advantage of digital photography is the availability of software to correct color problems. Because of the availability of software correction, photographers may become complacent and not optimize set-up for the photographs. In particular, the lack of adequate lighting and a tripod will lead to blurry pictures due to the combination of increased exposure time and camera movement. Another concern is the ability of those with the digital files to alter the photograph to promote their own agendas. Digital cameras have a very wide range of prices depending on their resolution and special features. Lower cost digital cameras may provide lower quality than a Polaroid, whereas expensive digital cameras can produce pictures equivalent to 35-mm film, especially single lens reflex digital cameras. Photographs obtained from cameras built into cellular phones are essentially cost-free, but provide relatively low resolution.

General Photography Guidelines

Regardless of the type of camera used, a number of general rules need to be followed to optimize photodocumentation. A photographic release form should always be signed by the patient before photographs are taken. If the patient is a minor, a parent or guardian must sign the photographic release. An identification code for the patient, the date, and a measuring scale need to be present on each photograph. Patient identification should use a code rather than the patient's name. Disposable paper scales with adhesive backing are commonly used within photographs. The patient's initials and the date are written on the scale. Ideally, the clinician will continue to use the camera at the same distance from the subject to better allow an eyeball comparison between photographs of the same wound. The single lens reflex system with interchangeable lenses offers the advantage of sufficient zoom for a range of wound size. A digital camera must have a sufficient optical zoom range to achieve the same result. Digital zoom is not useful as it simply reduces the size of photograph with a corresponding decrease in resolution. An alternative to using a scale in the photo is Polaroid grid film. The film provides a standardized grid size, provided that the camera is held at the proper distance from the wound. Achieving the proper distance is accomplished easily with the light-lock system. However, this system is inadequate for very large or small wounds. For small wounds the grid may obscure the wound rather than help. Large wounds may not fit the film if the camera is held at the standard distance.

For at least the initial evaluation, a photograph needs to be taken that allows the wounded body part to be identified. Although one may be tempted to fill the entire photograph with the wound, the quality of the surrounding skin and other contributing factors in the diagnosis or prognosis should be captured in the photograph. In many cases, wounds are slow to heal due to the condition of the surrounding skin; therefore, sufficient surrounding skin needs to be in the photograph. The patient's face, or anything else that could allow someone else to identify the patient, should not be in the photograph—unless the wound is located on the face. For wounds on the face, zoom enough to identify only what part of the face is involved and minimize the possibility of identifying the subject of the photograph.

Background needs to be considered when taking any type of photograph. In many cases, the background will consist only of the patient's intact skin. If a background other than the patient's skin exists, avoid white or yellow. These colors reflect too much light and will distort the color of the wound. Use blue or green drapes in these cases. Also avoid distracting objects within the photograph. Remove any equipment or personnel that might appear in the background. This problem is more likely to occur during the initial photograph showing the body part on which the wound is located. Carefully position the patient to allow the proper amount of light to strike the wound while attempting to optimize patient comfort. Insufficient or excessive lighting will obscure the details of the wound and colors will not be true. Avoid direct flash on the wound or flash too close to the wound. Excessive lighting or flash creates a bright picture with little contrast and inaccurate color. Be aware that direct flash will be reflected from moist surfaces. If flash is necessary, angle the camera so the flash is not reflected directly back toward the camera. Insufficient lighting will result in a dark picture with poor contrast and will also distort the color of the wound.

POTENTIAL PROBLEMS WITH DOCUMENTATION

Elements of documentation, although seemingly trivial, have the potential to create problems at any time in the future. Other clinicians may not be able to decipher the plan of care, its rationale, or its details. For example, not documenting the location and size of a tract may cause another clinician to miss it and fail to adequately irrigate it during a subsequent visit. A bad outcome such as sepsis or amputation, regardless of whether failure to adequately treat the wound contributed to the problem, could lead to a civil action seeking damages from the clinician or facility where the clinician practices. Inadequate documentation may lead to lack of reimbursement from a third-party payer.

Each note must include the date and time of the visit. Lack of date or time on each note can lead to denial of payment. Inaccurate measurement of wound dimensions, particularly when multiple clinicians measure a wound may give the impression of a wound that is fluctuating in size such that a trend toward healing or degeneration of the wound is obscured. The use of paper documentation requires handwriting. Often a hurried note leads to illegibility that may lead to errors in treatment and may aid the plaintiff's case in a lawsuit. Abbreviations may not be understood. Facilities generally provide a list of acceptable abbreviations. Although some items in the list of unapproved abbreviations may seem absurd, facilities attempt to follow recommendations from agencies such as the Joint Commission on Accreditation of Hospital Organizations (JCAHO). Most of the issues addressed by abbreviations are concerns about medication and surgical errors, but documentation rules must be applied equally to all clinicians, administrators, and technicians within the facility.

Although we would like to believe that our memories are flawless, as more time passes between a patient encounter and documentation, we become more likely to lose details. Ideally, documentation is done immediately following a patient encounter. Notes must be objective and accurate containing sufficient detail for any other clinician or payer to understand the patient's condition. Exaggerating improvement in a wound's quality or size may lead a payer to conclude that subsequent visits were unnecessary and to deny payment. Stating that the wound is worse than it is to obtain greater payment is fraudulent and could result in a number of severe penalties including dismissal, loss of practice privileges, demand for repayment, and fines. Clinicians must focus the reader of notes to the problems that persist during an episode of care. If one states that the wound is decreasing in size and the wound bed is red, moist, and granulating, but fails to mention that drainage is excessive, has a yellow/brown color, and the effluent from pulsed lavage within a tract is tan and opaque, requests for payment are likely to be denied. Another potential problem is the criticism of other clinicians. When writing a note, emphasize what needs to be done to resolve a problem that might have been caused by another clinician without explicitly stating that someone else did something wrong. For example, the scenario given at the beginning of the chapter of a referral with the diagnosis of cellulitis that was actually venous disease could be described simply in terms of the characteristics that led to the diagnosis of venous disease and not explicitly state that the referring diagnosis was wrong. Although what the patient states should be documented when it is pertinent, some patients will either deliberately or mistakenly provide incorrect information. If a patient is emphatic that another clinician did something wrong, remember that you were not present to confirm or deny what happened

between them. A patient may be trying to get you to take sides in a dispute. If you take sides with the patient in such a situation, you may find yourself in an uncomfortable situation in the future as a witness in a lawsuit or having destroyed a relationship with another clinician unnecessarily. Keep your notations as objective as possible; do not place blame on another individual for a patient's condition. To ensure completeness of notations, facilities may adopt a chart review procedure. An example of a wound care chart review tool is shown in Figure 17-14.

LEGAL ISSUES

Our system of law allows 2 types of litigation: criminal and civil. Criminal litigation involves violation of specific laws and prosecution by the local, state, or federal government. Criminal proceedings may result from fraudulent claims from third-party payers, assault, or battery. Although complaints of assault or battery against a patient are rare, excessive coercion perceived as a threat could be interpreted as assault and performing a procedure on a patient without informed consent could be interpreted as battery.

Civil complaints are most likely to occur when a bad outcome follows an episode of care. In the context of wound care, development of pressure ulcers, sepsis, or amputation of an affected body part might become a focus of a civil complaint. Informed consent and a good relationship between the clinician and patient decrease the probability of a civil complaint. Winning a judgment in a civil action is dependent on 4 elements that can be related to documentation. The first element is existence of a duty. If a clinician enters into an agreement to provide care to the patient, the first element is met. For example, a person who becomes a resident at a nursing home has entered into an agreement that the nursing home will provide an acceptable level of care. The nursing home now has a duty to that resident. The second element is breach of duty. Breach of duty could be either the omission of expected care or the commission of an act that harms a patient. Using the same example, failure to assess risk factors and provide interventions to prevent pressure ulcers represent breach of duty. The third element is injury caused by the breach of duty. Proximate cause between the breach of duty and harm to the patient must be proven. Proximate cause indicates a direct link between the breach of duty and injury. The plaintiff must show that the clinician's action or neglect was a substantial factor in the patient's injury, and that the injury would not have occurred without the clinician's negligence. Pressure ulcers caused by the lack of risk assessment and interventions to prevent them meet the third criterion. The fourth part is that actual damage occurred. Care given at a substandard level that does not harm the patient is not sufficient for winning

WOUND CARE CHART REVIEW TOOL

Indicators: Clients with wounds will be appropriately cared for as evidenced by the following indicators:
Threshold: Goal is 85% on all indicators
Sample size: 100% or 10 charts for clients with a wound per quarter
Year: _____
Quarter: Jan to Mar   Apr to Jun   Jul to Sep   Oct to Dec

	Yes	No	N/A
1. Wound assessment done on admission			
A. Integumentary portion of Outcome and Assessment Information Set (OASIS) filled out	___	___	___
B. Wound assessment sheet initiated	___	___	___
C. Braden scale value computed	___	___	___
D. Integumentary area of point of contact (POC) filled out			
1. If Braden score <12 "Potential for impaired skin integrity demonstrated by" filled out	___	___	___
2. Wounds described in "Problem" section by location, type, stage or partial/full thickness, and size in centimeter	___	___	___
3. Steps of wound care included on "communication with MD" line of OASIS and "perform" section of plan of care. Wound care orders match treatment section of wound assessment sheet, including whether caregiver will be taught	___	___	___
E. Orders for wound care on 485 (plan of care form) includes technique; products, frequency, whether any caregiver will be taught	___	___	___
F. 485 includes "consult to be done by certified wound, ostomy, continence nurse (CWOCN) within 2 weeks"	___	___	___
2. Consistent and accurate wound assessments and wound related teaching documented on skilled nurse visit (SNV) notes			
A. Wound described with each dressing change			
1. Wound bed described	___	___	___
2. Drainage described	___	___	___
3. Surrounding tissue described	___	___	___
4. Signs or infection noted and MD notified or "No s/s infection noted" documented	___	___	___
5. Patient response to wound care noted	___	___	___
6. Wound care steps described	___	___	___
7. Wound location and type described	___	___	___
B. Accurate wound measurements done weekly			
1. L x W x D measured in centimeters to tenths	___	___	___
2. Includes measurement of deepest undermining and where undermining is located	___	___	___
3. Wound described as outlined above in 2A	___	___	___
4. Current wound care described	___	___	___
5. SNV notes evidence of teaching regarding wounds, wound care, products, pressure prevention, and/or skin care as appropriate	___	___	___
3. All changes in wound care and/or frequency done are accompanied by an MD order and Coordination of Care note	___	___	___
4. All MD orders are signed and returned	___	___	___

Figure 17-14. Tool used to ensure complete documentation for home health visits. Developed by Megan Hughes, RN, CWOCN.

a lawsuit. If the lack of turning or proper positioning does not lead to pressure ulcers, no damages may be awarded. The plaintiff's attorney must prove with the preponderance of evidence that the defendant is responsible for damages suffered by the plaintiff. Damages may include lost wages, expenses (primarily, but not exclusively medical) incurred by the plaintiff, pain, and suffering that resulted from the defendant's negligent care. Monetary loss resulting from pressure ulcers and pain and suffering experienced by the nursing home resident represent damages sought by the plaintiff in this example.

The documentation of an initial evaluation establishes the duty of the clinician. Failure to provide informed consent, and to document the patient's condition and risk factors set the stage for problems later. Any patient behaviors that might cause a bad outcome should be documented as they are discovered. This information could come from a verbal account or observation of the patient. For example, document any alternative treatments that the patient is performing, eg, having a dog lick the wound, soaking in epsom salts, use of raw eggs, WD-40 (WD-40 Company, San Diego, CA) or Windex (S.C. Johnson & Sons, Inc., Racine, WI) on the wound. Also document whether the patient is compliant in home care. Objective evidence of noncompliance such as the condition of dressings and offloading devices should be documented. If a patient is apparently not performing regular dressing changes, cleansing the wound, or using offloading devices, the clinician should document this noncompliance as soon as it is discovered. In addition to documenting problems caused by the patient, also explicitly document any intervention to correct the patient's behavior. Changes in the wound's characteristics such as worsening quantity or quality of drainage, odor, or deterioration of the wound bed must be documented as they occur along with interventions to address them, including any communication of the patient's condition with other clinicians. For example, if a wound is healing slowly, then grayish drainage and an odor become apparent, communication with the patient's referring physician should be performed and documented.

A modification of the SOAP note has been suggested by Teichman as a means of clear documentation of informed consent. Teichman describes an acronym of SOOOAAP for Subjective, Objective, Opinion, Options, Advice, and Agreed Plan. Whereas subjective and objective are the same as in the SOAP format, the assessment part is broken down into 3 parts that lend themselves directly to the concept of informed consent. Opinion is used to emphasize that the clinician is using the available information to reach a conclusion about the patient's condition while lowering the expectation that a firm diagnosis can be offered to every patient. The options section details possible courses of action. Rather than spelling out a treatment plan that necessarily follows from the clinical diagnosis, options implies that the patient has been given all possible information on which a course of action can be based. The advice section describes what the clinician believes to be the optimal course of action. Finally, agreed plan emphasizes that the clinician and patient worked together to develop a plan of care. This subtle change in wording sends a strong message to any third parties that the patient was fully informed, options were discussed, and based upon the evidence available, the patient chose to follow this plan of care. This flow of information in the SOOOAAP note may be contrasted to a typical SOAP note in which the clinician appears to have all of the power in the relationship. If a negative outcome occurs, the perception of the clinician holding all of the power leads easily to the conclusion by a third party that the patient was a victim, thereby increasing the likelihood of litigation. In contrast, a note written with the elements of the SOOOAAP format shows that the patient was not only informed of the evidence, options, and advice, but was also a part of the decision process.

SUMMARY

Documentation is important for the obvious reason of maximizing reimbursement and avoiding civil judgments, but done well, it provides a road map for the episode of care. Information taken from the history section guides the physical examination and the combined information is assessed by the clinician to develop a diagnosis and prognosis. The diagnosis and prognosis, in turn, guide the plan of care. The plan of care includes communication and coordination of care, patient education, and direct interventions. The inability of the patient to adhere to the plan of care requires modification of patient education, changes in direct intervention, or the consultation of a social worker or other appropriate professional to manage resources so that the patient becomes able to adhere to the plan of care. The patient's lifestyle, work, school, or play also need to be accommodated in the plan of care. Photography can be used to communicate visual aspects of the wound that words might not. Documentation of pertinent characteristics of the patient and the patient's wound decrease the likelihood of denial of payment and civil litigation.

QUESTIONS

1. Why is documentation critical to a good outcome?
2. What is the role of documenting history?
3. How is this important with multiple clinicians working with the same patient?
4. How is physical examination related to history?

5. Explain how the physical examination might differ between a case with an obvious diagnosis and one without a clear diagnosis.

6. Contrast the subjective part of a SOAP note to the history and the objective part to the physical examination.

BIBLIOGRAPHY

Classen NS. The basics of medical photography. *Acute Care Perspectives*. 2000;8(2):7-11.

Levine JM, Savino F, Peterson M, Wolf CR. Risk management for pressure ulcers: when the family shows up with a camera. *J Am Med Dir Assoc*. 2008;9(5):360-363.

Teichman PG. Documentation tips for reducing malpractice risk. *Fam Pract Manag*. 2000;7(3):29-33.

Plan of Care

18

OBJECTIVES

- Discuss the relationship between physical impairments and plan of care.
- Discuss the relationships among impairments, functional limitations, and plan of care.
- Modify a plan of care based on upon impairments, functional limitations, and disability for prevention and healing of wounds.
- Set goals and determine appropriate outcomes for patients with various sets of abilities and disabilities, lifestyle, and resources.
- Discuss modifications of interventions necessary for the elderly patient.
- Describe prevention of skin injury in elderly persons.
- Discuss means of optimizing wound management in children.
- Determine when referral to other healthcare providers is appropriate.
- Determine appropriate topics and means of providing patient education.
- Utilize the *International Classification of Functioning, Disability and Health* model in development of a plan of care.

TERMINOLOGY OF THE DISABILITY MODEL

In years past, goals were set for a patient based on remediation of a documented impairment. For example, a deficit of range of motion would be remediated in terms of increased range of motion. Over time, however, the remediation of an impairment solely for the sake of remediation was questioned. Physical therapists were nudged in the direction of writing functional goals. As an example, shoulder range of motion would be improved to allow the patient to perform a task necessary to the individual's function in home, work, or community, such as dressing, operating machinery, and caring for children. Plans of care became hodge-podges of impairment and function-driven goals to be attained. Many clinicians either consciously or unconsciously began to incorporate the model of disablement into developing a plan of care. In November of 1997, the American Physical Therapy Association published the *Guide to Physical Therapist Practice*. A second edition was published in January of 2001. This document is based on the disablement model and directs the thought process of the clinician through impairment, functional limitation, and disability. The third edition will be based on the *International Classification of Functioning, Disability, and Health*, which is described at the end of this chapter.

Irion G.
Comprehensive Wound Management, 2nd ed. (pp 321-334)
© 2010 SLACK Incorporated

A given patient may be seen by a clinician at any point on the continuum from impairment, functional limitation, or disability. As defined in the *Guide,* impairment is a loss or abnormality of physiological, psychological, or anatomical structure or function; functional limitation is a restriction of the ability to perform at the level of the whole person, a physical action, activity or task in an efficient, typically expected, or competent manner; and disability is defined as the inability to engage in age-specific, gender-specific, or sex-specific roles in a particular context and physical environment. Placed in the context of the patient-clinician interaction, remediation of an impairment is not based on the impairment itself, but to overcome functional limitations and prevent disability. Interaction may also occur to allow the patient to adapt to functional limitations to prevent or minimize disability, or to retrain the patient for new roles following disability. In terms of wound management, the plan of care should not be focused on the "hole in the patient," but on the "whole of the patient." The outcome of the plan of care is ultimately to prevent or minimize functional limitations and disability secondary to integumentary impairments and to prevent secondary impairments. Secondary impairments result either directly or indirectly from another impairment. For example, the person placed on bed rest because of a neuropathic ulcer may develop cardiopulmonary complications caused by bedrest. Diminished cardiopulmonary function or cardiopulmonary disease would be a secondary impairment. Use of total contact casting or other means of keeping the patient ambulatory is an example of preventing secondary impairments. This is an excellent example of how two interventions—bedrest and total contact casting—may address the same impairment, but one intervention is superior due to the prevention of a secondary impairment. Often, wounds represent secondary impairments. Cardiopulmonary, musculoskeletal, or neuromuscular impairments resulting in immobility may cause integumentary impairments (wounds). For example, an individual with a spinal cord injury is at high risk for development of pressure ulcers. An important role of the clinician is to prevent these secondary integumentary impairments by identifying how the skin is placed at risk due to cardiopulmonary, musculoskeletal or neuromuscular impairments. The clinician then devises a plan of care to remediate the impairments that create the risk to the skin and prevent the secondary impairment manifesting itself as a wound.

COMPONENTS OF THE PLAN OF CARE

The plan of care is developed through the systematic process of examination, evaluation, diagnosis, and progno-

sis. Specific impairments are identified based on physical examination; and risks of functional limitations and disability are identified by evaluating the impact of the impairments on the patient's roles, lifestyle, home, resources, and available assistance. The clinician is responsible for taking a thorough history that may include general demographic information, social history, occupation/employment, growth and development, and living environment. In addition, the history of the current condition, current and prior functional status and activity level, current medications, past history of the current condition, past medical and surgical history, family history, health status, and social habits are considered in determining a diagnosis. Diagnosis is defined as a cluster of signs and symptoms, syndromes, or categories in the *Guide.* In contrast to the pathology-driven diagnostic categories used by physicians, the diagnoses described in the *Guide* are impairment-driven. Based on the history and diagnosis, a prognosis is developed. Prognosis as defined in the *Guide* includes the predicted optimal level of improvement in function and amount of time needed to reach that level. Prognosis may also include a prediction of levels of improvement that may be reached at various intervals during the course of therapy. The plan of care describes the interventions to be used, and the goals and outcomes of the interventions. In this model, goals refer specifically to remediation of impairments and outcomes related to minimizing functional limitations, optimizing health status, and preventing disability. The hope of clinicians is to prevent disability. Although not addressed specifically in the *Guide,* outcomes may be limited to minimizing disability, rather than preventing it. The plan of care may also include patient education, development of a maintenance program, and periodic reassessment of the maintenance program.

Procedural Interventions

With respect to skin integrity, actions required of the clinician include identifying the causes of wounds and how to prevent recurrence, identifying factors that interfere with healing, appropriately selecting and applying wound care products, appropriate debridement (if required), and selection of adjunctive therapies as indicated.

Fluid Balance

Healing is most effective if the wound microenvironment is optimized. This optimization includes maintaining an appropriate moisture level. A dry wound must be moistened and a heavily draining wound needs to be managed to either absorb excessive moisture or to decrease the cause of the copious drainage. Macromolecules produced in the wound, including glycosaminoglycans, fibronectin, collagen, and growth factors, need to be retained in the wound while acceptable levels of nonpathogenic organisms and protection from pathogens in the environment are achieved. An appropriate microenvironment is usually accomplished through the use of occlusive dressings that retain fluid in the wound while either absorbing or allowing evaporation of excessive moisture. Maintaining wound temperature near core body temperature produces optimal fibroblast replication. Wound moisture is particularly critical to allow the migration of epithelial cells, movement of enzymes, growth factors, and structural molecules through the wound. However, excessive moisture can cause maceration, injuring the source of epithelial cells needed to resurface the wound. Incontinence creates an even greater problem because of the acidity of urine and feces.

Allowing the wound to dry out was once encouraged as a means of preventing infection. However, this practice has been abandoned with research showing that dry wound beds impede wound healing. Although desiccated fibrin and blood act as a dressing to retain moisture below and keep out pathogens, scab formation slows epithelial cell migration as epithelial cells are forced to migrate deeply and through a dry environment. Scab formation is mainly an issue for wounds greater in diameter than a few millimeters. For narrow, especially linear wounds requiring minimal epithelial cell migration, scab formation is a minor issue. For superficial wounds, re-epithelialization can occur from appendages and wound edges. Re-epithelialization proceeds only from the edges of deeper wounds involving the full thickness of dermis; therefore, full-thickness wounds greater than a few centimeters in diameter may require operative repair. Full-thickness or deeper wounds fill with granulation tissue before re-epithelialization. A moist wound bed assists in migration and proliferation of fibroblasts as well as epithelialization.

Bacterial Balance

A second consideration is the issue of bacterial balance. Bacterial balance requires an understanding of infection, contamination, and colonization. All chronic open wounds are colonized by microbes, but clinicians should not be careless in maintaining cleanliness of the wound. Contamination of a wound may increase the risk of infection. Although the immune system and the balance of microbes may keep a given pathogen from proliferating in the wound, introduction of new bacteria or changing the environment of the wound may allow one bacterium to multiply rapidly and injure cells in the wound. Certain microbes may begin to digest the interstitial space producing cellulitis and spread subcutaneously forming sinus tracts and additional abscesses. Although occlusion promotes growth of cells needed for healing a wound, occlusion will also promote the growth of certain types of bacteria in the wound and, therefore, infected wounds should not be occluded. Grossly contaminated wounds and wounds suspected to be infected should be allowed, at least initially,

to heal by secondary intent until the wound is clean and stable. Any cavity in the tissue provides an environment conducive to bacterial overgrowth and prevents observation of the wound. Exposure to air and irrigation decrease bacterial count, but cause the wound to dry out, slowing healing. Therefore, the clinician must be ready to alter the treatment plan, depending on whether the goal is prevention/treatment of infection or promotion of granulation and epithelialization. Occlusive dressings are indicated when healing is to be promoted and the wound is not infected. Nonocclusive dressings are indicated in wounds that are infected or are at high risk for infection such as grossly contaminated wounds. Nonocclusive dressings should be used until the bacterial count is low enough to use occlusive dressings.

Drainage Management

The third consideration is the management of drainage. One aspect often neglected is the drainage caused by rough handling of wounds by the clinician or caregiver. By minimizing wound handling, inflammation is reduced. Inflammation caused by debridement, excess irrigation, and frequent dressing changes leads to edema, serous drainage, and slowed healing. One means of reducing drainage is to debride necrotic tissue as rapidly as possible. Protracted debridement with daily or even BID rough handling of the wound and the persistence of necrotic tissue promote inflammation and lead to drainage. A number of dressings are available to absorb a wide range of drainage. Alginate/hydrofiber and foam dressings can absorb moderate to maximum drainage longer than other dressings, allowing for less frequent changes. When inflammation and drainage have decreased to suitable levels, hydrocolloid sheets and semipermeable films can be used to retain an appropriate level of moisture for several days. Purulent drainage, however, is a clear sign to stop occluding the wound. Purulence should be absorbed with either gauze or alginate. Although aggressive sharp debridement is preferred, wounds may be filled with antibiotic-soaked gauze if other factors indicate. Another problem caused by chronic inflammation due to rough handling is the leakage of fibrinogen into the wound bed. Fibrinogen may be converted to fibrin on the wound surface, causing a hard yellow eschar to form on the wound surface. This type of eschar is particularly difficult to debride. Curettage, ultrasonic debridement, or enzymatic debriders may be used to clear this material from the wound. In a dry wound, moisture can be both added and retained by using amorphous hydrogel on the wound bed and an occlusive dressing. When retaining moisture in a wound, some moisture may run over the surrounding skin causing maceration. A moisture barrier cream or skin sealant can be effective in preventing maceration.

FORMULATING THE PLAN OF CARE

The plan of care needs to flow from the items discussed above. Given 2 patients with identical characteristics, 2 different plans of care are likely to be needed. Variances in the plan of care should be viewed as accommodations to the unique combinations of patient characteristics, including physical condition, cultural beliefs and behaviors, resources, and lifestyle. The plan of care needs to represent the optimum combination of appropriate wound care and the reality of how the plan interacts with the patient. Treatment planning may follow four basic decision points in addition to accommodations for circumstances beyond the characteristics of the wound. The 4 basic decision points are 1) presence, suspicion, or reasonable assumption of impending infection, 2) type of debridement suited to the patient and the wound, 3) depth of tissue loss, 4) management of drainage and surrounding skin.

Presence, Suspicion, or Reasonable Assumption of Impending Infection

When infection is known to be present, infection is suspected, or one may reasonably suspect that infection will occur, treatment decisions are directed primarily toward managing infection. Interventions directed toward eliminating infection may, in fact, slow wound healing. However, infection is sufficiently serious to warrant precedence over other aspects of wound management. Other aspects are not ignored; rather, potential conflicts in management of the different aspects of the wound are resolved by allowing certain aspects to take precedence. Infection can be managed in a number of ways. Critically important to bear in mind is the relationship between the presence of necrotic tissue and infection. Necrotic tissue provides a foothold for pathogenic bacteria that otherwise would remain under control on a relatively clean wound surface. Based on this principle, infection can be managed by sharp debridement or other means of rapid debridement. NPUAP recommends sharp debridement of pressure ulcers with impending infection. The American Diabetes Association recommends aggressive sharp debridement of neuropathic ulcers. In addition to use of sharp instruments, one may use pulsatile lavage, irrigation, or other forms of hydrotherapy to supplement removal of necrotic tissue and bacteria. Application of antibiotics or surface antiseptics may be appropriate for a small number of days, particularly for acute wounds at risk of infection because of gross contamination from gunshot wounds, motor vehicle, agricultural, and industrial accidents. Acute wounds, especially wounds that have not received care for several hours will need aggressive lavage, debridement, and possibly treatment with antibiotics. NPUAP recommends only a brief trial of surface treatment for pressure ulcers that fail to respond to optimal care. The American Diabetes Association, on the other hand, does not recommend surface treatment at all, instead calling for sharp debridement and parenteral antibiotics specifically selected for the identified pathogen.

Type of Debridement Needed

The second decision point is the type of debridement utilized. Several factors come into play. Factors may include economics of the healthcare setting, patient satisfaction, patient/caregiver skill, and clinician skill. Debridement is necessary for any wound with necrotic tissue. The type of debridement, however, needs to be determined based on a number of institutional, personal, and wound characteristics. In the acute care setting in which discharge is dependent upon the wound becoming clean and stable, rapid debridement is necessary. Some clinicians may choose to perform nonspecific mechanical types of debridement, often using hydrotherapy. Clinicians with the skill to perform sharp debridement can achieve a clean, stable wound much more rapidly than by using hydrotherapy alone. In many cases, especially with neuropathic ulcers, sharp debridement can be achieved in a single visit. The wound may need to be monitored and some further minor debridement may be necessary if discharge is pending completion of a round of intravenous antibiotic treatment. In many cases, however, the patient is now discharged to home with home health visits to complete a course of intravenous antibiotics. If clinician skill or patient preference dictates against sharp debridement, pulsatile lavage with concurrent suction may be a reasonable alternative. Whirlpool therapy, however, is generally not a reasonable alternative. Whirlpool therapy may be preferred for wounds with a large surface area requiring low level agitation and minor burns on extremities that require the cleansing of residues such as silver sulfadiazine. Soaking a wound to loosen necrotic tissue and pulling loose tissue with forceps once or twice a day is a common practice, but offers no advantage over sharp debridement or pulsatile lavage with concurrent suction. Whirlpool agitation is generally ineffective at debriding areas of subcutaneous involvement with undermining, tunneling, and sinus tracts, and risks contamination of wounds with flora from other submersed areas of the body. Within a limited depth of approximately 20 cm, flexible tips of pulsatile lavage units can readily reach these areas.

Whirlpool therapy should also be avoided for wounds due to venous disease. Edema is exacerbated by placing the limb in a dependent position with the thigh compressed against the edge of the tank and warm water increasing blood flow to the affected leg. In addition, the elevated temperature of typical whirlpool therapy increases the demand for blood flow without increasing flow in many cases of peripheral arterial disease and increases the risk of further tissue injury in thermal injuries and skin with diminished sensation. Fragile skin, especially in the elderly can be damaged by the agitation and maceration caused by soaking the extremity for 20 minutes.

When time frame is not critical or the quality of life is not dependent on rapid debridement of the wound, autolytic and chemical debridement are reasonable. However, the patient or a caregiver must be able to determine whether wound infection occurs. Infection demands immediate sharp debridement. In an outpatient or home health situation, a patient may express preference for autolytic or enzymatic debridement because of concern about pain or because of psychosocial factors. In a long-term care setting in which rapid debridement will not impact quality of life, the patient and clinician may agree to a more protracted but less invasive debridement procedure. For example, a bedfast individual with an open heel ulcer will not become ambulatory simply because of sharp debridement of the wound. On the other hand, a person who needs to be ambulatory and could be if not for a foot wound may decide on sharp debridement and total contact casting or one of its alternatives to become ambulatory sooner.

Depth of Tissue Loss

The third decision point is the presence of subcutaneous tissue loss, including undermining, tunneling, and sinus tracts. When infection is present, or debridement is ongoing, these tissue defects are typically filled with gauze material. Dressings moistened with either normal saline or an antibiotic solution are typically used. Packing strip with or without iodine may be used for tunnels and sinus tracts. Packing strip comes in various widths and usually needs to be fan-folded as it is placed in a tunnel or sinus tract. Although the cotton material may promote inflammation of the tissue in the wound, absorption of infectious drainage and preventing occlusion that promotes growth of bacteria take precedence. Of particular importance is preventing wounds from closing over subcutaneous defects. Ideally, a wound fills completely with granulation and re-epithelializes. However, some patients may re-epithelialize too rapidly. Patients may be pleased that the wound has closed, but occlusion of necrotic tissue and purulence beneath the skin is likely to lead to a skin abscess in the near future. Such wounds must be kept open with packing strip and irrigated as much as possible to allow the wound to granulate fully before it closes. Larger undermined areas and simple areas of subcutaneous loss may be filled with moistened 4 x 4 or 2 x 2 gauze sponges or bandage rolls until the risk of infection is minimized. Note, however, that gauze sponges and bandage rolls are not designed for packing wounds. Packing strip is specifically manufactured to prevent the shedding of fibers that is likely to occur when gauze sponges and bandage rolls are used for packing wounds. Because of its design, 2-inch iodoform is less likely to cause inflammation than a 2-inch bandage roll.

Once the wound is stable, nonirritating filling materials should be substituted. Alginates, hydrofibers, and combinations with collagen are good choices for filling these subcutaneous defects. Alginates and hydrofibers are available in both sheets and ribbons/ropes. These materials maintain their tensile strength while absorbing drainage and can be readily removed from the wound, even larger tunnels, and sinus tracts. Collagen present in the material is absorbed by the wound and may speed healing. A suitable secondary dressing needs to be placed over the wound based on the drainage and desired frequency of dressing change.

Management of Drainage

The fourth decision point is based on drainage and manipulation of the desired frequency of dressing change. With subcutaneous tissue loss, both a primary and secondary dressing are chosen. For a simpler full-thickness or partial-thickness wound, a primary dressing may be sufficient. The type of dressing chosen must be based on multiple factors, again based on the order of precedence discussed above: infection, debridement, subcutaneous involvement, and drainage. If a wound is infected and filled with gauze, a nonocclusive secondary dressing needs to be employed. Typical choices include bandage rolls, self-adherent gauze bandages, and abdominal pads taped over skin protectant. Bandage rolls may be used on any body part and can be fan-folded to increase absorption. Abdominal pads can be gently pulled back and retaped from one corner (or more if necessary) to inspect a wound. These absorbent materials may on occasion be used over materials such as alginates or hydrofibers to absorb copious drainage for a few days as inflammation resolves. An occlusive dressing is generally used over an occlusive type of wound filler (hydrogel, foam, alginate/hydrofiber); however, initially the drainage may overwhelm most occlusive dressings, requiring the use of some combination of abdominal pads, multiple gauze sponges, and bandage rolls.

When occlusion of the wound is appropriate, the quantity of drainage and characteristics of the patient and dressings must be considered. A desiccated wound can be rehydrated with amorphous hydrogel covered with a simple dressing, such as a semipermeable film. Light drainage from a partial-thickness or full-thickness wound without subcutaneous involvement may be managed with a semipermeable film. Hydrocolloids are the most occlusive wound dressing and are ideal for wounds that are clean and stable and therefore, only need to be protected. Ideally, the hydrocolloid dressing is left in place for 5 days or more. Depending on the drainage and extent of subcutaneous involvement, alginate, hydrofiber, or foam may be needed beneath the hydrocolloid sheet. The hydrocolloid dressing is changed at the desired interval of 5 to 7 days, or earlier if the dressing becomes white and swollen. Leaving an overhydrated occlusive dressing in place too long risks maceration of surrounding tissue. Hydrogel sheets are popular dressings for abrasions, and chemical and radiation burns due to their soothing effect. Water released from the hydrogel can macerate surrounding skin, and evaporation of water from the hydrogel dressing can allow the wound bed to desiccate if it is left in place too long. Foam dressing materials are good choices when a wound is ready for occlusion, but drainage is too heavy for hydrocolloid sheets. For a heavily draining wound with subcutaneous involvement, foam sheets can be placed into a wound as a primary dressing with a hydrocolloid secondary dressing. Composite dressings constructed of contact material surrounded with absorbent material and a waterproof exterior can also be used on this type of wound. Composite foam and film dressings may also be useful, but may not last for the number of days desired by the clinician. In addition to the characteristics of the dressing materials, the patient characteristics and wound location must be considered. A bulky dressing should not be placed on an area where it will catch onto clothing and shoes or other items in the environment. If the person will be showering, a film, foam, or hydrogel dressing will not stay in place. Hydrocolloid sheets are waterproof on the outside and if kept out of direct spray can last several days, even with showering. The decision points are summarized in Figure 18-1A through 18-1G.

Modifications for the Care of Aging Skin

Foremost, the choice of wound products to be used on the skin of the elderly must take into account the fragile nature of their skin. Moreover, because of decreased inflammation, greater risk of malnutrition and dehydration, the clinician must assume a longer period for healing. Therefore, dressings that need to be changed frequently or have strong adhesive must be used with care or avoided. Tape of any kind must be used judiciously. In particular, silk and plastic tape should not be used. Nontape alternatives such as stretch netting should be considered. When occlusive dressings are chosen, hydrocolloids and semipermeable films should be used only if nonadherent foam or hydrogel sheets are not practical. If films or hydrocolloid sheets are to be used, skin protectant needs to be placed on the surrounding skin. In addition, the absorbency of the dressing needs to be optimized. Although thin hydrocolloid sheets permit better visualization of the wound, thicker hydrocolloid sheets may be necessary to prolong time between changes. Filling the wound with an absorbent material such as alginate or hydrofiber can also prolong wearing time of hydrocolloid and semipermeable film dressings. When these dressings are removed, care must be taken to avoid injury to the skin. The skin should not be pulled with the dressing as it is removed. Gentle peeling of hydrocolloid sheets or stretching of a semipermeable film tangentially to the skin surface as the skin is held in place may reduce the risk of injury. In addition to selecting wound care products carefully, a number of other forms of skin protection should be considered. The skin of the elderly tends to become dry, brittle, and may fissure and tear with minor trauma. Therapeutic moisturizers may be necessary, especially during the winter or in low-humidity environments. Bed frames and rails should be inspected for sharp edges and padded as needed.

Cleansing of wounds of elderly persons needs to be done as gently as possible. Pulsatile lavage with suction may be done at a lower impact pressure or replaced by gentle irrigation as necessary. Mechanical damage and maceration can result from vigorous whirlpool therapy for cleansing or nonselective debridement. For many elderly patients, the clinician must consider the risks and benefits of different types of debridement. Frequently, orders are received for whirlpool and wet-to-dry dressings on the wounds of the elderly. Additives to the whirlpools or topical agents placed on the wound may cause severe injury to the wound or surrounding skin. Elderly patients in the terminal stage of an illness may not benefit from the full scale of options available from the clinician. The clinician must determine what benefits the patient will receive from any given intervention. Often, wound healing is not achievable due to the nutritional or cardiopulmonary status of the patient and goals are limited to reducing the risk of infection and managing drainage and odor of the wound. If sharp debridement provides no benefit, a treatment plan optimizing autolytic debridement can be appropriate.

Optimizing Wound Healing in Children

Compared with adults, children have a better outcome from laceration repair. Children are less likely to have wound infections (2.1% vs 4.1%) and have a better cosmetic outcome than adults. Lacerations in children are irrigated less frequently than those of adults (53% vs 77%) and more frequently scrubbed (50% vs 45%). Comparing the characteristics of wounds of children and adults, wounds are much more likely to occur on the head (86% vs 38%), to be linear, shorter, less likely to be contaminated, and more commonly caused by blunt trauma compared with adults. The greater prevalence of children's wounds on the highly vascular head may be responsible for the lower infection rate, rather than some intrinsic difference in wound healing between children and adults. Although children are believed to have a greater ability to heal than adults, several factors relevant to children

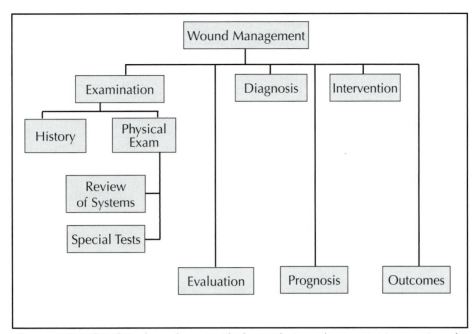

Figure 18-1A. The plan of care begins with data gathering. The examination consists of a history and physical examination with a review of systems and special tests used to rule in or rule out suspected causes of the wound. Following data gathering, the clinician undergoes a mental processing of the data. This process is called the evaluation. Based on the data, the clinician develops the impairment-driven diagnosis according to the processes described in the *Guide*. Although not necessary for every patient, the clinician may also seek to confirm or refute a pathology-driven diagnosis. The prognosis is developed based on the diagnosis and unique combination of circumstances of the patient derived from the history and physical examination. Interventions are devised based on the examination, diagnosis, prognosis, and patient preferences and resources. Appropriate outcomes are derived in consultation with the patient, family, caregivers, and other involved clinicians.

may slow healing. Children, especially neonates, have a greater surface area to body mass ratio and more difficulty in regulating body temperature than adults, which may impair healing. Young children, like elders, are at greater risk of malnutrition, especially in the presence of digestive disease or prematurity. Premature neonates have more fragile skin than full-term infants and, as such, are more susceptible to wounds due to weaker intracellular attachments. Due to the tremendous instrumentation required in the neonatal intensive care unit, premature infants are at great risk for cutaneous injury during handling. Moreover, multiple lines and equipment in conjunction with a lack of voluntary movement may place the neonate at risk of pressure ulcers from this instrumentation. In particular, infants are susceptible to occipital pressure ulcers due to the disproportionate head size. Risk factors for children in intensive care include age less than 36 months, ventricular septal defect (study involved children receiving open heart surgery), intubation longer than 7 days, and being in intensive care longer than 8 days. Infants are also at risk of skin injury secondary to persistent contact with urine and feces on the perineal skin.

PATIENT EDUCATION

The *Guide* specifically addresses patient education as one of the components of the therapist's interaction with a patient or client, in addition to procedural interventions, documentation, communication, and coordination of patient care. Each patient has a unique educational and lifetime learning background and level of self-efficacy. Some individuals are in a position of directly supervising and performing the bulk of their care, whereas others are completely dependent on others in developing and carrying out a plan of care. The clinician must, therefore, interview the patient, family, and caregivers to ascertain their levels of understanding of the process by which the wound developed and how to facilitate its healing. Topics for discussion include the etiology of the wound, rudimentary principles of wound healing, the purposes and mechanisms of action of any interventions, and expected outcomes. Most individuals will not be able to process all of this information at once and will need periodic reinforcement, including opportunities for the patient to discuss progress during each visit and to ask questions.

Figure 18-1B. Flow chart to evaluate etiology of a wound. Wounds are first divided into acute and chronic. Within the category of acute wounds, causes are divided into traumatic and surgical wounds of the type most likely to be referred to a clinician other than a surgeon. Within the category of chronic wounds, the subcategories of mechanical, vascular, and disease are given. Although many other causes of wounds exist, for the purpose of this flow chart, only the most common are demonstrated.

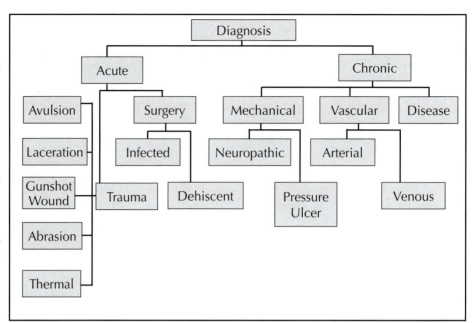

Figure 18-1C. Interventions for wound management consist of treating the "hole in the patient" and the "whole of the patient." Interventions for addressing the wound itself include debridement, cleaning, managing drainage, and optimizing the health of the skin surrounding the wound. To benefit the patient as a whole, the underlying cause of the wound is addressed and preventive measures are taken to prevent either recurrence of the wound or the development of new wounds elsewhere.

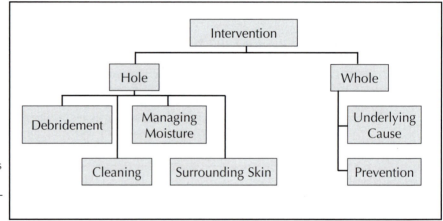

The clinician should also periodically assess the patient's or caregiver's cognitive (knowledge), psychomotor (ability to apply the knowledge), and affective (attitudes toward the process) learning.

COORDINATION AND COMMUNICATION

Each clinician has an ethical obligation to provide optimum care within the clinician's range of knowledge, skills, and abilities. As part of this, the clinician is ethically obligated to refer a patient to a clinician with the appropriate knowledge, skills, and abilities to provide optimal benefit for the patient. In the case of peripheral arterial disease, the patient obviously needs the services of a vascular surgeon. If a wound becomes infected or infection cannot be controlled by sharp debridement, referral to an infectious disease specialist or surgeon becomes necessary. If a wound requires more extensive debridement than can be managed without an operating room, requires general anesthesia, or if the patient has tunneling or sinus tracts that will need to be opened, referral to a surgeon is needed. If a clinician lacks skill at sharp debridement, this aspect of care needs to be turned over to a person who is skilled. If the clinician wishes to continue to see patients likely to need sharp debridement, the clinician should undergo appropriate training. Other potential situations requiring referrals include complicated cases of nutritional risk, management of incontinence, need for splints, adaptive or assistive devices, orthoses, prostheses, mobility or activity of daily living training, psychological counseling, assistance in obtaining financial resources and caregivers, vocational training, or creating a plan of care within constraints imposed by payers.

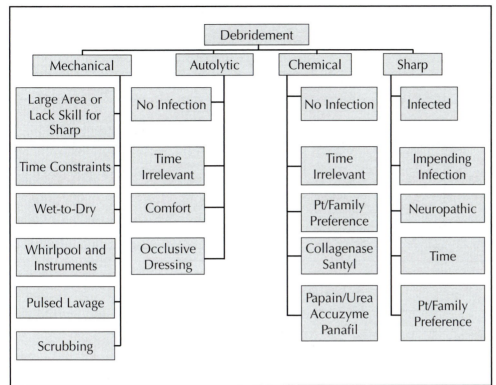

Figure 18-1D. Flow chart outlining the reasons and methods for debridement by the 4 basic means: mechanical, autolytic, chemical, and sharp debridement.

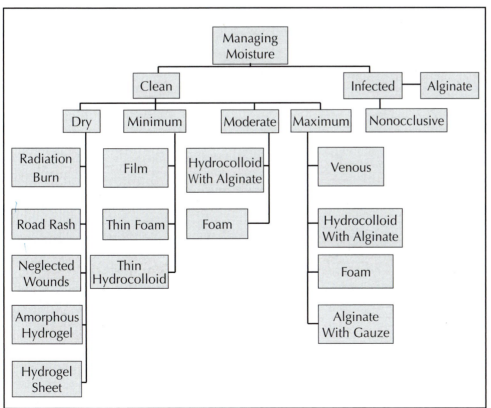

Figure 18-1E. Flow chart for managing drainage. The first division is into clean wounds and infected wounds, with only nonocclusive dressings or alginates as options. Clean wounds are categorized by the quantity of drainage. Selected examples of wounds typically observed to have different levels of drainage and types of primary dressings appropriate for the drainage are listed.

Figure 18-1F. Care for surrounding skin is divided into the categories of macerated and dry, and possible solutions for optimizing the moisture of the surrounding skin.

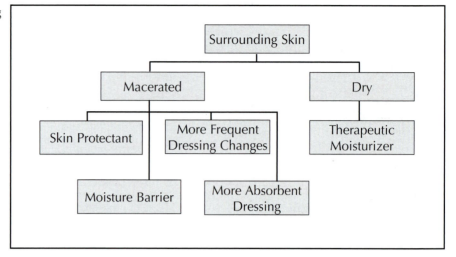

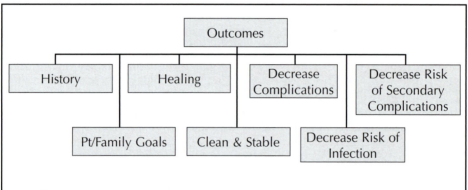

Figure 18-1G. Flow chart for development of outcomes and a select sample of them. Realistic outcomes are derived from understanding the patient's unique set of circumstances such as resources, lifestyle, and physical condition, as well as the goals of the patient, family, and caregivers. Possible outcomes range from complete healing to reducing the risk of secondary complications that would likely exacerbate the condition of a patient with terminal disease.

INTERNATIONAL CLASSIFICATION OF FUNCTIONING, DISABILITY AND HEALTH

International Classification of Functioning, Disability and Health (ICF) is a worldwide collaborative effort of the World Health Organization (WHO) to facilitate multidisciplinary healthcare. This system is an effort to provide common language regarding health that is meant to be understandable across nations, languages, disciplines, and is built on the Biopsychosocial Model. The first and second editions of the *Guide* are built on the disability model. The disability model was developed in an effort to encourage clinicians to consider more than a person's etiology in treatment planning. In contrast, the traditional medical model consists of obtaining a history and physical examination, performing a systems review, and conducting special tests

to aid diagnosis. Following diagnosis, medicine or surgery is used to treat the diagnosed disease using standard care. The primary emphasis encouraged through the use of the disability model is preventing the progression of an impairment to a disability, a disability to a handicap, or an impairment directly to a handicap. The disability model incorporates elements of a person's situation that may cause impairment to become a disability or a handicap, or cause a disability to become a handicap.

The disability model has several shortcomings. It does not explicitly direct clinicians to look at personal and environmental factors. It does not specify activities as important to a given person. It does not specify how well a person participates in activities, and it lacks a means of quantifying a person's condition or comparing data across clinicians, facilities, settings, or nations. Although the disability model is an improvement over the traditional medical model, its greatest shortcoming remains the non-

Table 18-1

World Health Organization's Definitions of Terms Used With the ICF Model[1]

Body Functions are physiological functions of body systems (including psychological functions).

Body Structures are anatomical parts of the body such as organs, limbs, and their components.

Impairments are problems in body function or structure such as a significant deviation or loss.

Activity is the execution of a task or action by an individual.

Participation is involvement in a life situation.

Activity Limitations are difficulties an individual may have in executing activities.

Participation Restrictions are problems an individual may experience in involvement in life situations.

Environmental Factors make up the physical, social, and attitudinal environment in which people live and conduct their lives.

---

uniform language clinicians use, even when framing the person's problems within the disability model. Neither the traditional medical model nor the disability model has a standard for coding personal and environmental factors, and they have no explicit means of communicating activities and participation. Instead, clinicians tend to develop their own language. Language disparity tends to worsen as one compares language used within a given facility by members of the same discipline, to different types of facilities, and to members of different disciplines. Disparity in language is likely to result in difficulty interpreting another clinician's documentation and time spent seeking clarification from him or her.

The purpose of creating ICF is facilitating the communication of clinicians within and between disciplines. It is also designed to be a systematic language acting as a basis for analyzing health statistics. As opposed to ICD codes, ICF codes are meant to be independent of etiology or healthcare provider. Improvements of the ICF model over the disability model include a greater emphasis on person's response to a given disease, a greater emphasis on patient-centered care, improved cross-discipline communication, and better integration with the biopsychosocial model. Within the framework of the ICF model, disability can mean physical, emotional, or social impairments manifesting themselves as limitations in activities and restrictions in participation. By its nature, the ICF model creates a patient-centered approach. The ICF model provides very specific definitions of terms commonly used in rehabilitation. The official WHO definitions of ICF terms are given in Table 18-1.

The ICF model operates under a small number of principles. Rather than drawing arbitrary distinctions between healthy and handicapped individuals, the model is based on the notion of a continuum of body structures, functions, activity limitations, and participation restrictions. For example, a person who cannot participate as a jockey in horse racing, as a professional basketball player, as a spelling bee competitor, or as an opera singer has some degree of impairment. A second major principle is that any specific impairment is equivalent without regard to its etiology (principle of equity/parity). A foot amputation resulting from trauma, arterial disease, infection, or congenital anomaly are treated identically within the model. In theory, the manner in which a person receives a wound is not directly germane to the person's condition or problems. Etiology might, however, have an indirect effect through what are termed contextual factors. For example, depending on the wound's etiology, a person's psychological response may differ, which in turn may affect any activity limitations or participation restrictions related to the altered body structure or function.

Contextual factors are divided into personal factors and environmental factors. Examples of personal factors given by the WHO include gender, age, other health conditions, coping style, social background, education, profession, past experience, and character style. According to the WHO, environmental factors include products and technology, natural environment and human-made changes to the environment, support and relationships, attitudes, services, systems, and policies. Using the ICF model places emphasis on relationships among the three core pieces of model—body structure/function, activities, and participation—and the effects of the contextual factors on them. Activities and participation are placed in nine specific categories: 1) learning and applying knowledge, 2) general tasks and demands, 3) communication, 4) movement, 5) self care, 6) domestic life areas, 7) interpersonal interactions, 8) major life areas, and 9) community, social, and civic life.

Within the ICF model, impairments are given capacity qualifiers and performance qualifiers to aid in communicating the person's condition. The capacity qualifier refers to the person's ability to actually execute a task or action under

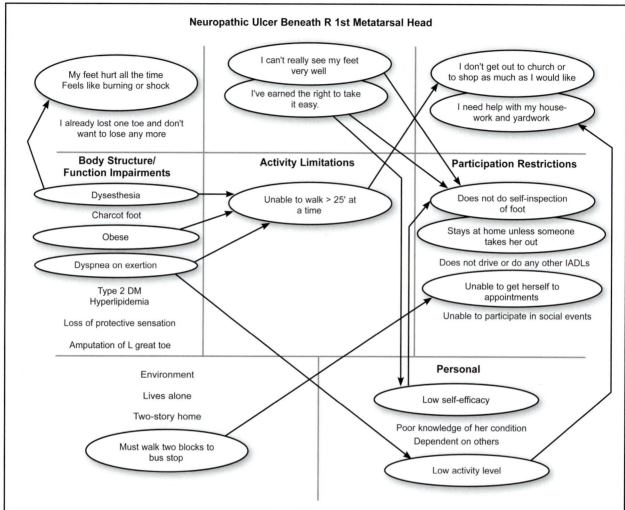

Figure 18-2. Using the ICF model to develop a plan of care. This tool is used to discover the patient's underlying problems so they can be addressed efficiently. The patient's participation restrictions were all traced to a small number of underlying problems (two of them are not linked in this example to improve the clarity of this figure). She did not perform self-inspection of her feet because of diabetic retinopathy and low self-efficacy. She stayed at home unless someone transported her, which led to missing healthcare appointments. She was obese, unable to walk more than 25 feet, had dyspnea on exertion, and complained of foot pain. Because of these physical problems, she had a low activity level and was unable to perform any IADLs. Finally, her low self-efficacy was caused by the negative impact of physical deterioration and isolation on her self-esteem. These basic problems led to a downward spiral of inactivity and physical and emotional decline. Underlying problems uncovered by this approach included the need for greater social support to improve her self-efficacy and to take her to healthcare appointments. Treatment of her dysesthesia pharmacologically has increased her willingness to perform activities on her feet, including physical therapy. Physical therapy has increased her mobility and broken the cycle of inactivity and physical deterioration. As a result of addressing these 3 problems, the patient now has the ability to get out of her home, participate in social events, do light shopping, and take better control of her health problems. Now she is less reliant on home care and has a much brighter outlook. As a result of these changes in addition to wound care, her neuropathic ulcer has healed and she is less likely to develop more ulcerations. As an exercise, finish connecting the remaining items on this figure. Then think back to a current or past patient and populate another grid until you are ready to use this tool with new patients.

ideal circumstances, whereas the performance qualifier communicates what the person actually does in his or her own environment. The use of personal assistance or assistive or adaptive devices is not material in terms of capacity. However, whether or not a person has access to assistance or equipment impacts his or her performance. According to this model, performance of an activity may be restricted by alterations in body structure or function, activity limitations, personal factors, or environmental factors. Note, however, as depicted in Figure 18-2, that arrows are drawn in both directions among body structure/function, activity limitations, and participation restriction. Arrows are also drawn from contextual factors to these 3 core entities. For example, if a person is given an offloading device, a walker, and personal assistance, he or she may be able to travel to healthcare providers, participate in activities related to wound care, and allow the neuropathic ulcer to heal.

Using the ICF Model as a Framework for Plan of Care

A person's needs and preferences are determined through a discussion of the person's problems and therapy goals and validated tools such as the SF-36 (Short-Form Health Survey). Components of the interview are open-ended questions with answers written in the person's own words. These questions are based directly on the ICF model, ie, which problems of the body functions are being experienced, which body structures are involved, what limitations of activities are being experienced, whether participation is being restricted in significant tasks or actions, and which environmental factors or personal factors are barriers or facilitators.

Following interviews and collection of data from standardized written tools, guided physical examinations are performed by relevant members of the healthcare team. Impairments are then placed into the three categories of 1) body structures/functions, 2) activities, and 3) participation. A form has been developed by Steiner et al specifically for the ICF model, which they termed the *Rehabilitation Problem-Solving Form* (RPS-Form). Alternatively, a simple 3-row grid with 3 columns in the first 2 rows and 2 columns in the third row can be created (Figure 18-2). The top row of the grid contains the interview and written data divided among the 3 core categories. The information obtained through physical examination is placed into the middle row within the appropriate 3 core categories. The third row consists of personal factors and environmental factors. The single clinician or preferably a healthcare team then looks for connections among the 8 blocks on the grid or the RPS-Form used. Circles and lines are drawn on the form to help visualize relationships among items in the 8 blocks. An assessment of any personal factors or environmental factors that might either cause or contribute to problems listed is made. Examining the completed form should cue clinicians to personal and environmental factors that might impact connections among items on the form or grid. Clinicians may identify facilitators that could be exploited or barriers that could be overcome with the availability of specific environmental factors. Hypotheses related to cause and effect for the person's problems and factors contributing to, rather than causing, the effects are developed and analyzed critically. When factors directly or indirectly responsible for any body structural or functional impairments, activity limitations, or participation restrictions are identified, a plan of care can be readily developed to address modifiable physical, personal, or environmental factors. The top section of the form or grid becomes useful in the reconciliation of differences between expectations of the patient and clinician. The patient may have expectations that are too high, too low, or misdirected, in the opinion of the clinician. The patient and clinician must then find a suitable solution to any conflicts in expectations. Reviewing the relationships using a visual tool with the patient directly may expedite any conflict resolution.

SUMMARY

The plan of care is a blueprint for interventions provided based upon the history and physical examination of the patient, a diagnosis of the cause of the wound, healing, and the prognosis for healing. It is modified based on a unique set of circumstances related to the patient's ability to follow through with the plan. Decision points include the need to treat infection, the type of debridement needed, filling subcutaneous defects, and managing drainage to optimize wound moisture while simultaneously maintaining the integrity of the surrounding skin. The skin of the elderly and neonate are at greater risk of injury due to anatomic and physiologic differences. Elderly skin has less contact area, decreased thickness and blood flow, and is vulnerable to tearing and bleeding. A number of risk factors for injury are present in neonates, especially premature infants. Decreased ability to regulate heat, potential for malnourishment, inability to reposition, and the presence of multiple lines and devices increases the risk of injury and slow healing. Both infants and the elderly need to be handled gently to avoid skin injury. The ICF model is described as a tool for treatment planning by identifying the relationships among physical impairments, activity limitations, participation restrictions, and personal and environmental factors.

QUESTIONS

1. How does the care setting affect the plan of care?
2. How might an immobile terminally ill patient's plan of care differ from an ambulatory person's plan of care for a foot wound?
3. What 2 critical functions do dressings perform in managing wound drainage?
4. What are critical reasons for performing sharp debridement?
5. Under what circumstances would sharp debridement not be performed?

6. What patient characteristics need to be considered in choosing a dressing that the patient will need to change at home?

7. Explain the greater risk of tearing and bleeding that occur in the skin of the elderly.

8. Describe steps that can be taken to minimize damage to the skin of the infant and elderly patient.

9. List risk factors for skin injury and slow wound healing commonly present in premature infants.

REFERENCE

1. Towards a Common Language for Functioning, Disability and Health ICF. Available at http://www.who.int/classifications/icf/training/icfbeginnersguide.pdf. Accessed September 9, 2009.

BIBLIOGRAPHY

American Physical Therapy Association. *Guide to Physical Therapist Practice. Physical Therapy.* 1997;77:1177-1619.

Gordon A, Kozin ED, Keswani SG, et al. Permissive environment in postnatal wounds induced by adenoviral-mediated overexpression of the anti-inflammatory cytokine interleukin-10 prevents scar formation. *Wound Repair Regen.* 2008;16(1):70-79.

Helgeson K, Smith AR. Process for applying the international classification of functioning, disability and health model to a patient with patellar dislocation. *Phys Ther.* 2008;88(8):956-964.

Hollander JE, Singer AJ, Valentine S. Comparison of wound care practices in pediatric and adult lacerations repaired in the emergency department. *Pediatric Emergency Care.* 1998;14:15-18.

Jette AM. Toward a common language for function, disability, and health. *Phys Ther.* 2006;86(5):726-734.

Malloy-McDonald MB. Skin care for high-risk neonates. *J Wound Ostomy Continence Nurs.* 1995;22(4):177-182.

Neidig JR, Kleiber C, Oppliger RA. Risk factors associated with pressure ulcers in the pediatric patient following open heart surgery. *Prog in Cardiovasc Nurs.* 1989;4(3):99-106.

Pieper B, Templin T, Dobal M, Jacox A. Prevalence and types of wounds among children receiving care in the home. *Ostomy Wound Manage.* 2000;46(4):36-42.

Steiner WA, Ryser L, Huber E, Uebelhart D, Aeschlimann A, Stucki G. Use of the ICF model as a clinical problem-solving tool in physical therapy and rehabilitation medicine. *Phys Ther.* 2002;82:1098–1107.

Verbugge L, Jette A. The disablement process. *Soc. Sci. Med.* 1994;38:1-14.

Regulations, Reimbursement, and Psychosocial Issues

OBJECTIVES

- Discuss Medicare and typical state licensing regulations relevant to wound management.
- Describe how to build a wound management team to optimize wound management.
- Discuss issues related to reimbursement for wound management services.

The issues discussed in this chapter, however contentious and subject to rapid and dramatic change, are important for a healthy practice that allows our patients and clients to benefit from our services. Unfortunately, a detailed description of what is optimal or even allowable in terms of reimbursement is likely to be outdated before many readers use this text. Changes occur due to federal legislation and rules dictated by government agencies such as the CMS. Prudence dictates that each facility have an individual responsible for analysis of the multitude of healthcare rules and regulations that may have an impact on reimbursement. Depending on the case mix of individual facilities, these issues may require adjustments of staffing. An attempt will be made to discuss general principles that are unlikely to change in the near future.

REGULATIONS

Regulation and reimbursement issues are often related. With Medicare as the largest third-party payer and other payers generally following the policies of CMS, regulations developed for CMS affect reimbursement profoundly. Pro bono cases are an important part of our social responsibility; however, when developing a plan of care, both wound care products and services rendered will need to be reimbursable in the vast majority of cases for the facility's own fiscal health. CMS expends nearly $400 billion per year for Medicare and Medicaid recipients. With such a large amount of money available, volumes of regulations are written in an attempt to use the available money most efficiently. CMS regulations themselves do not vary across states or among carriers or fiscal interme-

Irion G.
Comprehensive Wound Management, 2nd ed. (pp 335-348)
© 2010 SLACK Incorporated

diaries (companies contracted to manage Medicare Parts A and B), but the implementation of regulations may vary substantially such that services covered in one state, or by a certain CMS contractor may not be covered by another. Although only a small number of insurance companies serve as Medicare contractors, staff in different states may have different interpretations of a given Medicare rule and, within a given contractor, different personnel are likely to have different interpretations of the same rule. This situation is exacerbated by job turnover within these companies. Individuals working for the CMS contractors can be educated to understand the role of different interventions for various characteristics of a patient, but the loss of that employee forces the clinician to educate another. CMS attempts to improve uniformity by periodically distributing explicit instructions to their contractors on certain issues. Although the regulations often appear arbitrary and more favorable to specific settings and providers than to others, we must learn to work within these regulations while providing appropriate and fiscally responsible care.

Medicare requires the evaluation and interventions involved in wound management to be performed by appropriately trained and licensed individuals. In some cases, state laws may permit tremendous latitude in assigning personnel to direct patient care. Regardless of the letter of the law, ethical, moral, and risk management principles must be applied to staffing decisions. The potential risk of harming a patient can never be justified by assigning direct patient care to individuals lacking appropriate training or licensing, regardless of what individual state practice acts may allow. Moreover, fee schedules are based on the use of appropriate personnel; billing for direct patient care provided by an individual lacking the training specified by Medicare requirements could be ruled Medicare fraud and lead to severe consequences.

State licensing requirements generally become an issue on 2 points. First, does the patient have direct access to your services or must the patient be referred, usually through a family practitioner or other medical specialist? The second concern is how the state practice act for the different providers is written in terms of debridement. Individuals in each state need to determine current regulations for referral and sharp debridement. In general, physicians (including podiatrists), physician's assistants, and physical therapists are permitted to perform sharp debridement. Advanced practice nurses and other healthcare providers may be allowed within given states.

REIMBURSEMENT ISSUES

Charges for direct interventions generally eligible for reimbursement by CMS include those for evaluation, debridement, wound stimulation by high-volt pulsed current or pulsed electromagnetic field, and negative

pressure wound therapy. Only specific types of wounds are eligible for payment under debridement codes. These wound types are surgical wounds that must be left open to heal by secondary intention, infected open wounds, wounds caused by trauma or surgery, or wounds related to "complicating metabolic, vascular, or pressure factors."[1] This list covers the most common wounds discussed in Chapter 7 and nearly all of those produced by unusual causes as described in Chapter 16. Uncomplicated abrasions and lacerations are specifically excluded. CMS does not consider the use of treatments other than debridement, negative pressure wound therapy, and high-volt pulsed current and PEMF stimulation as medically necessary. Specific examples given by CMS as uncovered treatments are ultraviolet light, low intensity direct current, topical application of oxygen, and topical dressings with Balsam of Peru in castor oil.

The American Medical Association (AMA) working with CMS has developed a coding system for billing for services termed *common procedural terminology* (CPT). The term *CPT®* is a registered trademark of the AMA, who reserves all rights to the term *CPT* and the individual descriptions of each code. Because CPT is copyrighted material, only short descriptors of each code are allowed in publications other than the AMA's official annual publication, *CPT Current Procedural Terminology* and a monthly publication, *CPT Assistant*. Descriptions of individual CPT codes discussed in this text are not the complete official description, but the shortened version deemed acceptable by the AMA. Codes may be added, deleted, or descriptions of them modified on an annual basis by the AMA. Reimbursement amounts and requirements are also subject to change following notice by CMS. More complete descriptions and requirements for use of any given CPT code can be obtained from official AMA sources or from the Web sites of CMS contractors. HCPCS codes for supplies, equipment, and temporary or unusual situations are established by CMS. Three levels of HCPCS codes are in existence at the time of this writing. Level I includes the CPT codes, written by an AMA committee to aid in the administration of Medicare. Level II represents codes developed by CMS either on a temporary basis or to handle durable medical equipment, eg, specialty beds and surgical supplies such as wound dressings and compression bandages. Level III is developed to handle unique situations.

The original philosophy for CPT codes was that payment would be based on the service provided, rather than the provider. However, this philosophy has changed first with the codes for evaluation, which are now provider-dependent. Until 2000, debridement codes existed only under the surgical section of the codes. Sharp debridement had been paid to nonphysician providers under one of the surgical codes 11040-11044 by some CMS contractors, but others would not provide payment despite the ruling that Medicare payment for sharp debridement is allowed for physical therapists, podiatrists, physicians, and advanced practice nurses with specialized training. Payment under other plans or as part of a diagnosis-related group (DRG) may allow others to perform sharp debridement. The major problem with reimbursement under the surgical codes was the cost determined for reimbursing debridement as a surgical procedure and the absence of a code that reflected the lower cost of providing sharp debridement in a nonsurgical environment. In the revisions for 2001, CPT code 97601 for removal of devitalized tissue from wounds by selective debridement without anesthesia was implemented. Within the description for this code, examples of allowable means of debridement included both selective and nonselective means of debridement. Whirlpool, pulsatile lavage, and selective sharp debridement with scissors, scalpel, and forceps were given as examples. Reimbursement under this code bundled any topical applications, wound assessment, and instructions for ongoing care, per session, not the time spent performing the service. Moreover, for reimbursement, an evaluative component is expected with each session. The CPT code 97602 was created at the same time to designate nonselective debridement using procedures not requiring skilled services. Examples included simple cleaning or scrubbing with a 4 x 4.

New codes were implemented in 2005 for "active wound care management"[1] with a description implying selective debridement. The two codes 97597 and 97598 cover the same service, differing only in the size of the wound. Selective debridement of wounds with a surface area of 20 cm^2 or smaller is coded 97597; the same procedure for a wound with a surface area greater than 20 cm^2 is coded 97598. The payment for 97598 has been greater than 97597, but both have been increased to the same amount for 2008. None of the debridement codes are time-based. Payment is the same regardless of time spent, cost of dressings and other supplies applied, or the amount of assistance required to perform the service. However, ambulatory care patients seen in a physician-based clinic can be billed through office visit codes 99201-99215. The CPT codes 99201-99205 pertain to 5 levels of care for new patients with the descriptors problem focused, expanded, detailed, comprehensive, and high complexity assigned to these 5 codes respectively. Codes 99211-99215 are used for outpatient visits by established patients using the same 5 descriptors. Based on the time and other resources used for the office visit, 1 of the 5 levels for either a new or established patient is chosen. For example, a simple follow-up examination of a patient would be billed as 99211. Extensive, time-consuming debridement and use of expensive dressings could be billed as 99215. Other CPT codes that might be utilized in wound care are 16020, 16025,

and 16030 for debridement of partial-thickness burn injuries (small, medium, large) and codes 97605 and 97606 for negative pressure wound therapy.

With such a large number of claims being submitted, CMS monitors trends in an effort to optimize benefits for patients. When unusual trends develop such as the recent large increase in claims for selective and excisional debridement, the Office of the Inspector General has investigated. These investigations usually result in changes in the policies of CMS. In addition, CMS contractors may scrutinize claims. For example, Cahaba Government Benefit Administration (Medicare Part B carrier for Alabama, Georgia, and Mississippi) analyzed claims for 97597 and 97598. As a result, 88% of claims were denied. Of the bills submitted to them, $45,000 of $51,000 was denied. Although those filing claims may appeal, the better solution is to document in such a way that denials will not occur. Reasons given by Cahaba for denial included lack of physician certification or recertification, inadequate medical justification submitted, inadequate medical documentation submitted, the medical record did not verify that the services described by the code were provided, and lack of requested information. The specific issues identified by Cahaba included no documentation of wound measurements on the treatment or progress notes, documentation that the wound bed is clean with 100% granulation tissue, no documentation of tissue to be debrided, whirlpool billed on the same date as debridement, use of multiple units of 97597/97598 on the same date, no documentation of the method of selective debridement, billing for physical therapy evaluation in addition to 97597/8 without evidence of a complete evaluation of the patient beyond the wound, documentation that a nonselective method of debridement was used, lack of initial evaluation or wound assessment, use of whirlpool to clean wound, use of debridement codes for suture removal, lack of documentation of an open wound, lack of physician orders, and documentation that the wound was closed.

The 2 codes for active wound care management, 97597 and 97598 are limited to removal of necrotic tissue with the expectation that the procedure can be done selectively (selective debridement). The type of tissue or time spent on the procedure are not part of the description. The distinction between codes 97597 and 97598 is based strictly on an arbitrary size of 20 cm^2. Code 97597 is used if the computed surface area of length x width as described in wound assessment is 20 cm^2 or less, and for wounds greater than 20 cm^2, code 97598 is used. When billing for debridement, codes for excisional debridement (11040 series) and selective debridement (97597-8) cannot be used on the same day. An appropriate use of both sets of codes would be excisional debridement by a surgeon on one day, followed by selective debridement no sooner than the next day by a physical therapist, advanced practice nurse, or physician's assistant. For 2008, a category III CPT was developed for "low frequency, noncontact, nonthermal ultrasound."[1] This code 0183T does not guarantee payment by specific CMS contractors. For codes of this nature, clinicians must determine whether CMS or other insurers will pay for submissions under this code. If payment is received from the CMS contractor, the amount would be essentially the same as that for "active wound management."[1]

Codes in the 11040 series pertain to surgical excision of tissue as a means of debridement and will generally require anesthesia and an operating or special procedures room. The codes for selective debridement are to be used by physicians when the service performed is the same as that provided by a physical therapist or nurse. If anesthesia is not used and a surgical debridement code is billed, payment is denied. An operative report is required for surgical procedures such as excisional debridement and application of living skin equivalents. The number of surgical excisions reimbursed on a single wound will be limited to a much lower number than selective debridement procedures. Currently, this limit is 5 per year for any combination of codes 11043 and 11044; however, additional payments may be obtained if a valid argument for medical reasonableness can be presented.

A nonselective debridement procedure code is available (97602), but it is considered a nonskilled service. It originally had no payment associated with it. It was later given a substantially lower value, but for 2008 has been assigned the same value as 97597 and 97598. The application of wet-to-dry dressings, enzymatic debriders, and scrubbing are included under this code. Some CMS contractors may consider whirlpool therapy to belong in this category and deny payment if a bill for whirlpool is submitted under codes 97597 or 97598.

Codes are available for foot care (CPT codes 11055-7) and nail care (CPT codes 11720 and 11721), but foot care is generally considered to be a maintenance service and will not be covered by Medicare except under specific circumstances elaborated by CMS under its Routine Foot Care policy (ARA-02-043). This policy lists many appropriate conditions that might become foot-threatening without appropriate foot care. Conditions include diabetes mellitus and a large number of other neuropathic and metabolic diseases. Routine foot care includes nail debridement, but nail debridement is included in the exceptions granted under the Routine Foot Care policy for systemic conditions.

CMS defines nail debridement as a "significant reduction in the thickness and length of the nail to the tolerance of the patient with the aim of allowing the patient to ambulate without pain."[1] This definition is then further qualified by stating that simple trimming by cutting or grinding is not considered debridement. Superficial fungal infections that do not cause significant symptoms are not covered. If the patient is nonambulatory, CMS will only cover nail debridement of mycotic nails resulting in pain, or secondary infection that results from dystrophic nails.

Medicare covers foot exams including associated treatment once every 6 months for eligible individuals with a documented loss of protective sensation if the patient has not been seen by a "foot care specialist"[1] within this 6 month period. CMS requires diagnosis of loss of protective sensation to be established by standardized testing with the 5.07 monofilament including 5 sites on the plantar surface of each foot. The full 10-point exam endorsed by the American Diabetes Association is not required. The criterion of the American Podiatric Medicine Association is considered acceptable. This criterion requires failure to detect the 5.07 Semmes-Weinstein monofilament at 2 or more sites out of 5 tested on either foot. Examination required by CMS includes patient history and a minimum of visual inspection of the feet, monofilament testing, examination of foot structure, biomechanics, vascular status, and the need for special footwear. Patient education, local care of superficial wounds, debridement of callus, and trimming and debridement of nails are included in the payment for the semiannual visit. A large number of qualifiers are included in the policies covering foot care and nail debridement. The reader is directed to the CMS Web site to view these details.

If callus removal is performed during a selective debridement procedure, payment is only provided through 97597 or 97598. An additional submission for payment under 11055-7 will be denied. Similarly, if only callus removal is performed, a claim for selective debridement will be denied. Therefore, the additional resources needed for callus removal are absorbed by the clinic performing the selective debridement. Due to the restrictive nature of CPT codes available, a clinic visit for a 10 cm^2 neuropathic ulcer that includes 45 to 60 minutes of wound and callus debridement will be reimbursed at a lower rate than a 15 minute procedure on a 22 cm^2 wound. Specific indications and limitations for debridement CPT codes and guidelines for their use are listed verbatim in Tables 19-1 and 19-2.

Medicare regulations related to electrical stimulation and pulsed electromagnetic field (G0281 and G0329) require that a period of "appropriate standard wound care has been tried for at least 30 days and there are no measurable signs of healing."[1] The phrase "appropriate standard wound care" is vague, but implies that CMS has the right to deny coverage if documentation does not support the expected level of care. Similarly the phrase "no measurable signs of healing" is vague. Failure of wound dimensions to decrease is unlikely to satisfy requirements. The quality of the wound must also be considered. Documented evidence of decreased bioburden, improved quality of surrounding

Table 19-1

CMS Indications and Limitations of Coverage and Medical Necessity

Indications:

Chronic wound care is generally necessary for the following types of wounds:

- Second and third degree burn wounds
- Surgical wounds that must be left open to heal by secondary intention
- Infected open wounds, induced by trauma or surgery, or associated with complicating metabolic, vascular, or pressure factors
- Open or closed wounds complicated by necrotic tissue and eschar
- Wounds that have various factors that complicate normal healing, such as subcutaneous fluid and blood collections that require specialized drains or devices

Limitations:

1. There must be a documented plan of care with goals and follow-up by the patient's attending physician. Follow-up by the physician should be at least weekly during the first 4 weeks of therapy and at appropriate intervals thereafter (usually less frequently). There must be clearly documented evidence of the progress of the wound's response to treatment at each physician visit. At a minimum, this documentation would include wound size, wound depth, presence or absence of obvious signs of infection, presence or absence of necrotic or devitalized tissue, and state of the patient's nutrition.
2. Cornerstones of decubitus ulcer and chronic foot ulcer management include relief of pressure, control of infection, and appropriate debridement. The treatment plan in the care of such wounds must ensure appropriate attention to relief of pressure and control of infection.
3. Debridements of the wound(s), if indicated, must be done judiciously and at appropriate intervals. Debridement of a wound more than once daily in the early stages of chronic wound care (approximately the first 1 to 2 weeks of care) would be rare.
4. Debridement more than 3 times a week in the intermediate stages (approximately the second through fourth weeks of care), or more than approximately weekly thereafter would also be considered to be rare occurrences. When debridements are done, the debridement notes must document the level of tissue removed (ie, skin, full or partial thickness, subcutaneous tissue, muscle, and/or bone), the method used to debride (ie, hydrostatic vs sharp vs abrasion methods), and the character of the tissue before and after debridement.
5. When the only wound care service provided is the non-surgical cleansing of the ulcer site, with or without the application of a surgical dressing, do not use debridement codes.
6. When wound care reaches a point that it can be done by the patients themselves or by their caregiver, the wound has reached a "maintenance care" level. Maintenance care is not covered by Medicare other than the evaluation and management services of the physician attending the patient.
7. Wound care complicated by factors that require other adjunctive interventions, such as hyperbaric oxygen therapy or bilaminate skin substitutes will have the medical necessity limitations outlined in the Local Coverage Determinations for these services. Other adjunctive services to chronic wound care such as skin autografts, allografts, or xenografts are covered on a medically reasonable and necessary basis.
8. Various methods of promoting wound healing have been devised over time. Physicians and health care providers must understand that many of these methods are expensive and unproven by valid scientific literature, and would be considered investigational. Investigational treatments are non-covered by Medicare as not medically necessary. The patient can be requested to pay for investigational treatment under waiver of liability provisions of Medicare law, but an advance beneficiary notice must be obtained for the beneficiary to be liable for such payment.

continued

Table 19-1

CMS Indications and Limitations of Coverage and Medical Necessity (continued)

9. Platelet derived formula containing growth factors intended to treat non-healing wounds (eg, Procuran) are addressed in the Coverage Issue Manual 45-26 as a non-covered service. Other systems of treatment that are based on the principal of using a platelet derived formula to enhance or augment healing are also felt to be addressed by this coverage issue non-coverage. There is a lack of sufficient published data to determine the safety and efficacy and hence will be non-covered until such data is available.
10. For services performed on or after April 1, 2003, Medicare will cover electrical stimulation for the treatment of wounds only for chronic Stage III or Stage IV pressure ulcers, arterial ulcers, diabetic ulcers and venous stasis ulcers. All other uses of electrical stimulation for the treatment of wounds are not covered by Medicare. Electrical stimulation will not be covered as an initial treatment modality.

The use of electrical stimulation will only be covered after appropriate standard wound care has been tried for at least 30 days and there are no measurable signs of healing. If electrical stimulation is being used, wounds must be evaluated periodically by the treating physician, but no less than every 30 days by a physician. Continued treatment with electrical stimulation is not covered if measurable signs of healing have not been demonstrated within any 30-day period of treatment. Additionally, electrical stimulation must be discontinued when the wound demonstrates a 100% epithelialized wound bed.

http://www.arkmedicare.com/provider/medpola/ara02025.asp. Accessed 10/26/09.

Table 19-2

CPT Debridement Code Utilization Guidelines Given by CMS

1. Debridements of the wound(s) must be done judiciously and at appropriate intervals. It is rarely necessary to debride a wound more than once daily in the early stages of chronic wound care (approximately the first 1 to 2 weeks of care), more than 3 times a week in the intermediate stages (approximately the second through fourth weeks of care) or more than approximately weekly thereafter.
2. When wound care reaches a point the patients can reasonably do it themselves or by their caregiver, the wound has reached a "maintenance care" level. Such maintenance care is not covered by Medicare other than the evaluation and management services of the physician attending the patient.
3. The CPT code selected should report the level of debrided tissue (eg, partial thickness skin, full thickness skin, subcutaneous tissue, muscle and/or bone), not the extent, depth, or grade of the ulcer or wound. For example, use CPT code 11042 if only necrotic skin and subcutaneous tissue are debrided, even though the ulcer or wound might extend to bone.

http://www.arkmedicare.com/provider/medpola/ara02025.asp. Accessed 10/26/09.

skin and wound bed within 30 days prior to initiation of electrical stimulation for wound healing is likely to lead to denial of payment. Additionally, CMS will deny any claims for electrical stimulation once the wound bed is 100% re-epithelialized. Also note that CMS will only cover electrical stimulation for chronic wounds, specified as "…stage III and IV pressure ulcers, arterial ulcers, diabetic ulcers, and venous stasis ulcers."[1]

The use of infrared devices in the forms of infrared, near-infrared light, or heat is no longer a covered Medicare benefit as of October 2006. This decision by CMS includes the Warm-up device (Augustine Medical, Inc., Eden Prairie, MN) designed to maintain wound temperature and monochromatic infrared energy (MIRE). Although MIRE has been proposed as a treatment for pain and sensory loss associated with diabetic and other forms of neuropathy, CMS has ruled that these devices are not medically necessary to treat any covered conditions. A list of CPT codes considered to be wound management is given in Table 19-3.

Table 19-3

CPT® Codes Considered as Wound Care by CMS

- 11040 Debride skin, partial
- 11041 Debride skin, full
- 11042 Debride skin/tissue
- 11043 Debride tissue/muscle
- 11044 Debride tissue/muscle/bone
- 16020 Dress/debride p-thick burn, s
- 16025 Dress/debride p-thick burn, m
- 16030 Dress/debride p-thick burn, l
- 97597 Active wound care ≤20 cm^2
- 97598 Active wound care >20 cm^2
- 97602 Wound(s) care non-selective
- 97605 Neg press wound tx, ≤50 cm^2
- 97606 Neg press wound tx, >50 cm^2
- G0281 Electrical stimulation (unattended), for pressure factors
- G0329 Electromagnetic therapy, for chronic wounds

Codes are subject to change on an annual basis. Refer to current CPT manuals and descriptions for actual patient billing.

CPT® is a trademark of the American Medical Association.

Current Procedural Terminology © 2009 American Medical Association. All rights reserved.

The descriptions appearing in this publication are the acceptable short versions. Please consult an official CPT publication for complete descriptions.

http://www.trailblazerhealth.com/Tools/Local%20Coverage%20Determinations/Default.aspx?id=2897&DomainID=1

A large number of CPT codes are now available for skin replacement and skin substitute application. This number reflects the increasing technologic advancements and types of skin replacements. Different ranges of CPT codes are available for different combinations of living, non-living, allografts, xenografts, and acellular matrix products. The use of these codes requires a physician to harvest the graft (as appropriate) and care for the donor site. Application of the skin replacement/substitute requires surgical fixation. This fixation may include staples, sutures, or adhesive. Use of a wound dressing to hold the material in place does not meet the requirements for use of the CPT codes. A range of CPT codes for each type of material is used to delineate the site and the size of the skin substitute. When billing for application of these materials, concurrent billing for surgical debridement (11040-11042) or creation of a recipient site (15000) is not allowed.

A trend for CMS is the incorporation of supplies necessary for performing a task into the payment for a given CPT code. This is termed *bundling*. When billing, one must be aware of what supplies are bundled. Billing for both the task and the supplies or for individual tasks covered by a code is termed *unbundling*. The use of a code that pays a higher rate than the code that CMS considers appropriate for the level of care provided is termed *upcoding*. Both unbundling and upcoding are considered forms of fraud by CMS.

CMS requires a discount on procedures that are bilateral in nature. Specifically noted by CMS is application of an Unna's boot (29580). Instead of paying double for an application of 2 Unna's boots (one on each leg), CMS pays 50% for the second procedure. Substantial documentation of the need for 2 separate applications on different days might be acceptable once, eg, a diagnosis of venous disease on the second leg was made later. Subsequent visits would require bilateral application whenever medically feasible.

Outpatient or home services performed under the physician's supervision fall under the "incident-to"[1] rule. The incident-to rule applies to part B of Medicare and is paid to the physician as if the physician were performing the care. This rule does not apply to inpatient hospitals, skilled nursing facilities, and hospital outpatient departments. The incident-to rule requires that the services rendered are "integral"[1] parts of the physician's professional service, a normal part of the patient's plan of care, the physician performs the initial service, and the physician remains actively involved in the patient's care. These requirements imply that the incident-to services are rendered on an established patient with an established plan of care in place. Services provided by nonphysicians under this rule must be either those that are commonly not billed individually or are billed under the physician's charges such as dressing changes and application of enzymatic debriders that would otherwise be performed by the physician as part of the charge. Those allowed to perform "incident-to"[1] services must be considered employees of the physician, whether directly employed or contracting with the physician. The relationship between the person rendering the incident-to services and the physician must be part of the documentation. The physician must be nearby, eg, in the same office suite, but does not need to be present in the room where treatment is being provided. In addition, individual nonphysicians working for physicians may bill under their own NPI (National Provider Identifier) for services within their scopes of practice under specific circumstances. These services must be those that would be payable to a physician for the same service, the provider must have his or her own NPI, and state laws and regulations must be met. If these conditions are met, the physician is not required to be present. However, CMS pays at a lower rate if the nonphysician's NPI is used for billing.

Although Medicare covers a large portion of expensive technology and supplies to facilitate wound healing, co-payments for office visits, procedures, and supplies obtained from DME suppliers are required. Co-payments for expensive dressings and procedures may discourage the patient or clinician from using them. Not collecting the co-payment as an incentive for the patient to utilize services is not allowable; both clinics and DME suppliers are required to "make every effort"[1] to collect co-payments. Failure to do so can result in punitive action from CMS, which could include decreased payments, suspension from participating in CMS programs, or even exclusion. Higher co-payments must be considered during treatment planning. Patients may be willing to incur costlier co-payments per visit if they can heal more rapidly, and save money compared with a more protracted course of treatment. In addition to co-payments, clinicians must consider the possibility of capped benefits. Patients will be required to pay for services that exceed capped amounts. Congress has required CMS to cap therapy services, but has also put into effect numerous rules for exceptions, which may change as

Congress acts on legislation. Although clinicians should keep track of caps on services by CMS, they must also be mindful of caps imposed by private insurers for patients with coverage other than Medicare or Medicaid.

ICD-9 Codes

To receive reimbursement under debridement codes, a limited number of ICD-9-CM codes may be used for the patient's diagnosis (at this time, much of the world is using ICD-10 and ICD-11 is under development). Software is used to determine whether the CPT codes used for billing are appropriate given the ICD-9 code used for a patient's diagnosis. If an appropriate ICD-9 code is not present, automatic denial of claims will occur for CPT codes 11040, 11041, 11042, 11043, 11044, 16020, 16025, 16030, 97597, 97598, 97605, and 97606. These ICD-9 codes consist mainly of the 707 series for chronic wounds and 870 series for open wounds. Other allowable diagnoses for payment under CPT codes related to wound management are gas gangrene, atherosclerosis of the "native arteries of the extremities," lower extremity venous disease, skin infection, necrotizing fasciitis, and gangrene. More restrictive codes must accompany claims for a physical therapy evaluation. Acceptable ICD-9 codes for reimbursement of the physical therapy evaluation to occur along with payment for selective debridement include burns (second or third degree), pressure ulcers, and chronic ulcers of the lower extremities.

MEETING MEDICARE DOCUMENTATION REQUIREMENTS

Based on current regulations, 3 key items are needed to satisfy Medicare requirements for documentation: medical necessity, progress, and progress relative to the resources used. The first item to document is whether the patient's condition justifies the level of care given. The patient's conditions, including any complicating factors that weigh in the choice of intervention, should be included. In addition to documenting the need, the documentation should support the interventions based on what is likely to occur if the intervention is not done, that the appropriate person is carrying out the intervention, and the likelihood of the intervention being successful. For example, a necrotic wound that is either infected or at risk for infection justifies the intervention of sharp debridement by a physical therapist, advanced practice nurse, podiatrist, or physician. The risks of spreading infection, failure to heal, and possible amputation should also be discussed. Moreover, if more frequent outpatient visits are needed due to limited ability of the patient or patient's caregivers to care for the wound, documentation should be provided to support the greater number of visits. Addition of electrical stimulation

Table 19-4

Medicare Documentation Requirements for Debridement Codes

1. Documentation supporting the medical necessity should be legible, maintained in the patient's medical record, and must be made available to Medicare upon request.
2. There must be a documented plan of care with goals and follow-up by the patient's attending physician present in the patient's medical record.
3. Likewise, in the patient's medical record, there must be clearly documented evidence of the progress of the wound's response to treatment at each physician visit. This documentation at a minimum should include wound size, wound depth, presence or absence of obvious signs of infection, presence or absence of necrotic or devitalized tissue, and state of the patient's nutrition.
4. When debridements are done, the debridement notes must document the level of tissue removed (ie, skin, full or partial thickness; subcutaneous tissue; muscle; and/or bone), the method used to debride (ie, hydrostatic vs sharp vs abrasion methods), and the character of the wound before and after debridement.

http://www.arkmedicare.com/provider/medpola/ara02025.asp. Accessed 10/26/09.

needs to be supported by documented lack of healing despite appropriate wound management for a minimum of 30 days.

The second item to document is how well the patient is responding to the intervention. Patient response to treatment needs to be described in progress reports. A brief mention that the patient is responding well to treatment is not sufficient. The documented progress should be related directly to the desired outcomes or goals listed on the initial evaluation. The documentation should indicate objective measures of improvement including the removal of necrotic tissue, appearance of the wound bed, drainage, and wound dimensions. Descriptions indicating improved healing or potential for healing such as improvement of the surrounding skin may be necessary. Simple wound measurements may not be sufficient to capture the true improvement in a wound's condition, especially early in the treatment plan, as wounds may actually increase in size with debridement.

The third item to document is whether the resources used are appropriate for the progress observed. If the treatment plan fails to produce progress, an explanation of why this happened and steps to overcome impediments, including a change in treatment plan, need to be documented. For example, if the patient is unable or unwilling to perform required dressing changes or compression therapy, a brief narrative explaining complications and defining a new course needs to be written. All 3 of these issues will be supported more readily by photographic documentation. Exact wording for Medicare documentation requirements from one CMS contractor is given in Table 19-4.

By today's standards, the ability to bill CMS for services requires a computerized billing system and indi-

viduals trained in using the software. For example, regulations for billing from an outpatient clinic require the entry of several codes to describe the service performed. In addition to the CPT code, debridement or negative pressure wound therapy codes used for services provided by a clinician other than a physician, the appropriate therapy modifier is to be attached (GP for physical therapy, GO for occupational therapy, GN for speech). Other codes used for billing when services are provided in a hospital outpatient setting under the outpatient prospective payment system include therapy revenue codes to receive payment under the Medicare Physician Fee Schedule. Software termed the *Integrated Outpatient Code Editor* then determines the appropriate Ambulatory Payment Classification.

Dressings and Topical Medications

Under the rules of Ambulatory Payment Classification, the cost of any dressings or topical agents used is bundled into the payment for the procedure performed. If the patient has received any dressings or medications for home use, these are not to be used for outpatient therapy. Additionally, the use of free samples distributed to a clinic is not allowed. If the only procedure performed is cleansing and reapplication of an enzymatic debrider, code 97602 may be used. The active wound care management (selective debridement) codes are not to be used in this situation. Code 97602 is only to be billed once per visit, not per wound treated. Regardless of the number of the wounds receiving this service, only one charge of 97602 is allowed for a given day.

Although dressing changes themselves are not billable, dressing materials as well as chemical debriders for patients to use at home are billed under the appropriate HCPCS code. Under Medicare Part B, surgical/wound dressings (primary and secondary) are covered under specific criteria: the dressings are medically necessary for the treatment of a wound caused by, or treated by a surgical procedure or when debridement of a wound is medically necessary. Dressings are not covered for stage I pressure ulcers or first degree (superficial) burns. No payment is given for skin sealants or barriers, skin cleansers or irrigating solutions or solutions used to moisten gauze, topical antiseptics and topical antibiotics, or enzymatic debriding agents. Orders must be signed by a healthcare practitioner (see above) with the type of dressing, size, number used each time, frequency of dressing change, and expected duration. New orders are required if a new dressing is added and if the quantity increases. A new order is also required every 3 months for each dressing used. DMERC (durable medical equipment regional carrier) regulations provide utilization guides; therefore, the frequency of dressing change should match these guidelines when ordered. The guidelines are listed in Table 12-5. You should consult your DMERC for current DMERC guidelines.

An issue newly determined by CMS relates to the use of silver-containing dressings. CMS has ruled that coding for silver-containing dressings will be based on the materials and features of the dressing as they would be for any other dressing, regardless of the presence of silver. Therefore, dressings must be billed to the DMERC based on the existing HCPCS code definitions. Payment for any additional cost associated with the presence of silver is not allowed. For materials designed specifically to deliver silver to the wound, but that do not meet any of the DMERC's definition for any types of dressing, the product is billed with HCPCS code A9270. This specific code does not result in payment as this code is used for noncovered items or services. Some agencies have attempted to obtain payment by billing under HCPCS code A4649, surgical supply, miscellaneous for silver-containing dressing. CMS has ruled that this code should not be used for dressings containing silver.

TAG F-314

New regulations have been developed to motivate healthcare facilities to reduce costs. CMS will no longer pay for any additional costs due to specific complications occurring during hospitalization. These include infections associated with bladder catheterization, vascular access, and median sternotomy. Other problems included in this directive are blood incompatibility, air embolism, falls, pressure ulcers, and objects left in a patient's body after surgery. Congress has given CMS the latitude to add other complications to the list. Of particular interest is the need to document any pressure ulcers present within 48 hours

of admission to a facility. Costs associated with development of pressure ulcers not documented as present within this 48-hour time span will not be paid by CMS. The regulation specific to pressure ulcers is labeled F-314 by CMS. Specifically, it states, "Based on the Comprehensive Assessment of a resident, the facility must: a) ensure that a resident that enters the facility without pressure sores does not develop pressure sores unless the individual's clinical condition demonstrates that they were unavoidable; b) promote the prevention of pressure ulcer development; c) promote the healing of pressure ulcers that are present (including prevention of infection to the extent possible); and d) prevent development of additional pressure ulcers."[1]

COST-EFFECTIVENESS

This topic is often uncomfortable for clinicians and a seemingly endless battleground between clinicians and administrators. Several studies have indicated, however, that optimal wound care is often more cost-effective than lower cost per visit alternatives (see Bolton et al). For example, Bolton shows a range of 53% to 615% greater costs of care to use gauze dressings on various types of ulcers compared with clinically more prudent choices of hydrocolloid dressings (see his Table 4). Frequently, the argument for a given type of intervention is based on the cost of materials and not the cost of labor or the likelihood of attaining goals set for the intervention. The cost of a single application of gauze is much less than a hydrocolloid sheet, but the cost of applying gauze to a wound 3 to 4 times daily for 5 days is much greater than the single application of a hydrocolloid sheet. Even the cost of materials thought to be cheaper can become much greater depending on the frequency of dressing changes and the quantity of gauze used for each dressing change. Secondly, the larger picture of direct and indirect costs of wound care needs to be analyzed for the different possible options. Direct costs include the materials for primary and secondary dressings, materials used for wound cleansing, debridement, and dressing change such as bottles of saline, additional gauze, gloves, gowns, masks, shoe covers, tape, and labor involved in these activities including cost of set up and cleaning, especially when considering whirlpool therapy. Large quantities of water, cost of filling tanks, disinfecting tanks, and quality checks on infection control can become very high relative to other aspects of wound management. Other equipment may include pressure relief/reducing devices, operating room time, surgical procedures, and pharmacy. Potential indirect costs include prolonged treatment (increased inpatient days, increased home health, or outpatient visits), loss of days of work by the patient, treatment of complications of slower healing, costs of waste disposal driven higher by more frequent dressing changes, and the potential for litigation if a suboptimal plan is followed. One common example is the comparison of whirlpool therapy with pulsed lavage. Although the cost for materials for pulsatile lavage is greater than whirlpool, the much greater cost in clinician's time and possibly slower achievement of the same outcome, can make whirlpool therapy much more expensive. Another example is the provision of sharp debridement. One visit for sharp debridement may be more expensive than a single visit for hydrotherapy for debridement, but the faster outcome from sharp debridement can make the cost per outcome achieved much lower for selective sharp debridement compared with using hydrotherapy and disposable or resterilizable instruments to remove small amounts of necrotic tissue over the course of several days. Although each clinical unit must make its own decisions regarding cost-effectiveness of treatments, the issues of quality of life must be taken into account along with the more typical issues of decreased wound size, pain relief, debridement, and risk or frequency of infection.

WOUND MANAGEMENT TEAMS

Successful management of patients with wounds, especially those managed by DRGs, requires coordination, communication, and cooperation. Teams in an acute care facility typically consist of a physician, physical therapist, clinical dietician, and wound ostomy continence nurse. Some facilities may include occupational therapists and other personnel. Each individual on the team plays an important role due to the unique training of the individual within his or her discipline and the individual's experience. The key to success is to determine ahead of time what responsibilities each member of the team will have. Waiting until the program is underway to assign responsibilities is likely to create hard feelings within the group, perhaps creating a siege mentality and dividing the group. Members need to elaborate what their individual skills are clearly and with what patient populations the individual clinician is familiar. Flow charts designed from this information allow each clinician on the team to determine the next step in the sequence and to refer, when necessary, to a different discipline.

A common pitfall is the assumption of hierarchical knowledge within the team. One individual is unlikely to have all of the knowledge, and skills of the other clinicians. Optimal staffing would include a sufficient number of clinicians of different disciplines and specializations such that any given patient could be seen by a member or combination of members of the wound care team with the appropriate knowledge and skills for each situation. Any patient would, therefore, receive all of the necessary evaluations, education, and direct interventions leading to optimal care. A team is likely to have several members who have substantially overlapping knowledge or abilities along with a smaller number with highly specialized skills.

Every team requires a leader to be functional. The team leader is not necessarily a physician, but should be a person with the vision, passion, commitment, and interpersonal skills necessary for the team to be functional. In many clinics the team leader is a physical therapist, nurse, or dietician who has the respect of the other team members and other key leaders of the facility. This person is most likely the person who recognizes how to weed out inefficiency and improve patient satisfaction without creating a stressful environment. A preliminary team representing typical disciplines needs to be assembled and the perceived roles of members of each discipline need to be shared with the other members. Often members of one discipline understand very little of the training and experience of other members. Preliminary flow charts identifying the roles of each member of the wound care team should be designed by a small number of members of the team and submitted for approval by the team as a whole. Attempts to design flow charts by the entire team are unlikely to be fruitful. A subgroup of more than 4 to 5 individuals is likely to bog down on details, whereas a group smaller than 3 is likely to miss details. Sharing the work of the subgroup with the entire development team is used to improve the product. Turf battles may still arise, therefore, one of the first agenda items on such committees is a series of team building exercises and establishment of rules of conduct for the meetings. Agreeing to a consensus process as opposed to a majority process may improve the workings of the group as well. When a flow chart is developed, review of previous cases or hypothetical ("paper") patients can be used to identify any modifications needed. Several rounds of this exercise may be necessary to fine tune the processes of the team.

In putting the actual team together, team leaders must recognize that the presence of too many or too few members from a given discipline can create an unhealthy environment and the destructive nature of the development of cliques. Any perception of a subgroup of the team 'ganging up' will quickly destroy objectivity and undermine any trust built within the group. Meetings of the development committee need to be scheduled regularly with an optimal interval. Often weekly meetings are used. This time allows individual work to be accomplished between meetings and meaningful reflection to occur. Longer intervals cause members to lose focus and allow other events to take precedence over the work of the committee. In any environment, but especially in a DRG environment such as acute care hospitals in which the length of stay may be determined by the effectiveness of the team, cost effectiveness of the team is important. Generally, the DRG environment encourages facilities to discharge patients as rapidly as possible, which may require continued care following discharge. Lack of coordination of patient care and the wait for orders to be written may delay discharge or result in premature patient discharge. Often continued care is necessary in the form of home health, outpatient physical therapy, or inpatient rehabilitation. For this reason, case managers should be members of the team. Having a wound care team in place with autonomy is more likely to result in timely and appropriate level of care. In facilities without well-defined teams, conflicts are common. Individual physicians may write orders for out-dated, inappropriate, or inefficient treatment plans. When approached about revising their orders, some physicians may become defensive or hostile. Conflicts may also arise from the multiplicity of physicians involved with individual patients. A primary care physician, general surgeon, orthopedic surgeon, endocrinologist, infectious disease specialist, internal medicine specialist, and others may be involved in the care of a patient with a wound. Without authority of the wound care team to manage the patient's wounds, different physicians may write conflicting plans, or none of the physicians may actually take responsibility for the wounds. Therefore, all physicians who may be involved in patients with wounds must be willing to refer patients to the team without any micromanagement. The referring physician's input is important to the team's ability to develop and execute a plan of care, but they must be free of constraints placed on them by individual physicians.

SUMMARY

The execution of a plan of care must take into account a number of nonpatient issues: legal limits on personnel performing services, CMS regulations, and the payment provided by CMS and other payers for services. CMS rules are tremendously complex with a seemingly endless list of acronyms applied to different types of facilities and providers. Billing CMS for services requires a working knowledge of ICD-9 and CPT codes, dedicated software, and personnel. One must learn what is included in CPT codes used and whether CMS considers the service provided under the CPT code as medically necessary for a given ICD-9 code. Failure to utilize codes correctly could result in unbundling and upcoding, which can then lead to punitive action by CMS. CMS services are contracted to a number of private companies with employees that may interpret CMS regulations differently. A good working relationship with the contractor can greatly reduce the possibility of denial of payments. CMS contractors and healthcare service providers can work together to ensure that patients are receiving the most appropriate care and that fair reimbursement is paid. Cost-effectiveness of care and development of wound care teams are necessary to optimize care and fiscal responsibility. Cultures of individual facilities can undermine the autonomy of wound

care teams and disrupt morale to the point of the team disbanding. Overcoming a facility's culture can become an overwhelming task, requiring a strong leader with support from the highest levels of the facility's administration for patients to receive optimum care.

QUESTIONS

1. Explain how the use of a $7 hydrocolloid dressing may become more cost effective than the use of wet-to-dry gauze sponges.
2. Define the terms *unbundling* and *upcoding*. Explain how this can happen with manual charge entry.
3. Explain the relationship between CPT and ICD-9 codes and the need for coding experts and computerized data entry.
4. What are the 3 cornerstones of documentation of wound intervention to ensure CMS payment for services?
5. Under what circumstances will payment for electrical stimulation be given by CMS? How does CMS language regarding continued payment for wound care limit the possibility of ever becoming eligible to receive payment for using electrical stimulation?

REFERENCES

1. CMS Manual System Department of Health & Human Services (DHHS). Available at http://www.cms.hhs.gov/Transmittals/downloads/R1279cp.pdf. Accessed September 9, 2009.

BIBLIOGRAPHY

Application of Bioengineered Skin Substitutes: Ulcers (of Lower Extremities) – 4S-134AB-R1. http://www.trailblazerhealth.com/Tools/Local%20Coverage%20Determinations/Default.aspx?id=2865&DomainID=1. Accessed July 30, 2009.
Bolton LL, van Rijswijk L, Shaffer FA. Quality wound care equals cost-effective wound care: a clinical model. *Adv Wound Care*. 1997;10:33-38.
CMS Manual System Department of Health & Human Services (DHHS). Available at http://www.cms.hhs.gov/Transmittals/downloads/R1279cp.pdf. Accessed September 9, 2009.
http://www.arkmedicare.com/provider/medpola/ara02025.asp. Accessed August 27, 2009.
http://www.cms.hhs.gov/MCD/overview.asp. Accessed August 27, 2009.
http://www.cms.hhs.gov/QuarterlyProviderUpdates/. Accessed August 27, 2009.
http://www.cms.hhs.gov/Transmittals/01_overview.asp. Accessed August 27, 2009.
http://www.medicare.gov/Coverage/Home.asp. Accessed August 27, 2009.
http://www.medicare.gov/MedicareEligibility/Home.asp. Accessed August 27, 2009.

Hyperbaric Oxygen (HBO) Therapy - 4M-30AB. http://www. trailblazerhealth.com/Tools/Local%20Coverage%20Determin ations/Default.aspx?id=2881&DomainID=1. Accessed July 30, 2009.

Non-Covered Services – 4Z-18AB-R1. http://www.trailblazerhealth. com/Tools/Local%20Coverage%20Determinations/Default. aspx?id=2949&DomainID=1. Accessed July 30, 2009.

Panting G. How to avoid being sued in clinical practice. *Postgrad Med J.* 2004;80:165-168.

Physical Medicine and Rehabilitation, Outpatient - 4Y-22AB-R2. http://www.trailblazerhealth.com/Tools/Local%20Cover age%20Determinations/Default.aspx?id=2962&DomainID=1. Accessed July 30, 2009.

Pub. 100-07; Transmittal 4 Date: November 12, 2004. SUBJECT: Guidance to Surveyors for Long Term Care Facilities http:// www.cms.hhs.gov/transmittals/downloads/R4SOM.pdf Accessed 8/27/09. (Tag F-314)

Routine Foot Care/Mycotic Nail Debridement – 4P-7AB-R1. http:// www.trailblazerhealth.com/Tools/Local%20Coverage%20De terminations/Default.aspx?id=2884&DomainID=1. Accessed July 30, 2009.

Wound Care - 4S-150AB-R1. http://www.trailblazerhealth.com/ Tools/Local%20Coverage%20Determinations/Default. aspx?id=2897&DomainID=1. Accessed July 30, 2009.

Appendix:
Wound Care Resources

ORGANIZATIONS

- Alliance of Wound Care Stakeholders. http://www. woundcarestakeholders.org/
- APTA Section on Clinical Electrophysiology and Wound Management. http://www.aptasce-wm.org/
- American Professional Wound Care Association (APWCA). http://www.apwca.org/
- Amputee Coalition of America. http://www.amputee-coalition.org/
- Association for the Advancement of Wound Care (AAWC). http://www.aawconline.org/; http://advancingthepractice.aawconline.org/
- National Pressure Ulcer Advisory Panel (NPUAP). http://www.npuap.org/
- Undersea & Hyperbaric Medical Society (UHMS). http://uhms.org/
- Wound, Ostomy and Continence Nurses Society. http://www.wocn.org/
- Wound Healing Society. http://woundheal.org/

CERTIFICATIONS

- American Academy of Wound Management. http://www.aawm.org/ Multidisciplinary accreditation in wound management.
- National Alliance of Wound Care (NAWC). http://www.nawccb.org/ National wound care credentialing.
- Wound Care Plus. http://www.woundcareplus.net/ Education and certification in wound care.
- Wound Ostomy Continence Nursing Certification Board (WOCNCB). http://www.wocncb.org/

EDUCATIONAL MEETINGS

- Clinical Symposium on Advances in Skin & Wound Care (affiliated with Lippincott Williams & Wilkins, publishers of Advances in Skin & Wound Care)
- Symposium of Advanced Wound Care. http://www.sawc.net/ (official meeting site for the AAWC)

Irion G.
Comprehensive Wound Management, 2nd ed. (pp 349-350)
© 2010 SLACK Incorporated

8888888

- Wound Care Congress. http://www.woundcarecongress.com/

JOURNALS

- *Advances in Skin & Wound Care.* http://www.woundcare-journal.com/
- *American Journal of Infection Control.* http://www.ajic-journal.org/
- *Journal of the American Podiatric Medical Association.* http://www.japmaonline.org
- *Journal of Wound Care.* http://www.journalofwoundcare.com/
- *Journal of WOCN.* www.jwocnonline.com
- *Open Access Journal of Plastic Surgery.* http://www.eplasty.com/
- *Podiatry Today.* www.podiatrytoday.com
- *Wound Repair and Regeneration.* http://www.wiley.com/bw/journal.asp?ref=1067-1927
- *WOUNDS.* www.woundsresearch.com

EDUCATIONAL WEB SITES

- Hooked on Evidence. http://www.hookedonevidence.org/ Website developing database of research evidence on effectiveness of physical therapy interventions

- Lab Tests Online. http://www.labtestsonline.org/ Information on interpretation of lab test results and listing of lab tests appropriate for given conditions.
- National Guideline Clearinghouse. http://www.guidelines.gov/ Searchable database of clinical guidelines, including those related to skin and wound care.
- The Quality Management Consulting Group. http://www.qmcg.com/Publications/ (Information regarding CMS and CPT)
- Ostomy Wound Management. http://www.o-wm.com/
- RxList. The Internet Drug Index. http://www.rxlist.com/script/main/hp.asp
- Wound Care Information Network. http://medicaledu.com/
- World Wide Wounds. http://www.worldwidewounds.com/
- The Wound Care Institute Inc. http://www.woundcare.org/
- Wound Care Education Institute. http://www.wcei.net/ Educational site associated with the National Alliance of Wound Care.
- The Wound Institute. Healthpoint, Ltd. Clinical Education. http://www.thewoundinstitute.com

Index

N

Q

R

S

WAIT

...There's More!

SLACK Incorporated's Health Care Books and Journals offers a wide selection of products in the field of Physical Therapy. We are dedicated to providing important works that educate, inform, and improve the knowledge of our customers. Don't miss out on our other informative titles that will enhance your collection.

Integumentary Essentials: Applying the Preferred Physical Therapist Practice Patterns[SM]
Marilyn Moffat PT, DPT, PhD, FAPTA, CSCS;
Katherine Biggs Harris PT, MS
160 pp, Soft Cover, 2006,
ISBN 13 978-1-55642-670-4, Order# 46704, **$50.95**

This text answers the call to what today's physical therapy students and clinicians are looking for when integrating the *Guide to Physical Therapist Practice* as it relates to the integumentary system in clinical care. This text will integrate the parameters of the *Guide*, as it relates to the integumentary system, into the practice arena, that not only covers the material but also allows for a problem-solving approach to learning for educators and students.

Quick Reference Dictionary for Physical Therapy, Second Edition
Jennifer Bottomley PhD[2], MS, PT
624 pp, Soft Cover, 2003,
ISBN 13 978-1-55642-580-6, Order# 45805, **$39.95**

This is the perfect, pocket size companion for school, clinical affiliations, preparation for the licensure exam, and physical therapy practice. This resource provides quick access to more than 3,000 words and their definitions that are encountered on a day-to-day basis. There are 39 appendices included in this user-friendly, handy reference.

Cardiovascular/Pulmonary Essentials: Applying the Preferred Physical Therapist Practice Patterns[SM]
Marilyn Moffat PT, DPT, PhD, FAPTA, CSCS;
Donna Frownfelter DPT, MA, CCS, FCCP, RRT
328 pp, Soft Cover, 2007,
ISBN 13 978-1-55642-668-1, Order# 46682, **$58.95**

Musculoskeletal Essentials: Applying the Preferred Physical Therapist Practice Patterns[SM]
Marilyn Moffat PT, DPT, PhD, FAPTA, CSCS;
Elaine Rosen PT, DHSc, OCS, FAAOMPT;
Sandra Rusnak-Smith PT, DHSc, OCS
448 pp, Soft Cover, 2006,
ISBN 13 978-1-55642-667-4, Order# 46674, **$58.95**

Neuromuscular Essentials: Applying the Preferred Physical Therapist Practice Patterns[SM]
Marilyn Moffat PT, DPT, PhD, FAPTA, CSCS;
Joanell Bohmert PT, MS; Janice Hulme MS, PT, DHSc
320 pp, Soft Cover, 2008,
ISBN 13 978-1-55642-669-8, Order# 46690, **$58.95**

Gait Analysis: Normal and Pathological Function
Jacquelin Perry MD
556 pp, Hard Cover, 1992, ISBN 13 978-1-55642-192-1,
Order# 11923, **$81.95**

Patient Practitioner Interaction: An Experiential Manual for Developing the Art of Health Care, Fourth Edition
Carol M. Davis EdD, PT, MS, FAPTA
304 pp, Soft Cover, 2006,
ISBN 13 978-1-55642-720-6, Order# 47204, **$47.95**

Complementary Therapies in Rehabilitation: Evidence for Efficacy in Therapy, Prevention, and Wellness, Third Edition
Carol M. Davis DPT, EdD, MS, FAPTA
432 pp, Hard Cover, 2009,
ISBN 13 978-1-55642-866-1, Order# 48661, **$55.95**

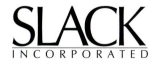